Diagnostic Criteria Handbook

in

HISTOPATHOLOGY

Diagnostic Criteria Handbook

in

HISTOPATHOLOGY

A Surgical Pathology *Vade Mecum*

by

Paul J. Tadrous
MB BS MSc PhD MRCPath

Histopathology Unit, CRUK, London, UK

BICENTENNIAL
1807
WILEY
2007
BICENTENNIAL

John Wiley & Sons, Ltd

Other Wiley Editorial Offices

John Wiley & Sons Inc., 111 River Street, Hoboken, NJ 07030, USA

Jossey-Bass, 989 Market Street, San Francisco, CA 94103-1741, USA

Wiley-VCH Verlag GmbH, Boschstr. 12, D-69469 Weinheim, Germany

John Wiley & Sons Australia Ltd, 33 Park Road, Milton, Queensland 4064, Australia

John Wiley & Sons (Asia) Pte Ltd, 2 Clementi Loop #02-01, Jin Xing Distripark, Singapore 129809

John Wiley & Sons Canada Ltd, 6045 Freemont Blvd, Mississauga, Ontario, L5R 4J3, Canada

Wiley also publishes its books in a variety of electronic formats. Some content that appears in print may not be
available in electronic books.

Anniversary Logo Design: Richard J. Pacifico

Library of Congress Cataloging-in-Publication Data:

Tadrous, Paul Joseph.
    Diagnostic criteria handbook in histopathology : a surgical pathology vade mecum / by Paul J. Tadrous.
        p. ; cm.
    Includes bibliographical references and index.
    ISBN 978-0-470-51903-5 (alk. paper)
        1. Histology, Pathological–Handbooks, manuals, etc.   2. Pathology, Surgical–Handbooks, manuals, etc.
    3. Diagnosis, Surgical–Handbooks, manuals, etc.   4. Histology, Pathological–Examinations, questions, etc.
    5. Pathology, Surgical–Examinations, questions, etc.   6. Diagnosis, Surgical–Examinations, questionss, etc.
    I. Title. [DNLM: 1. Diagnosis, Differential–Handbooks. 2. Pathology, Surgical–methods–Handbooks.
    3. Histological Techniques–methods–Handbooks. WO 39 T122d 2007]

    RB30.T33 2007
    616.07'583–dc22   2007024036

British Library Cataloguing in Publication Data

A catalogue record for this book is available from the British Library

ISBN 978-0-470-51903-5 (H/B)

Typeset in 10/12 Times New Roman by Aptara Inc., New Delhi, India
Printed and bound in Great Britain by CPI Antony Rowe, Chippenham, Wiltshire.

Disclaimer

While every effort has been made to ensure the information in this book is accurate and timely, there is always the possibility that errors have been made or that medical opinion has changed since the time of writing. The author cannot accept any liability for damages of any kind resulting from the use of information received from this book.

Dedication

I dedicate this book to the memory of my father, Mr Joseph Zaki Tadrous, who sadly passed away at the age of 84 in March 2007.

Contents

Please note that full-colour versions of all figures within Chapter 4, and also figures 5.3, 8.1, 11.3, 14.1, 16.1, 17.1 and 23.1 can be found in the colour plate section of this book

Preface

This book presents criteria for histopathological diagnosis in list form for rapid access. It covers diagnostic surgical pathology, cytology, autopsy practice, histological technique, lab management, RCPath guidance and UK Law relevant to histopathology. Trainees and consultants in diagnostic practice and those needing a quick refresher in preparation for professional exams (such as the MRCPath) should find this book a useful companion.

While at the microscope, the pathologist will often be able to suggest a limited list of conditions in the differential and may need a reminder of the diagnostic criteria of those conditions in order to decide on the preferred option. One may go to a standard diagnostic text for this purpose but there is almost invariably a lengthy few paragraphs of prose to read in order to glean the required morphological points. These words are not wasteful when learning about a condition for the first time as one needs a substantial background of information to appreciate the condition in its context.

However, most pathologists will have already read a full account of most conditions and just need to be reminded of the major points for diagnosis. These points are what this book aims to provide as an aid to rapid acquisition of diagnostic criteria and salient information on management, Law and technique. It is not intended as an initial source text and is not a substitute for reading a full account in specialist reference texts. This is not a comprehensive account of pathology – no attempt is made to cover very basic material and some of the rarer entities are pointed to via references. This book focuses on:

- *diagnostic criteria* for each condition;
- *immuno profiles* of normal cells, tissues and pathological entities where this is helpful;
- *criteria for malignancy* in otherwise benign lesions e.g. what makes a malignant SFT? What are the criteria for malignancy in a pilomatricoma? When should you be worried with an ameloblastoma and when does MGUS become myeloma?
- *differential diagnoses* with notes on distinguishing features e.g. how do you distinguish Kaposi's sarcoma from Kaposiform haemangioendothelioma or mucoepidermoid carcinoma from adenosquamous carcinoma or epithelioid haemangioendothelioma from epithelioid angiosarcoma or an atypical adenomatous hepatocellular nodule from hepatocellular carcinoma?
- *definition of terms* and quantities needed for diagnosis. For example, what are the size and mitotic count criteria for placing GISTs into malignancy risk categories? What is the definition of vertical and radial growth phases for melanoma? What constitutes an inadequate cervical smear? How big must a focus of atypical adenomatous hyperplasia be before it is considered bronchioalveolar carcinoma? What makes a lymph node metastasis a micrometastasis and how does this differ from 'isolated tumour cells present'? Many of these have important management implications;
- *grading, scoring, classification and staging* criteria for tumours and non-neoplastic conditions (e.g. transplant rejection, hepatitis, ER and PgR receptor status, spermatogenesis, etc.). No attempt has been made to reproduce the TNM staging system as the UICC book is an excellent handy reference which all pathologists working with tumours should have. Some aspects of TNM have, however been included in this book where it emphasises certain practical points (e.g. in Chapter 4: Cut-Up and Reporting Guidelines). A separate Grading Index page is provided for rapid access to the various schemes (see page xxv);
- *dating* criteria for endometria, myocardial infarction, thrombi and villi (following intra-uterine death);
- *normal values and ranges* e.g. for PM weights, placental weights, weight ratios, mitotic counts, etc;
- *laboratory methods* are covered from a pathologist's perspective;
- *laboratory management* (health and safety, UK legislation and government initiatives, budgetary control, Clinical Governance, etc.) and summary guidance from the RCPath *National Datasets for Reporting Cancers*, cut-up, autopsy practice and reporting major types of specimen together with handy *anatomical diagrams*;
- *frozen section diagnosis* –a separate 'Frozen Section Index' (see page xxvi) points to advice for per-operative diagnosis in all the chapters for rapid access to this information;
- *mnemonics and general advice* in exam technique are offered for MRCPath exam candidates.

This book bridges the gap between specialist diagnostic texts (with their reams of context) and study books for trainees (with their reams of aetiology, pathogenesis and molecules) by presenting diagnostic information in practical detail – but without the padding.

PJT, London, 2007

Acknowledgements

The support of the Pathological Society of Great Britain and Ireland in helping to get this book to press is gratefully acknowledged. I would like to thank all my colleagues, both junior and senior, who contributed to this book by answering my queries and by giving me questions to answer. A special thanks to all the pathologists who answered my specific questions regarding topics in their own field while I was researching this book – this was often in response to queries I had over individual patient's cases as well as specifically for the book. They include (in alphabetical order – and apologies for anyone I may have missed): Dr Emyr Wyn Benbow, Dr Ashish Chandra, Prof H. Terry Cook, Prof Amar P. Dhillon, Prof Cyril Fisher, Prof Andrew M. Hanby, Prof Alec J. Howie, Prof Stefan G. Hübscher, Prof Günter Klöppel, Dr Jay H. Lefkowitch, Dr Iain Lindsay, Dr Neil J. Sebire, Prof Neil A. Shepherd, Prof Sami Shousha, Prof Ian C. Talbot, Prof Rosemary A. Walker and Prof Clive A. Wells. Thanks are also due to Dr Caroline Brodie who proofread early drafts of some of the chapters and gave helpful feedback. Thanks also to all those who made their libraries and collections available to me, including Dr Ann Sandison, Dr Josephine Wyatt-Ashmead, Dr Neil J. Sebire, Dr Alan W. Bates, Dr Michael T. Sheaff, Dr Malcolm Galloway and Dr Juan Piris. Finally, I would like to thank all the staff at John Wiley & Sons for their helpfulness and skill in taking this book from manuscript to press.

Abbreviations and Symbols

!	indicates a potential pitfall	3YS	3 year survival
#	fracture	5YS	5 year survival
&	and	10YS	10 year survival
∴	therefore	AAC	Advisory Appointments
→	'leading to', 'which leads to', 'which could lead to', 'resulting in', 'gives rise to'		Committee(s) (for consultants)
		AAFB	acid-alcohol-fast bacilli/bacillus
		AAH	atypical adenomatous hyperplasia
↑	increased, increases, higher, hyper, raised, expanded, enlargement	AAN	atypical adenomatous nodule (liver)
		Ab(s)	antibody (antibodies)
↓	decreased, decreases, lower, hypo, lowered, reduced, suppression, deficiency	AB	alcian blue
		ABC	'aneurysmal bone cyst' or 'Achievable standards, Benchmarks for reporting and Criteria for evaluating cervical cytology' or 'avidin-biotin complex'
↑↑	greatly increased		
α_1ACT	α_1-antichymotrypsin		
α_1AT	α_1-antitrypsin		
αSMA	alpha smooth muscle actin	ABDPAS	alcian blue diastase PAS stain
γGT	γ-glutamyl transferase	ACC	adrenocortical carcinoma
μ	micrometer	ACE	angiotensin converting enzyme
μCa^{2+}	microcalcification(s)	ACEI	ACE inhibitors
/	'or', 'divided by' or 'per'	AChE	acetylcholinesterase
+	and, plus, with	ACIS	adenocarcinoma *in situ*
+/	'and or'	ACP	Association of Clinical Pathologists
++	'lots thereof'	ACS	acute chest syndrome
+ve	positive	ACTH	adrenocorticotrophic hormone
+vity	positivity	AD	autosomal dominant
−ve	negative	AdCC	adenoid cystic carcinoma
−vity	negativity	ADH	atypical ductal hyperplasia or additional duty hours
±	'with or without', 'may have/show'		
±ve	positive or negative	ADI	AIDS-defining illness/illnesses
≤	'less than or equal to', 'at most'	ADP	acute diffuse proliferative (GN)
<	'less than', 'fewer than', 'less common(ly) than'	ADPCKD	autosomal dominant polycystic kidney disease
≪	much less than	AEC	3-amino-9-ethylcarbazole
≥	'more than or equal to', 'at least'	AFE	amniotic fluid embolism
>	'greater than', 'more than', 'more common(ly) than'	AFIP	(USA) Armed Forces Institute of Pathology
≫	much greater than	AFP	alpha-fetoprotein
≠	'not', 'does not equal', 'which is not the same as'	AFX	atypical fibroxanthoma
		Ag(s)	antigen(s)
=	'is equal to', 'which is the same as', 'synonymous with'	AIDS	acquired immunodeficiency syndrome
≈	'is approximately equal to', 'which is similar to', 'almost identical to'	AIH	autoimmune hepatitis
		AIHA	autoimmune haemolytic anaemia
∝	'is proportional to', 'depends on', 'is related to', 'correlates with'	AIN	anal intra-epithelial neoplasia
		AIP	acute interstitial pneumonitis
°	degree(s)	AITCL	angioimmunoblastic T-cell lymphoma
∅	diameter		
[i(...)]	isochromosome..., e.g. [i(7q)]	AK	actinic keratosis (! do not confuse with KA)
1°	primary		
2°	secondary	AL	Amyloid (light chain type)
3°	tertiary	ALC	anti-liver cytosol Abs
3βOHSD	3-β-hydroxysteroid dehydrogenase	ALCL	anaplastic large cell lymphoma
3D	3-dimensional	ALD	alcoholic liver disease
5-HT	5-hydroxy tryptophan	ALH	atypical lobular hyperplasia

ALIP	abnormal location of immature precursors (lesion)	BLAG	benign lymphocytic angiitis and granulomatosis
ALK	anaplastic lymphoma kinase (=ALK-1)	BM	basement membrane
ALKM	anti-liver / kidney microsomal Abs	BMI	body mass index (= weight in Kg ÷ [height in m]^2), normal is 18.5–25
ALL	acute lymphoblastic leukaemia	BMS	biomedical scientist
ALP	alkaline phosphatase	BMTx	bone marrow transplant(ation)
ALT	alanine aminotransferase	BNA	borderline nuclear abnormalities
AMA	anti-mitochondrial Ab(s)	BNC	borderline nuclear changes (= BNA)
AMACAR	α−Methylacyl CoA racemase (P504S) also called AMACR	BNLI	British National Lymphoma Investigation
AMD	age-related macular degeneration	BO	Barrett's oesophagus
AML	acute myeloid leukaemia	BOO	bladder outflow obstruction
AMLS	amyotrophic lateral sclerosis	BOOP	bronchiolitis obliterans organising pneumonia
ANA	anti-nuclear Abs		
ANCA	anti-neutrophil cytoplasmic Abs	BP	blood pressure
APC	antigen presenting cell	BPH	benign prostatic hypertrophy
APR	abdominoperineal resection	BPOP	bizarre parosteal osteochondromatous proliferation
APT	anatomical pathology technician (= mortician)		
APUD	Amine Precursor Uptake and amino acid Decarboxylation	BRIC	benign recurrent intrahepatic cholestasis
AR	'autosomal recessive' or 'androgen receptor'	BSG	British Society of Gastroenterology
		BTA	bladder tumour Ag
arch.	architecture	BTTP	British testicular tumour panel
ARDS	adult respiratory distress syndrome	Bx	biopsy
ARF	acute renal failure	BXO	balanitis xerotica obliterans
ARVD	arrythmogenic right ventricular dysplasia	c282y	the haemochromatosis amino acid substitution
ASAP	atypical small acinar proliferation	CA	carcinoma (either alone or at the end of a subtype e.g. adenoCA = adenocarcinoma)
ASAPUS	atypical small acinar proliferation of uncertain significance		
ASC	adenosquamous carcinoma	CA1	*cornu Ammonis* region 1 = Sommer's sector of hippocampus
ASGP-R	anti-asialoglycoprotein receptor Abs	Ca^{2+}	'calcium' or 'calcification'
ASH	alcoholic steatohepatitis	CAA	congophilic amyloid angiopathy
ASMA	anti-smooth muscle auto Abs	CAA	coloanal anastomosis (not used in this book)
ASPS	alveolar soft part sarcoma		
assoc^d	associated	CABG	coronary artery bypass graft
AST	aspartate aminotransferase	CAE	chloroacetate esterase
ATN	acute tubular necrosis	CAH	chronic active hepatitis
AV	atrioventricular	CALLA	common ALL Ag (= CD10)
AVM	arteriovenous malformation	CAM	congenital adenomatoid malformation
B&L	Bernatz and Lattes classification		
BA	biological agent(s)	CAM5.2	Carol A. Makin 5.2 cytokeratin antibodies to CK8 and CK18
BAC	bronchioalveolar carcinoma		
BAL	bronchioalveolar lavage	CAPD	chronic ambulatory peritoneal dialysis
BAUS	basal (cell/layer) abnormalities of un-determined significance	CAPSS	columnar cell alteration with prominent snouts and secretion
BCC	basal cell carcinoma		
BCDA	basal crypt dysplasia-like atypia	CASTLE	carcinoma showing thymus-like elements
BCG	bacille Calmette-Guérin		
BCL	B-cell lymphoma (= Bcl)	CAVG	coronary artery vein graft
BCP	basal cell papilloma (= SK)	C-C	central to central
BCS	Budd-Chiari syndrome	Cb	centroblast
BD(s)	bile duct(s)	CBD	common bile duct
BFH	benign fibrous histiocytoma	cbs/wb	ratio of brain weights post-fixation = (cerebellum + brainstem) ÷
BJP	Bence-Jones Protein		

	(cerebrum + cerebellum + brainstem)
CC	collagenous colitis
Cc	centrocyte
CCAM	congenital cystic adenomatoid malformation
CCC	clear cell carcinoma
CCF	congestive cardiac failure
CCL	columnar cell lesions
CCST	Certificate of Completion of Specialist Training (see also CCT)
CCSTA	clear cell sarcoma of tendon and aponeuroses
CCT	Certificate of Completion of Training (successor to the older CCST)
CD	'cluster of differentiation' or 'condenser diaphragm'
CDC	communicable disease control
CDLE	chronic discoid lupus erythematosus
cDNA	complementary DNA
CDSC	communicable disease surveillance centre of the HPA
CEA	carcinoembyonic antigen
CEMD	confidential enquiry into maternal deaths
CERAD	consortium to establish a registry for Alzheimer's disease
CF	cystic fibrosis
CFA	cryptogenic fibrosing alveolitis
CFV	cresyl fast violet
CgA	chromogranin A
CgB	chromogranin B
CGIN	cervical glandular intraepithelial neoplasia
CGL	chronic granulocytic leukaemia
CHAI	Commission for Healthcare Audit and Inspection = 'the Healthcare Commission' (formerly CHIMP)
ChC	choriocarcinoma
CHIMP	Commission for Healthcare Improvement (now called CHAI)
CIBD	chronic (idiopathic) inflammatory bowel disease
CIN	cervical intraepithelial neoplasia
circ.	circumscribed
CIS	carcinoma *in situ*
CJD	Creutzfeldt-Jakob disease
CK	cytokeratin
CLH	chronic lobular hepatitis
clin.	clinical (features) / clinically
CLL	chronic lymphocytic leukaemia
CM	complete hydatidiform mole
CMF	cyclophosphamide, methotrexate and fluorouracil
CML	chronic myeloid leukaemia
CMML	chronic myelomonocytic leukaemia
CMT	core medical training

CMV	cytomegalovirus
CNI	calcineurin inhibitor(s)
CNS	central nervous system
COC	combined oral contraceptive
COP	cryptogenic organising pneumonia
COPD	chronic obstructive pulmonary disease
COPMED	Conference of Postgraduate Medical Deans (www.copmed.org.uk)
COREC	Central Office for Research Ethics Committees (part of the NPSA)
COSHH	Control of Substances Hazardous to Health regulations 2002
CPA	Clinical Pathology Accreditation
CPAM	congenital pulmonary airway malformation
CPC	clinicopathological correlation
CPD	continuing professional development
CPH	chronic persistent hepatitis
CPPD	calcium pyrophosphate deposition disease
CPR	cardiopulmonary resuscitation
CR	Congo red
CREST	Calcinosis, Raynaud phenomenon, oEsophageal dysfunction, Sclerodactyly and Telangiectasias
CRF	chronic renal failure
CRM	circumferential margin
CSF	cerebrospinal fluid
CSL	complex sclerosing lesion
CT	computed tomography
CTD	connective tissue disease(s)
Cu	copper
CuBP	copper binding protein
CUSA	cavitron ultrasonic surgical aspirator
CVA	cerebrovascular accident
CVID	common variable immuno-deficiency
CVS	cardiovascular system
cx	cervix / cervical
cytol.	cytological
d.p.	decimal places
d/dg	differential diagnosis
DAB	3,3′- diaminobenzidine
DAD	diffuse alveolar damage
DAPI	4′,6-diamino-2-phenylindole
DCIS	ductal carcinoma *in situ*
DCT(s)	distal convoluted tubule(s)
DD	diverticular disease
def^n	definition
DEJ	dermoepidermal junction
del.	deletion
DF	dermatofibroma
DFSP	dermatofibrosarcoma protruberans
DGH	district general hospital
DH	dermatitis herpetiformis
DIC	disseminated intravascular coagulation
diff	differentiated

DIP	desquamative interstitial pneumonitis	ETTL	enteropathy-type TCL (= EATL)
DLB	dementia with Lewy bodies	EV	epidermodysplasia verruciformis
DLBCL	diffuse large B-cell lymphoma	EVG	elastic van Gieson
DM	diabetes mellitus	EWTD	European Working Time Directive 93/104/EC 1998
dmin	double minutes		
DoH	Department of Health	F	female (unless otherwise specified)
DOPA	dihydroxyphenylalanine	F/U	follow-up
DPAS	diastase periodic acid Schiff	F1	Foundation year 1
DPN	deep penetrating naevus	F2	Foundation year 2
DPX	Kirkpatrick & Lendrum's distrene, phalate and xylene mountant	FA	fibroadenoma
		FAA	formol acetic alcohol
DSRCT	desmoplastic small round cell tumour	FAB	French-American-British
DU	duodenal ulcer(s)	Fab	'fragment Ag binding' of an immunoglobulin (Ig = Fab + Fc)
DUB	dysfunctional uterine bleeding		
E.coli	Escherichia coli	FAP	familial ademomatous polyposis
EAA	extrinsic allergic alveolitis	FATWO	female adnexal tumour of probable Wolffian origin (= TPWO)
EAE	experimental autoallergic encephalomyelitis		
		FB	follicular bronchiolitis
EAM	external auditory meatus	Fc	'fragment crystallisable' (part of the immunoglobulin's constant 'tail')
EAMF	elastin associated microfilament protein		
		FCH	fibrosing cholestatic hepatitis
EATL	enteropathy-associated T-cell lymphoma (see also ETTL)	FCL	follicular lymphoma (old name = follicle centre cell lymphoma)
EBA	epidermolysis bullosa acquisita	FD	fibrous dysplasia
EBMT	endocervical-type borderline mucincous tumour	FDC	follicular dendritic reticulum cell(s)
		FDE	fixed drug eruption
EBNA	EBV nuclear antigen	Fe	iron
EBV	Epstein-Barr virus (= HHV4)	FFI	familial fatal insomnia
EC	enterochromaffin	FHx	family history
ECF	extracellular fluid	FIGO	international Federation of Obstetrics and Gynaecology
ECG	electrocardiogram		
ECL	enterochromaffin-like	FISH	fluorescent in situ hybridisation
EDTA	ethylene diamine tetra-acetic acid	FNA	fine needle aspiration
EED	erythema elevatum diutinum	FNCLCC	Fédération Nationale des Centres de Lutte Contre le Cancer
EEG	electroencephalogram		
EGFR	epidermal growth factor receptor	FOB	faecal occult blood
EM	electron microscopy	FOBt	faecal occult blood test
EMA	epithelial membrane antigen	FPS	fee-paying services
EMH	extramedullary haemopoiesis	FS	frozen section
EMM	erythema multiforme minor	FSGN	focal segmental glomerulonephritis
EMU	early morning urine sample	FSGS	focal segmental glomerulosclerosis
EORTC	European Organisation for Research into the Treatment of Cancer	FSH	follicle stimulating hormone
		FTSTA	fixed term specialty training appointment
eos.	eosinophil(s)		
ePR	electronic Patient Record	FVIIIRA	factor 8-related antigen (i.e. von Willebrand factor)
EQA	external quality assurance		
ER	oestrogen receptor	FXIIIa	Factor 13a (clotting cascade)
ERCP	endoscopic retrograde cholangiopancreatography	G1, G2, G3	grades 1 to 3
		GA	granuloma annulare
ERPC	evacuation of retained products of conception	GAF	Gomori's aldehyde fuchsin
		GANT	gastrointestinal autonomic nerve tumour
ERS	European Respiratory Society		
esp.	especially	GAVE	gastric antral vascular ectasia
ESR	erythrocyte sedimentation rate	GB	gall bladder
ESTSCLE	endometrial stromal tumour with sex cord-like elements	GBM	'glioblastoma multiforme' (or 'glomerular basement membrane' in the literature – but not in this book)
ET	essential thrombocythaemia		
et seq.	'and sequelae'	G-CSF	granulocyte colony stimulating factor

GC	giant cell(s)		HG	hazard group(s)
GCT	giant cell tumour		HGF	herpes gestationis factor
GFAP	glial fibrillary acidic protein		HGP	horizontal growth phase
GFR	glomerular filtration rate		HH	hiatus hernia
GH	growth hormone		HHV4	human herpes virus 4 (= EBV)
GHRH	growth hormone releasing hormone		HHV8	human herpes virus type 8 (= KSHV)
GI	gastrointestinal		histol.	histology
GIP	giant cell interstitial pneumonitis		HIV	human immunodeficiency virus
GIST	gastrointestinal stromal tumour		HL	Hodgkin lymphoma
GIT	gastrointestinal tract		HLA	human leukocyte antigen
GLUT1	glucose transporter protein 1		HLO	*Helicobacter*-like organism
GM-CSF	granulocyte/monocyte colony stimulating factor		HME	hereditary multiple exostoses
			HMFG	human milk fat globule-associated antigen (types 1 and 2)
GMC	General Medical Council			
GN	glomerulonephritis		HMW	high molecular weight
GnRH	gonadotropin releasing hormone (gonadorelin)		HNPCC	hereditary non-polyposis colorectal carcinoma (mutator phenotype)
GO	galactose oxidase		HOCM	hypertrophic obstructive cardiomyopathy
GOJ	gastro-oesophageal junction			
GORD	gastro-oesophageal reflux disease		HPA	Health Protection Agency (incorporates the former PHLS)
GOS	galactose oxidase Schiff			
GP	general practitioner		HPC	haemangiopericytoma
GPI	general paralysis of the insane		hpf	high power field
GS	glomerulosclerosis		hPL	human placental lactogen
GSS	Gerstmann-Stäussler-Sheinker syndrome		HPV	human papilloma virus
			HRCT	high resolution CT
GU	genitourinary		HRG	Healthcare Resource Group
GVHD	graft *vs*. host disease		HRT	hormone replacement therapy
GVHR	graft *vs*. host reaction (in the skin)		HS	hereditary spherocytosis
H&E	haematoxylin and eosin		HSE	Health and Safety Executive
H/RS	Hodgkin or Reed-Sternberg (cell/s)		HSP	Henoch-Schönlein purpura
			HSR	homogeneously staining regions
HA	non-molar hydropic abortion		HSV	herpes simplex virus
HAART	highly active anti-retroviral therapy		HSWA	Health and Safety at Work Act 1974
HAV	hepatitis A virus		HT	hypertension
Hb	haemoglobin		HTA	'hyalinising trabecular adenoma' or 'Human Tissue Authority'
HB	hepatitis B (used as a combining form e.g. HBeAg for hepatitis B 'e' antigen)			
			HTLV-1	human T-cell lymphotrophic virus 1
HBP	hepatitis B surface protein		HTT	hyalinising trabecular tumour
HBV	hepatitis B virus		HUS	haemolytic uraemic syndrome
HC	Hassall's corpuscle(s)		HUT	hyperplasia of usual type
HCA	hepatocellular adenoma(s)		HVG	haematoxylin van Gieson
HCC	hepatocellular carcinoma		Hx	history
hCG	human chorionic gonadotrophin		HX	histiocytosis X
HCV	hepatitis C virus		i.m.	intestinal metaplasia
HCW	health care worker		IATA	International Air Transport Association
HD	Hirschprung's disease			
HDAC8	histone deacetylase 8		IBMS	Institute of Biomedical Science
HDV	hepatitis delta agent		IBMT	intestinal-type borderline mucinous tumour
HEFCE	Higher Education Funding Council of England			
			IC	indeterminate colitis
HELLP	haemolysis, elevated liver enzymes, low platelets		ICD	infection control department
			ICF	intracellular fluid
HEPA	high efficiency particulate air		ICH	intra-cranial haemorrhage
HER2	*Human EGFR 2* (=c-erbB-2)		ICRS	Integrated Care Record Service
HEV	hepatitis E virus		ID	identification
HFE	haemochromatosis gene		IDA	iron deficiency anaemia

IDC	'infiltrating ductal carcinoma (of the breast)' or 'interdigitating dendritic reticulum cell(s)'
IDDM	insulin-dependent diabetes mellitus
IEL	internal elastic lamina
IELs	intraepithelial lymphocytes
IEM	inborn error(s) of metabolism
IF	immunofluorescence
IFS	International Fellowship Scheme
Ig	immunoglobulin
IHD	ischaemic heart disease
ILC	infiltrating lobular carcinoma (of the breast)
IM	infectious mononucleosis
IMA	inferior mesenteric artery
immuno	immunohistochemistry
incl.	including
inflam^n	inflammation
inflam^y	inflammatory
inter alia	'amongst other things'
IP	interstitial pneumonitis/pneumonia
IPAA	(proctocolectomy with) ileal pouch anal anastomosis
IPF	idiopathic pulmonary fibrosis
IPMN	intraductal papillary mucinous neoplasm
IPSID	immunoproliferative small intestinal disease
IPX	*immunoperoxidase (immunostain)*
IQC	internal quality control
IRDS	immune reconstitution disease syndrome
IRMA	intraretinal microvascular anomalies
irreg.	irregular
ISH	*in situ* hybridisation
ISN	International Society of Nephrology
ISHLT	International Society for Heart and Lung Transplantation
ISSVA	International Society for the Study of Vascular Anomalies
ITGCNU	intratubular germ cell neoplasia unclassified type
ITP	immune thrombocytopaenic purpura
IUCD	intrauterine contraceptive device
IUD	intra-uterine death
IUGR	intra-uterine growth restriction
IVC	inferior vena cava
IVDA	intravenous drug abuser(s)
Ix	investigated or investigation(s)
JPAC	Joint Planning Advisory Committee
KA	keratoacanthoma (! do not confuse with AK)
KF	keratosis follicularis
Ki-67	a nuclear prolif^n-assoc^d Ag found in microwell Nō 67 at Kiel University
KS	Kaposi Sarcoma
KSHV	Kaposi Sarcoma-associated Herpes Virus (= HHV8)
L&H	lymphocytic and histiocytic Hodgkin's cells
l.p.	*lamina propria mucosae*
lab(s)	laboratory (laboratories)
LAD	left anterior descending artery
LAM	lymphangiomyomatosis
LBC	liquid-based cytology
LC	lymphocytic colitis
LCA	leukocyte common Ag
LCirc	left circumflex coronary artery
LCIS	lobular carcinoma *in situ*
LCV	leukocytoclastic vasculitis
LDHL	lymphocyte-depleted HL
LE	lupus erythematosus
LEL	lymphoepithelial lesion(s)
LESA	lymphoepithelial sialadenitis
LFB	luxol fast blue
LFT	liver function test(s)
LGV	lymphogranuloma venerium
LH	luteinising hormone
LI	labelling index (e.g. of Ki-67)
LIP	lymphoid interstitial pneumonitis
LM	conventional light microscopy
LMC	left main coronary artery
LMP	EBV latent membrane protein or last menstrual period
LMW	low molecular weight
LN(s)	lymph node(s)
LNp	lymphadenopathy
LOH	loss of heterozygosity
LP	lichen planus
LPD	luteal phase defect
LPHL	lymphocyte predominant HL
LPL	lymphoplasmacytic lymphoma
LRCHL	lymphocyte-rich classical HL
LREC	local REC
LRT	lower respiratory tract
LV	left ventricle
LVF	left ventricular failure
LVH	left ventricular hypertrophy
LVm	left ventricular mass
LyP	lymphomatoid papulosis
M	male (unless otherwise specified)
M.	*Mycobacterium*
M-H	Müller-Hermelink (classification of thymomas)
Mϕ	macrophage(s)
m.m.	*lamina muscularis mucosae*
macro	macroscopically
MADEL	Medical And Dental Education Levy
MAI	mycobacterium avium intracellulare
malig.	malignant / malignancy
MALT	mucosa-associated lymphoid tissue
MAP-2	microtubule-associated protein 2
max.	maximum
mCEA	monoclonal CEA
MCL	mantle cell lymphoma

MCLNS	mucocutaneous LN syndrome of Kawasaki	MSA	muscle specific actin (e.g. clone HHF-35, *not* the same as αSMA)
MD	maternal death(s)	MSB	Martius Scarlet Blue
MDA	minimal deviation carcinoma	MSU	mid-stream urine sample
MDBT	multidisciplinary bereavement team	MTAS	Medical Training Application Service
MDM	multidisciplinary team meeting		
MDS	myelodysplastic syndrome	MTC	medullary thyroid carcinoma
MDT	multidisciplinary team	MTD	malignant teratoma differentiated
MEA	multiple endocrine adenopathy	MTI	malignant teratoma intermediate
MEC	mucoepidermoid carcinoma	MTO	medical technical officer
mega(s)	megakaryocyte(s)	MTT	malignant teratoma trophoblastic
MEN	multiple endocrine neoplasia	MTU	malignant teratoma undifferentiated (embryonal carcinoma)
MESA	myoepithelial sialadenitis		
meso	mesothelioma	Mx	management
mets	metastases	MZ	marginal zone
MF	mycosis fungoides	MZL	marginal zone lymphoma
MFD	metaphyseal fibrous defect	n	superscript 'n' at the end of a word denotes the 'ion' ending e.g. $excret^n$ for excretion
MFH	malignant fibrous histiocytoma		
MG	myasthenia gravis		
MGA	microglandular adenosis	NA	nephrogenic adenoma
MGG	May Grünwald Giemsa	NAFL	non-alcoholic fatty liver
MGH	microglandular endocervical hyperplasia	NAI	non-accidental injury
		NASH	non-alcoholic steatohepatitis
MHC	major histocompatibility complex	NB	if italic = '*Nota Bene*' ('note well'); otherwise = 'neuroblastoma'
MHSWR	Management of Health and Safety at Work Regulations 1999		
		NBT	nitro-blue tetrazolium
MI	myocardial infarction	NCCG	non-consultant career grade
MIDD	renal non-amyloidotic monoclonal immunoglobulin deposition disease	NCEPOD	National Confidential Enquiry into Perioperative Deaths (role now subsumed by NICE)
micro	microscopically		
min.	minimum	NCI	National Cancer Institute (USA)
MMC	Modernising Medical Careers	NCR	nucleocytoplasmic ratio
MMMT	malignant mixed Müllerian tumour	NE	neuroendocrine
MMP-2	matrix metalloproteinase 2	NEC	neuroendocrine carcinoma(s)
MMR	measles, mumps and rubella vaccine	NET	neuroendocrine tumour(s)
		NF	neurofibroma
MN	mucosal neuroma	NF-1	neurofibromatosis type 1
MND	motor neuron disease	NF-2	neurofibromatosis type 2
MNG	multi-nodular goitre	NGF	nerve growth factor
MNOH	multi-nodular oncocytic hyperplasia	NHL	non-Hodgkin lymphoma
mod	moderate	NHS	National Health Service (of the UK)
MP	Member of Parliament	NHSBSP	NHS Breast Screening Programme
MPD	myeloproliferative disorder(s)	NHSCSP	NHS Cervical Screening Programme
MPET	Multi-Professional Education and Training levy	NHSFT	NHS Foundation Trust (in the UK)
		NICE	National Institute for Health and Clinical Excellence
MPGN	membranoproliferative GN		
MPNST	malignant peripheral nerve sheath tumour	NICH	non-involuting congenital haemangioma (see also RICH)
MPO	myeloperoxidase	NIDDM	non-insulin-dependent diabetes mellitus
MPS	mucopolysaccharides		
MPVFD	massive perivillous fibrin deposition	NK	natural killer
MRC	Medical Research Council	NLPHL	nodular lymphocyte-predom. HL
mRNA	messenger RNA	NMET	non-medical education and training
MREC	multi-centre REC	NMP22	nuclear matrix protein 22
MRI	magnetic resonance imaging	Nõ.	number
MRN	macro regenerative nodule	NOF	non-ossifying fibroma
MRSA	methicillin resistant *Staph.aureus*	NOS	not otherwise specified
MS	multiple sclerosis	NPC	nasopharyngeal carcinoma

NPI	Nottingham Prognostic Index	PDGFRα	platelet-derived growth factor receptor alpha
NPSA	National Patient Safety Authority		
NPV	negative predictive value	PDP	personal development plan
NRH	nodular regenerative hyperplasia	PE	pulmonary embolism
NSA	necrotising sarcoid angiitis	PECAM-1	platelet endothelial cell adhesion molecule 1 (= CD31)
NSAID	non-steroidal anti-inflammatory drug(s)		
		PEComa	perivascular epithelioid cell tumour
NSE	neuron-specific enolase	PEH	pseudoepitheliomatous hyperplasia
NSEst	non-specific esterase	PEL	primary effusion lymphoma
NSF	National Service Framework	periph	peripheral
NSGCT	non-seminomatous germ cell tumour	PET	pre-eclamptic toxaemia
NSHL	nodular sclerosis HL	PFI	Private Finance Initiative
NSIP	non-specific interstitial pneumonitis	PFIC	progressive familial intrahepatic cholestasis
NSR	National Spine Record		
NST	no special type	PGL	progressive generalised lymphadenopathy
NTN	National Training Number		
OA	osteoarthritis	PGP 9.5	protein gene product 9.5
occ.	occasional(ly)	PgR	progesterone receptor
OCP	oral contraceptive pill	PHAT	pleomorphic hyalinising angiectatic tumour
OF	osteitis fibrosa		
OFC	osteitis fibrosa cystica	PHLS	Public Health Laboratory Service (now subsumed into the HPA)
OH	alcohol		
OKT3	therapeutic anti-CD3 Ab	PID	pelvic inflammatory disease
oligo	pertaining to oligodendrocytes or their tumours	PIN	prostatic intraepithelial neoplasia
		P-J	Peutz-Jeghers
OLT	orthotopic liver transplant	PI	performance indicator
OMEE	oxyphilic metaplasia of the endocervical epithelium	PLAP	placental alkaline phosphatase
		PLAT	paraganglioma-like 'adenoma' of the thyroid
ONS	Office of National Statistics		
OOP	out of phase	PLC	*pityriasis lichenoides chronica*
OP	organising pneumonia	pleom.	'pleomorphism' or 'pleomorphic'
OSCE	objective structured clinical exam	PLEVA	*pityriasis lichenoides et varioliformis acuta*
OSPE	objective structured pathology examination		
		PLGA	polymorphous low grade adenoCA
PA(s)	'programmed activity(activities)' or 'pernicious anaemia'	PM	'post mortem' or 'Pagetoid melanocytosis'
PAL	pyothorax-associated lymphoma	PMC	pseudomembranous colitis
PALS	periarteriolar lymphoid sheath	PMD	placental mesenchymal dysplasia
PAMRAG	pseudoactinomycotic radiate granules	PMETB	Postgraduate Medical Education and Training Board
PAN	polyarteritis nodosa	PMF	progressive massive fibrosis
PanIN	pancreatic intra-epithelial neoplasia	PMHx	past medical history
PAP	peroxidase anti-peroxidase	PML	progressive multifocal leucoencephalopathy
Pap	Papanicolaou stain		
pap.	papillary	PMN	polymorphonuclear neutrophil(s)
PAS	periodic acid Schiff	PMO	pseudomyxoma ovarii
PASH	pseudoangiomatous stromal hyperplasia	PMP	pseudomyxoma peritonei
		PMR	polymyalgia rheumatica
PBC	primary biliary cirrhosis	PNET	peripheral neuroectodermal tumour
P-C	portal-to-central	PNS	peripheral nervous system
PB	peripheral blood	PNST	peripheral nerve sheath tumour
PbR	Payment by Results	POD	post-ovulatory day
pCEA	polyclonal carcinoembryonic Ag	POEMS	polyneuropathy, organomegaly, endocrinopathy, monoclonal gammopathy and skin changes
PCP	*Pneumocystis carinii* pneumonia		
PCT(s)	'porphyria cutanea tarda' or 'proximal convoluted tubule(s)' or 'primary care trust(s)'		
		POP	progestagen only pill
		P-P	portal-to-portal
PCV	post-capillary venule	PP	pancreatic polypeptide

PPH	postpartum haemorrhage	RF	renal failure
PPNAD	primary pigmented nodular adrenocortical disease	RhA	rheumatoid arthritis
		RICH	rapidly involuting congenital haemangioma (see also NICH)
PPV	Positive Predictive Value		
PR	*per rectum*	RIDDOR	Reporting of Diseases and Dangerous Occurrences at Work Regulations
PRAD1	PaRathyroid ADenoma 1 (= Bcl-1)		
pRb	retinoblastoma protein (= p105)	RMC	right main coronary artery
predom.	predominantly	RMS	rhabdomyosarcoma
PRHO	pre-registration house officer	RPC	rapidly progressive crescentic (glomerulonephritis)
PRL	prolactin		
prog.	prognosis	RPE	retinal pigment epithelium
prolif.	proliferative	RPOC	retained products of conception
prolif^n	proliferation	RPS	Renal Pathology Society
prom.	prominent	RR	relative risk
PRV	polycythaemia rubra vera	RS	Reed Sternberg (cells)
PSA	prostate specific antigen	RSV	respiratory syncytial virus
PSAd	pleomorphic salivary adenoma(s)	RTA	renal tubular acidosis
PSAP	prostate-specific acid phosphatase	RV	right ventricle
PSC	primary sclerosing cholangitis	RVH	right ventricular hypertrophy
PSS	progressive systemic sclerosis	RVm	right ventricular mass
PSTT	placental site trophoblastic tumour	Rx	therapy or treatment
PT(s)	portal tract(s)	S.H.I.P.	SLE, HSP, infective endocarditis, microscopic polyarteritis, (diseases associated with some forms of glomerulonephritis)
PTA	phosphotungstic acid		
PTAH	phosphotungstic acid haematoxylin		
PTC	papillary thyroid carcinoma		
PTCL-U	peripheral TCL – unspecified	SA	sino-atrial
PTFOL	post-traumatic fibro-osseous lesion	SADS	sudden adult death syndrome
PTH	parathyroid hormone	SAH	subarachnoid haemorrhage
PTHrP	PTH-related polypeptide	SAP	serum amyloid P
PTLD	post-transplant lymphoproliferative disorder	SARS	severe acute respiratory syndrome
		SBRCT	small blue round cell tumour
PUD	peptic ulcer disease	SCAP	syringocystadenoma papilliferum
PUJ	pelviureteric junction	SCC	squamous cell carcinoma(s)
pulm.	pulmonary	SCD	sudden cardiac death (or 'serious communicable disease(s)' but not in this book)
PUNLMP	papillary urothelial neoplasm of low malignant potential		
		SCJ	squamocolumnar junction
PUWER	Provision and Use of Work Equipment Regulations	SCLE	subacute cutaneous LE
		SCTAT	sex cord tumour with annular tubules
PV	*per vaginam*		
PVNS	pigmented villonodular synovitis	SD	'spongiotic dermatitis' or 'standard deviation'
q.v.	'which see'		
QA	quality assurance	SE	standard error (of the mean)
R&D	research and development	SEMS	superficial epithelioid malignant Schwannoma
radiol.	radiological (features)		
RAI	Banff liver Tx rejection activity index	SETTLE	spindle and epithelioid tumour with thymus-like elements
RB	respiratory bronchiole		
RBC	red blood cells / cell	SF-1	nuclear steroid factor 1
RBILD	respiratory bronchiolitis-associated interstitial lung disease	SFT	solitary fibrous tumour
		SHA	strategic health authority
RCC	renal cell carcinoma	SHO	senior house officer
RCC MA	renal cell carcinoma marker / antigen (also PN-15 or 66.4C2)	SI	small intestine
		SIDL	solid intraduct lymphoid proliferation
RCP	Royal College of Physicians	SIDS	sudden infant death syndrome
RCPath	Royal College of Pathologists	SIFT	service increment for teaching
rea.	rearrangement	SIFTR	service increment for teaching and research
REC	Research Ethics Committee		
resp.	respiratory		
retic	reticulin	sig.	significant

SK	seborrhoeic keratosis (= BCP)	Thy1-5	thyroid FNA scoring notation
SLA(s)	'service level agreement(s)' *or* 'soluble liver antigens'	TI	terminal ileum
		TJ	trans jugular
SLE	systemic lupus erythematosus	TLA	transmural lymphoid aggregates
SLP	soluble liver proteins (CK 8 & 18) (also called SLA)	TMA	thrombotic microangiopathy
		TMJ	temporomandibular joint
SLVL	splenic MZL with circulating villous lymphocytes	TNM	the UICC Tumour, lymph Nodes and Metastases staging system for cancers, sometimes followed by a number indicating which edition e.g. TNM5 or TNM6
SMA	'superior mesenteric artery' or 'spinal muscular atrophy'		
SMC	smooth muscle cell		
SmCC	small cell carcinoma	TPN	total parenteral nutrition
SMILE	stratified mucinous intraepithelial lesion	TOP	termination of pregnancy
		TORCH	toxoplasma, rubella, CMV, HSV
SMV	superior mesenteric vein	TORi	target of rapamycin inhibitor(s)
SN	sentinel node	TPWO	tumour of probable Wolffian origin (= FATWO)
SNOMED	systematized nomenclature of medicine		
		TRAP	tartrate-resistant acid phosphatase
SNOP	systematized nomenclature of pathology	TRIC	trachoma and inclusion conjunctivitis
		TS	tuberose sclerosis
SOP(s)	standard operating procedure(s)	TSH	thyroid stimulating hormone
SPA(s)	supporting professional activity/ies	tTG	tissue trans-glutaminase
SPD	subcorneal pustular dermatosis	TTP	thrombotic thrombocytopaenic purpura
spp.	species		
SpR	specialist registrar (see also StR)	TTTS	twin to twin transfusion syndrome
SPRU	special pathogens reference unit of the HPA	TURBT	trans-urethral resection of bladder tumour
SRUS	solitary rectal ulcer syndrome	TURP	trans-urethral resection of prostate
SSC	secondary sclerosing cholangitis	TV	tubulovillous
SSPE	subacute sclerosing panencephalitis	Tx	transplant
ST#	StR Training post at the appropriate year/level indicated by the number # e.g. ST1 for a year 1 StR	UC	ulcerative colitis
		UICC	Union Internationale Contre le Cancrum
STA	Specialist Training Authority of the Medical Royal Colleges	UIP	usual interstitial pneumonitis
		undiff	undifferentiated
STAH	sub-total abdominal hysterectomy	UoA	'Unit of Application' for specialty training posts in the UK (this is usu. equivalent to a region or Deanery but histopathology is a UoA unto itself)
Staph.	*Staphylococci/us/al*		
StR	specialty registrar (see also SpR)		
Strep.	*Streptococci/us/al*		
STUMP	smooth muscle tumour of uncertain malignant potential		
		UOQ	upper outer quadrant
SUDEP	sudden unexpected death in epilepsy	URT	upper respiratory tract
SV40	simian vacuolating virus 40	usu.	usually
SVC	superior vena cava	UTI	urinary tract infection
SWAG	Specialist Workforce Advisory Group	UTROSCT	uterine tumour resembling ovarian sex cord tumour (see also ESTSCLE)
Sx	symptoms	UV	ultraviolet
T4	CD4 +ve T-cell	VAIN	vaginal intra-epithelial neoplasia
T8	CD8 +ve T-cell	vCJD	new variant Creutzfeldt-Jakob disease
TB	tuberculosis (tubercle bacillus)		
TCC	transitional cell carcinoma(s)	VdW	van der Waals forces
TCL	T-cell lymphoma	VEGF	vascular endothelial growth factor
TCRF	trans-cervical resection of fibroid	VG	van Gieson
TDLU	terminal-duct lobular unit	VGP	vertical growth phase
Tdt	terminal deoxynucleotidyl transferase	VHF	viral haemorrhagic fever(s)
		VHL	von Hippel Lindau syndrome
TEM	tuboendometrioid metaplasia	*vide infra*	'see below'
TEN	toxic epidermal necrolysis	*vide supra*	'see above'

VIN	vulval intraepithelial neoplasia	WG	Wegener's Granulomatosis
viz.	'namely'	WHAFFT	worrisome histological alterations
VMAT-2	vesicular monoamine transporter 2		following FNA of the thyroid
vMC	von Meyenburg Complex(es)	WHO	World Health Organisation
VOD	veno-occlusive disease	WLE	wide local excision
VSD	ventriculoseptal defect	WT1	Wilms' tumour 1 (gene / Ab)
VZV	varicella-zoster virus	XL	X-linked (heredity)
w.r.t.	with respect to	YST	yolk sac tumour
WCC	white cell count	ZE	Zollinger-Ellison
WDC	Workforce Development	ZF	zona fasciculata
	Confederation	ZG	zona glomerulosa
WDHA	watery diarrhoea, hypokalaemia and	ZN	Ziehl Neelsen
	achlorhydria syndrome	Zn	zinc
WDTC	well-differentiated thymic carcinoma	ZR	zona reticularis

General Bibliography and Suggested Reading

At the end of each chapter the bibliography lists sources for the information in this book and gives suggestions for further reading. Because some sources have contributed to most chapters, I list them here rather than repeat them at the end of every chapter:

Fletcher, C.D.M. (ed) (2000) *Diagnostic Histopathology of Tumors*, 2nd edn, Churchill Livingstone, London. [3rd ed. 2007]

Frisman, D.M., http://www.immunoquery.com/(accessed March 2007)

Mills, S.E., Carter, D., Greenson, J.K., Oberman, H.A., Reuter, V.E. and Stoler, M.H. (eds) (2004) *Sternberg's Diagnostic Surgical Pathology*, 4th edn, Lippincott Williams & Wilkins, Philadelphia.

MacSween, R.N.M. and Whaley, K. (eds) (1992) *Muir's Textbook of Pathology*, 13th edn, Edward Arnold, London.

Weidner, N., Cote, R.J., Suster, S, Weiss, L.M. (eds) (2003) *Modern Surgical Pathology*, 1st edn, Saunders, Philadelphia.

I have also drawn on the following series (in addition to other journals and publications of official organisations). References to the specific articles are given at the end of each chapter:

Recent Advances in Histopathology

Progress in Pathology

Current Diagnostic Pathology

Pathology journals: *Histopathology; American Journal of Surgical Pathology; American Journal of Clinical Pathology; Modern Pathology; Journal of Clinical Pathology; Journal of Pathology,* etc.

Visit the Book's Web Site
www.pathbook.com

The problem with paper textbooks is that they go out of date as soon as the manuscript leaves the author. In order to counteract this I have set up a users' web site with the intention that updates can be made available and any errata corrected as they are found. The web site has the added advantage of allowing all the readership to contribute their comments and suggestions for improvements and additions.

Below is shown one of the pages from the site.

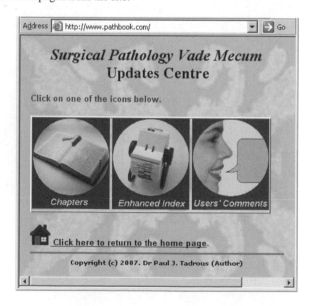

Index to Grading and Classification Systems

Neoplasia

Reader's Index

Use this space to make your own handy reference / bookmark list

Topic	Page

1. Advice for Exam Candidates

Introduction

There is no 'secret' or 'technique' that will ensure success in the MRCPath exam and by far the best way to prepare is to do lots and lots and lots of routine diagnostic and autopsy work in as many busy general and specialist hospitals as you can over the years of your training. You should attend one of the major **diagnostic histopathology courses** and one of the major cytopathology courses close to your exam because they help fill gaps in your knowledge and give you confidence. Going over slide collections is tempting but is often not very helpful because slide collections are made up of fascinomas whereas the exam is made up of routine surgicals.

The examiner is looking for evidence that you will be a **safe** and **effective** pathologist when left to your own devices. *Safe* means that you know your limitations (know when to refer or defer) and have a mature approach to diagnosis i.e. you make diagnoses based on a combination of multiple factors: clinical, constellations of morphological criteria, ancillary results, etc. with due consideration of appropriate differentials and with regard to the consequences of your decisions. Diagnosis by picture-matching or putting undue emphasis on a single feature is not appropriate for consultant-standard candidates. *Effective* means you have sufficient knowledge and experience to be able to make a confident diagnosis in the majority of the cases – anyone can muddle through by sitting on the fence or referring every case – but this can cause harm by means of delayed diagnosis (= delay in getting appropriate treatment) or by causing the patient to undergo unnecessary repeat diagnostic clinical procedures.

As a trainee, try to avoid the comfort of staying in one institution for longer than 18 months. Moving around gives you a broader vision, you learn new 'tricks' from new colleagues and new ways of approaching the same conditions. This builds **breadth of experience** rather than depth – and both are important.

It is vitally important to ensure that you **keep good timing** – many have failed because they haven't given themselves time to answer all the questions or study all the cases. Take every opportunity you get to do mock exams and ensure that you are strict with yourself over timing. Take a watch or clock with you to the exam (but not one with an audible alarm). You are also well advised to check in advance the quality and build of the microscope available in the centre and consider taking your own instrument to the exam: making diagnoses in the pressure of the exam is stressful enough without having to fiddle with an unfamiliar objective turret, field of view, focus mechanism and maladjusted illumination system.

In diagnostic practice, **knowledge** (of what diseases exist and what criteria define them) is more important than a visual memory for pictures. The histopathology of any one disease entity is defined by the presence of a set of morphological ($\pm$ clinical) criteria. Because any one or more of these criteria may dominate in a given instance of that disease, the overall histological *picture* may look dramatically different to a picture of the same disease occurring in another patient – the criteria for making that diagnosis, however, are the same. This is why *pattern matching* for diagnosis is potentially dangerous (pattern matching is only useful to recognise the presence or absence of any individual morphological criterion) and that is why this book concentrates on defining diagnostic criteria rather than illustrations of 'typical lesions'. Knowledge is built up over the years by getting into a habit of reading, teaching and doing. Knowledge is just as important for the practical exam as it is for the written exam – and even more so for real life diagnostic practice. A suggested reading list is given in the 'General Bibliography' of this book (see page xxiv).

There follows some general advice on approaching the practical aspects of the MRCPath exam. The exam is in the process of changing as postgraduate medical education in the UK also undergoes restructuring towards 'run through' training with a defined curriculum and competency-based assessments. The moves are towards standardisation, centralisation and modularisation. In particular the autopsy component has been separated off from the main exam as autopsy training becomes more specialised. Gynae cytology may eventually also become a separate module. For details of the latest exam structures and what's expected of candidates see the documents posted on the RCPath website, www.rcpath.org.uk.

At the end of this chapter I suggest a small (and incomplete) list of conditions you should always think about before arriving at a diagnosis (the 'Never Forget Group') and finally, for the desperate, I provide a list of mnemonics found throughout this book.

The Diagnostic Slides

Short Surgical Pathology Cases (usu. 20 cases)
- You get 9 minutes to write a structured report for each one: ① description, ② diagnosis, ③ clinical comment. You don't need all three for straightforward cases (obviously, ② is essential).
- Avoid lists of stains – if you feel the need for further stains or procedures always state why each stain is needed and what you would expect to see (i.e. how it will help you decide amongst the differentials). In the set of 20 surgical short cases it would be unusual to put in a case that needs lots of extra stains / procedures to arrive at a preferred diagnosis (this is the point of the long cases).
- Avoid lists of differentials and always attempt to give a preferred diagnosis. If your confidence level in your preferred diagnosis is low, say so, and discuss the most likely alternatives with reasons for and against. It is highly frowned upon for a differential to span the benign – malignant divide. This is clinically a useless position for a pathologist to maintain. If you are really stuck in this decision it may be a case you will have to 'refer for second opinion' but you can't do this too often (see below).
- Use formal language in your reports without anecdotes or use of 'note style' writing. For example: 'On this section alone my preferred diagnosis is X rather than Y. However, my degree of confidence is not high and, given the importance of making the distinction between X and Y in this case, I would like to . . .' [continue, for example, with one of the following]:
  - ➤ '. . . examine further levels to look for [state the features that will help]'
  - ➤ '. . . perform a Congo red for amyloid to substantiate the H&E findings'
  - ➤ '. . . refer the case for a second opinion'
  - ➤ '. . . further sub-classify the lesion by making reference to a major dermatopathology textbook [or, better still, state a precise reference]'.
- An exam pass-standard candidate should be able to give a preferred or definite diagnosis for most of the 20 cases (*at least* 17 of the 20 as a general rule of thumb).

Long Surgical Pathology Cases
- These will be something like a renal, bone marrow trephine or liver biopsy with special stains or a tumour with special stains. Special stains may include tinctorial, immuno & EM ± macro photo.
- Compose a formal and structured report as you would normally do in routine practice. Give your preferred diagnosis ± a limited differential with reasons (as described for the short cases above).
- Show the examiner that you are able to interpret the significance of the special stains: positivity, negativity, strength / grade and distribution / pattern of staining, artefactual changes, etc.
- You may get an unexpected result in the specials – the examiners are trying to see how you cope, e.g. a probable follicular lymphoma with a negative CD10 stain.
- You may get an impossibly difficult case – this is deliberate and you are not expected to give the diagnosis but the examiner wants to see how you handle something you can't do. This will be where your experience and judgement – or lack of it – will really show.

Cytology
- Gynae short cases: at the end of your report you should give an appropriate recommendation for management based on the patient's age and previous smear history. State if inadequate and why.
- Non-gynae short cases should result in clear and unambiguous results. State if inadequate and why.
- For the long cases bear in mind problems of interpreting special stains and ensure you have the necessary controls.
- Make sure you are aware of (and familiar with) the common pitfalls: atrophic smear *vs.* severe dyskaryosis, decoy cells in urine *vs.* malignant cells, etc., etc., etc.

The *Viva Voce* and Macroscopic Pathology exam

- Display effective communication skills: address the questioner, look them in the eye, don't mumble, use clear expressive and articulate language, don't waffle and don't fight.
- If you don't know the answer to a question be honest and up-front. Say you don't know about that particular thing but what you do know is. . . [something closely related to the question] – and let the examiner stop you if they want to. Don't use 'politician speak' or weasel words to try and 'fool' the examiner: the examiner will not be fooled – and neither will they be impressed.
- The *viva* is part of an OSPE with a strict marking scheme so you cannot use it to admit 'mistakes' you made in the practical (∴ there's no point discussing the cases with your fellow candidates).

The Autopsy

General
- This will be done on a separate day to the rest of the exam and possibly at a different centre.
- You will be allowed up to 3 hours to conduct the autopsy (excluding presentation and write-up).
- Review the notes and *consent form* and write a summary: age, date of death, clinical history.
- Conduct a risk assessment (use the local form / questionnaire where available).
- Ask the examiner about arrangements for contacting clinicians / students to attend the presentation.
- Discuss any special requirements anticipated (e.g. X-rays for neonates, microbiology, FS facilities).
- Do not criticise the instruments – although ask for others if required.
- On external examination: check identity, check for LNp and – ! – remember to check the back of the body.
- Health and safety is very important, slackness here can easily fail you:
  - ➤ maintain an orderly instrument layout and demonstrate safe handling of them
  - ➤ be clean and tidy at all times
  - ➤ do not leave pools of blood in the body cavities – rinse and sponge out.

Evisceration
- Consider taking ascitic fluid for culture if there is intra-abdominal sepsis.
- Remember to check for pneumothorax.
- The MTO may remove the cranium but you could be expected to remove the brain.
- Remove the diaphragm intact by cutting it flush with the thoracic wall.
- After removing the organs, clean the inside and outside of the body and check the inside of the rib cage for fractures (haemorrhage) and check for scoliosis / crush fractures of the spine.
- Ask if it is routine to remove the femur. [*NB*: This is not expected in the current MRCPath exam.]
- Ask if you are expected to fix the brain (the preferred option) or dissect it fresh.

Organ Systems
- Show the examiner you have a good-quality dissecting technique: open both iliac veins down to the femorals at the level of the great saphenous vein; keep the pericardium (and display it); assess the skull thickness for Paget's disease; don't spill gastric contents or bile (open these structures into containers); don't leave part of the right atrium behind (you will have trouble demonstrating the SA node when asked). Also, it is generally not good if the examiner opens the 1st part of the duodenum for you to reveal the ulcers you missed! Remember the carotid and *vertebral* arteries (at least inspect the intracranial portions of the vertebrals [the current MRCPath doesn't require a full dissection]).
- Show that you can think of things relevant to the clinical history or PM findings: remember the lymph nodes, bone marrow and tonsils in patients with lymphoproliferative disease; be prepared to comment on the renal arteries in someone with HT; take CSF by syringe from the 3rd / 4th ventricle for microbiology if there is reason to suspect meningitis or brain abscess.
- Show you have a good knowledge base: know your normal weights and measures, be prepared to discuss specialist dissection techniques and their indications (inflation of the lungs, vertebral arteries, conducting system, middle ear, etc.), issues of health and safety, consent and the Law (e.g. the Human Tissue Act, the Coroner's rules and when to refer a case to the Coroner), macro staining methods (for MI, amyloid, iron, etc.), toxicology, the future of autopsy (minimally invasive, radiologically assisted, sub-specialised, etc.), mortuary design and other topical issues.

Presentation and Writing a Report
- Periodically clean, dry and arrange the organs and instruments during the presentation.
- Start with the history then, in order: cause of death in ONS format → predisposing pathology → other major findings → trivia. Avoid lists of negatives. Demonstrate good interpretative skills.
- Be slick (e.g. you should be able to demonstrate the coronary arteries swiftly) and point specifically to pathology with a probe. Your manual dexterity (throughout the autopsy) is part of the assessment.
- Demonstrate good communication skills and show a good rapport with the clinicians.
- After presentation write the report and block index (ask the examiner for details – some may allow you to dictate). Remember to put the cause of death in the ONS format (for those over 28 days old) and do not use modes of dying as a substitute for a cause of death (see Chapter 25: Autopsy).

The Frozen Sections Exam

- Give a clear and unambiguous answer that will help the management – not a detailed report / diagnosis.
- If you are really stuck, you may 'defer to paraffin' but do this once too often and you will fail. Although in real life there is the possibility of requesting further levels on a FS or more tissue from the surgeon, the cases chosen for the exam are unlikely to require this.
- Remember FS artefacts (e.g. the lack of lacunar cells in NSHL or Orphan Annie nuclei in PTC) and be prepared to mention the possibility and utility of imprint cytology.

The 'Never forget' Group

Don't make a diagnosis until you've considered the following – the mnemonic, 'CAMMeLS', will help you to remember:
- **C**hemotherapy / radiotherapy / inflammatory atypia
- **A**myloid
- **M**elanoma (1° / 2°)
- **M**etastatic / 2° carcinomas (e.g. RCC metastatic to mucosae, skin or bone)
- **L**eukaemia: CLL, chloroma / 'granulocytic sarcoma' (AML / CGL)
- **S**arcoid / Crohn's (incl. extra-intestinal Crohn's) / reaction to malignancy: when faced with true epithelioid granulomas

Mnemonics

Mnemonic Index

Condition/entity	Mnemonic	Chapter
'Never forget' group of diseases	CAMMeLS	Chapter 1: Advice for Exam Candidates
Atheroma (complications of)	CUT	Chapter 6: Vascular
Abbreviated list of T-cell / NK lymphomas:	THE PSALM	Chapter 10: Lymphoreticular
Morphological types of myoepithelial cells:	SPEC	Chapter 11: Alimentary Tract
Neuroendocrine cell tumours:	EDGE	Chapter 11: Alimentary Tract
Causes of malabsorption:	FIDLES BV	Chapter 11: Alimentary Tract
Drug effects in the small bowel	VACU	Chapter 11: Alimentary Tract
Drug effects in the large bowel	PUMICE	Chapter 11: Alimentary Tract
Hepatocellular carcinoma variants:	PC STAGS	Chapter 12: Liver, Biliary Tract and Pancreas
Nephrotic and nephritic syndromes:	POH / OHO	Chapter 15: Renal Medicine
Causes of 2° membranous GN:	SIND	Chapter 15: Renal Medicine
Causes of 2° FSGN:	S.H.I.P.	Chapter 15: Renal Medicine
Causes of nephrotic syndrome	DASHIN	Chapter 15: Renal Medicine
Infiltrating lobular carcinoma of the breast:	CAST	Chapter 18: Breast
MEN 1 (Wermer's syndrome):	All the 'P's	Chapter 19: Endocrine
Painful lumps in skin / subcutis:	TEABAGSPEND	Chapter 20: Skin
Leukocytoclastic vasculitis (associations):	MAID	Chapter 20: Skin
Blistering diseases of the skin:	PErHEPS	Chapter 20: Skin
Distribution of bullous pemphigoid:	WOLF	Chapter 20: Skin
Epidermolysis bullosa acquisita (associations):	ABC	Chapter 20: Skin
Carcinomas metastatic to bone:	The 5 'B's	Chapter 22: Osteoarticular
Albright's syndrome:	All the 'P's	Chapter 22: Osteoarticular
Sarcomas positive for cytokeratins (CK):	PEARLS	Chapter 21: Soft Tissues
Malignant fibrous histiocytoma (MFH):	MAGIC Skin	Chapter 21: Soft Tissues
Kaposi sarcoma (clinical types):	CELTA	Chapter 21: Soft Tissues
Kaposi sarcoma (classical type):	WIELDA	Chapter 21: Soft Tissues
Kaposi sarcoma (endemic type):	SMACS	Chapter 21: Soft Tissues
Kaposi sarcoma (lymphadenopathic type):	RAW	Chapter 21: Soft Tissues
Kaposi sarcoma (transplant associated):	LAFS	Chapter 21: Soft Tissues
Kaposi sarcoma (AIDS associated):	MDM	Chapter 21: Soft Tissues
Causes of shock	CHAOS	Chapter 25: Autopsy

Bibliography

Stamp, G.W.H. and Wright, N.A. (1990) *Advanced Histopathology*, 1st edn, Springer-Verlag, Berlin & Heidelberg.

Weir, J., Benbow, E.W. and McMahon, R.F.T. (2004) How to pass and how to fail the MRCPath in histopathology part 2, *ACP News* (Winter 2004), 39–43.

Web sites

www.rcpath.org.uk (accessed April 2006) *MRCPath Part 2 examination – Autopsy module: Guidelines for examiners and candidates* (2004), Royal College of Pathologists.

2. Histological Techniques

Köhler Illumination

Köhler Illumination for Photography and Image Analysis

Setting up the microscope for Köhler illumination
For even illumination and optimum contrast do the following.

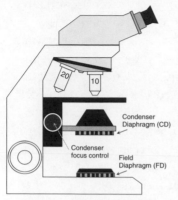

Condenser
Diaphragm (CD)

Condenser
focus control   Field
Diaphragm (FD)

FIGURE 2.1 Controls relevant to Köhler illumination

1. Put a specimen on the stage, fully open both the field diaphragm (FD) and the condenser diaphragm (CD) and focus the image at low power (e.g. ×10 or the lowest power at which full field illumination is achieved without the need to 'flip down' part of the condenser lens system. This is because the full set of condenser optics is needed for the following steps).

2. Close the FD and adjust the condenser focus control (! not the main microscope focus control) until you see a sharp image of the FD.

3. Centre the image of the FD by adjusting the condenser centration screws usu. found near the base of the condenser. Some microscopes have a locking screw which must be loosened before adjusting the centration screws. It should be re-tightened when centration is complete.

4. Adjust the FD aperture such that its image just disappears beyond the field of view. As the aperture of the FD is increased you may find it easier to make fine adjustments to the condenser centration.

5. Now adjust the CD aperture to match the numerical aperture of the objective. This may be done by either a direct or indirect method:
➤ Direct method: remove one of the eyepieces and look down at the aperture of the objective with your eye ≈ 5–10cm away from the eyepiece holder tube. Adjust the CD until its boundary is just within the aperture of the objective.
➤ Indirect method: leave the eyepieces in place and look at the specimen. Slowly close the CD until a slight drop in image brightness is first perceived.

6. Adjust brightness and colour-balance using the illumination power control or filters only – do not adjust the diaphragms or condenser focus because this will alter image quality / sharpness. For imaging work, note that a change of objective or any of the controls above will alter the amount of light getting through to the imaging device – so re-calibration / re-metering will be necessary.

7. Whenever you change objective you should repeat steps 4 and 5 above to match the new field of view and objective numerical aperture. If you change the slide you may also need to repeat steps 1 and 2 because the preparation may be of slightly different optical thickness. [*NB*: low power objectives may require some modification of the condenser such as swinging a lens out or, with very low power (≤ ×2) the condenser may have to be removed altogether or the CD fully opened or a condenser diffuser inserted.]

Köhler Illumination in Diagnostic Practice
The above method is unnecessary for day-to-day work and may have disadvantages (e.g. any spec of dust on filters over the FD may be constantly in the field of view causing an irritating distraction). Thus most pathologists set up their microscope as described above once only and then leave the CD open to that extent which is appropriate for the highest power objective commonly used (usu. ×40 or ×63), only opening it further if they go to a higher power (e.g. ×100 oil immersion). Leaving the CD open like this has negligible detrimental effects for direct viewing at lower power objectives. It is also common to keep the condenser in a slightly de-focused position in order to get dust particle images blurred enough so as to be unnoticeable. The FD is usu. left completely open at all times. Precise Köhler re-adjustment may, however, be necessary when using very high power lenses e.g. looking for bacteria in Gram, ZN or CFV preparations.

Diagnostic Criteria Handbook in Histopathology: A Surgical Pathology Vade Mecum by Paul J. Tadrous
Copyright © 2007 by John Wiley & Sons, Ltd.

Counting Mitotic Figures and Ki-67 Proliferation Labelling Index

- Only include definite mitoses in metaphase/anaphase (furry chromosomes and no nuclear membrane).
- Scan the section for the most mitotically active area and start the count at that field. In some tumours – e.g. breast – you must count at the growing edge of the tumour (not the centre).
- For counts per 10hpf there are two methods:
    1. count 3 or 4 sets of 10 fields and give the highest count;
    2. count 100 hpf and divide the count by 10.
- For counts per 50hpf count the nõ. of mitoses in 50 hpf.
- An hpf usu. means a ×40 objective with a standard wide field ×10 eyepiece. You should state the area (e.g. in mm^2) or diameter (in mm) of your hpf whenever giving a mitotic count in a report.
- Mitotic count decreases with time from excision to fixation (up to 50% fewer if >12 hours) so are usu. higher in frozen sections *cf.* paraffin sections.
- For Ki-67, use the most active area and either ① count the nõ of +ve nuclei in 2000 tumour cells and divide by 20 to give a % or ② give the nõ of +ve tumour cell nuclei per 10 hpf.

Fixation

Formaldehyde
- Covalently cross-links peptides to inhibit degradation and 'fix' structure
- A standard fixative as 4 % aqueous saline solution (=10 % formalin) cheap and widely available
- Good membrane structural preservation for LM (and, to a lesser extent, EM)
- Good Ag preservation when combined with Ag retrieval methods (heat, protease, washing, sonic)
- Slow tissue penetration rate (≈500 μ/hour) with even slower optimal fixation rate (≈80 μ/hour) because it takes time for the cross-links to form even when formalin is present
- Induces fluorescence in biogenic amines (e.g. noradrenaline and melanin precursors) / alters the fluorescence properties of other native tissue structures
- Some aqueous molecules / antigens (Ags) can diffuse out of the tissue
- If not buffered, varying pH can cause varying artefacts, such as nuclear shrinkage and hyperchromasia and variable cytoplasmic staining intensity
- Can form birefringent formalin pigment in bloodied areas
- Increases the weight of specimens (sometimes by almost 10%)
- The volume of fixative should be ≥ 10× the specimen volume for adequate fixation

Alcoholic Fixatives
- Disrupts hydrophobic bonds → denatures tertiary structure leaving 1° and 2° structure intact
- Examples include: 70% ethanol, Carnoy's (=ethanol, chloroform, acetic acid – excellent for fixing tissue inks onto specimens at cut-up), formol alcohol, etc.
- Faster tissue penetration *cf.* formalin (∴ good for cytology / rapid process / FS post-fixation)
- Better preservation of large peptide Ags and less induced autofluorescence (∴ good for some IF)
- Better preservation of nucleic acids (with Carnoy's)
- Worse preservation of membrane structure ∴ sometimes combined with acetone (which has better membrane-preserving properties but worse Ag preservation) e.g. for cytology
- Can show worse differential tissue shrinkage artefacts *cf.* Formalin

Bouin's
- An example of a combination fixative, ingredients: picric acid, formaldehyde, acetic acid
- Advantages:
    - ➢ stains tissue yellow ∴ easy to find LNs or embed small fragments (e.g. brain Bx)
    - ➢ good nuclear detail (e.g. spermatocytic seminoma)
    - ➢ small antigens are less soluble → enhanced sensitivity on immuno (e.g. AFP)
    - ➢ good for fixing India ink onto specimens prior to cutting
- Disadvantages:
    - ➢ degrades RNA and DNA ∴ not good for ISH / PCR / Feulgen cytometry
    - ➢ causes undue differential shrinkage (e.g. glomeruli)
    - ➢ picric acid is explosive when dry ∴ can't use as a fixative in ordinary processors
    - ➢ more expensive than formalin
    - ➢ some Ags don't survive the acid fixation or they show altered staining patterns (e.g. prostate lumenal cell +vity for the protein product of c-erbB-2 [= the proto-oncogene of type 2 EGFR, also known as HER2, the rat equivalent being *neu*]).

Additives to Standard Fixatives
- E.g. mercurials (obsolete due to health and safety), aprotinin and zinc
- These enhance peptide antigenicity by inhibiting natural tissue proteases thereby hindering autolysis

Effects of Fixation on Staining
- Fat retention: osmium / dichromates > formalin / glutaraldehyde $\gg$ acetone / OH
- Protein retention: formalin / glutaraldehyde > osmium / dichromates > acetone / OH
- Enzyme activity: acetone / OH > formalin / glutaraldehyde
- Different methods alter the acidophilia:basophilia balance between tissue structures
- Fe is leached out by acid fixatives
- Effects of resin embedding: tissue and Ag occlusion, dye retention (e.g. due to hydrophobicity)
- Formalin reduces colour contrast of many trichrome methods – use Bouin's fixative (alternatively pre-treat formalin-fixed tissues with picric acid and trichloroethylene)

Hard Tissues

Decornification
- Softens tough keratinous tissues e.g. toe-nail
- Phenol (outmoded due to health and safety)
- Commercial alternatives available

Decalcification
- Acids or Ca^{2+} chelating agents – often mixed with formalin for combined decalcification/fixation
- Strong acids (e.g. nitric) are rapid but give worse cytological and antigenic preservation
- Weak acids (e.g. formic) are a good compromise between speed and Ag preservation
- Chelators (e.g. EDTA) are the slowest but give best Ag / enzymic preservation
- surface / superficial decalcification: bathe the cut-surface of a wax tissue block in HCl

Assessing when Decalcification is Complete
- Standard time – uniform specimens (e.g. trephine Bx) may be known to decalcify within a set time for a given decalcification agent and can be standardised for any given lab
- X-raying specimens: expensive and has additional health and safety requirements for operators
- Chemical tests of residual Ca^{2+} in the decalcification fluid: when changing the fluid, add ammonia and ammonium oxalate to the spent fluid. If CaOH precipitates out (fluid turns cloudy) the specimen needs more decalcification → add fresh decalcification fluid.

Undecalcified Sections
- Sections of bone can be cut with a diamond knife and ground down to histological thinness
- This allows routine staining (usu. with von Kossa or Goldner's method – p. 11) and assessment of calcification front and osteoid seam thickness for assessing metabolic bone diseases e.g. osteomalacia

Staining (Principles)

Dye Nomenclature
- Mordanted dyes are dyes complexed to metal ions. The metal ion forms a covalent bond with the tissue thus cementing (mordanting) the dye in place e.g. iron haematoxylin (celestin blue) is used in HVG because VG is an acidic counterstain and will complex with and remove ordinary haematoxylin
- Acid dyes are those whose coloured species are anionic e.g. eosin
- Basic dyes are those whose coloured species are cationic e.g. methylene blue or alum haematoxylin (by means of its Al^{3+} mordant)
- Neutral dyes: both the anion and cation are coloured e.g. the Romanowsky mixture (p. 10)

Immunohistochemical Methods

Labelling Technologies
1. Fluorophore: very sensitive and can be used for quantitation if used with a direct method but fluorescence fades with time so no good for permanent preparations

2. Enzyme: reacts with a chromogenic additive to give a permanent dye and is sensitive due to enzymatic amplification but this makes it less useful for quantitative studies

3. Radioisotope: requires a development procedure which can be lengthy and has extra lab health and safety requirements. Can give a permanent reaction product and may be used for quantitative studies with the right methods

4. Colloidal gold: allows immuno for EM. Different sized gold particles can be used as separate markers for different Ags thereby making multiple Ag staining possible on the same section

Antibody layering methods

- Direct methods: labelled 1° Ab applied to tissue. Fast and good stoichiometry for quantitative studies but insensitive so tend to be used with IF. Limited repertoire – you need a labelled Ab for each Ag. Enzymatic labelling is possible with commercial methods that use a polymer-labelled 1° Ab (allows many enzyme units to attached to each 1° Ab).

- Indirect 2 step: unlabelled 1° Ab applied first, then labelled 2° Ab. More sensitive (multiple 2° Abs can bind to each 1°) so allows enzymatic methods. Expanded repertoire as may use the same species specific 2° Ab for a range of unlabelled 1° Abs to different Ags. Too many stoichiometric variables assoc^d with multiple binding over the two layers make this unsuitable for quantitative analyses of stain intensity.

- Indirect 3 step, e.g. the ABC method: unlabelled 1° Ab, then biotin-labelled 2° Ab, then enzyme-labelled avidin layer – creates a huge avidin-biotin complex (ABC) around each 1° Ab containing many enzyme molecules. Very sensitive permanent reaction but not quantitative (w.r.t. intensity) and problems re endogenous biotin may cause false +ve if not properly blocked (this is one good reason to inspect tissue specific *negative* controls with every run). Other 3-layer methods exist.

Methodological considerations

- Some Ags require certain fixation to be detected by certain Abs (or must be unfixed-frozen tissue).
- Some Ags require appropriate 'antigen retrieval methods' of pre-treatment to be detectable on routine preparations. These include:
  - ➤ heat (usu. in a microwave / pressure cooker with a salt solution)
  - ➤ enzymatic digestion (e.g. trypsinisation)
  - ➤ washing (prolonged washing in water can 'undo' some of the effects of formalin)
  - ➤ ultrasound (a sonic bath is rarely used in diagnostic practice).
- Co-staining the same section for 2 or 3 Ags (or rarely more) is possible using different coloured chromogen reactants for each reaction but these are technically demanding and not routinely used.
- Peroxidase-based enzymatic methods require endogenous tissue peroxidase to be blocked to avoid false +ve staining (one more good reason to inspect tissue-specific negative controls).

In Situ Hybridisation (ISH)

- This may be done on routine paraffin sections and cDNA probes may locate DNA or RNA targets.
- The probes may be tagged with fluorophores (FISH), enzymes for chromogenic detection or radioisotopes.
- Fluorescent labels are quick (because there is no chromogen development step) and are easier to use for double-labelling methods but the fluorescence fades so the preparations are not permanent.
- Chromogen labels give a permanent preparation and no need for fluorescence microscope.
- DNA ISH can detect chromosomal anomalies in interphase cells e.g. HER2 amplification in breast carcinoma May also be used for chromosome counting using α-satellite probes (e.g. ploidy analysis or using Y-chromosome for confirmation of male / female cell origin).
- ISH for mRNA can detect if a cell is *producing* certain peptides (*cf.* merely *containing* them as may occur by phago/pinocytosis) by looking for the peptide's specific mRNA e.g.:
  - ➤ κ and λ light chains for confirmation of clonal restriction in lymphomas
  - ➤ albumin – only present in cells with hepatocellular or hepatoid differentiation.

Staining (Practice)

Some Common Staining Methods and Stain Reaction Results

Rapid H&E method for frozen sections

1. Fix in formol-acetic alcohol (FAA) for 30 seconds. } (Alternatively, dewax and rehydrate
2. Rinse in distilled water. } if using a paraffin section)

3. Lillie-Mayer's (or Harris) Haematoxylin for 2 minutes.
4. Rinse in distilled water.
5. Rinse ('blue') in alkaline (Scott's) tap water solution for 30 seconds.
6. Rinse in tap water.
7. 1% eosin for 1 minute.
8. Rinse in tap water.
9. Dehydrate (graded alcohols), clear (xylene) and mount (e.g. in DPX).

Papanicolaou
See p. 353

Romanowsky Stains (e.g. May Grünwald ± Giemsa)
Uses methanolic methylene blue and eosin (or azure B & eosin)

van Gieson
Nuclei	-	blue/black
Collagen	-	red
Bilirubin	-	green
Other	-	yellow

Masson's trichrome:
Nuclei	-	blue/black
Collagen/osteoid	-	blue or green (and birefringent)
Muscle, RBC, fibrin	-	red

Martius scarlet blue (MSB)
Nuclei	-	blue/black
Collagen	-	blue
Muscle, RBC	-	red
Fibrin	-	yellow → red → blue (with age)

Movat's pentachrome
Nuclei and elastic	-	black
Collagen and retic	-	yellow
Mucin/ground substance	-	blue
Fibrinoid/fibrin	-	intense red
Muscle	-	red

- May be useful for visualising bronchial and vascular structure in the lung

Lendrum's phloxine tartrazine alcian green
Nuclei and elastic	-	blue / black
Collagen and retic	-	yellow
Mucin/ground substance	-	green
Fibrinoid / fibrin	-	yellow
Muscle	-	yellow
Keratin	-	red
Viral inclusions	-	red
Russell bodies	-	red
Paneth cells	-	red
RBC	-	orange / red

- May be used to detect mucin and squames in the lungs of perinates as evidence of meconium aspiration
- Also used for detecting viral inclusion bodies (! d/dg other red blobs listed)

Silver stains
- A redox reaction causes metallic silver grains to precipitate onto tissue structures thereby turning them black. The reaction may (argyrophil) or may not (argentaffin) require an exogenous reducer.
- Examples include: Gallyas (for neuronal processes), Grimelius (for argyrophil chromogranin A granules e.g. in MTC and foregut carcinoids), methenamine silvers for bugs (e.g. Grocott) and BM (e.g. Jones), Gordon and Sweets' (for reticulin) and argentaffin stains (for biogenic amines/aldehydes).

Phosphotungstic acid haematoxylin (PTAH)
- PTA is colourless. It works by blocking haematoxylin from binding certain tissue components. Its differential tissue distribution is due to different diffusion times in various tissue components according to its large molecular size. PhosphoMolybdic Acid is similar. They are used in various trichrome methods e.g. MSB
- Muscle striations (e.g. contraction band necrosis in MI, some myopathies)
- Fibrin (esp. for dating thrombi – early = yellow, medium = red, very old = blue by the MSB method)

- Granules of parietal cell carcinoma
- Granules of salivary gland tumours: ⟶ oncocytic granules are PTAH +ve and DPAS −ve
- cilia   ⟶ acinic cell granules are PTAH −ve and DPAS +ve
- myelin and glial cells

Tissue Components

Alkaline phosphatase (ALP)
- Stained using 'naphthol AS-BI' with 'fast red TR' → stable red deposits at sites of ALP activity
- If air-dried fresh imprints are not available, tissue can be fixed in formol calcium and embedded via a low temperature process (e.g. *LR Gold* resin embedding) to preserve ALP (and other enzyme) activity
- ALP is seen in endothelia, PMN, chondrocytes engaged in endochondral ossification and osteoblasts

Amyloid
- Eosinophilic with H&E and strong variable reaction with DPAS
- Congo red (apple-green birefringence on 8μ thick sections) – most specific tinctorial method
- Sirius red (similar to Congo red)
- Thioflavin T or S (green/yellow/blue fluorescence $\propto$ filter set) – can be used with paraffinised tissue; more sensitive *cf.* Congo red but less specific: +ve in fibrinoid, granules of mast cells and Paneth cell and myeloma-related renal tubular proteinaceous casts
- Lugol's iodine for macro specimens: purple staining (turns blue on addition of weak sulphuric acid)
- EM: unbranched 10nm thick fibrils (sandwich of two dense strands with a central pale strand) in random tangles. Fibrils are often straight. Occasional small bundles are seen
- Immuno: SAP (generally), tau protein (cerebral amyloid e.g. Alzheimer's), other specific components e.g. A4(β) in cerebral congophilic angiopathy and Alzheimer's, prion proteins in CJD, κ or λ light chains in AL, β_2-microglobulin in dialysis-related joint amyloid, etc.

Basement membranes
- These contain collagen IV and a carbohydrate rich (proteoglycan) matrix and will thus stain with PAS, methenamine silver (another oxidation-aldehyde method) or immuno for collagen IV

Bone/osteoid in undecalcified sections
- von Kossa's silver nitrate method will show mineralised bone as black with osteoid as red
- Goldner's stain contains more dyes and gives better colour contrast and cytological detail (mineralised bone = green, cartilage = purple, osteoid = reddish orange)

Calcium
- von Kossa stains the phosphates commonly assoc^d with calcium
- Alizarin red stains the calcium itself

Carbohydrates
- PAS staining sensitive to diastase is specific for glycogen and starches (diastase contains amylases that break the α-1:4 links in the polymer to produce mono and di-saccharides that dissolve out of the section. (see p. 12 under 'Mucins' for the basis of the PAS reaction)
- *NB*: glove starch gives a 'Maltese cross' birefringence similar to cholesteryl ester crystals (d/dg)

Catecholamines (the chromaffin reaction)
- Method: ① fix a thin slice of fresh tissue in potassium dichromate salt-containing formalin solution, ② look for brown pigmentation (granular and diffuse) in the cytoplasm of cells in an unstained section after paraffin embedding (false −ve results occur if the tissue is not immediately [<1–2 hours] fixed).
- +ve in the chromaffin paraganglia (the adrenal medullae and groups of cells within or abutting the ganglia of the sympathetic and splanchnic nerves/plexuses e.g. para-aortic organ of Zukerkandl near the IMA origins and many dispersed smaller cell groups not forming macroscopic 'organs').
- −ve in the non-chromaffin paraganglia (chemoreceptors of the carotid bodies, aortic bodies and *glomus jugulare tympanicum*). Also negative in most adrenaline-containing nerves because the test is insensitive and requires high concentrations of adrenaline to be +ve.
- Formalin-induced fluorescence is an alternative (more sensitive) method for catecholamines

Collagens
- Type I has many cationic groups that will stain with acid dyes e.g. eosin, van Gieson, Masson's trichrome, MSB, picrosirius red (stoichiometric, birefringent and fluorescent). Orange birefringence.
- Type III (reticulin) fibres contain argyrophil reactive groups in a carbohydrate matrix ∴ will be demonstrable by silver methods (e.g. Gordon and Sweets') and PAS (esp. in frozen sections) which do not stain the collagen itself.
- specific collagen types may be stained by immuno (e.g. type IV for BM – *vide supra*)

Elastic tissue

- Elastic fibres contain two elements in varying proportion (according to the age of the fibres):
    1. hydrophobic elastin protein (upto 90% with age)
    2. elastin-assoc[d] microfilament protein (EAMF) which is rich in disulphide bonds and carbohy-drate moites (dominant component in young fibres)
- EOSIN – elastic fibres are acidophilic, congophilic and refractile (but not birefringent *cf.* collagen)
- ORCEIN (and Victoria blue) is a hydrophobic dye with steric complementarity to elastin and with numerous aromatic groups. This stains elastin protein by Van der Waals bonding (mutual hydrophobicity brings the two together, the aromatic groups provide electrons for VdW bonding). Orcein stains elastin, copper-assoc[d] protein (CuBP), hepatitis B surface protein (HBP) and ceroid pigment. The strength of orcein staining for these three components is variable between brands and goes off with time after make-up of the solution esp. if older than 2 weeks. CuBP is not stained by some natural orceins but is usu. stained by synthetic orceins and HBP staining may be weaker with some synthetic orceins (see Kirkpatrick, 1982, for more details).
- DPAS will stain the carbohydrate moietes of the EAMFs (good for young fibres)
- VERHOEFF Staining solution: alcoholic haematoxylin, Lugol's iodine and $FeCl_3$. The iodine and ferric chloride oxidise the S-S bonds in the EAMFs into sulphonic acids which then bind the 'basic' dye haematoxylin. Haematoxylin usu. binds nucleic acids but the high electrolyte concentration of the Verhoeff staining solution prevents this. Verhoeff is less sensitive to fine fibres.
- WEIGART'S RESORCIN(OL) FUCSHIN – this is a commonly used E in EVG and is less technically demanding than Verhoeff. Weigart's mechanism of action is incompletely understood.

Lipids

- Neutral lipids ('fats') should be sought in unfixed frozen tissue – although formalin does not leech out fats (unless fixation is prolonged), processing through solvents to paraffin does.
- Hydrophobic Sudan III ('oil red O') & IV stain fats red. Sudan Black B is less specific
- Oil red O also stains submicronic polyethylene particles in paraffin-processed tissue
- Toluidine blue and methylene blue may be used as a −ve stain for fats (show up as unstained globules)
- Birefringence is seen with some crystalline lipids e.g. 'Maltese cross' pattern of cholesteryl esters
- Other lipids can be stained by various histochemical techniques (refer to specialist texts)

Mucins

- ALCIAN BLUE (a basic dye) is a synthetic complex of phalocyanin and Cu. It binds the carboxyl groups of sialic acid or sulphated sugars via electrostatic forces such that altering the pH of the reaction can result in selective staining of various acid mucins (mucopolysaccharides) as follows:
    ➢ pH 0.5: strongly sulphated mucins (e.g. chondroitin / keratan sulphate)
    ➢ pH 1.0: sulphated acid mucopolysaccharides
    ➢ pH 2.5: acid mucopolysaccharides
    ➢ pH 2.5: pre and post hyaluronidase: connective tissue mucin (hyaluronic acid).
- HALE's COLLOIDAL IRON: stains acid mucins dark blue by a Perls' stain on colloidal iron adsorbed to tissue polyanions ∴ beware false +ve staining due to tissue haemosiderin. It is more sensitive *cf.* AB (so may also show ↑ background staining). In normal kidney, staining of tubular epithelium indicates high background staining while failure of glomerular epithelium to stain implies too weak a reaction.
- PERIODIC ACID SCHIFF (PAS): Periodic acid breaks the C-C bond in 1:2 *cis*-glycols of monosac-charides, converting the glycol groups to dialdehydes. The aldehydes then react with Schiff's reagent to produce a magenta dye. Sialic acids exist in several forms. Some contain O-acetyl groups at certain positions which results in loss of the 1:2 *cis*-glycol groups and hence PAS negativity (e.g. colonic sialic acid mucins). KOH saponification removes the O-acetyl groups and unmasks the *cis*-glycols. Thus colonic mucin can be distinguished by PAS ± saponification. However, the mucins in many colonic cancers revert to the non-O-acetylated form.
- MUCICARMINE: Acidic, non-sulphated mucins (epithelial acid mucins) and Cryptococcus capsule. Specific but not sensitive ∴ not used as a general mucin stain. Red product.
- GALACTOSE OXIDASE SCHIFF: GO converts 1:2 *cis*-glycol groups in galactose and N-acetyl galac-tosamine into dialdehydes hence the GOS reaction shows gastric columnar cell mucins.
- SULPHATED MUCINS *vs.* CARBOXYLATED (SIALO-) MUCINS: Basic aniline dyes such as orcein and aldehyde fuchsin bind to sulphate groups in mucins without a prior oxidation step. Gomori's aldehyde fuchsin (GAF) combined with alcian blue (Spicer and Meyer's method) can be used to distinguish sulphated (purple) from carboxylated (blue) mucins. The high iron diamine/AB method stains sulphated mucins brown/black and carboxylated mucins blue ∴ has a more distinct colour contrast but it uses more hazardous reagents.

- **IMMUNOHISTOCHEMISTRY**: is more specific so can distinguish between upregulated glycocalyx material *vs.* mucin (both of which are PAS +ve):
  - MUC1 (EMA): meningioma, plasma cells, T-cells, skin adnexal sweat gland tumours, Ki-1 anaplastic large cell lymphoma, mesothelial cell membrane, adenocarcinoma. This is also found in normal breast and infiltrating ductal carcinoma NST
  - HMFG1 and HMFG2 (to the protein core of MUC1)
  - MUC2, MUC5AC and MUC6: gel-forming mucins associated with mucincous carcinoma and mucocoele-like lesions of the breast (that have a better prognosis *cf.* the non-gelling MUC1 associated with IDC NST).

Myelins
- Normal myelin:
  - LFB: copper phalocyanine stains myelin cyan
  - Heidenhain – myelin stains blue/black
  - PTAH – both myelin and astrocyte fibrils stain blue
- Degenerate myelin (Marchi stain):
  - degenerate myelin stains black, normal myelin light brown
  - it is an osmium tetroxide method (potassium chlorate pre-Rx prevents the osmium from being taken up by the normal myelin so only the degenerate myelin is stained black)

Nucleic acids
- DNA and RNA: haematoxylin and any cationic dye (also stain mucins) incl. pyronin (ordinary LM or fluorescence) and acridine orange (fluorescent); propidium iodide (red fluorescence, stoichiometric)
- DNA: DAPI and Hoescht 33342 (blue fluorescence), methyl green, Feulgen (blue, stoichiometric)
- RNA: methyl green + pyronin mixture: the methyl green preferentially binds DNA thereby blocking DNA binding of pyronin (red) that ∴ binds preferentially to RNA. Hoescht or DAPI may be used instead of methyl green if fluorescence is preferred (Hoescht is a vital dye)

Skeletal muscle
See Table 13.3 on p. 188.

Pigments

Bile pigments (and meconium pigment)
- Green with HVG
- Biliverdin is green but may be masked by eosin – use a lightly nuclear stained section
- Bile pigments are not autofluorescent (*cf.* lipofuscin)
- Fouchet's method: all bile pigments are oxidised (by ferric chloride and trichloroacetic acid) to green biliverdin and blue cholecyanin

Formalin pigment (and malarial pigment = haemozoin)
- Birefringent (unlike d/dg carbon)
- Removed by picric acid pre-treatment (unlike d/dg carbon)
- Malarial pigment is essentially the same as formalin pigment and may obscure the parasites

Iron (ferric iron by Perls' Prussian blue reaction)
- Ferric Fe as haemosiderin is soluble in acidic solutions, hence it leeches out in decalcified specimens
- Some tightly bound Fe is not stainable (unless unmasked by H_2O_2) e.g. haemoglobin / myoglobin
- Metallic Fe or rust (iron oxide) is negative
- Sections are treated in a solution of HCl and potassium ferrocyanide
- The HCl unmasks the protein bound ferric iron and allows it to react with the potassium ferrocyanide to produce Prussian blue (= ferric ferrocyanide)

Lipofuscin
- Green by Giemsa
- DPAS, orcein and Victoria blue +ve (esp. the earlier, less mature forms i.e. ceroid pigment)
- Autofluorescence on unstained sections
- Red by long ZN
- Blue by long Schmorl's

Melanin
- Melanin is a strong reducing agent. Thus it can reduce ammoniacal silver solutions (! explosive when dry) to form metallic silver without an exogenous reducing agent (*argentaffin* reaction). Masson's method is an argentaffin reaction using Fontana's silver solution.

- Melanin will produce Prussian blue by reducing ferricyanide to ferrocyanide in the presence of ferric salts – the Schmorl's reaction.
- Schmorl's reaction is also seen with lipofuscins, NE granules and bile pigments but melanin, may be *bleached* by strong oxidising agents ∴ perform Schmorl's ± prior bleaching.
- Formaldehyde-induced fluorescence of melanin precursors in early melanosomes is also not specific as other biogenic amines fluoresce.
- The DOPA reaction detects tyrosinase (= DOPA oxidase) – use postfixed frozen sections; may be negative in mature melanosomes.

Exogenous pigments

- Carbon – usu. appears black without staining and is not birefringent
- Tattoo – black, cobalt blue, other colours
- Heavy metals – argyrosis / argyria (silver), chrysiasis (gold), mercury, etc.

Micro-organisms

See also Chapter 23: Infection and Immunity.

- Gram: crystal violet is taken up by the peptidoglycan in the cell walls of both Gram +ve and −ve bacteria but the thicker wall of Gram +ve bacteria retain the dye in the diffing stage leaving the Gram −ve to stain only with the nuclear counterstain (neutral red)
- ZN *et al*: hot carbol fuchsin is taken up by mycobacteria and is retained by them even after the acid-alcohol diffing stage (hence AAFB). The Fite stain has less stringent diffing (*Nocardia, M. Leprae*)
- Silver methods: not just for fungi / spirochaetes. A Warthin-Starry / Dieterle is more sensitive for mycobacteria than ZN and can also stain all bacteria including those difficult to stain with Gram (*Legionella, Rochalimaea, H. pylori*, etc.)
- Fluorescence: auramine-O, rhodamine and Papanicolaou (mycobacteria), calcofluor white (fungi)
- Mucicarmine: capsule of *Cryptococcus* and cell wall of Blastomyces but does not stain Histoplasma
- Intrinsic melanin: Cryptococcus, some moulds
- Giemsa: protozoa, *Pneumocystis, Histoplasma*
- *H. pylori* stains: modified Giemsa → blue, cool Carbol fuchsin methods (McMullen's Gimenez) → magenta, Nissl's cresyl fast violet (CFV) → blue, silver stains → black, acridine orange → orange yellow fluorescence, immuno → colour depends on chromogen

Diagnostic Immunohistochemistry

Cytokeratins

- (As with all immuno) every rule has exceptions ∴ need clin. and morphological context ± a panel of Abs including non-CK ones. Hence, only strong and diffuse (many cells) +vity should be regarded as 'positive' as many tumours / tissues can show focal / weak staining
- CKs are numbered 1–20, the lower the CK number the higher the molecular weight
- AE1/AE3 reacts with CK 2,4,6,8,10,14,16 and CK 5,9,15,19 ⎫ broad
- MNF116 reacts with CK 6,8 and CK 5,17,19 ⎬ spectrum
- LP34 reacts with CK 5,6,18 ⎫ high molecular
- 34βE12 reacts with CK 1,5,10,14 + ? others ⎬ weight (HMW)
- CAM5.2 reacts with CK 8,18   } low molecular weight (LMW)
- In general:
  - ➤ LMW CK react to immature / simple (non-stratified) epithelia e.g. glandular
  - ➤ HMW CK react to mature / stratified / squamous epithelia ± basal / myoepithelial cells
- CK7:
  - +ve: endothelial cells, some vascular and myometrial smooth muscle cells, endocervix, endometrium, ovary (serous, endometrioid and transitional and mucinous tumours), normal prostate lumenal cells, TCC, breast incl. Paget's disease, thymic carcinoma, pulmonary adenocarcinoma, normal alveoli, mesothelium, pancreatic duct adenocarcinoma, some salivary and sweat gland carcinoma, fibrolamellar HCC, normal biliary epithelium and biliary metaplastic hepatocytes, some NE cells and tumours (except most SmCC), thyroid follicular cells (and follicular and papillary tumours), renal collecting duct cells, 80% of cholangiocarcinoma, 20% of carcinoma metastatic to the liver
  - −ve: some SCC, 80% of HCC (except fibrolamellar), 20% of cholangiocarcinoma, adrenocortical carcinoma, carcinoma of the Ampulla of Vater, normal pancreatic acini, sex cord / stromal tumours of the ovary, gastric intestinal metaplasia

±**ve**: cervical SCC, gastric carcinoma, colonic adenocarcinoma (85% are −ve), cholangiocarcinoma, some NE tumours, SmCC, epithelioid haemangioendothelioma, prostatic carcinoma,
RCC (chromophobe > papillary > conventional)

- CK20:

  +**ve**: Merkel cell CA, colorectal CA, pancreatic CA, gallbladder CA, TCC, breast papillary tumours,
  mucinous tumours (breast, colorectum, ovary), endocrine and NE cells, normal gastrointestinal epithelium, some salivary gland SmCC (but not other 1° sites)

  −**ve**: SmCC (except of salivary gland), SCC, RCC, prostatic CA, mesothelium, normal breast /
  sweat / salivary glands, biliary and pancreatic ducts, alveoli, renal collecting duct cells

  ±**ve**: pulmonary adenocarcinoma, breast IDC of NST

- 34βE12 is said to be one of the best markers for squamous differentiation in poorly diff SCC. TCC is
  ±ve (more likely to be +ve if heat Ag retrieval is used cf. enzyme digestion). PTC is +ve cf. hyalinising
  trabecular tumour (−ve).

- CK8 and CK18 (CAM5.2) stains hepatocytes and wide variety of simple epithelia (incl. biliary epithelium) and some non-epithelial tissues e.g. LN reticulum cells, subserosal cells, ALCL, myeloma,
  melanoma, Schwannoma, muscle tumours, angiosarcoma., MFH, meningioma

- CK7 and CK19 stain biliary epithelium but usu. not hepatocytes. CK19 stains 10% of HCC, 50%
  of cholangiocarcinoma, 15% of carcinoma metastatic to the liver, many simple epithelia, dermal
  basal cells, mesothelium, PTC (strong diffuse +vity) cf. follicular thyroid lesions (focal +/ peripheral +vity) incl. hyalinising trabecular tumour (usu. −ve) but >50% of benign thyroids are
  +ve.

- CK5/6 stains prostatic basal cells; for ADH see p. 258; 1° pulmonary adenocarcinoma are usu. −ve
  but SCC +ve; mesothelioma +ve; mesothelial cells +ve (e.g. in LN inclusions), TCC ±ve

Immunostaining melanotic lesions

- Use of Azure B as counterstain (instead of haematoxylin) turns melanin cyan leaving DAB as brown
- Peroxidase-based Ab systems may also be developed with alternative chromogens such as 3-amino-
  9-ethylcarbazole (AEC – red but carcinogenic) or 4-chloro-1-naphthol (dark blue). These are both
  soluble in alcohol so the sections need to be counterstained with (e.g.) methyl green, air-dried and
  aqueous-mounted. These are also 10 to 20 times less sensitive detection methods cf. DAB
- ALP-based Ab systems (if available) may be developed with 'Fast Blue BB' or 'Fast Red'
- Bleaching the melanin before immunostaining can alter the antigenicity of many Ags

S100 protein (Dimers of α and β subunits)

Positive normal structures

- Present in ≈ all cells (and may stain all cells if unfixed tissue is used); nuclear +/ cytoplasmic staining
- Schwann, perineural and myoepithelial cells, glia, melanocytes, (some neurons are α-subunit +ve)
- β-subunit +ve in IDC and Langerhans cells; α-subunit +ve in Mφ (e.g. in LN tingible bodies / sinuses)
- Cartilage, skeletal muscle, adipocytes, mast cells; sparse spindle cells in healing wounds
- Folliculostellate cells (anterior pituitary), posterior pituicytes (β-subunit), paraganglial sustentacular
  cells, fetal adrenal neuroblasts (but not phaeochromocytes), thyroid follicular cells (±ve)
- Some Leydig, Sertoli and granulosa cells
- Some ductal epithelial cells in the breast, salivary glands and sweat glands
- Some acinar epithelial cells in sweat glands and peribronchial serous glands

Some positive pathological lesions (there are many more than those listed here)

- Melanoma (! small cell variant can be −ve), oligodendroglioma (often GFAP −ve), astrocytomas, NB
- Histiocytosis X (CD1a +ve), Rosai-Dorfman disease (CD1a −ve), IDC sarcoma
- soft tissue tumours: Schwannoma (incl. granular cell tumour), MPNST, CCSTA, liposarcoma / lipomas,
  chordoma, chondroma, chondrosarcoma and some synovial sarcoma and alveolar soft part sarcomas
- Some Leydig, Sertoli and granulosa cell tumours; ovarian carcinomas and FATWO
- Microglandular adenosis of the breast (*epithelial* cells) but not tubular carcinoma
- 50% of invasive carcinoma and Paget's disease of the breast and ≈ all phyllodes (epithelial component)
- Salivary gland carcinomas: PLGA, salivary duct carcinoma, signet ring carcinoma, AdCC
- 30% of Merkel cell carcinomas show +vity of variable extent
- Many thyroid carcinomas (follicular, papillary and medullary) – α-subunit more commonly than β

HMB45 (gp100)

- Some melanomas (desmoplastic ones are often −ve esp. in deep spindle cells, but S100 is usu. +ve),
  Spitz naevi, DPN and all blue naevi (benign or malignant) (for more details, see Chapter 20: Skin)
- Benign junctional melanocytes/nests and anal melanocytes in squamous and transitional zones
- Atypical/congenital/hormonal naevi can be +ve but other typical benign naevocytes are −ve

- Activated melanocytes (in healing wounds, overlying dermal tumours, adjacent to melanomas, etc.)
- Sugar tumour of the lung
- Angiomyolipoma   } These are PEComas (see p. 326)
- Lymphangioleiomyomatosis
- Melanotic Schwannoma
- Others: some ovarian steroid cell tumours; most tumours arising in TS
- Macrophages are −ve for HMB45
- Artefactual +vity may be seen in plasma cells / lymphomas / carcinoma due to cross-reactivity of clone contaminants or stromal/inflammatory cells due to artefact of mercurial fixation

Melan-A (MART 1 gene, Ab clone A103)

- Melanocytes (see Chapter 20: Skin) and some PEComas, sex cord/stromal and adrenocortical tumours

CD10 (CALLA)

- PMN, normal follicle B-cells, ALL (not AML), FCL, Burkitt's, some DLBCL, AITCL
- Stromal cells of endometrium (stromal tumours and endometriosis) and phyllodes tumours
- Myoepithelial cells (breast and salivary)
- Prostate epithelium and Gartner's duct epithelium (cervix)
- Renal tubule and glomerular cells and clear cell and papillary rcc (but not most chromophobe)
- Liver: canalicular pattern (like pCEA)

CD99 (O13 / MIC-2)

- Ewing's / PNET (+ve for Fli-1 by immuno – most other childhood SBRCTs are −ve)
- Synovial sarcoma (also shows the triad of Bcl-2, CK and EMA[1] +ve)
- $\approx \frac{1}{3}$ of osteosarcomas (not confined to the small cell type) and $\approx 25\%$ of mesenchymal chondrosarcoma
- 50% of Merkel cell carcinoma (but 90% are +ve for Fli-1 immunostaining)
- Lymphoblastic leukaemia / lymphoma (CD10 and / or CD45 +ve, Tdt +ve)
- Solitary fibrous tumour (together with Bcl-2 and CD34 and is morphologically not a SBRCT)
- Sex cord tumours and the sex cord elements in UTROSCT and ESTSCLE
- CD99 +vity is strong evidence *against* neuroblastoma in the d/dg of SBRCTs

CD117 (c-kit)

- GIST (strong, diffuse cytoplasmic with membranous accentuation)
- Myofibroblasts (cytoplasmic blob) and their lesions e.g. fibromatosis (but not inflammatory myofibroblastic tumour) esp. the Dako™ A4502 clone that also stains some SFTs (weak and patchy)
- Germ cells (± membranous accentuation), seminoma and ITGCNU
- Myeloblasts, AML, erythroid and megakaryocyte precursors (but usu. not lymphoid), ALCL, RS cells
- Mast cells (± membranous accentuation) and their proliferations
- Melanocytes (± membranous accentuation) and melanomas
- Endothelial cells (fetal), angiosarcoma, Kaposi sarcoma (focal), HPC and PEComa
- Other sarcomas: DFSP, well diff liposarcoma (sclerosing subtype), clear cell sarcoma, Ewing's, FDC sarcoma
- Breast epithelial cells and phyllodes tumours (sub-epithelial stromal cells)
- Other epithelia (salivary, sweat gland, renal tubular) and carcinomas e.g. SmCC, AdCC, endometrial adenocarcinoma and thymic carcinomas (but not thymomas)
- Some gliomas

Other CD antigens

See pp.107–108.

TTF-1 (nuclear staining)

- Lung (80% of adenocarcinoma are +ve *cf.* 20% of SCC)
- Thyroid follicular cells
- SmCC of any 1° site (but Merkel cell carcinoma is −ve)
- all other sites / tumours are usu. −ve (esp. with clone 8G7G3/1 but clone SPT24 may focally stain colonic adenoCA and some clones may rarely stain ependymoma or other adenoCA e.g. gastric, endometrioid [incl. prostatic ductal], serous, papillary nasopharyngeal, etc.)

WT1 (nuclear staining)

- Wilms' tumour (epithelium and blastema)
- $\approx 50\%$ of AML (but is −ve in ALL)

---

[1] EMA (+ve in epithelial and spindle elements) helps differentiate synovial sarcoma from MPNST, fibrosarcoma and EMA −ve carcinomas

- Metanephric adenoma
- DSRCT and some RMS
- Associated with androgen insensitivity if +ve in prostate carcinoma (using the C19 Ab to the C-terminus)
- Ovarian serous tumours incl. carcinoma (70% have >50% of cells +ve) but usu. not uterine serous CA (only 8% of cases have >50% of cells +ve); endometrioid CA of ovary or uterus are ≈ all −ve
- Ovarian TCC (not bladder)
- Some endometrial stromal tumours
- Mesothelium / mesothelial tumours
- Sertoli cells (mature and immature) and some sex cord and stromal tumours of the gonads
- *Cytoplasmic staining* is seen in glioblastoma, melanoma, sarcomas and many carcinomas

Vimentin (in epithelial cells)
- Endometrial glands and carcinomas
- ±ve in ovarian *non-serous* neoplasms (incl. mucinous and endometrioid), −ve in serous
- Thyroid carcinomas: follicular, PTC (100%), medullary (60%)
- Salivary gland: salivary duct carcinoma, PLGA, carcinoma *ex* PSAd
- Myoepithelial carcinoma
- Carcinosarcoma and spindle cell carcinoma
- Adrenocortical tumours
- (Melanoma)

The D2-40 antibody to the surface membrane oncofetal protein M2A
- M2A is found on testicular germ cells (= aggrus). The podoplanin Ab recognises the same protein
- 99% specific for lymphatic endothelium (−ve for most blood vascular endothelia)
- +ve in KS, Schwannoma, many benign and malig. spindle cell tumours (−ve in sarcomatoid mesothelioma)
- Mesothelial cells and epithelioid mesothelioma (but not d/dg serous carcinoma of peritoneum / ovary)
- Craniopharyngiomas, chondroma and chondrosarcoma (but not d/dg chordoma)
- Immature brain (cerebral cortex, cerebellar outer Purkinje layer, germinal matrix, ependyma, meninges)
- Brain tumours: haemangioblastoma, anaplastic ependymoma, glioblastoma, germinoma, meningiomas & choroid plexus papilloma & carcinoma (but not d/dg metastatic adenocarcinoma)

Some Immunohistochemical Panels for Differential Diagnosis
- These are typical profiles but exceptions occur and depend on Ab clone and technique
- −ve usu. means <10% of cases stain +ve with that Ab.
- See also specific chapters for other profiles (e.g. ovary, endometrium, mesothelioma, etc.)

Gastric glandular tumours
- +ve: AE1/AE3, EMA, CEA, CK19 (80%), CA-19.9 (70%)
- ±ve: CK7, CK20, CA-19.9
- −ve: WT1, TTF-1, CK17, ER, PgR, GCDFP15, CA-125

Pancreatic exocrine glandular tumours
- +ve: CK7, CK17, CK19, CA-19.9, CEA, HER2 (>80%), mesothelin   ⎫ ≈ $\frac{1}{3}$ are CK7+ve,
- ±ve: CK20 (≈ 50% of cases are +ve), CA-125, CD138 (≈ $\frac{1}{3}$ are +ve)   ⎬ CK20 −ve & 5% are
- −ve: WT1, TTF-1, ER, PgR, GCDFP15, PSA, AMACAR, vimentin, S100   ⎭ CK7−ve, CK20 +ve

Colorectal carcinoma
- +ve: CK20, CEA, AMACAR (>80%), CD138, CK19, CA-19.9 ⎫ ≈ none are CK7+ve, CK20 −ve
- ±ve: CK7 (15–20%), mesothelin ($\frac{1}{3}$), S100 (20%), CK17 ($\frac{1}{3}$) ⎭ and 80% are CK7−ve, CK20+ve
- −ve: HER2 (<15%), TTF-1, PSA, vimentin, CA-125 (10%), uroplakin

Breast carcinoma (ductal and lobular)
- +ve: CK7, CK19, CAM5.2
- ±ve: GCDFP15, ER, PgR, S100 (25%), CK19 (60%), CK17, CK20
- −ve: CK20 (10% of cases are +ve), WT1, TTF-1, CA-19.9 (10% are +ve), CA-125, mesothelin
- *NB*: GCDFP15 is −ve in lung, endometrial and ovarian adenoCA (See p. 259 for Paget's disease)

SCC
- +ve: 34βE12 (even in poorly diff. tumours), CK14, CK5/6 ⎫ Markers of squamous differentiation in
- ±ve: CK7   ⎬ other tumours (e.g. TCC) also include:
- −ve: CK20   ⎪ MAC387 (to myelomonocytic L1 Ag),
                                                                                       ⎭ CK10,14,19 & caveolin 1

Urothelial differentiation / TCC

There is no single Ab specific for TCC but +vity for all / most of the following is suggestive:

- Uroplakin III (said to be −ve in TCC of the ovary but +ve in urological TCC) – although highly specific *cf.* other organs, only ≈ 50% of invasive urothelial TCC stain +ve
- CK7 and CK20 both +ve (but +vity decreases with increasing TCC grade and prostatic carcinoma +vity increases with increasing Gleason grade)
- CA-19.9 (also +ve in pancreaticobiliary, gastric, colorectal ± other carcinomas)
- Thrombomodulin: useful in d/dg prostatic / RCC because these are both ≈ always −ve but ! other carcinomas are +ve for thrombomodulin incl. breast, SCC, lung adenoCA, mesothelioma and angiosarcoma
- CK5/6 (becomes −ve in poorly diff TCC) and p63
- 34βE12 (with heat Ag retrieval) is useful in d/dg prostatic adenocarcinoma (but not ASC or SCC of prostate or elsewhere or adenocarcinoma of breast or colon because these may all be +ve)
- Monoclonal CEA, +ve though not sensitive in TCC, is helpful in d/dg prostatic carcinoma (−ve) but polyclonal CEA has higher +vity rates in both TCC and prostatic carcinoma so doesn't help
- For CIS, see pp. 219–220.

Prostatic neoplasia

- Loss of basal cell layer by CK5/6 and p63 (also LP34 / 34βE12 and P-cadherin) – but HMW CK staining gets weaker / more patchy with ↑ fixation and small/atrophic glands at periphery of lobules and some higher Gleason grade (e.g. 3+4) carcinoma cells are +ve (so use morphology to distinguish)
- Epithelial (lumenal) cell positivity for AMACAR:
  - ➢ positivity defined as strong staining – visible on < ×10 objective – in cells with H&E features of malig. with any of the following patterns: circumferential, apical, diffuse cytoplasmic or granular .
  - ➢ staining is unaffected by radioRx / anti-androgen Rx or inflammation
  - ➢ focal, weak, non-circumferential staining may occur in occasional benign glands
  - ➢ high grade PIN is +ve and partial atrophy can be +ve ⎫ hence the need to interpret
  - ➢ *most* cases of AAH are −ve / weak focal (8% are +ve) ⎭ AMACAR with a basal cell marker
  - ➢ nephrogenic adenoma can be +ve (! and is −ve for basal cells) – use morphology and PSA
  - ➢ atrophy, basal cell hyperplasia and seminal vesicle cells are negative
  - ➢ also +ve in other carcinomas (oesophageal, colorectal, urothelial, lung, ovarian, breast), lymphoma, melanoma and normal cells in other organs
- PSAP and PSA are selective but not specific to prostatic epithelial cells, especially if there is only focal / weak staining. Polyclonal PSA is more sensitive for prostate *cf.* monoclonal in the d/dg of TCC
- PSAP can stain carcinoids and pancreatic islet cell tumours as well as the tissues / tumours listed below for PSA. Both PSA and PSAP are −ve in seminal vesicle / ejaculatory duct epithelium
- PSA staining is +ve in: (*NB:* the polyclonal Ab appears to be more sensitive without loss of specificity)
  - ➢ 90% prostatic carcinoma – high grade more likely to be −ve ⎫ *NB:* the result is sensitive
  - ➢ 50% PSAd (Pleomorphic Salivary Adenomas) ⎪ to Ab dilution so you may
  - ➢ 25% salivary gland carcinomas ⎬ need to perform PSA
  - ➢ 10% each for bladder and gastric cancers ⎭ staining at multiple titrations
  - ➢ melanoma, colonic CA, breast CA, pancreatic acinar cell CA and tumours of Skene's glands
  - ➢ normal / benign tissues: perianal glands, urachal remnants, cystitis cystica, seminal vesicles and other urogenital glands (male bulbo-urethral [Cowper's] and female peri-urethral [Skene's])

Immunohistochemistry of myoepithelial / basal cells

- HMW CK (CK5/6, 34βE12 or LP34) ⎫ These are also +ve
- P-cadherin (cell-cell border +vity) ⎬ in basal cells e.g. of
- p63 (nuclear stain) – also +ve in AdCC / pleomorphic adenoma, *etc.* ⎭ the prostate
- p63 is also +ve in monophasic sarcomatoid / metaplastic carcinoma of the breast (most of which are also CK +ve)
- Smooth muscle myosin (less myofibroblast staining than αSMA) ⎫ These stain *myoepithelial*
- Calponin (less myofibroblast staining than αSMA) ⎪ cells (as opposed to
- S100 and GFAP ⎬ basal cells)
- CD10 (also +ve in some stromal cells) ⎪
- CK14 (also +ve in some epithelia) ⎭
- CK 8/18 (CAM5.2) is −ve

Immunohistochemistry of mast cells and plasma cells

See p. 100.

Serum Levels of Some Markers Also Used in Immunohistochemistry

CA-19.9 (normally <40 kU/l)

- A carbohydrate antigen to Lewis blood group factor ($\therefore$ CA-19.9 is −ve in the 5% of the population who are Lewis$^{-/-}$ − no matter what cancer or other condition they may have)
- ↑ (in decreasing percentage) in carcinomas of the pancreas, biliary tract, stomach and liver
- ↑ (in a smaller percentage) in benign conditions of the above (except biliary tract)
- ↑ also in: breast, gynae (cervix / ovary), kidney, thyroid and lower GI tumours and germinomas

CA-125 (normally <35 kU/l)

- ≈ 25% of ovarian carcinomas do not give ↑ levels
- Not specific for serous ovarian carcinoma if below 1000 kU/l
- Mucinous ovarian carcinoma gives levels in the low hundreds
- Other causes of ↑ CA-125 (usu. ≪200 kU/l):
  - ➤ other gynae site tumours: leiomyoma, carcinoma of Fallopian tube / cervix / endometrium
  - ➤ other 1° site carcinoma (colon, breast, lung, pancreatic, biliary), mesothelioma and Krukenberg
  - ➤ non-neoplastic gynae: early pregnancy, endometriosis, PID, menstruation
  - ➤ non-neoplastic non-gynae: liver cirrhosis, pancreatitis and any cause of serosal irritation / inflam^n
  - ➤ miscellaneous: some CTD, endocrinopathies and in <2% of normal women.

PSA (normally <5 μg/l; half-life is 2 days)

- Normal levels are seen in upto 20% of prostatic CA; otherwise log(serum level) ∝ tumour volume
- ↑ in 1–5% of tumours of the lung, kidney and those stated above (under 'Prostatic Neoplasia')
- ↑ in benign GU disease (incl. orchitis, nephritis, urethritis, acute urine retention and BPH)
- ↑ in benign non-GU disease of CVS, liver, lung and general infections / endocrine / CTD
- transient ↑ after fingering (2× normal) or needling (60× normal) the prostate

AFP (normally <10 kU/l; 1kU = 1μg; half-life is upto 1 week)

- 10–35% of HCC / hepatoblastomas do not give raised levels
- ↑ In other tumours: MTU, YST, pancreaticobiliary, gastric, lung, breast, some sarcomas
- Non-neoplastic (usu. <400 kU/l): hepatitis/cirrhosis, liver trauma, benign familial ↑AFP, fetal defects
- Some IEM (esp. tyrosinosis) can give very high levels (>400 kU/l)
- Glypican-3 (GPC3) is a newer oncofetal protein that may be used in immuno and serology for HCC

CEA (normally <10 μg/l, half-life is 2 days):

- ↑ in cancers of endoderm-derived organs: GIT, pancreas, liver, lung (SmCC and non-SmCC)
- ↑ in other cancers: breast, gynae
- Upto 35–50% of all the above cancers do not give raised levels
- ↑ (but not by much) in benign / inflammatory conditions of these organs (incl. smoking)

Bibliography

Al-adnan, M. Williams, S., Anderson, J., Ashworth, M., Malone, M. And Sebire, N.J. (2006) Immunocytochemical nuclear positivity for WT1 in acute myeloid leukaemia. *Journal of Pathology*, **210** (Suppl.), 62A.

Al-Hussaini, M., Stockman, A., Foster, H. and McGluggage, W.G. (2004) WT-1 assists in distinguishing ovarian from uterine serous carcinoma and in distinguishing between serous and endometrioid ovarian carcinoma. *Histopathology*, **44**, 109–105.

Ananthanarayanan, V., Pins, M.R., Meyer, R.E. and Gann, P.H. (2005) Immunohistochemical assays in prostatic biopsies processed in Bouin's fixative. *Journal of Clinical Pathology*, **58** (3), 322–324.

Bancroft, J.D. and Stevens, A. (eds.) (1996) *Theory and Practice of Histological Techniques*, 4th edn, Churchill Livingstone, New York.

Bishop, A.E. and Polak, J.M. (1993) Modern histological imaging methods, in *Surgical Endocrinology*, 1st edn (eds J. Lynn and S.R. Bloom.), Oxford University Press Ltd, Oxford, pp. 93–104.

Bonin, S., Petrera, F., Rosai, J. and Stanta, G. (2005) DNA and RNA obtained from Bouin's fixed tissues. *Journal of Clinical Pathology*, **58** (3), 313–316.

Carvalho, S., Silva, A.O., Milanezi, F. *et al.* (2004) c-KIT and PDGFRA in breast phyllodes tumours: overexpression without mutation. *Journal of Clinical Pathology*, **57** (10), 1075–1079.

Chorny, J.A. and Barr, R.J. (2002) S100-positive spindle cells in scars a diagnostic pitfall in the re-excision of desmoplastic melanoma. *American Journal of Dermatopathology*, **24** (4), 309–312.

Chu, P.G. and Weiss, L.M. (2002) Keratin expression in human tissues and neoplasms. *Histopathology*, **40** (5), 403–439.

Dabbs, D.J. (ed) *Diagnostic immunohistochemistry*, 1st edn, Churchill Livingstone, New York.

Leong, A.S-Y, Cooper, K. and Leong, F.J.W.M. *Diagnostic antibodies for immunohistochemistry*, 2nd edn, Greenwich Medical Media, London.

Evans, A.J. (2003) α-Methylacyl CoA racemase (P504S): overview and potential uses in diagnostic pathology as applied to prostate needle biopsies. *Journal of Clinical Pathology*, **56** (12), 892–897.

Evennett, P.J. (1995) Light microscopy, in *Image Analysis in Histology: Conventional and Confocal Microscopy*, 1st edn (eds R, Wootton, D.R. Springall and J.M. Polak.), Cambridge University Press Ltd, Cambridge, pp. 134–150.

Fisher, C. (2005) Gastrointestinal stromal tumours, in *Recent Advances in Histopathology*, vol. 21 (eds M. Pignatelli and J. Underwood.), The Royal Society of Medicine Press, London, pp. 71–88.

Helander, K.G. (1999) Formaldehyde binding in brain and kidney: A kinetic study of fixation. *The Journal of Histotechnology*, **22** (4), 317–8.

Jass, J.R. (1996) Origins of. . . mucin staining. *Journal of Clinical Pathology*, **49** (10), 787–790

Kahn, H.J., Marks, A., Thom, H. and Baumal, R. (1983) Role of antibody to S100 protein in diagnostic pathology. *American Journal of Clinical Pathology*, **79** (3), 341–347.

Kakar, S., Muir, T., Murphy, L.M., Lloyd, R.V. and Burgart, L.J. (2003) Immunoreactivity for Hep Par 1 in hepatic and extrahepatic tumours and its correlation with albumin in situ hybridization in hepatocellular carcinoma. *American Journal of Clinical Pathology*, **119**, 361–366

Kiat-Hon Lim, T., Teo, C., Giron, D.M. *et al.* (2007) Thyroid transcription factor-1 may be expressed in ductal adenocracinoma of the prostate: a potential pitfall. *Journal of Clinical Pathology*, **60** (8), 941–943.

Kirkpatrick, P. (1982) Use of orcein in detecting hepatitis B antigen in paraffin sections of liver. *Journal of Clinical Pathology*, **35**, 430–433.

Lau, S.K., Prakash, S., Geller, S.A. and Alsabeh, R. (2002) Comparative immunohistochemical profile of hepatocellular carcinoma, cholangiocarcinoma, and metastatic adenocarcinoma. *Human Pathology*, **33**, 1175–1181.

Leverton, K.E. and Gullick, W.J. (1998) Growth factor receptor gene mutations and human pathology, in *Progress in Pathology*, vol. 4 (eds N. Kirkham and N.R. Lemoine.), Churchill Livingstone, Edinburgh, pp. 215–239.

Lombart, B., Monteagudo, C., López-Guerrero, J.A. *et al.*(2005) Clinicopathological and immunohistochemical analysis of 20 cases of Merkel cell carcinoma in search of prognostic markers. *Histopathology*, **56**, 622–634.

Lopez-Beltran, A., Requena, M.J., Alvarez-Kindelan, J. *et al.* (2007) Squamous differentiation in primary urothelial carcinoma of the urinary tract as seen by MAC387 immunohistochemistry. *Journal of Clinical Pathology*, **60** (3), 332–335.

Martignoni, G., Pea, M. and Brunelli, M. *et al.* CD10 is expressed in a subset of chromophobe renal cell carcinomas. *Modern Pathology*, **17**, 1455–1463.

Matsukita, S., Nomoto, M., Kitajima, S. *et al.* (2003) Expression of mucins (MUC1, MUC2, MUC5AC and MUC6) in mucinous carcinoma of the breast. *Histopathology*, **42** (1), 26–36.

Millward, E.J. and Heatley, M.K. (2003) Cytokeratin immunostaining profiles in diagnostic pathology, in *Recent Advances in Histopathology*, vol. 20 (eds D. Lowe and J.C.E. Underwood.), Royal Society of Medicine Press Ltd, London, pp. 17–28.

Moss, E.L., Hollingworth, J. and Reynolds, T.M. (2005) The role of CA-125 in clinical practice. *Journal of Clinical Pathology*, **58** (3), 308–312.

Mount, S.L. and Cooper, K. (2001) Beware of biotin: a source of false positive immunohistochemistry. *Current Diagnostic Pathology*, (September) **7** (3), 161–167.

Nakamura, Y., Kanemura, Y., Yamada, T. *et al.* (2006) D2-40 antibody immunoreactivity in developing human brain, brain tumors and cultures neural cells. *Modern Pathology*, **19** (7), 974–985.

Nakatsuka, S., Oji, Y, Horiuchi, T., *et al.* (2006) Immunochemical detection of WT1 protein in a variety of cancer cells. *Modern Pathology*, **19**, 804–814.

Nishimura, R., Yokose, T. and Mukai, K. (1997) S-100 protein is a differentiation marker in thyroid carcinoma of follicular cell origin: an immunohistochemical study. *Pathology International*, **47** (10), 673–679.

Penman, D., Downie, I. and Roberts, F. (2006) Positive immunostaining for thyroid transcription factor-1 in primary and metastatic colonic adenocarcinoma: a note of caution. *Journal of Clinical Pathology*, **59** (6), 663–664.

Polak, J.M. and Van Noorden, S. (2003) *Introduction to Immunocytochemistry*, 3rd edn, BIOS Scientific Publishers, Oxford.

Rassidakis, G.Z., Georgakis, G.V., Oyarzo, M., Younes, A. and Medeiros, L.J. (2004) Lack of c-kit (CD117) expression in CD30+ lymphomas and lymphomatoid papulosis. *Modern Pathology*, **17**, 946–953.

Reis-Filho, J.S. and Schmitt, F.C. (2003) p63 expression in sarcomatoid/metaplastic carcinomas of the breast. *Histopathology*, **42** (1), 94–95.

Rindi, G., Azzoni, C., La Rosa, S. *et al.* (1999) ECL cell tumor and poorly differentiated endocrine carcinoma of the stomach: prognostic evaluation by pathological analysis. *Gastroenterology*, **116** (3), 532–542.

Rosai, J. (ed) (2004) *Rosai and Ackerman's Surgical Pathology*, 9th edn, Mosby, Edinburgh.

Rotimi, O., Cairns, A., Gray, S., Moayyedi, P. and Dixon, M.F. (2000) Histological identification of *Helicobacter pylori*: comparison of staining methods. *Journal of Clinical Pathology*, **53** (10), 756–759.

Sarkady, E. and Benbow, E.W. (2007) TTF-1 reactivity in colorectal adenocarcinoma. *Journal of Pathology* (Suppl.) (poster p20 at the Winter Meeting, 3–5th January 2007 UCL, in press).

Silva, E.G. and Balfour Kraemer, B. (1987) *Intraoperative Pathologic Diagnosis. Frozen section and other techniques*, 1st edn, Williams and Wilkins, Baltimore.

Skordilias, K. and Howatson, A.G. (2003) The diagnostic challenge of paediatric small round cell tumours, in *Progress in Pathology*, vol. 6 (eds N. Kirkham, N.A. Shepherd.), Greenwich Medical Media Ltd, London, pp. 1–27.

Symmers, W. St. C (ed) *Systemic Pathology*, Vol. 4, 2nd edn (1978), Churchill Livingstone, London.

Takahashi, K., Isobe, T., Ohtsuki, Y. *et al.* (1984) Immunohistochemical study on the distribution of alpha and beta subunits of S-100 protein in human neoplasm and normal tissues. *Virchows Archiv B*, **45** (4), 385–396.

Tillyer, C.R. (1994) The clinical biochemistry of neoplasia, in *Scientific Foundations of Biochemistry in Clinical Practice*, 2nd edn (eds) D.L. Williams and V. Marks, Butterworth-Heinemann Ltd., Oxford, pp. 161–188.

Trejo, O., Reed, J.A. and Prieto, V.G. (2002) Atypical cells in human cutaneous re-excision scars for melanoma express p75NGFR, C56/N-CAM and GAP-43: evidence of early Schwann cell differentiation. *Journal of Cutan Pathology*, **29**, pp. 397–406.

Ulbright, T.M., Amin, M.B. and Young, R.H. (1999) Tumors of the testis, Adnexa, spermatic cord and scrotum, in *Atlas of Tumor Pathology Fascicle No. 25*, 3rd series, Armed Forces Institute of Pathology, Washington DC.

Varma, M. and Jasani, B. (2005) Diagnostic utility of immunohistochemistry in morphologically difficult prostate cancer: review of current literature. *Histopathology*, **47**, 1–16.

Wheater, P.R., Burkitt, H.G. and Daniels, V.G. (1987) *Functional Histology: A text and colour atlas*, 2nd edn, Churchill Livingstone, Edinburgh.

Winn, W.C. Jr. (2000) Demonstration of infectious agents in tissue. *Current Diagnostic Pathology*, **6** (2), 84–92.

Yamauchi, N., Watanabe, A., Hishinuma, M. *et al.* (2005) The glypican-3 oncofetal protein is a promising diagnostic marker for hepatocellular carcinoma. *Modern Pathology*, **18**, 1591–1598.

Web sites

Histotechnical Protocols of the University of Nottingham Medical School Division of Histopathology www.nottingham.ac.uk/pathology/default.html (accessed March 2007).

Histotechnical Protocols of the University of Bristol School of Vetinary Science Pathology Department www.bristol.ac.uk/vetpath/cpl/lablinks.html (accessed March 2007).

Protocols Online www.protocol-online.org/ (accessed March 2007).

'Antibody and Beyond' web site: www.antibodybeyond.com/ (accessed March 2007).

Vyberg, M. and Moll, R. 'Cytokeratins in diagnostic histopathology. Dako information sheet.' www.dakocytomation.co.uk/ (accessed July 2004).

3. Laboratory Management

Health & Safety

Aims of a Lab Health & Safety Policy
- Identify and assess any risks   (risk assessments for infection, chemical and other hazards)
- Take appropriate precautions   (building design, protective clothing, storage, waste, etc.)
- Prepare and publish local rules   (SOPs and rules for porters, domestic staff, visitors, etc.)
- Ensure everyone is aware of them   (induction for new staff, regular fire lectures, etc.)

Hazard Groups (HG) for Biological Agents (BA)
- HG1. BA unlikely to cause human disease in immunocompetent people (e.g. *Aspergillus*)
- HG2. BA that can cause disease but is unlikely to spread to the community and effective Rx/prophylaxis is available (e.g. MRSA, *Actinomyces*, *Clostridia*, HSV / HPV)
- HG3. BA that can cause severe disease / spread to community but effective Rx/prophylaxis is available (e.g. TB, *Salmonella typhi*, *Brucella*, anthrax, Q-fever, HBV, HCV, HIV, SARS, CJD)
- HG4. BA that cause severe disease, are likely to spread and no effective Rx/prophylaxis (e.g. rabies, smallpox and VHFs such as ebola and Lassa fever)
- The above 'definitions' are a general guide only and have exceptions (e.g. there is no effective Rx for CJD, but this is still classified as HG3) ∴ always check the official classificat^n for a particular bug
- The term 'serious communicable diseases' (SCD) refers to BA in ≈ HG3 + HG4

Legislation and Regulations

Health and Safety at Work Act 1974 (HSWA)
- Employers must protect and prepare staff
- Employees must: ➢ take care, for themselves and others
                    ➢ co-operate with employers.

Management of Health and Safety at Work Regulations 1999 (MHSWR)
- Risk assessments
- SOPs
- Appoint helpers
- Employees must report risks

Control of Substances Hazardous to Health Regulations 2002 (COSHH)
- Risk assessments for all chemicals and infective materials used in lab
- Employers must: ➢ provide free vaccines
                    ➢ keep health records on employees dealing with (or potentially exposed to) HG3/4 agents.

Reporting of Diseases and Dangerous Occurrences at Work Regulations (RIDDOR)
- Report all major diseases or dangerous occurrences
- Keep an in-house record of *all* injuries and adverse events

European Working Time Directive 93/104/EC 1998 (EWTD)
- No-one shall be required to work > 48 hours per week

Other regulations to be aware of:
- Fire precautions in the workplace
- Manual handling
- Display screen equipment
- Provision and Use of Work Equipment Regulations (PUWER)
- Ionising radiation regulations (e.g. for the use of Faxitron® machines and the like)
- Regulations for the use and disposal of radioisotopes (e.g. for radioactive sentinel LNs)
- Noise at work, electricity at work, first aid at work

Diagnostic Criteria Handbook in Histopathology: A Surgical Pathology Vade Mecum by Paul J. Tadrous
Copyright © 2007 by John Wiley & Sons, Ltd.

The Transport of Specimens
- Documentation must comply with The Labelling, Transport and Reception of Specimens Regulations (1985). Advice is available on the Royal Mail web site (www.royalmail.co.uk)
- For high risk infective specimens, packaging must conform to the latest edition of the IATA Dangerous Goods Regulations for infectious substances packaging instruction UN602. See HPA guidance notes available at URL www.hpa.org.uk/cepr/specialpathogens/SPRU_brochure.pdf
- Some things that *cannot* be sent by regular Royal Mail:
  - clinical / medical waste
  - alcoholic solutions over 70% / flammables / aerosols
  - some radioactive materials
  - poisons / HG4 and some HG3 agents
- To send wet medical diagnostic samples by Royal Mail (max. 50ml of fluid) use the Royal Mail SafeBox$^{®}$ (see Royal Mail web site for details) otherwise a maximum of 50ml/50gm sample can be sent (within UK only) by ensuring certain minimum packaging standards are adhered to e.g.:
  - it is kept in a leak-proof container
  - surrounded by sufficient absorbent material to absorb all the fluid
  - with an outer container strong enough to contain any part of the specimen should it break
  - plus other requirements of appropriate health and safety standards (contact Royal Mail).
- Do not use taxis / public transport to transport clinical specimens

The Post Mortem Room – autopsies on high risk cases (HG3 / HG4)
- All staff must be fully trained
- Limit the nõ. of people present in the autopsy room to the minimum required
- Only the *pathologist* should open/eviscerate/handle organs
- Use a 'circulator' (clean assistant) for recording / photographing / using phone, etc.
- Follow correct disposal / cleaning procedures for tissues, instruments, consumables and surfaces
- For more specific guidance see Autopsy chapter and RCPath publications
- A *risk assessment* should be conducted before any PM to identify if there a risk of a BA, what is its HG, etc. Standard risk assessment forms should be available locally for these purposes.

The Clinical Laboratory – Factors to Consider
- Dealing with spillage and contamination
- Regulation of formalin levels: adequate ventilation and regular checks (chemosensitive badges / formaldemeters)
- Protection of culture stocks / securing the lab (ID cards, combination locks, etc.) – more relevant for microbiology labs and follows toughened anti-bioterrorism regulations
- Description of laminar air-flow safety cabinets and other equipment
- Correct storage of flammable liquids (i.e. in lockable metal flammable cupboards) / gasses
- Autoclaving and correct disposal of samples / waste

Conditions of Employment – Factors to Consider
- Checks before employment (e.g. disability questionnaire, exposure to infections, criminal records)
- Checks on employment (e.g. vaccinations, baseline health check / serum storage for HIV, etc.)
- Checks during employment (e.g. regular respiratory function tests for anyone working with glutaraldehyde)

Workforce-Related Issues

The 'New Deal' for Doctors in Training and New Contract for Junior Doctors
Unsocial hours and poor working conditions of juniors resulted in junior doctors' representatives negotiating a new work and pay structure with the UK Government called the 'New Deal' in 1991, features of which included the following:
- Limits were placed on the nõ. of hours that could be worked and on working at antisocial times
- Minimum requirements for rest periods were agreed
- Minimum standards were agreed regarding available accommodation
- Catering facilities must meet availability and quality standards
- Safety and security in the workplace must be assured

- Management heads must submit regular (e.g. 6 monthly) statements to the Trust Executive indicating how well their posts comply with these standards
- The new junior's contract abolishes ADHs and replaces this with a 'banding supplement' i.e. a fixed payment which is a percentage of the basic salary. The amount of this payment is determined by the degree of compliance of the post to New Deal working hours and falls within one of 3 'bands' (with sub-bands).

New Consultants' Contract (for NHS consultants in England)
- The only contract to be offered to new NHS appointees from October 2003
- Consultants must agree a Job Plan with their clinical head (head of department or clinical director) in terms of direct clinical care Programmed Activities (PAs), Supporting Professional Activities (SPAs), additional responsibilities (e.g. Trust committees), external duties (i.e. off-site additional responsibilities such as RCPath committees) and fee-paying services (FPS e.g. Private, Coronial and Category 2 work[1]: PA = 4 hours, equivalent to 1 session ($\approx$ half a normal working day)
  SPA = 4 hours for administration, audit, teaching, research, appraisal, CPD, etc.
- There must be (at least) annual review of this job plan as part of consultant appraisal. Appraisal also includes agreement on (and review of progress in) a personal development plan (PDP) for CPD
- The contract for clinical academics with honorary consultant status is along the same lines but many (e.g. 50%) of the PAs and SPAs are funded via academic sources. There will be joint appraisal (with both Trust and University appraisers present)
- Consultants cannot be required to work >48 hours(= 12 PAs) per week for the NHS but may opt out of the EWTD to work longer *in a self-employed capacity* (e.g. private practice) provided this does not affect their ability to do their NHS work
- Certain criteria must be satisfied if a consultant is to be granted *pay progression* (i.e. increment of salary for the next year(s) upto a maximum ceiling over 20 years). These criteria mostly relate to how well a consultant has stuck to their agreed Job Plan and satisfactory participation in appraisal.
- Locum service (of any duration) is credited towards seniority and recognised for pay progression *starting from* the first job that is $\geq$6 months duration and subject to Job Plan review (e.g. appraisal).
- FPS may be undertaken provided all NHS commitments are fulfilled as a priority. If FPS are done during PA time then the consultant must offer to work an additional PA for the NHS
- Flexible working (as encouraged in the DoH policy framework *Improving Working Lives*, 2000) means that some PAs / SPAs may be done at home e.g. letter writing / preparing audit presentations
- *NB*: work from home is subject to RCPath guidelines that state:
  - confidentiality must be maintained by the use of timed-out password protection, etc.
  - transporting irreplaceable specimens (e.g. cervical smears) must be done by courier or staff
  - appropriate working conditions and equipment must be available (e.g. quiet, uninterrupted, etc.)
  - the service must be audited and PM slides must not be stored longer than needed for diagnosis

The Changing Role for Biomedical Scientists incl. 'Agenda for Change'
- Low pay and low job satisfaction lead to problems with recruitment and retention of BMSs
- The DoH suggested the need for a single pay and promotion scale (or 'spine') which allows BMSs (and nurses, etc.) to progress through a variety of routes (not just going into management) which include opportunities for extending their skills as Advanced Practitioners, nurse endoscopists, nurse consultants, BMS in cut-up, etc. This new pay structure and career progression system is the subject of what the DoH terms the '*Agenda for Change*' (2007)
- Advanced practitioners in cervical cytology take on an independent diagnostic role but RCPath guidelines state that they must work with at least 2 consultants doing cytology to have someone to show difficult cases to.
- BMS role in cut-up is supported by the RCPath in the light of a favourable report of a joint RCPath / IBMS working party 1 year pilot scheme over 10 hospitals however:
  - this is delegation not independent practice $\therefore$ consultant is still responsible and must have the final say as to what, if anything, gets delegated to a BMS, however senior
  - training of junior doctors must not be compromised
  - a consultant must preview and review all specimens cut-up by a BMS (but this initial safeguard was not always adhered to in the pilot and its recommendation appears to be being relaxed)

---

[1] Category 2 work incl. cremation fees and things done for insurance reports, etc.)

  ➤ there is a need for a standardised training and exam structure for BMSs in cut-up
  ➤ there is a need for funding to: ☞ supplement cut-up BMS salaries;
                                         ☞ replace BMS time in the lab with new recruits;
                                         ☞ fund equipment such as digital cameras
  ➤ to succeed there needs to be wide acceptance by consultants
- The Joint Working Party now offer a 'Diploma of Extended Practice in Histological Dissection' for BMSs in cut-up who follow an approved training program with log book portfolio and exam

Medical Workforce Planning in Histopathology
- It is important to ensure that the supply of trained pathologists meets future requirements
- Deaneries control, monitor (and fund) the nõ. of current training posts via the NTN system
- Workforce monitoring to detect trends is important in forward planning. One way to do this is by monitoring AACs (via the RCPath representative on the AACs) and another is by direct surveys which the RCPath Medical Workforce Department conducts
- NHS Workforce Development Confederations (WDCs – local branches of the NHS Workforce Group and Executive Committee):
  ➤ help conduct workforce monitoring at a local level (all professions – not just Drs)
  ➤ plan workforce targets and liaise with local Human Resources departments and Deaneries
  ➤ negotiate and manage contracts with suppliers of training schemes
  ➤ manage practice placements for HEFCE and NHS-funded students
  ➤ control and distribute government funds for education and training via the MPET levy (includes MADEL, NMET and SIFT).
- The RCPath has provided updated guidance on how to calculate work-load figures so that departments can calculate the no. of consultants they need to cope with their workload:
  ➤ workload figures are now expressed as sessional (PA) maxima (not yearly) because Job Plans differ w.r.t. the nõ. of clinical PAs worked
  ➤ numerical work weights are used instead of nõ. of cases as cases vary in complexity
  ➤ workload matrices are provided for each specimen type which codify the macro and micro work into numbers 0, 1, 3, 5 and 10. Add these two scores to get the weight for that specimen
  ➤ autopsies are graded as low (1.5 hours), medium (3 hours) and high (6 hours) input (times include ancillary tests and writing the report)
  ➤ a score of 10 units per hour (40 per PA) is considered appropriate. A whole-time NHS consultant should work 7.5 PA (minus 1.5 PA per MDM or patient-related SPA) per week and should work 40 weeks per year
  ➤ if working much more than this consider a work-load management strategy: keep a diary; eliminate unnecessary specimens of 'limited or no clinical value'; use BMSs in cut-up; form a 'waiting list' by triage and prioritisation of specimens, etc.
- The SWAG has superseded the JPAC as the body which recommends changes to the numbers of training posts in various specialties in response to anticipated need
- Government initiatives: the International Fellowship Scheme (IFS) was launched in 2002 to give over-seas doctors the chance to work in the UK as consultants for two-year fellowships. There are also controversial plans to introduce a 'sub-consultant' grade where limited autonomous practice would be performed by doctors of shorter duration training than full consultants (and on lower pay)

'Modernising Medical Careers', 'The Calman Report', the PMETB and Training Issues
- Undergraduate teaching in pathology is becoming less prominent in the 'New Curriculum'
- *'Modernising Medical Careers'* is a project from the Learning and Policy Development Section of the DoH, launched in 2003, which aims to:
  ➤ establish a two stage (usu. two-year) Foundation Program of training after graduation admin-istered via regional 'Foundation Schools' to which new medical graduates apply
    ☞ F1 year is equivalent to PRHO and has a structured curriculum with assessments based on the GMC's *'The New Doctor'* document (PMETB/GMC, 2007). Success in F1 results in full registration with the GMC and progression to F2.
    ☞ F2 is equivalent to 1st year SHO. There will also be defined aims and assessments to gauge successful completion of F2 (which entitles the Dr to apply for an StR or CMT post). This takes care of 'the lost tribe' (of SHOs) as discussed in *'Unfinished Business'* (Donaldson, 2002) and fulfils the pledge in *'The NHS Plan'* (DoH, 2000) to reform SHO training

in line with recommendations from *'A Health Service of all the Talents: Developing the NHS workforce'* (DoH, 2000) which emphasised the need for workforce planning and modernising training across the NHS.

> ➤ 'streamline training' at StR level and implement 'competency-based criteria' for assessment
> ➤ develop career pathways that enable flexible working and career breaks
> ➤ develop and encourage academic career paths

- In the past, under and overestimates of the nõ. of trainees led to backlogs of senior registrars or staff shortages at consultant level. Hence the *Calman Report* (1993) advised a system of structured training, combining registrar and senior registrar into one Specialist Registrar (SpR) grade with a staged and monitored (appraised) progression to complete specialist training. On completion, a doctor is awarded a CCT by the PMETB and is eligible be put on the Specialist Register of the GMC (before 2006, a CCST awarded by the STA of the Medical Royal Colleges was the equivalent entry route to the Specialist Register).
- In 2007 the SHO and SpR grades were merged into a single Specialty Registrar (StR) grade for each specialty (and each specialty has its own curriculum for training approved by the PMETB)
- The Postgraduate Medical Education and Training Board (PMETB) has replaced the STA and it:
  > ➤ prescribes standards for drawing up postgraduate training curricula
  > ➤ sets principles for assessment of postgraduate training
  > ➤ is responsible for quality assurance of training programmes via the relevant Royal College
  > ➤ is responsible for certifying that a Dr has completed specialist training.

Clinical Governance and Research Governance

- Clinical governance is a framework for clinical practice, management and accountability designed to protect patients by monitoring and continually improving the standard and effectiveness of healthcare.
- The monitoring activities include:
  > ➤ continuing audit cycles against defined standards (benchmarking)
  > ➤ annual appraisal for staff
  > ➤ implementation of risk management systems including error logging
  > ➤ regular inspections from the CHAI (also known as the Healthcare Commission)
  > ➤ quality control procedures (including IQC)
- The continual improvement activities include:
  > ➤ a system for closing the loop on audit (implementing any beneficial changes identified)
  > ➤ personal development programmes for staff (CPD, life long learning)
  > ➤ lesson learning from complaints and adverse clinical incidents recorded via risk assessment
  > ➤ implementing evidence-based practices including advice from the NICE
  > ➤ quality assurance activities (including EQA)
- Departmental / divisional clinical governance meetings should be held regularly (e.g. monthly) to ensure the above is being performed and to take decisions based on information from error logs, audit results, etc.
- A 'risk management' policy involves: ① recording errors, ② analysing their causes and ③ making changes to the system to: a) prevent errors and b) minimise their impact on patient care
- Research Governance is similar but aimed at ensuring responsible research practices. This involves ensuring that appropriate peer review and ethical approval is obtained for any research project in advance of the research taking place (this usu. also involves getting prior approval from your hospital's R&D department before you can apply to the REC: see www.nres.npsa.nhs.uk). Issues relating to consent, the Human Tissue Act and the Data Protection Act also need due consideration

See Chapter 25: Autopsy for aspects of consent, the Human Tissue Act and the application of clinical governance to autopsy practice. See below for the Data Protection Act.

Aspects of Budgetary Control

- Departments should receive monthly budget statements (from the directorate's financial officer)
- Departments should hold monthly budget meetings with Heads of department to discuss the budget: Are we overspending / underspending? Is it a consistent trend? Do we need to do anything to cut expenditure to meet the end of year targets?
- Only a restricted nõ. of people should have the authority to sign purchase orders

- Collect work weight data regularly so that accurate costing of departmental activities can be calculated for use in billing purchasers
- Attend yearly budget meetings with the trust board where one can put forward annual spending figures and predict usage by department / purchaser for the forthcoming year so that Pathology's proportion of any commission can be accurately updated
- Procure Service Level Agreements (SLAs) for regular outside work (SLAs provide a contract which guarantees payment for services rendered and defines sanctions for service failures)
- For *ad hoc* work use an order nõ. system so that price can be agreed in advance to avoid the external department's finance office denying all knowledge of the work and refusing to pay.
- Funding for new developments in the service (e.g. setting up a diagnostic molecular pathology lab) may be secured by putting together a 'business case proposal' setting out the arguments for the new venture in collaboration with the clinical teams that would benefit and the benefits to patients, waiting times, NHS long term cost cuts, etc. The proposal is tendered to the Trust Executive together with proposals from other departments for consideration and the successful bids are put to the SHA for funding.
- Typical sources of income and sinks of expenditure of a histopath department are shown in the figure. The details are subject to new government initiatives e.g. 'Payment by Results' (PbR – *vide infra*)

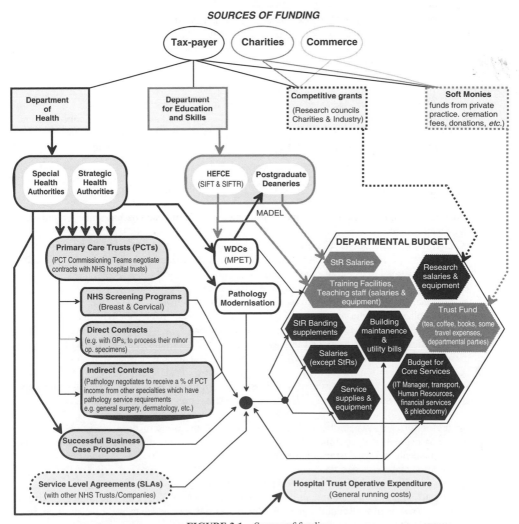

FIGURE 3.1   Source of funding

- In 2005 the UK government specified 'National Tariffs' (i.e. standard price tags for most in-patient, outpatient and A&E procedures adjusted for local costs and wage levels and with 'top-up' additional payments for some clin. specialties) so that Trusts receive ≈ 75% of their income as 'Payment by Results'

('results' being the volume of each such procedure they undertake) rather than payment according to historical budgets or inflated price-tags procured through 'skilful' local negotiating.

- Trusts are free to spend any surplus Tariff money they get due to 'efficiency' (e.g. if they can do a hip replacement for less than Tariff price, they keep the change) thus PbR is said to 'incentivise efficiency' and favour shorter hospital stays.
- Services excluded the Tariff system are subject to locally negotiated contracts: e.g. critical care, dialysis, direct access pathology, chemo/radioRx, community/mental health/rehab services, etc.

Pathology Modernisation

- Pathology services should aim to cut duplication by adopting a 'spokes and hub' lab structure (i.e. a 'managed network') ± some outsourcing to private companies (= 'Independent Sector Procurement')
- Hub (usu. a central teaching hospital) for routine work and specialised services
- Spokes (peripheral labs in outer sector hospitals) for emergency services (e.g. frozen section, cross-matching, clinical chemistry) and some specialised services (e.g. neuropathology in a centre doing neurosurgery).
- May save money by having specialised expensive equipment (and staff) at one site only, but . . .
- . . . may cost more (monies are available from the DoH Pathology Modernisation Team via the NHS Modernisation Agency, supported by the National Pathology Modernisation Group, applying the *National Framework for Pathology Service Improvement,* McClure and Barnes, 2005) due to the:
  - ➤ need for compatible IT across the network to avoid unnecessary repeat of tests just because staff can't look up the results done in another hospital
  - ➤ need for an effective, dedicated transport system for specimens ± staff
  - ➤ sharing of staff between sites that can lead to inefficient use of staff time e.g. a consultant and BMS go to a peripheral site to do a frozen section and end up waiting around for the specimen to arrive when they could be doing other things if they were at their own site.

External Quality Assurance (EQA)

- EQA schemes serve to maintain and improve performance by education and performance surveillance.
- An EQA scheme involves:
  - ➤ circulating slides of typical work-load standard (avoiding extremes of simplicity / obscurity)
  - ➤ the submission of diagnostic opinions (in coded anonymised form where the identifying codes are only known to a central scheme secretary)
  - ➤ a participants' meeting where participants discuss all the cases
  - ➤ personal feedback letters sent in confidence to each participant.
- Extensive consultation on the cases should be avoided – it makes personal performance statistics meaningless if an individual's response is the consensus opinion of the whole department
- A 'certificate of participation' is issued to participants if they take part in at least two out of three consecutive EQAs. The certificates are useful for CPD, appraisal and CPA inspections
- EQA schemes are a requirement for laboratory accreditation by CPA UK Ltd.
- EQA organisers must set up EQA schemes with advice from the RCPath EQA Steering Committee that also reviews each scheme annually. This is a requirement for an EQA scheme to be recognised by CPA UK Ltd.
- Scoring: the no. of cases a pathologist gets 'right' could be the basis of their score. The 'correct' diagnosis must not rest on the opinion of one 'expert' – it is usu. defined as the consensus diagnosis. When all respondents' scores are ranked in order, those who fall in the bottom 2.5% may be considered to have 'failed' in that round of CPA
- Performance surveillance – action points for defining persistently poor performance:
  - ➤ first action point: two failures in three consecutive rounds of EQA (or one clinically serious failure) results in a 'Dear colleague' letter which must be responded to by the recipient offering an explanation. This is still anonymised
  - ➤ second action point: same as first but this time failure to participate is included as a 'failure'. This results in an investigation by the chairman of the Histopathology National Quality Assurance Advisory Panel which may result in satisfactory resolution or the matter will be passed on to the Professional Standards Unit of the RCPath for further action.

Clinical Audit

- One audit cycle / loop involves: the monitoring of current practice → compare current practice to set standards → identify bottlenecks / areas for improvement → results inform changes in practice (= 'closing the loop' because the cycle is now repeated – i.e. audit should be continuous)
- Data for audit is gathered from: lab computers, IQC, EQA, request forms, reports, audit forms, questionnaires, re-examination of a sub-set of specimens, monthly budget statements, invoices, etc.
- Why do audit?   ➢ Clinical Governance (linked to quality assurance, risk management and PDPs)
  - ➢ to meet the requirements of CPA, Cancer Peer Review, CHAI, Monitor, PbR, etc.
  - ➢ for CPD (education, appraisal and revalidation)
  - ➢ funding and time should be built into job descriptions (as SPAs)
  - ➢ ± help from: local Audit Offices, RCPath College Audit Committee.
- Some examples of what may be audited:
  - ➢ requests (appropriateness, sufficiency of clinical information, etc.)
  - ➢ reports (content / utility and compare to RCPath Standards and Datasets)
  - ➢ quality of cut-up
  - ➢ correlation (with cytology / haematology / clin. chemistry / clin. outcome)
  - ➢ turnaround times (routine, urgent, FS, autopsy, etc.; identify bottlenecks)
  - ➢ cost per test
  - ➢ clinical care (e.g. Mortality Meetings where PM reports inform clinical practice).

The Calman-Hine Report, Cancer Networks and MDTs

The Calman-Hine Report 1995
- The report delivered a framework for cancer care that aimed to make high standards of care uniformly available to all patients eliminating the 'postcode lottery' of cancer outcome measures.
- It proposed the concept of 'cancer networks' made up of PCTs, cancer units and cancer centres with clearly defined referral and follow-up policies.
- Cancer units were seen as, typically, DGHs with expertise to diagnose and treat the most common cancers. A 'lead clinician' should be appointed for each unit to co-ordinate cancer services.
- Cancer centres were seen as large central / teaching hospitals which could treat and manage all cancers common and uncommon. These centres would normally be the only locations to provide certain specialist serves across the network e.g. radiotherapy.
- Anatomical site-specific specialisation should occur and be expanded esp. in centres but also in units. Surgical specialisation and nurse specialists were specifically mentioned in the report but now specialisation in histopathology too is becoming more the norm.
- They emphasised the importance of multidisciplinary team (MDT) working and the collection of statistics through cancer registration, both of which were already taking place to some extent.

Implementation of Calman-Hine w.r.t. Histopathology
- The establishment of multidisciplinary teams (MDTs) comprising:
  - ➢ lead clinician (could be any of the medical members of the MDT)
  - ➢ histopathologist, surgeon, radiologist, oncologist, nurse ± others e.g. physiotherapist
  - ➢ MDT co-ordinator: sets up multidisciplinary team meetings (MDMs), assembles patient-lists for distribution to pathology / radiology, etc. so they can get reports ready, records outcomes of meetings, collects patient notes.
- Pathologists working in cancer units / centres will take part in regular (usu. weekly) MDMs where cancer patients' radiology, pathology, surgical, oncological and nursing management and follow up are reviewed and further management decisions made and recorded.
- The RCPath have developed National Datasets for cancer reporting for anatomical site-specific cancers which:
  - ➢ aim to make the standard of examination of cancer specimens uniform across the UK
  - ➢ aim to facilitate cancer registration
  - ➢ state that all pathologists reporting cancer should take part in appropriate EQA schemes
  - ➢ state that there should be a 'lead pathologist' for each specialty in each department who is responsible for co-ordinating and ensuring the uniform application of the dataset standards. This has fuelled the drive towards specialisation in pathology.

- Implementation of Calman-Hine via the DoH '*NHS Cancer Plan*' (2000) has made new monies available for cancer networks which may be used e.g. for purchasing teleconferencing equipment to allow MDMs with staff across hospital sites. This may also help fund pathology e.g. the need for a new consultant histopathology post to deal with the increased work-load from new surgical consultants.
- Cancer Peer Review: to ensure National Cancer Standards (including cancer network standards on e.g. waiting times) are being met there will be annual Cancer Peer Review inspections of regional services. This may take the form of a series of interviews (by the Peer Review Panel) of the MDT members and local chiefs of service. An MDT should prepare an operational policies folder containing all protocols and SOPs (for histopathology, policies may include:
    - a) staging must be recorded according to the RCPath National Datasets standards
    - b) a designated pathologist must attend the MDMs
    - c) facilities must be available to store slides and blocks for an appropriate time
    - d) the lab must have appropriate accreditation).
  The Peer Review Panel may ask questions arising from their prior study of this folder.

Freedom of Information Act, Data Protection Act, Pathology Reports and Caldicott Guardians

Freedom of Information Act 2000
- Subject to specific exclusions, anyone has the right to receive any type of recorded information (incl. emails, minutes, etc.) held by public authorities within 20 days of them requesting it.
- Although enacted from 1st January 2005, the Act is retrospective.
- Exclusions include requests relating to: audit functions, criminal investigations, living persons (i.e. subject to the DPA), commercial sensitivity or if the information is available elsewhere.
- Enquiries must be in writing and are usu. dealt with via the Chief Executive's office.

Data Protection Act 1998 (DPA)
- Replaces and updates the Data Protection Act 1984 which concentrated on electronic data
- Now any personal data held on any type of file system including paper, electronic or otherwise is covered by the Act
- The data must be stored securely with safeguards to ensure security and avoid unauthorised access
- Any data acquired must be done with prior informed consent with mention of what data is to be stored and for what purposes it is to be used
- The data must be dealt with according to 'fair processing' rules e.g.:
    - ➢ no more data must be recorded than is required for the stated purposes
    - ➢ the data must not be stored for longer than the stated purposes require
    - ➢ data should not be used for any other purpose without specific consent
    - ➢ data must not be released to another party except in a few well-defined circumstances (e.g. to prevent or detect crime).
- A designated local *data controller* must be nominated to oversee the Act is followed in collecting, storing and processing of the data. The data controller must be registered on the Public Register of Data Controllers by the Information Commissioner (the statutory body overseeing the register)
- The subject has the right to see their data except where the data was given by a third party in confidence (e.g. a reference) or where disclosure would unavoidably identify a third party

RCPath Guidance on the Handling of Pathology Reports
- This is a partial summary only – see the report for full details and section on Storage and Disposal below
- Reports are part of the patient's record so must be stored and processed in accordance with the DPA
- Avoid using phone / fax / email for results due to lack of security e.g. verification of the identity of the recipient(s) and that the location of the receiving fax machine is in a confidential place, etc.
- Report information should only be given:
    - ➢ to the clinician who made the request
    - ➢ to the clinician's delegates
    - ➢ to others involved in the clinical care where the information is relevant to their clinical decisions.
    - ➢ to relevant authorities for reporting a notifiable disease
    - ➢ to relevant authorities when it is in the public interest

> to others with the expressed consent of the patient
> to the patient via Trust procedures (according to the patient's right under the DPA)
> to the patient directly where the clinician has agreed the patient may know their results e.g. to take appropriate action according to the monitoring of a previously diagnosed condition (but if the results show new information it should be communicated via the clinician).

The Caldicott Report 1997 and Caldicott Guardians
- Dame Fiona Caldicott was asked to examine the use of medical records by non-patient care staff (e.g. for national statistics). She recommended, *inter alia*:
  > information may be used but must first be 'de-identified' by removing the name and address and replacing this with NHS nõ. and postcode
  > a network of patient data 'guardians' should be established throughout the NHS to safeguard the protection and oversee the use of patient data in the NHS
  > only release information when absolutely necessary and give the minimum necessary with access limited via a 'need to know' basis.
- Potential problems with the Caldicott recommendations include:
  > NHS 'Trace' system allows name and address to be found from NHS nõ.
  > postcode and age is sufficient to identify most people (except those in communal addresses).
- A Caldicott Guardian must be appointed at each NHS institution (e.g. PCT / Trust) and must:
  > be a senior member of the health care or managerial staff
  > have their name and contact address held on the National Register of Caldicott Guardians
  > be involved in developing protocols governing the acceptable use of patient-identifiable data within their organisation including the interaction with regional and local ethics committees and the approval of IT system security protocols
  > develop and review protocols for transfer of patient identifiable information to third parties such as the Child Support Agency and for statistical purposes.

Storage and Disposal of Pathological Specimens and Reports

- Tissue blocks and slides should be incinerated (after minimum storage periods) in opaque containers.
- Human material should be separated from clinical waste and have separate incineration events.
- Fetuses *born dead* <24/40 may be incinerated as above but parents should be given the choice of other disposal options (cremation / burial) e.g. via a consent form. Stillbirths >24/40 or any fetus born alive <24/40 are defined as 'human remains' and are thus subject to death certification and disposal law (so cannot be incinerated as surgical waste).
- Tissue may be returned to the patients at their request provided:
  > hospital authorities are satisfied with the proposed disposal / storage methods
  > written notice of any hazards assoc[d] with the material are also given
  > the minimum storage period is served unless the tissue is not related to the medical record.
- Tissue may be handed over to a police / law-enforcement officer provided (*NB:* exceptions apply):
  > the officer's identity is confirmed (ask for ID card and nõ. and record these ID details)
  > the officer shows either informed consent for the patient or the order of a judge (make a copy)
  > you ensure the officer's health and safety and patient's confidentiality w.r.t. packaging, etc.
- Minimum storage periods are (*NB:* 'permanently' = at least 30 years):
  > wet tissue: 4 weeks after the final report is issued
  > paraffin blocks and material for EM/DNA analysis: permanently or lifetime of patient (DNA and PM tissue/slides require consent / Coronial instruction – see Chapter 25: Autopsy)
  > histology / cytology slides incl. FS: 10 years (permanently for abnormal cervical smears)
  > records relating to IQC, CPA and inspections: 10 years
  > histology / autopsy reports, museum catalogues, patient-related correspondence, SOPs, images made as part of the diagnostic process [not solely for communicat[n] e.g. MDTs]: permanently
  > request forms: 1 month after the final report is issued (permanently if they contain original diagnostic or clinical information)
  > day books / specimen receipts, EQA records, telephoned advice logs: two years
  > research records / data: anonymised or destroyed six months after final publication of results (data may be kept for 10 years to refute fraud allegations and must be kept for ≥15 years if part of a trial for new therapies. The DPA provisions must be adhered to in these cases).

- No record (tissue, report or notes) older than 1660 should be destroyed.   } separate laws govern
- No record pre-dating the NHS (dated ≤ 1948) should be destroyed.   } these two issues

Screening Program Management

Definition of Important Statistics
- Sensitivity = true test +ve cases / All[2] those with the disease
- Specificity = true test −ve cases / All those without the disease
- Predictive value of a positive test result = true test +ve cases / All who tested +ve   (=PPV)
- Predictive value of a negative test result = true test −ve cases / All who tested −ve   (=NPV)
- The predictive values depend on the prevalence of the disease in a population in addition to the characteristics of the test method
- False positive rate = false test +ve cases / All those with the disease
- False negative rate = false test −ve cases / All those with the disease

Breast Screening Program (UK)
- Three-yearly mammography is offered to women aged 50–70 years
- Details on the calculation of the above stats w.r.t. breast histology and cytology are given in the NHSBSP Publication nõ. 50 (2001) with additional stats e.g. 'absolute sensitivity' (= nõ. of C5 and B5 results as numerator) *vs.* 'complete sensitivity' (= nõ. of non-negative results as numerator)
- Stats are calculated by screening program computer systems given the biopsy and histology results
- Individual pathologists should regularly audit their own PPVs and other stats
- Annual returns of stats are made via forms KC62 (completed by breast screening units) and KC63 (completed by health authorities)

Cervical Screening Program (UK)
- Women are offered their first smear at age 25, then 3 yearly till 49, then 5 yearly till 64.
- Details of definitions for individual screener and laboratory stats (such as sensitivity, PPV, etc.) are given in the ABC document and form part of the annual returns (submitted on form KC61).
- Each laboratory must keep its own performance continually under review by measuring and auditing these statistics monthly in minuted departmental meetings.
- Labs must aim to keep their performance to the achievable standards set out in the ABC document.
- Annual returns of screening statistics from each laboratory must be provided via form KC61. This includes biopsy histology as well as cytology results and screening statistics such as PPV.
- Information provided by the cervical screening service also contributes to the annual returns on sexual health (form KC60) by providing information on the nõ. of major and minor smear abnormalities and genital infections (HSV, HPV, *Trichomonas*, etc.)

Bowel Cancer Screening Program (UK)
- Two-yearly, all NHS registered people aged 60–69 are sent an FOBt kit with foil-wrap return envelope.
- The person mails the completed test to 1 of 5 centres (called 'hubs') to read the results.
- ≈ 2% will be 'strong +ve' and invited to attend nurse clinic at the hub where endoscopy is offered.
- If patient accepts then endoscopy is arranged at their local 'screening centre'.
- If endoscopy is unsuitable then alternatives are considered (barium enema or virtual colonoscopy).
- If the FOBt is weak +ve or spoilt a retest is requested. If −ve, repeat in two years.

Some Other Topics Relevant to Management

- Appraisal: includes 360° peer review (i.e. getting formal feedback from those on the receiving end of your services), competency-based, objectives-based and trait-based appraisal. Keep an appraisal portfolio for the purposes of revalidation.
- Revalidation – requirement of the GMC for continued license to practise. The GMC may inspect a doctor's evidence of keeping up-to-date over any five-year period. For most hospital doctors' evidence of satisfactory participation in appraisal is sufficient. See www.gmc-uk.org/register/licensing/index.asp
- Professional standards and sub-standard performance issues. See GMC documents 'Good Medical Practice' (see also the RCPath version of this) and 'Duties of a Doctor' (regularly updated on the

---

[2] The word 'All', in these definitions, refers to all who were tested, regardless of the test result.

GMC's website, www.gmc-uk.org), and the RCPath guidance document on dealing with substandard performance. Know the requirements of the RCPath CPD scheme (e.g. must make annual returns and accrue $\geq$ 250 CPD points per 5 year period)

- CPA UK Ltd laboratory accreditation procedures: register with CPA $\rightarrow$ comply with the ($>$40) CPA standards $\rightarrow$ receive CPA inspectors $\rightarrow$ full/conditional/deferred accreditation
- The NHS Purchaser/ Provider contracting process and the role of 'market testing' in pathology (i.e. the process of getting management consultants to receive bids from local and outside providers to see whether an alternative supplier of pathology services could be more efficient / effective)
- Team-building: good communication (inclusivity, regular meetings), departmental outings, etc.
- The National Spine is the proposed UK-wide IT network infrastructure of the NHS which is being developed to allow healthcare staff anywhere to access medical details about patients (held in National Spine Records – NSRs). It forms the basis of the Integrated Care Record Service (ICRS – the nationally networked version of the current local electronic Patient Record or ePR). SNOMED / SNOP coding is to be an integral component of the ICRS so these codes should be used accurately
- Government policy statements e.g. *Hospital Medical Staffing: Achieving a Balance* in 1986 created the 'staff grade' as an NCCG post to alleviate the backlog of trainees – held for years in junior posts – because of the lack of full consultant vacancies. This latter created problems as staff grade doctors were not trained to (post-Calman) CCT level so could not upgrade to full consultants as more posts became available and could not move to European posts either (this situation was alleviated when NCCGs were later allowed to compete for StR positions). *The Health of the Nation* (1992–1997) was an attempt to address major issues in public health by focusing on five areas (IHD/stroke, cancer, mental illness, sexual health, accidents) setting targets and objectives that guided subsequent government policies. *The New NHS: Modern, dependable* is a Labour White Paper (DoH, 1997) stating goals for replacing the Conservative's 'internal market' with 'integrated care' (equalise standards of care across the country, reduce beurocracy, etc.). *The NHS Plan* (DoH, 2000) sets out the governments priorities (over 10 years) for investing the extra resources it pledged in the March 2000 budget statement. This includes goals for more beds, better quality catering, more doctors and nurses with reformed training arrangements, cleaner wards, updated IT, shorter waiting times and *The NHS Cancer Plan* (DoH, 2000) for implementing the Calman-Hine Report recommendations. The NHS Plan abolishes and supersedes *The Patient's Charter* originally published by the Conservatives in 1991
- National Service Frameworks (NSFs) are documents detailing targets and standards for individual disease categories e.g. diabetes, cancer, mental health, renal diseases, etc.
- Star ratings system: NHS hospitals may be awarded 0–3 stars according to how well they adhere to certain targets called Performance Indicators (PIs) set by the CHAI. PIs are categorised as Key Targets (e.g. waiting times in A&E), Patient Focus targets (e.g. patient questionnaire responses), Clinical Focus targets (e.g. post-operative death rates) and Capacity Targets (e.g. record-keeping, working conditions for staff)
- Foundation hospitals: NHSFT status is an option for 3 star hospitals which allows them to raise local funds, set individual pay scales and have more local control of other managerial decisions. They are authorised and regulated by an Independent Regulator (called 'Monitor')
- NHS Confederation: A body (with local branches e.g. the London NHS Confederation) that has representatives from all organisations of the NHS (SHAs, PCTs, Hospital Trusts, Ambulance Trusts, Mental Health Trusts, Care Trusts, etc.). The confederation lobbies Parliament and MPs on behalf of its members and facilitates sharing of information between its members. See http://www.nhsconfed.org/ (accessed August 2007)

For other NHS issues see: http://www.nhs.uk/england/aboutTheNHS/default.cmsx (accessed August 2007).

- The GMC publishes a document called *Management for Doctors* explaining the duties and standards expected of doctors in management roles. Find it online under the 'management guidance / ethical guidance' link in the 'Standards' section of the GMC web site (www.gmc-uk.org)
- Aspects of employment law relating to non-discrimination e.g. issues of accessibility and building design and achieving 'positive about disabled people' status as an employer (from the Employment Service – now part of JobCentrePlus) by making and demonstrating certain specific commitments (e.g. to interview any disabled applicant for a job if they fulfil the minimum criteria, to make every effort to retain staff who subsequently become disabled, etc.). Also 'equal opportunities' (male/female), racial equality and meeting certain management standards such as 'Investors in People' which requires the use of development plans (for individuals and teams), taking action to implement these plans

(guaranteed study-leave arrangements, etc.) and review / evaluation of the effectiveness and outcome of such measures. See:

> www.eoc.org.uk   (Equal Opportunities Commission)
> www.cre.gov.uk   (Commission for Racial Equality)
> www.drc-gb.org   (Disability Rights Commission)
> www.jobcentreplus.gov.uk   (see Employer's pages)
> www.investorsinpeople.co.uk   (Investors in People)

Bibliography

Anderson, T.J. (1989) Breast cancer screening: principles and practicalities for pathologists. *Recent Advances in Histopathology*, **14**, 43–61.

Calman, K. (1993) *'The Calman Report': Hospital doctors. Training for the future: the report of the Working Group on Specialist Medical Training*. DoH, London.

Calman, K. and Hine, D. (1995) *A Policy Framework for Commissioning Cancer Services*. London: DoH. Available at: www.dh.gov.uk/assetRoot/04/01/43/66/04014366.pdf (accessed March 2007)

Department of Health (1997) *The New NHS, Modern, Dependable*. HMSO, London. Available at: www.archive.official-documents.co.uk/document/doh/newnhs/newnhs.htm (accessed March 2007)

Department of Health (2000) *A Health Service of all the talents: Developing the NHS workforce*. DoH, London. Available at: www.dh.gov.uk/assetRoot/04/08/02/58/04080258.pdf (accessed March 2007)

Department of Health (2000) *Improving Working Lives Standard*. DoH, London. Available online at: http://www.dh.gov.uk/en/Publicationsandstatistics/Publications/PublicationsPolicyAndGuidance/DH_4010416 (accessed August 2007)

Department of Health (2000) *The NHS Cancer Plan: A plan for investment, a plan for reform*. DoH, London. Available at: www.dh.gov.uk/assetRoot/04/01/45/13/04014513.pdf (accessed March 2007)

Department of Health (2000) *The NHS Plan: A plan for investment, a plan for reform*. DoH, London. Available at: www.dh.gov.uk/en/Policyandguidance/Organisationpolicy/Modernisation/DH_4082690 (accessed March 2007)

Department of Health (2004) *Modernising Pathology Services*. DoH, London.

Department of Health and Social Security (1986) *Hospital Medical Staffing: Achieving a balance*. DHSS, London.

Department of Health and Social Security (1992) *The Health of the Nation: A strategy for health in England*. HMSO, London.

Donaldson, L. (CMO) (2002) *Unfinished Business: Proposals for reform of the senior house officer grade – a paper for consultation*. DoH, London. Available online at: www.dh.gov.uk/assetRoot/04/01/88/08/04018808.pdf (accessed March 2007)

du Boulay, C. (2003) Error trapping and error avoidance in histopathology, in *Recent Advances in Histopathology*, vol. 20 (eds D. Lowe and J.C.E Underwood). Royal Society of Medicine Press Ltd, London, pp. 103–113.

Health & Safety Executive (2003) *Safety in Health Service Laboratories: Safe working and the prevention of infection in clinical laboratories*. HSE, London.

Health & Safety Executive (2003) *Safety in Health Service Laboratories: Safe working and the prevention of infection in the mortuary and post-mortem room*. HSE, London.

Health & Safety Executive Information Sheet HSIS1 (1998) *The Reporting of Injuries, Diseases and Dangerous Occurrences Regulations 1995: Guidance for employers in the healthcare sector*. HSE, London.

Health & Safety Executive (1998) *Manual Handling in the Health Services*. HSE, London.

Health & Safety Executive (1995) *Glutaraldehyde and You*. HSE, London.

Joint Royal College of Pathologists and Institute of Biomedical Science Working Group (2004) *The Implementation of the Extended Role of Biomedical Scientists in Specimen Description, Dissection and Sampling, Final Report*. Royal College of Pathologists, London.

McClure, J. and Barnes, I. (2005) *National Framework for Pathology Service Improvement*. Available online at: http://www.pathologyimprovement.nhs.uk/documents/key_documents/Pathology_Framework05.pdf (accessed August 2007).

Medical Protection Society (1998) Clinical Governance: essential ingredients. *Casebook*, **12**, 9–10.

National Co-ordinating Group for Breast Cancer Screening (1995) *Pathology Reporting in Breast Cancer Screening*, 2nd edn. NHSBSP, London. Available online at: www.cancerscreening.nhs.uk/breastscreen/index.html (accessed March 2007).

Non-operative diagnosis subgroup of the National Co-ordinating Group for Breast Cancer Screening (June 2001) *Guidelines for Non-operative Diagnostic Procedures and Reporting in Breast Cancer Screening. NHSBSP Publication No. 50*. 1st edn. NHS Breast Screening Programme, London.

Price, A. (Chair) (2001) *The Royal College of Pathologists' Working Party Report: Draft guidelines for the involvement of biomedical scientists in the dissection of specimens and selection of tissues*. Royal College of Pathologists, London.

Royal College of Obstetricians and Gynaecologists (2005) *Good Practice No. 5: Disposal Following Pregnancy Loss Before 24 Weeks Gestation*. RCOG, London. Available online at: http://www.rcog.org.uk/resources/public/pdf/goodpractice5.pdf (accessed August 2007).

Royal College of Pathologists (2005) *Histopathology of Limited or No Clinical Value*. 2nd edn. RCPath, London. Available online at: www.rcpath.org/resources/pdf/HOLNCV-2ndEdition.pdf (accessed April 2005).

Royal College of Pathologists (2005) *Guidelines on Staffing and Workload for Histopathology and Cytopathology Departments*. 2nd edn. RCPath, London. Available online at: www.rcpath.org/resources/pdf/GuideHistoCytoWorkload0605.pdf (accessed April 2005).

Royal College of Pathologists and IBMS (2006) *Guidelines on the Release of Specimens and Data to the Police and Other Law Enforcement Agencies*. RCPath, London. Available online at: http://www.rcpath.org/resources/pdf/G040Guidelines_onrelease_specimensdatatopoliceOCT06v3.pdf (accessed August 2007).

Royal College of Pathologists (2006) *Guidance for Histopathologists / Cytopathologists on Reporting at Home*. 2nd edn. www.rcpath.org/resources/pdf/G017-GuidanceForHisto-CytoOnReportingAtHomeFINAL.pdf (accessed March 2007).

Royal College of Pathologists (1998) *Recommendations for the Development of Histopathology/ Cytopathology External Quality Assessment Schemes*. RCPath, London. www.rcpath.org/resources/pdf/G012-RecsForDevpmtOfHisto-CytoEQASchemes.pdf (accessed July 2004).

Royal College of Pathologists (1996) *Clinical Audit in Pathology: Histopathology*. RCPath, London. Available online at: www.rcpath.org.uk (accessed July 2004).

Royal College of Pathologists (2002) *Advice Relating to the Ownership, Storage and Release of Pathology Results – Revised Guidelines*. RCPath, London.

Royal College of Pathologists and IBMS (2005) *The Retention and Storage of Pathological Records and Archives*. 3rd edn. RCPath, London. Available online at: www.rcpath.org.uk (accessed July 2006).

Royal College of Pathologists (2002) *Interim Guidelines for the Disposal of Tissue, Blocks and Slides from Biopsies and Surgical Resections*. RCPath, London.

Stephenson, T. (2004) Con-tract or intractable con?; Pathology-specific problems of implementing the New Consultant Contract. *ACP News* (Autumn) 11–15.

UK Parliament (1988) *Data Protection Act 1988*. HMSO: London. Available at: www.hmso.gov.uk/acts/acts1998/19980029.htm#aofs (accessed March 2007).

Web sites

NHS Cervical Screening Publications (2000) *Achievable Standards, Benchmarks for Reporting and Criteria for Evaluating Cervical Cytology ('The ABC Document')*. 2nd edn. NHSCSP, London. http://www.cancerscreening.nhs.uk/cervical/publications/cc-02.html (accessed August 2007).

Dark, G. Trainee forum of CancerWeb: www.cancerweb.ncl.ac.uk/cancerweb/trainees/doc/tr-auth.html (accessed March 2007).

Department of Health Guidance on the EWTD: http://www.dh.gov.uk/en/policyandguidance/humanresourcesandtraining/workingdifferently/Europeanworkingtimedirective/index.htm (accessed August 2007).

Department of Health notes on the Junior Doctor's Contract: http://www.dh.gov.uk/en/Policyandguidance/Humanresourcesandtraining/Modernisingpay/Juniordoctorcontracts/DH_4053873 (accessed March 2007).

Department of Health policy framework: *Agenda for Change*. www.dh.gov.uk/en/Policyandguidance/Humanresourcesandtraining/Modernisingpay/Agendaforchange/index.htm (accessed March 2007).

Department of Health Notes on the *Caldicott Report*. http://www.dh.gov.uk/en/Publicationsandstatistics/Publications/PublicationsPolicyAndGuidance/DH_4006467 (accessed August 2007).

Department of Health Notes on the Consultants Contract: www.dh.gov.uk/en/Policyandguidance/Humanresourcesandtraining/Modernisingpay/Consultantcontract/index.htm (accessed March 2007).

Modernising Medical Careers Project. www.mmc.nhs.uk (accessed March 2007).

New Deal information from the DHSSPS, Northern Ireland: www.dhsspsni.gov.uk/scujuniordoc-2 (accessed March 2007).

New Implementation Support Group NHS Scotland: www.newdealsupport.scot.nhs.uk/introduction.htm (accessed March 2007).

NHS National Service Frameworks: www.dh.gov.uk/en/Policyandguidance/Organisationpolicy/Modernisation/DH_4082690 (accessed March 2007).

The Information Commissioner web site. www.ico.gov.uk (accessed March 2007).

4. Cut-Up and Reporting Guidelines

Applied Anatomy

Brain

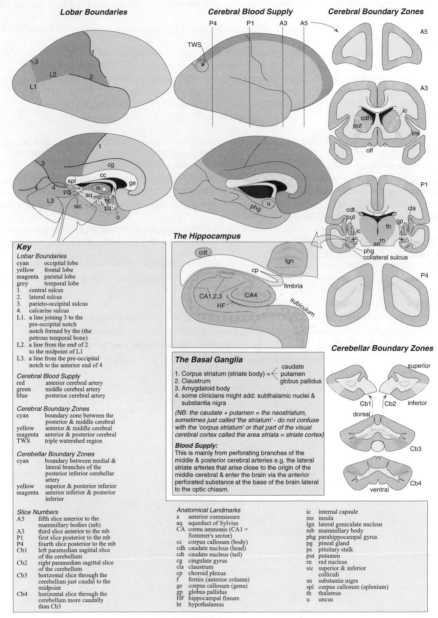

FIGURE 4.1　Brain

- Charcot's 'artery of cerebral haemorrhage' refers to the lenticulostriate branches of the middle cerebral that enter the anterior perforated substance and supply the external capsule and basal ganglia.
- Cerebral cortex terminology: apart from some regions considered phylogenetically old (olfactory and hippocampal), the cortex has six layers and is called *neocortex = isocortex = homogenetic* cortex

Diagnostic Criteria Handbook in Histopathology: A Surgical Pathology Vade Mecum by Paul J. Tadrous
Copyright © 2007 by John Wiley & Sons, Ltd.

Eyes

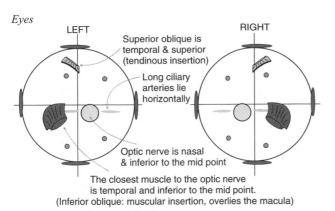

For orbital exenterations, the caruncle and lower lid punctum (which may be probed to find the nasolacrimal duct margin) identify the medial aspect; longer lashes and a fold identify the upper lid.

TABLE 4.1 Normal values for a globe

globe ⌀ (X,Y,Z)	22–23 mm
optic nerve ⌀	4 mm
corneal ⌀ (X)	12 mm
corneal ⌀ (Y)	11 mm
iridocorneal angle	454° (>30°)

Superior oblique is temporal & superior (tendinous insertion)

Long ciliary arteries lie horizontally

Optic nerve is nasal & inferior to the mid point

The closest muscle to the optic nerve is temporal and inferior to the mid point.
(Inferior oblique: muscular insertion, overlies the macula)

FIGURE 4.2   Eyes (orientation and measurements)

Neck

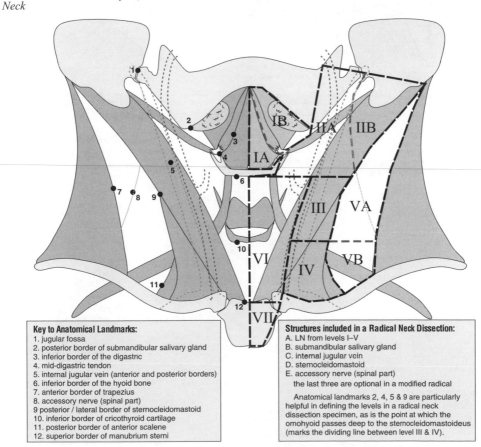

Key to Anatomical Landmarks:
1. jugular fossa
2. posterior border of submandibular salivary gland
3. inferior border of the digastric
4. mid-digastric tendon
5. internal jugular vein (anterior and posterior borders)
6. inferior border of the hyoid bone
7. anterior border of trapezius
8. accessory nerve (spinal part)
9 posterior / lateral border of sternocleidomastoid
10. inferior border of cricothyroid cartilage
11. posterior border of anterior scalene
12. superior border of manubrium sterni

Structures included in a Radical Neck Dissection:
A. LN from levels I–V
B. submandibular salivary gland
C. internal jugular vein
D. sternocleidomastoid
E. accessory nerve (spinal part)
   the last three are optional in a modified radical

   Anatomical landmarks 2, 4, 5 & 9 are particularly helpful in defining the levels in a radical neck dissection specimen, as is the point at which the omohyoid passes deep to the sternocleidomastoideus (marks the dividing line between level III & IV).

FIGURE 4.3   Neck dissection (Lymph node Levels I–VII)

- Nodal *groups* (for TNM) are: 1 = IA, 2 = IB, 3–5 = perijugular parts of II–IV, 6 (peri-accessory nerve, spinal part) = VA, 7 (supraclavicular) = VB + part of IV, 8 = VI, [9–12 do not correspond to levels] 9 (retropharyngeal), 10 (parotid), 11 (buccal / facial), 12 (mastoid + occipital)
- The 'posterior triangle group' comprises level VA + VB (≈groups 6 + 7)

Neck (Surface anatomy of the carotid sheath)
- Trace a line from the sternoclavicular joint to the midpoint between the angle of the mandible and tip of the mastoid process.
- Beneath this line lie the carotid artery, the internal jugular vein, the deep cervical lymph nodes and the vagus nerve.

Larynx and Pharynx

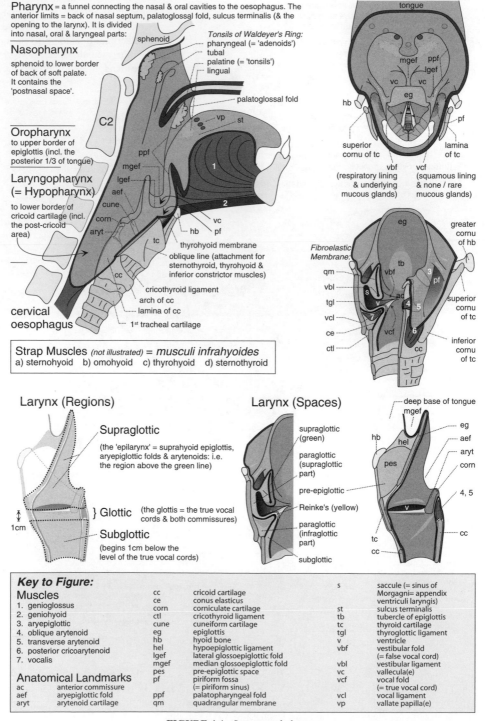

FIGURE 4.4 Larynx and pharynx

Notes on the larynx

- The larynx extends from the epiglottis to the bottom of the cricoid cartilage. The epiglottic, corniculate and cuneiform cartilages are elastic type (the others are hyaline).
- The *vestibule* is that part of the lumen of the larynx proximal to the true cords.

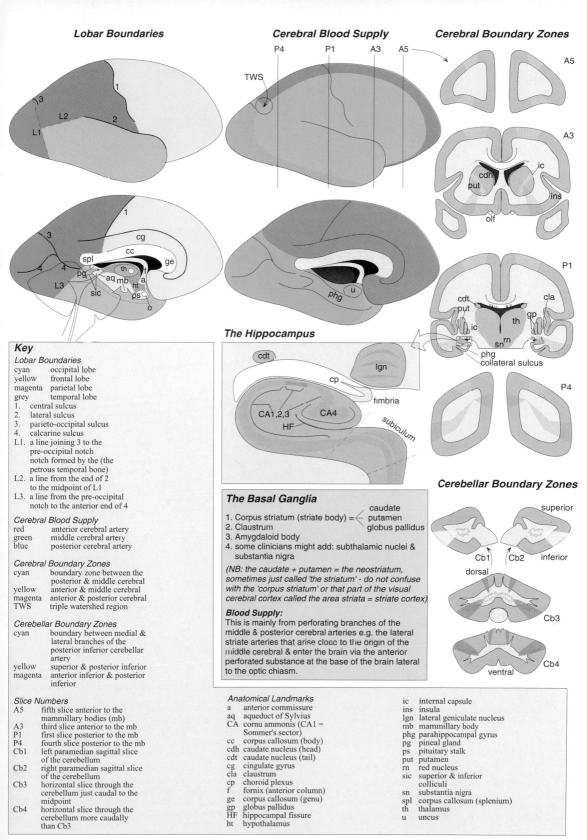

FIGURE 4.1

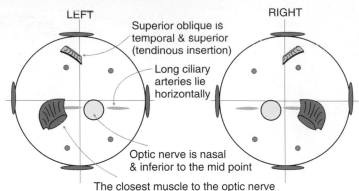

Superior oblique is temporal & superior (tendinous insertion)

Long ciliary arteries lie horizontally

Optic nerve is nasal & inferior to the mid point

The closest muscle to the optic nerve
is temporal and inferior to the mid point.
(Inferior oblique: muscular insertion, overlies the macula)

FIGURE 4.2

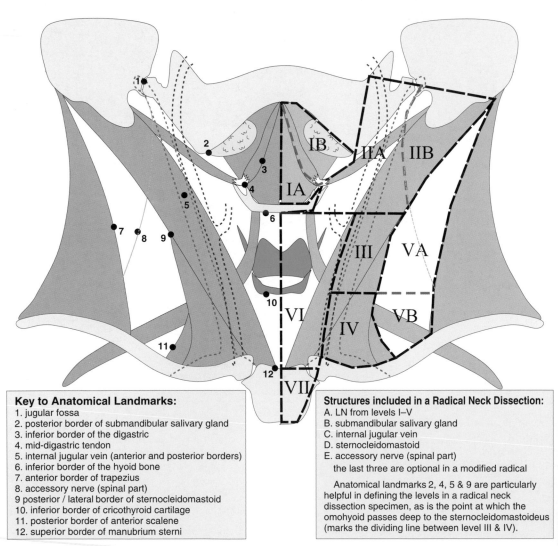

Key to Anatomical Landmarks:
1. jugular fossa
2. posterior border of submandibular salivary gland
3. inferior border of the digastric
4. mid-digastric tendon
5. internal jugular vein (anterior and posterior borders)
6. inferior border of the hyoid bone
7. anterior border of trapezius
8. accessory nerve (spinal part)
9 posterior / lateral border of sternocleidomastoid
10. inferior border of cricothyroid cartilage
11. posterior border of anterior scalene
12. superior border of manubrium sterni

Structures included in a Radical Neck Dissection:
A. LN from levels I–V
B. submandibular salivary gland
C. internal jugular vein
D. sternocleidomastoid
E. accessory nerve (spinal part)
  the last three are optional in a modified radical

  Anatomical landmarks 2, 4, 5 & 9 are particularly helpful in defining the levels in a radical neck dissection specimen, as is the point at which the omohyoid passes deep to the sternocleidomastoideus (marks the dividing line between level III & IV).

FIGURE 4.3

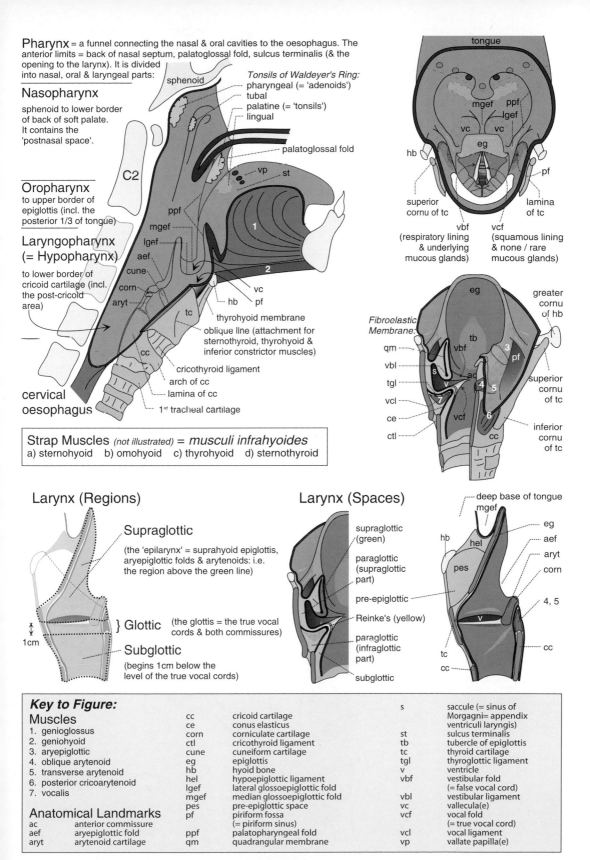

FIGURE 4.4

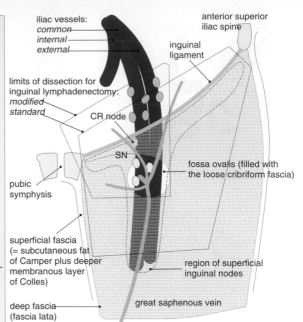

Points to Note:
- The femoral artery begins as the continuation of the external iliac at the midpoint between the anterior superior iliac spine & pubic symphysis.
- The fossa ovalis here refers to the saphenous opening in the fascia lata.
- The external iliac nodes are shown in grey.
- The deep inguinal nodes (in the fossa ovalis) are shown in yellow and one is constant, labelled as 'CR Node', at the medial high point of the femoral vein (= Cloquet's node of Rosenmüller).
- The superficial inguinal nodes lie near Colles' fascia, are arranged in vertical & horizontal groups and total upto 25. The lateral part of the horizontal group receive lymph from the lower back. The region marked 'SN' is where the sentinel nodes of penile CA are found.
- The modified lymphadenectomy field is that of Catalona and is a saphenous vein-sparing method with fewer complications used prophylactically in clinically node negative patients - but may be converted to the standard radical dissection if positive nodes are found (incl. by the use of frozen section).

iliac vessels:
common
internal
external

anterior superior iliac spine

inguinal ligament

limits of dissection for inguinal lymphadenectomy:
modified
standard

CR node

SN

pubic symphysis

fossa ovalis (filled with the loose/cribriform fascia)

superficial fascia (= subcutaneous fat of Camper plus deeper membranous layer of Colles)

region of superficial inguinal nodes

deep fascia (fascia lata)

great saphenous vein

FIGURE 4.5

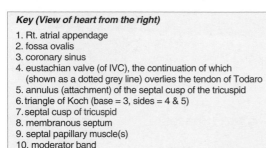
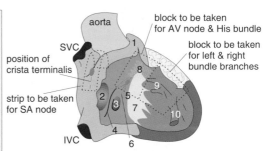

Key (View of heart from the right)
1. Rt. atrial appendage
2. fossa ovalis
3. coronary sinus
4. eustachian valve (of IVC), the continuation of which (shown as a dotted grey line) overlies the tendon of Todaro
5. annulus (attachment) of the septal cusp of the tricuspid
6. triangle of Koch (base = 3, sides = 4 & 5)
7. septal cusp of tricuspid
8. membranous septum
9. septal papillary muscle(s)
10. moderator band

aorta

block to be taken for AV node & His bundle

block to be taken for left & right bundle branches

SVC

position of crista terminalis

strip to be taken for SA node

IVC

FIGURE 4.6

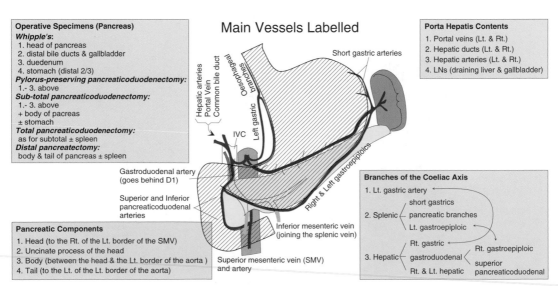

Operative Specimens (Pancreas)
Whipple's:
1. head of pancreas
2. distal bile ducts & gallbladder
3. duedenum
4. stomach (distal 2/3)
Pylorus-preserving pancreaticoduodenectomy:
1.- 3. above
Sub-total pancreaticoduodenectomy:
1.- 3. above
+ body of pacreas
± stomach
Total pancreaticoduodenectomy:
as for subtotal ± spleen
Distal pancreatectomy:
body & tail of pancreas ± spleen

Main Vessels Labelled

Hepatic arteries
Portal Vein
Common bile duct

Oesophageal branches

Short gastric arteries

IVC
Left gastric

Right & Left gastroepiploics

Gastroduodenal artery (goes behind D1)

Superior and Inferior pancreaticoduodenal arteries

Inferior mesenteric vein (joining the splenic vein)

Superior mesenteric vein (SMV) and artery

Porta Hepatis Contents
1. Portal veins (Lt. & Rt.)
2. Hepatic ducts (Lt. & Rt.)
3. Hepatic arteries (Lt. & Rt.)
4. LNs (draining liver & gallbladder)

Pancreatic Components
1. Head (to the Rt. of the Lt. border of the SMV)
2. Uncinate process of the head
3. Body (between the head & the Lt. border of the aorta)
4. Tail (to the Lt. of the Lt. border of the aorta)

Branches of the Coeliac Axis
1. Lt. gastric artery
2. Splenic
   - short gastrics
   - pancreatic branches
   - Lt. gastroepiploic
3. Hepatic
   - Rt. gastric
   - gastroduodenal
   - Rt. & Lt. hepatic
   - Rt. gastroepiploic
   - superior pancreaticoduodenal

FIGURE 4.7

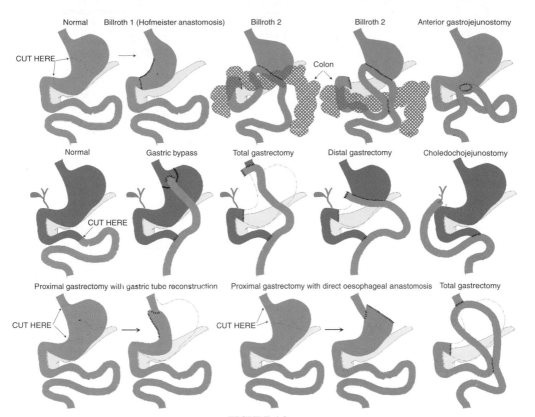

Normal   Billroth 1 (Hofmeister anastomosis)   Billroth 2   Billroth 2   Anterior gastrojejunostomy

CUT HERE

Colon

Normal   Gastric bypass   Total gastrectomy   Distal gastrectomy   Choledochojejunostomy

CUT HERE

Proximal gastrectomy with gastric tube reconstruction   Proximal gastrectomy with direct oesophageal anastomosis   Total gastrectomy

CUT HERE   CUT HERE

FIGURE 4.8

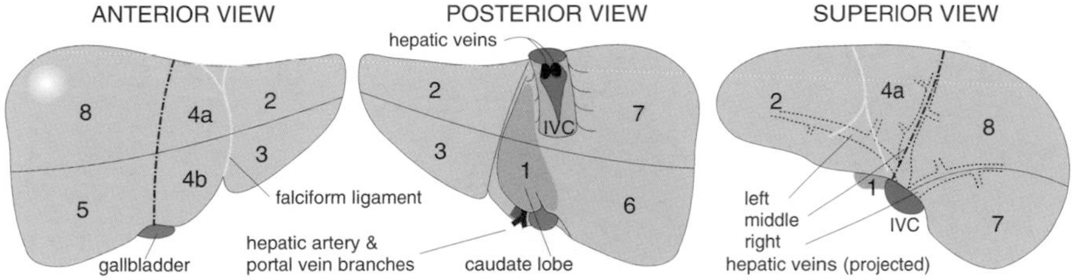

ANTERIOR VIEW   POSTERIOR VIEW   SUPERIOR VIEW

hepatic veins

8 4a 2

4b

3

5   falciform ligament

gallbladder

hepatic artery &
portal vein branches

2   7

IVC

3

1

6

caudate lobe

4a

2   8

1

left
middle
right

IVC

7

hepatic veins (projected)

FIGURE 4.9

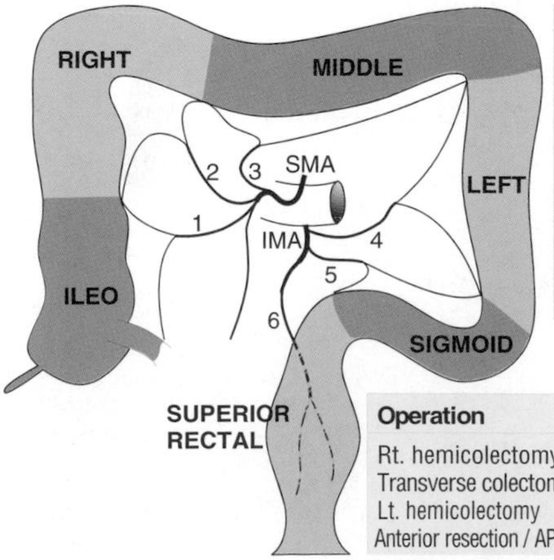

RIGHT   MIDDLE

2 3 SMA

LEFT

1

IMA 4

ILEO

5

6

SIGMOID

SUPERIOR
RECTAL

Key to Arteries:

1. ileocolic
2. right colic
3. middle colic
4. left colic
5. sigmoid
6. superior rectal

NB: The IMA arises ≈ 4 cm
above the aortic bifurcation
and may be small.

Operation	Vascular Ties
Rt. hemicolectomy	ileocolic, Rt. colic ± mid colic
Transverse colectomy	midcolic ± Lt. colic
Lt. hemicolectomy	Lt. colic, sigmoid, ± superior rectal
Anterior resection / APR	superior rectal

FIGURE 4.10

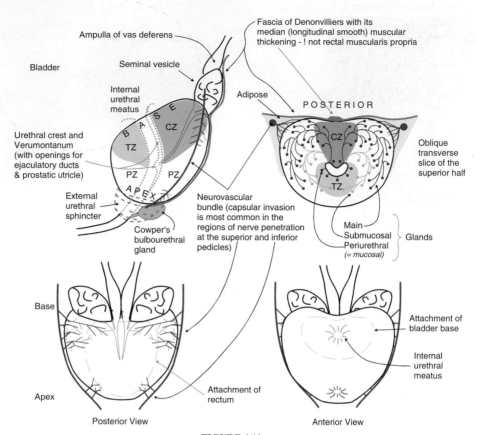

FIGURE 4.11

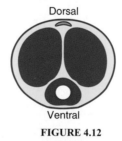

FIGURE 4.12

UTERUS ANTEROLATERAL VIEW

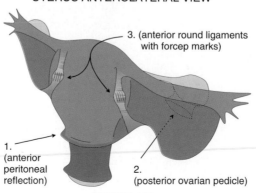

FIGURE 4.13

Layers of the Normal Chorion & Amnion

Intertwin Membranes

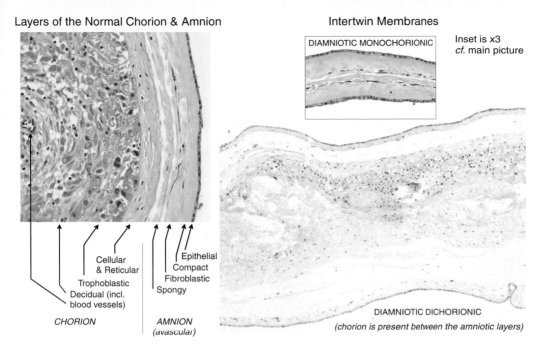

DIAMNIOTIC MONOCHORIONIC

Inset is x3
cf. main picture

Epithelial
Compact
Fibroblastic
Spongy

Cellular
& Reticular
Trophoblastic
Decidual (incl.
blood vessels)

CHORION

*AMNION
(avascular)*

DIAMNIOTIC DICHORIONIC
(chorion is present between the amniotic layers)

FIGURE 5.3

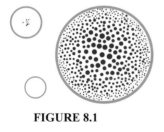

FIGURE 8.1

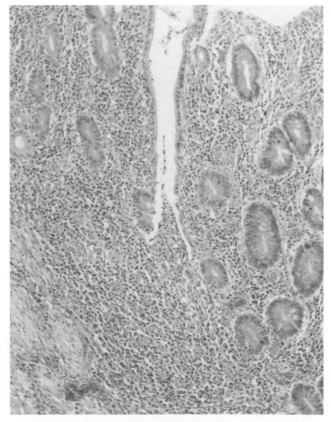

FIGURE 11.3

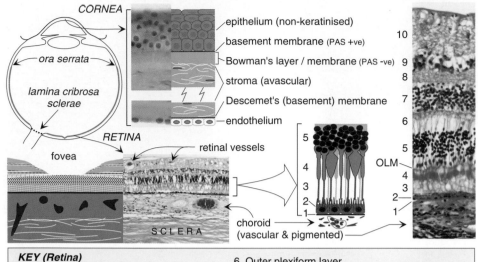

CORNEA

ora serrata

lamina cribrosa sclerae

— epithelium (non-keratinised)
— basement membrane (PAS +ve)
— Bowman's layer / membrane (PAS -ve)
— stroma (avascular)
— Descemet's (basement) membrane
— endothelium

10
9
8
7
6

RETINA

retinal vessels

fovea

5
4
3
2
1

OLM
5
4
3
2
1

choroid
(vascular & pigmented)

SCLERA

KEY (Retina)

1. Bruch's (basement) membrane
2. Retinal pigment epithelium (RPE)
3. Layer of rods & cones (outer segment)
4. Layer of rods & cones (inner segment)
5. Outer nuclear layer

6. Outer plexiform layer
7. Inner nuclear layer
8. Inner plexiform layer
9. Ganglion cell layer (scant to many nuclei thick)
10. (Optic) Nerve fibre layer (with retinal vessels)
OLM = Outer limiting membrane

FIGURE 14.1

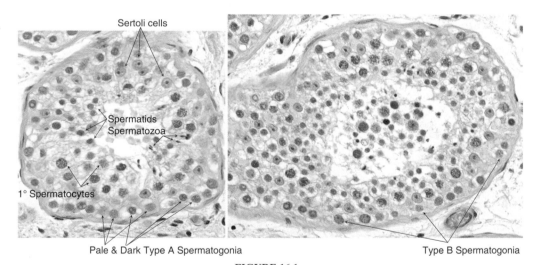

Sertoli cells

Spermatids
Spermatozoa

1° Spermatocytes

Pale & Dark Type A Spermatogonia

Type B Spermatogonia

FIGURE 16.1

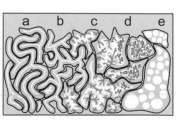

a b c d e

FIGURE 17.1

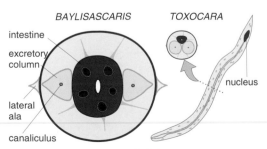

BAYLISASCARIS   *TOXOCARA*

intestine
excretory column

lateral ala

canaliculus

nucleus

FIGURE 23.1

- The term 'glottis' refers to the true vocal cords and space between them (called the *rima glottidis*).
- The laryngeal *spaces* are based on the natural fibroelastic membrane and lymphatic territories that are relevant to the local spread of tumour. The fibroelastic membranes (akin to the muscularis mucosae in other sites) mark the boundary between mucosa and submucosa and penetration of this membrane by tumours limited to the true cord contraindicates local ablation Rx.
- The laryngeal *regions* are for description of tumour subsite and distribution. The lower limit of the glottic region is not universally agreed but one should state if a glottic tumour extends > 1cm below the true cord (= 'glottic tumour with subglottic extension') and distinguish these from tumours that are entirely subglottic (i.e. no true cord involvement).

Axilla (Lymph node levels)

- I (low axilla and intramammary): low axillary LN lie below and lateral to the pectoralis minor
- II (mid axilla) lie superficial and deep to the pectoralis minor
- III (apical axilla region) lie above and medial to the pectoralis minor. The actual apical nodes lie just lateral to the 1st rib below the axillary vein
- Other named regions are: internal mammary, infraclavicular (= subclavicular) and supraclavicular
- All the above count as locoregional LN for breast carcinoma by TNM6 *if they are ipsilateral*

Inguinal Lymphadenectomy

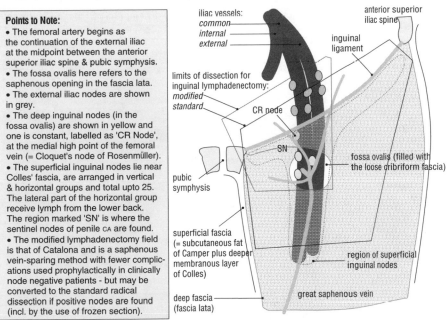

Points to Note:
- The femoral artery begins as the continuation of the external iliac at the midpoint between the anterior superior iliac spine & pubic symphysis.
- The fossa ovalis here refers to the saphenous opening in the fascia lata.
- The external iliac nodes are shown in grey.
- The deep inguinal nodes (in the fossa ovalis) are shown in yellow and one is constant, labelled as 'CR Node', at the medial high point of the femoral vein (= Cloquet's node of Rosenmüller).
- The superficial inguinal nodes lie near Colles' fascia, are arranged in vertical & horizontal groups and total upto 25. The lateral part of the horizontal group receive lymph from the lower back. The region marked 'SN' is where the sentinel nodes of penile CA are found.
- The modified lymphadenectomy field is that of Catalona and is a saphenous vein-sparing method with fewer complications used prophylactically in clinically node negative patients - but may be converted to the standard radical dissection if positive nodes are found (incl. by the use of frozen section).

FIGURE 4.5   Inguinal lymphadenectomy

Heart: Conducting system

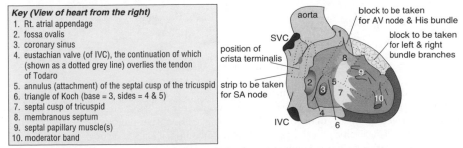

Key (View of heart from the right)
1. Rt. atrial appendage
2. fossa ovalis
3. coronary sinus
4. eustachian valve (of IVC), the continuation of which (shown as a dotted grey line) overlies the tendon of Todaro
5. annulus (attachment) of the septal cusp of the tricuspid
6. triangle of Koch (base = 3, sides = 4 & 5)
7. septal cusp of tricuspid
8. membranous septum
9. septal papillary muscle(s)
10. moderator band

FIGURE 4.6   Heart: Conducting system

For the dissection method, block-taking and relevant bibliography, see pp. 389–390.

Upper GI Anatomy

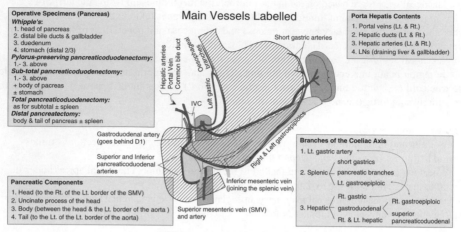

FIGURE 4.7   Upper GI anatomy

- The minor duodenal papilla, when present, is 2cm proximal to the ampulla of Vater ± a little anterior
- The Lt gastric artery is most commonly involved with gastric ulcers; the gastroduodenal with DU

Surgical alterations

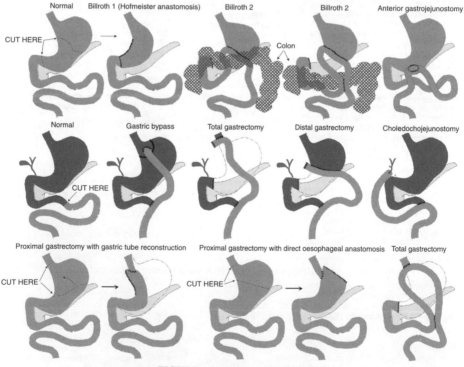

FIGURE 4.8   Surgical alterations

- The Billroth distal gastrectomies have many modifications e.g. Hofmeister anastomoses only allow a patent lumen near the greater curve part of the cut stomach while Polya anastomoses allow lumenal continuity over the whole length (a Polya Billroth 2 also tends to have a retrocolic anastomosis).
- The middle row shows some procedures for which a Roux-en-Y jejunal anastomosis is used.
- A pyloroplasty is often performed with proximal gastrectomies.
- A jejunal pouch (e.g. 'U'-shaped) may be used to restore continuity after proximal or total gastrectomy.
- A segment of colon or jejunum may be used to reconstruct after a high oesophagogastrectomy.

Liver (Segmental anatomy)

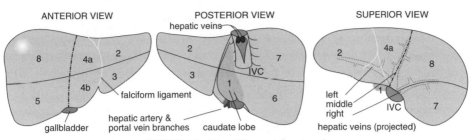

FIGURE 4.9　Liver (Segmental anatomy)

- Although Rt and Lt *lobes* are defined by the falciform ligament; *segments* are vascular compartments useful for planning surgery and are precisely defined for any individual by pre-op radiology.
- The bold broken line in the figure joins the left side of the groove for the IVC to the mid-part of the gallbladder fossa and divides the liver into left and right *hemilivers*.
- The falciform ligament divides the left hemiliver into segments 4 and 2+3.
- The caudate lobe is segment 1.

Lower GI Anatomy (blood supply)

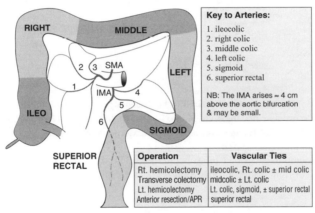

FIGURE 4.10　Lower GI anatomy (blood supply)

- Some lesions (e.g. carcinoids) may be categorised according to the part of the gut they arise in using embryonic terminology as: foregut, midgut, hindgut, tailgut. The first 3 correspond to those parts of the adult GIT supplied by the coeliac axis, SMA and IMA.
- The tailgut (a diverticulum of the hindgut under the tail-root of some animals) may persist to form a *tailgut cyst* (multilocular *retrocaecal hamartoma* with smooth muscle in the wall and a variable lining from columnar to transitional/squamous) or adenocarcinoma.

Kidney (Hilar structures)
- The renal vein is (usu.) the most anterior structure (anterior to the renal arteries and pelvis/ureter).
- The renal artery usu. has three branches at the pelvis – two go anterior to the pelvis/ureter and 1 posterior.
- The renal sinus is that part of the pelvis lateral to the hilar plane, its fat envelops the collecting system and abuts the renal cortex without an intervening fibrous capsule.
- Invasion (incl. microscopic invasion) of the sinus fat by carcinoma constitutes stage pT3a.
- The sinus contains muscular tributaries of the renal vein, gross invasion of which by carcinoma constitutes stage pT3b (renal vein involvement).

Urinary Bladder
- The superior posterior aspect is covered by serosa.
- The urethral aspect is tapered.

Prostate

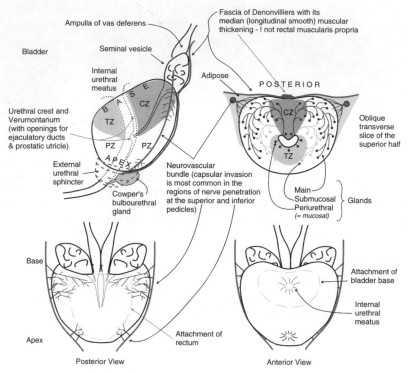

FIGURE 4.11   Prostrate

- For TNM staging the prostate may be divided into Lt. and Rt. halves (= 'lobes') ignoring the anatomical middle lobe as a distinct entity; involvement of the external sphincter urethrae (striated muscle) or bladder neck (smooth muscle) = pT4.
- pT2b (tumour restricted to >1/2 of 1 lobe) is interpreted as >50% volume by some (in which case it is vanishingly rare) or tumour linear dimension >1/2 of the lobe's linear dimension by others.

Penis

- Specimens may be distorted by disease and fixation artefact.
- The most dorsal aspect contains the *dorsal vein* overlying the paired *corpora cavernosa*, the latter enclosed in a thick fibrous coat – the *tunica albuginea corporum cavernosum*.
- The urethral is most ventral and surrounded by the *corpus spongiosum* invested in a thinner *tunica albuginea corporis spongiosi*.
- The spongiosum overshoots the cavernosa and expands to cover the distal cavernosa in the form the conical *glans penis*. Its oblique basal rim, the *corona glandis*, overhangs the shaft and the groove between the shaft and corona is the *coronal sulcus*. The obliquity is such as to allow the dorsal corona to be more proximal than the ventral part.
- The overlying skin contains a sub-dermal dartos smooth muscle layer with Buck's vascular fibroelastic fascia separating this muscle from the tunica albuginea of the 3 corpora.

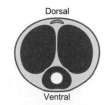

FIGURE 4.12   Penis

Uterus (Orientation)

- There are three main landmarks, some of which may not be present in every specimen):
    1. the peritoneal reflection is higher anteriorly (bladder) than posteriorly (pouch of Douglas)

UTERUS ANTEROLATERAL VIEW

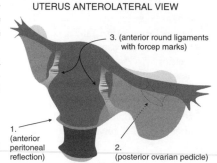

FIGURE 4.13   Uterus

2. the ovarian pedicles (or ovaries if present) are on the posterior surface of the broad ligament
3. the round ligaments are anterior (these usu. have forceps marks imprinted on them as the surgeon grasps the uterus and pulls it forward by the round ligaments during an abdominal hysterectomy).

Specimen Handling and Reporting Guidelines

Interpretation of LN Metastases w.r.t. the TNM6 Classification
- Tumour in a LN is considered LN +ve whether it got there by metastasis or direct extension
- Tumour deposit without residual LN structure is LN +ve if it has a smooth outline consistent with the form of a LN (else = vascular +/ discontinuous tumour spread). In the UK this is controversial (2007) and some (e.g. GI pathologists) advocate continued use of the TNM5 rule based on size not contour (*viz.* a deposit >3mm ⌀ in a lymph draining region is a LN metastasis, if ≤3mm = discontinuous 1° tumour spread and is included in the pT category). See also Neck Dissection below
- Tumour nodules in a LN that are >2mm in max. dimension are LN +ve with no further qualification
- If ≤2mm but >0.2mm = 'micrometastasis': use the 'mi' qualifier, e.g. pN1(mi), only if there are none bigger
- If ≤0.2mm then = 'isolated tumour cells' (ITC) and staged as pN0(i+)[1]
- The ITC concept is also valid for the pM classification in bone marrow (pM0(i+))
- That ITC results in a pN0 stage is controversial in the UK (2007) so some advocate adding a comment like 'this would previously have been called pN +ve'
- In some pN stages, size of the LN metastasis is important (not the size of the whole LN)
- LN mets distant to the *regional* lymph drainage fields are included in the pM category (not pN)
- Use of pTNM implies a resection sufficient to assess the most extreme scores

Central Nervous System (CNS)
- Record volume of sample and nature of procedure (incl. whether CUSA was used)
- Decalcify bony fragments and consider samples for glutaraldehyde (EM) or freezing (molecular genetics) if CPC suggests an unusual tumour.
- Lobectomy: give anatomical description, bread-slice coronally (5mm intervals), record presence/extent of necrosis and comment if there is margin / meningeal involvement
- Blocks: embed all if small/stereotactic biopsies else take sufficient blocks to document tumour heterogeneity, invasion across anatomical boundaries and margins
- Margin status should not be described as 'clear' for most 1° CNS tumours except for intact meningioma resections
- Reporting: give tumour type and WHO grade (there is no TNM staging because CNS tumours infiltrate diffusely and rarely metastasise; however, describe if anatomical boundaries are breached: into bone, through pia into subarachnoid space, meningioma invading brain or dura/bone, etc.)
- Brain smears: place a tiny piece of fresh sample (≤1mm³) onto a slide, squash gently with a second slide on top until it forms a thin layer then sweep the top slide over the first to produce the smear. Fix in alcohol and stain with H&E (cytoplasmic detail) or 1% toluidine blue (good nuclear detail)

Muscle Biopsy (Non-neoplastic)
- 1–2 pieces received fresh (sutured to a stick while *in situ* +/ laid out on card to avoid contraction and to preserve orientation). Site is usu. deltoid or quadriceps.
- ≈1mm³ taken to glutaraldehyde for EM (longitudinal sections)
- ≈0.5 × 0.5 × 2cm snap frozen (unfixed) for transverse sections for LM (! avoid ice crystal artefacts)
- Routine stains: H&E, PAS, myosin ATPase (various pH), NADH, Sudan Black, Gomori trichrome
- Others as indicated: dystrophins, spectrin, myosins, phosphorylase, cytochrome oxidase, etc.
See table 13.3 on p. 188 for interpretation of these stains.

Peripheral Nerve Biopsy (Non-neoplastic)
(See p. 389, under '*Nerves for ? Neuropathy*'.)

---

[1] or pN0(mol+) if tumour cells were detected by non-morphological methods e.g. flow cytometry

Eye
- The terms 'inner' [or 'internal'] and 'outer' [or 'external'] refer to 'towards the centrepoint of the globe' (the centre of the vitreous) and 'towards the surface of the globe' respectively.
- Measure globe (length and ⌀), pupil ⌀ and optic nerve length.
- The vortex veins are harvested and embedded (longitudinally) with the cut end (margin) of the optic nerve in a standard cassette.
- After transillumination via the cornea (to mark the base of any tumour) or via the optic nerve (to examine the cornea/iris), the globe is cut into three slices ('calottes') where the cuts pass 1mm into the corneal limbus – either horizontal (for macular lesions), vertical (for glaucoma / cataract assessment) or oblique – with the middle calotte containing the pupil, iris, lens, optic nerve and main bulk of any tumour. Each calotte is embedded in a separate deep cassette. However, this is not always optimum with some tumours so the specimen should be cut so as to yield the following information:
  - ➢ for iris melanoma radial extent (in terms of clock hours) and extension (ciliary body, sclera and extraocular) is important for staging
  - ➢ for ciliary body and choroidal melanoma the largest basal diameter (in mm or optic disc diameters) and maximum height of the tumour (in mm or diopters) are important for T stage. Penetration of the sclera with extraocular extension and vascular invasion (including vortex vein) are important but penetration of Bruch's membrane is irrelevant (unlike with retinoblastoma)
  - ➢ for retinoblastoma tumour height, distance from tumour base to fovea and optic nerve, retinal detachment, subretinal deposits (penetration of Bruch's membrane) ± choroidal / scleral invasion or orbital (extra-ocular) spread, optic nerve invasion (Magramm gade 1 = prelaminar, 2 = upto and including the lamina cribrosa, 3 = beyond it, 4 = optic nerve margin involved), deposits in the vitreous (seeding) should be distinguished from true multifocality (>1 deposit within the retina), vitreous extension to contact the lens, deposits in ciliary body / iris / anterior chamber
  - ➢ for exenterations, measure skin margins, ink superior/inferior halves and nasolacrimal duct margin (sample this margin and the optic nerve margin), remove and decal any bone, then bread slice in vertical sections 1cm thick (first and last cuts should just avoid the eyeball).

Temporal Artery Biopsy for ? Arteritis
- Cut the biopsy into 2mm long transverse slices.
- Embed all the slices *en face* and request levels and EVG.

Head and Neck (SCC and Other Types of Carcinoma)

Clinical data
The surgeon should:
- ➢ orientate the specimen (and pin-out a neck dissection, marking the major LN levels)
- ➢ give the clinical TNM stage and state whether prior therapy was given
- ➢ specify the side and op-type e.g. neck dissection – selective / radical / modified radical.

Biopsies
- State if dysplasia or vascular invasion is present in addition to tumour characteristics.

Main resection (general)
- Some advocate decalcification of specimens with soft tissue *in situ* before dissection.
- Measure (mm) max. depth and ⌀ of tumour. Tumour depth is measured from the level of surface of the surrounding, uninvolved, mucosa (extrapolated/interpolated if there is ulceration/fungation).
- Take 1 block per cm ⌀ of tumour (plus margins, uninvolved mucosa, thyroid, etc.)
- Tumour type, extent, and subsite (e.g. supraglottic, glottic, transglottic or infraglottic – see Figure 4.4)
- Grade (by worst area) – well / moderately / poorly diff
- Pattern of invasive front: cohesive/non-cohesive (non-cohesive = strands <15 cells wide/single cells)
- Distance to margins (mucosal and soft tissue) <1mm = 'involved', >5mm = 'clear', else = 'close'
- Invasion of:
  - ➢ vessels
  - ➢ nerves (esp. if beyond the invasive front of the main tumour)
  - ➢ bone (distinguish erosion of cortex from invasion of intertrabecular spaces)
- Dysplasia (presence, degree, distance to margins)

Laryngectomy
- If it will not disrupt the tumour, a longitudinal posterior midline incision may be made to assess tumour extent – otherwise, leave the specimen intact.
- Some advocate sharp dissection to remove the hyoid (to avoid decalcifying the whole specimen) with examination of the soft tissue thus exposed and histology of the hyoid only if that tissue is involved. The UK National Dataset advises whole decalcification followed by serial 5mm transverse slicing.
- Assess the caudal and anterior (tongue base) *submucosal* margins (as well as mucosal) by sagittal sections.
- State if (and where) tumour has perforated the cartilages with extralaryngeal soft tissue spread.
- State if tumour has crossed the midline.
- State what other structures are present (e.g. parathyroids) and examine as appropriate.

Maxilla, mandible, sinuses and other specimens
See Slootweg, 2005

Neck dissection
- For each level state: nõ. of LN present and nõ. of LN involved and whether extracapsular spread (if extracapsular spread approaches a surface of the specimen, ink that surface and block such as to estimate distance of / involvement by tumour).
- Measure size of largest metastasis (for TNM).
- For matted LN state the max. dimension of the mass and its level.
- Ignore TNM6 rule and call a LN metastasis if there is a deposit in a lymph drainage field (call it 'discontinuous spread' only if it is <10mm from the 1° and there is no residual LN structure).
- State if vascular invasion is seen (= poor prognostic).
- Take blocks of other structures involved by tumour (salivary gland, sternomastoid, jugular vein).

*Oesophageal Tumours (incl. Siewert & Stein Type 1 Adeno*CA*)*

Biopsies
- Type of cancer and depth of invasion (state if submucosal tissue is present and whether it is invaded)
- Presence of dysplasia or the metaplasia of Barrett's oesophagus

Resections macro
- Length of oesophagus (state if pinned prior to fixation) and any stomach
- Tumour site relative to GOJ / highest peritoneal reflection: if >50% above = oesophageal (if exactly at the junction then = oesophageal if SCC/SmCC/undiff CA but = gastric if adenocarcinoma)
- Tumour max. ∅, length, distance to margins and whether polypoidal or not
- Always take both proximal and distal margins (circumferential *en face* method preferred)
- Location of any LN found (e.g. coeliac *vs.* other perigastric)

Resections micro
- Tumour type and grade (well, moderately or poorly diff – by worst area)
- Depth (incl. level) of invasion (TNM) and if CRM is involved (i.e. <1mm clearance) [*NB:* CRM clearance can't be assessed if the surgeon has dissected LN from it separately]
- Serosal surface involvement (distinguish pleura from gastric serosa)
- Vascular invasion
- Total nõ. of any LNs found as well as nõ involved by tumour
- Presence of dysplasia or the metaplasia of Barrett's oesophagus

*Gastric Carcinoma (incl. Siewert & Stein Type 3 Adeno*CA *and some Type 2)*
- Specify gastrectomy type: total, partial (proximal/distal), oesophago; measure length of components
- Normally open along anterior greater curve (but avoid tumour and any gastrojejunostomy line)
- Tumour: size (max. ∅), distance to margins, Borrmann type (polypoid / fungating / ulcerated *vs.* diffuse)
- Tumour site incl. Siewert and Stein type for peri-cardiac adenocarcinoma (Type: ① midpoint of tumour is 1–5cm above the anatomical cardia; ② from 1cm above to 2cm below the cardia; ③ 2–5cm below the cardia). 'Anatomical cardia' = the most proximal limit of the gastric rugae[2] (or highest peritoneal reflection).
- ≥3 blocks from tumour + all LN; take margin blocks parallel to the margin (esp. at oesophageal end) + take adventitial CRM if tumour goes near the lower oesophagus

---

[2] *NB:* Siewert & Stein defined these types of adenocarcinomas using *endoscopic* and *radiological* localisation

- Type (adeno/other), class (by Laurén), grade (poor/other – by worst area), vasc. invasion (lymph and blood)
- Depth:[3] into subserosa = pT2b, penetration of serosa = pT3 (not invading other organs, else = pT4)

Liver (for 1° HCC or Metastatic Carcinoma)

Macro
- Measure, incise and drain gallbladder, weigh; capsule intact? any adherent structures?
- Serial 1cm slicing in 'CT-plane' if practicable; distance of tumour(s) to all margins
- Note number, size and site of all tumours ± satellites (= nodules <10mm ∅ surrounding a larger tumour) ± vascular invasion
- Tumour blocks: HCC → ≥3; mets → 1 from each met (more if neoadjuvant Rx given)

Micro
- Tumour type (and grade if HCC), margin and LN status, background liver
- PT vascular invasion requires the identification of a residual lumen and endothelium

Exocrine Pancreas, Bile Ducts and Ampulla of Vater

Macro
- Ink, open duodenum; some recommend slicing the pancreas prior to fixation
- Note named structures e.g. vessels
- Record specimen dimensions and lengths (incl. ducts)
- Tumour size and site (head / body / tail / whole / Ampulla / bile ducts) incl. multicentricity
- Spread to other structures: LN, portal vein
- Distance to margins: duodenal +/ gastric, ducts, pancreatic (transection, retroperitoneal, medial[4])
- LN groups: bile duct, infrapyloric (regional to head tumours only), pancreaticoduodenal (anterior/posterior), pancreatic (superior/inferior), pancreatic tail and splenic hilum (not regional to head tumours), coeliac (not regional to body/tail tumours); [Note: tumours <2cm ∅ are unlikely to be node +ve]

Micro
- Tumour type and grade (according to worst area – see p. 176)
- Margins (as above) or anterior pancreatic capsule invasion / extension
- Local spread (pT stage is that of TNM5):
  - ➤ perineural
  - ➤ (pT3): duodenum, Ampulla, bile ducts, peripancreatic fat
  - ➤ (pT4): stomach, colon, spleen, large named vessels (portal, superior mesenteric or common hepatic)

Appendix (for Carcinoid)
- Tumour subtype, size (</>2cm), clearance at base, LN involvement, invasion of mesoappendix or onto serosal surface, vascular invasion and perineural invasion may all influence further Mx

Colorectal Carcinoma
- Macro (rectal only):
  - ➤ relation to anterior peritoneal reflection (and distance to dentate line if APR)
  - ➤ grade the CRM plane as: ① mesorectal (bulky, no coning, no defect deeper than 5mm); ② intramesorectal (coning to levators, moderate bulk but irregular, no muscularis propria visible); ③ muscularis propria (not bulky / deep defects with muscularis visible)
- A margin is considered 'involved' if tumour (main, separate deposit or in a LN or any vessel) extends to 1mm from it
- If the tumour is a poorly diff / infiltrative subtype then proximal and distal margins / doughnuts should be sampled for histology (even if the tumour is >3cm clear macroscopically)
- Extratumoural deposit ≥3mm = 'LN +ve' (in TNM6, only if form and smooth outline are consistent with a LN else = 'vascular invasive deposit' V1 if micro only / V2 if visible macroscopically)

---

[3] 'early gastric cancer' = pT1 (limited to mucosa/submucosa) i.e. not muscle invasive (pT2a) or beyond
[4] The medial pancreatic margin (= 'SMV margin') is the fatty tissue deep to the head – it is the plane dissected off the superior mesenteric vein / portal vein and superior mesenteric artery

- Serosal involvement does NOT imply incomplete *excision* (because it is *not* a surgical margin)
- pT3 or greater: measure the greatest extent of extramural extension
- pT4 = serosal breach (pT4b) or adjacent organ spread (pT4a) *including* colon to colon (by way of the serosa – so may be pT4 a and b) or direct spread into the levator striated muscles
- pM1 includes non-regional LN mets (e.g. para-aortic)[5]
- Extramural vasc. invasion = tumour cells in endothelial-lined space with blood *or* muscle
- Use ypTNM if previous chemo/radioRx and decide if response to neoadjuvant Rx is 'complete', 'marked' (tumour epithelium identified with difficulty) or 'not-marked'
- High risk subgroup of Dukes B CA has any of the following: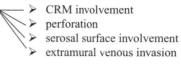
  - ➤ CRM involvement
  - ➤ perforation
  - ➤ serosal surface involvement
  - ➤ extramural venous invasion

Lymphoma

Cases where referral to a haematopathologist is advisable:
- All paediatric lymphomas, any TCL, ? Burkitt's or lymphomas assoc[d] with immunosuppression
- Where the distinction between reactive and neoplastic is blurred (e.g. in AITCL or some FCL)
- Any which have atypical morphology or immuno or where distinction between types is difficult (e.g. lymphocyte depletion HL *vs.* ALCL or CLL *vs.* MCL)

Specimen handling and reporting
- Specify site and use a standard fixation regimen (helps standardise immuno results).
- Remember to look for hilar LN and splenuncula in splenic resections.
- Cut thin sections and use WHO classification (use immuno, even if H&E seems obvious).
- An H&E, PAS, retic, Giemsa on one block may help (± Perls' for trephines).
- For trephine involvement specify type of lymphoma present.

Lung (for Cancer)

Biopsies
- Confirm if it is cancer and, if so, whether it is small cell / non-small cell type.
- Only attempt to sub-classify further if definite features are present ('report only within your limits').

Resections
- Inflate lung with formalin (if bronchus is blocked you can inject the parenchyma with a needle).
- Sample bronchial and vasc. margins then slice longitudinally down bronchi or multiple transverse cuts or sagittally.
- Describe site according to bronchopulmonary segmental anatomy
- Blocks: ≥3 of tumour (block all if ≤2cm ∅) and ≥3 of uninvolved lung and others
- LN: ➤ describe separately sent LN according to their station
  - ➤ N1 nodes are in the lung
  - ➤ N2 nodes are outside the hilar pleural envelope e.g. peribronchial or mediastinal.
- Use the WHO classification for tumours (see Chapter 8: Respiratory and Mediastinum)
- Visceral pleural invasion is defined as tumour breaching the superficial elastic layer (the pleura has a characteristic double elastic layer which differentiates it from fibrosis ∴ use EVG)

Features to note re staging
- Largest tumour ∅ (= pT3 if >3cm)
- Distance of invasive tumour to the bronchial resection margin
- Whether the tumour is in the main bronchus or a lobar / more distal bronchus (if in main bronchus, distance from carina determines stage: pT2 if >2cm, pT3 ≤2cm and pT4 if invading the carina itself – may need CPC to stage)
- Is there >1 tumour in the same lobe as the 1° (= pT4) or a deposit in a different lobe (= pM1)?
- Is there invasion of pleura (= pT2), mediastinal pleura (= pT3) or mediastinal soft tissues (= pT4) ?
- Does any assoc[d] 'atelectasis' or obstructive pneumonia extends to the hilar region (= pT2) or involve the entire lung (= pT3) ?
- Is there a cytology positive pleural effusion (= pT4) ?

---

[5] Peritoneal deposits away from the 1° site are classified as 'pM1 PER' but make sure your oncologist knows that this does not imply distant haemoatogenous/lymphatic mets

Lung (for Non-neoplastic Occupational Disorders / Pneumoconioses)
- Examine externally for pleural plaques, hilar LN, etc. and note size and nõ of lesions.
- Inflate the lung with formalin via the main bronchus to fix.
- Slice sagittally at 1–2cm intervals and prepare one wholemount (Gough-Wentworth) section [protocol for this can be found in Gibbs and Attanoos (2000) – see Bibliography]
- Asbestos body concentration can vary 10-fold depending on site so, for each lung, sample at least 4 (non-tumour) blocks: apex of upper and lower lobe + base of lower lobe + main bronchus with LN.
- Include pleura in some of the blocks and sample any focal lesions.
- Describe and quantitate 1° and 2° dust foci, interstitial fibrosis and emphysema (for grading systems see p. 85, and Gibbs and Attanoos, 2000)

Skin Cancers
- Specify type, site and 3-dimensions and ink the margins
- Fusiform / ellipse excision: bread slice,[6] embed max. 1 slice per cassette for malignant melanoma or 2 slices for SCC / BCC; embed polar ends with your cut face down (to be sectioned first)
- Re-excision Bx: treat such as to be able to comment on completeness of excision of the scar
- Measure peripheral and deep margins to nearest whole mm if >1mm clearance, else state '<1mm' (if involved record as '0 mm'); state measures for invasive and *in situ* components in SCC/melanoma
- Comment on neural / vascular invasion

BCC
- Type (nodular (NST), superficial multicentric, inflammatory / morphoeic, micronodular, etc.)
- Moderately / severely atypical squamous component present
- pT stage $\propto$ diameter and whether invades muscle / cartilage / bone (= pT4)

SCC
- Type (NST, spindle, acantholytic, verrucous, desmoplastic, pseudoangiosarcomatous, etc.)
- Grade: well / mod. / poorly / undifferentiated (see p. 284)
- Clark level (but some clinicians may find this confusing so local protocols may not require it)
- Tumour thickness (from beneath keratin layer)
- pT stage as for BCC

Malignant melanoma
- Type (lentigo maligna, superficial spreading, nodular, acral lentiginous, desmoplastic, neurotropic, naevoid [i.e. symmetrical, cytologically homogeneous and minimal stromal reaction], etc.)
- Macro: nodule present, pigment, border
- Growth phase (VGP / HGP) – defined in Chapter 20, p. 291
- If VGP → mitotic count per 10hpf and tumour lymphocytic response (brisk, non-brisk, absent)
- Ulceration (incl. ∅ of ulceration)
- Presence of:
    a) regression
    b) microsatellites
    c) a benign naevus component

> A microsatellite, defined by T.J. Harrist *et al.* (1984), is a nest (>0.05mm ∅) in the reticular dermis, subcutis or vessels beneath the main tumour and separate from it [by ≥0.5mm according to the RCPath Dataset].

- Clark level and Breslow thickness to 2 d.p. of a mm (from beneath the keratin layer or ulcer base ignoring appendigeal sheath extension of melanoma); *NB:* Clark level only adds significant prognostic information for thin melanomas (i.e. Breslow thickness ≤0.75 mm) that usu. have an excellent prognosis.
- pT stage $\propto$ depth and ulceration

Frozen Sections and Mohs' Micrographic Surgery
- FS is not usu. done on skin cancer (and should normally be avoided in melanoma)
- Mohs' surgery (the pathology is usu. done by the surgeon – a dermatologist trained in pathology):
    ➤ usu. done for BCC / SCC which is recurrent, ill-defined or in an anatomically sensitive site
    ➤ is an iterative surgical procedure involving mapped excision of a lesion with FS of all margins and re-excision of involved areas at the same sitting.

Renal Biopsies (Medical/Transplant)
- Put Bx in saline immediately after taking it and look for glomeruli with a dissecting microscope.
- Under the dissecting microscope, divide into three pieces: 1mm of glomerulus-containing cortex for EM (glutaraldehyde), 2mm of glomerulus-containing cortex for IF (place in special transport medium

---

[6] For a very large circular Bx, cruciate-type sampling is acceptable; for a very small Bx (<5mm) with no clear lesion, embedding whole is acceptable.

or surround in a viscous medium [e.g. Tissue-Tek® O.C.T. compound] and snap freeze is isopentane slush) and the rest for routine LM (formalin).
- A separate portion for IF may be omitted if the lab uses immunoperoxidase for immuno.
- Dividing the Bx for IF/EM may be omitted in the early (≤6 months) post Tx period for ?rejection unless there are unusual findings or ?development of GN in the graft (*de novo* or recurrent).
- If EM is considered essential but glomeruli are not identifiable (as is often the case in chronically diseased kidneys), take a 1mm piece from both ends of the Bx into glutaraldehyde.
- Other variations on handling depend on the clinical questions asked – CPC is required.

Kidney (Adult Renal Tumours)
- Dissect and examine the hilar structures – some do this by serial *en face* slices – prior to slicing to fix (partial slicing, avoiding transection of the hilum, is acceptable if the specimen is to be fixed first).
- Specify side and size of kidney – is it a radical or partial (nephron-sparing) nephrectomy?
- Tumour: size (3D incl. max. ∅), location, type and grade; blocks ≥ 1 per cm max. ∅, include adjacent necrosis (is it coagulative tumour necrosis, hyaline necrosis or therapeutic embolisation infarction?)
- Sample any hilar / other LNs (need ≥ 8–10 nodes for reliable staging of pN0; use TNM6 criteria)
- State if adrenal is present and serially slice and sample it – identify if tumour invades into it by direct extension (= pT3a) or as isolated foci (= pM1)
- Sample vascular resection margins (some take a block through the hilum)
RCC
- Renal vein involvement must be sought macroscopically (confirm by microscopy) – pT3b includes the main renal vein, its segmental tributaries with muscular media and the IVC below the diaphragm.
- Perirenal fat: *infiltration* = cellular infiltration without a capsule (NOT just bulged into).
- Renal sinus fat: cellular infiltration (as defined above) = pT3a (microvascular invasion in this fat, as elsewhere, does not affect the stage – but document it). Tumour blocks should include ≈ all the renal sinus – tumour interface.
- Is there invasion of adjacent organs or beyond Gerota's fascia (the perirenal fatty dissection plane)?
- Is there invasion of the collecting system? (does not affect TNM but record it).
- Serially slice the tumour (look for white solid areas – ?sarcomatoid).
- Serially slice the kidney (look for synchronous tumours) and sample uninvolved kidney.
TCC
- Take distal resection margin of ureter, examine the pelvis for synchronous tumours and sample for CIS.
- Seek invasion of renal parenchyma or peripelvic fat (pT3) or perirenal fat via renal parenchymal invasion (pT4).
- The size of LN mets are important for TNM staging (not just the nõ.)

Urinary Bladder

Biopsies
- Punch Bx (specify how many and sites), TURBT (specify weight and *either* embed all *or* ≈ 4 blocks to include likely muscle/solid areas – if microscopy shows pT1 or no muscle, embed more +/ do levels).
- Specify tumour presence, type, grade and level of invasion (pT stage upto 'at least pT2a' i.e. tumour infiltrates thick cohesive muscle bundles – not the thin separated fibres of the muscularis mucosae).
- Specify whether or not there is flat CIS or invasion of prostatic / urethral tissue.
Cystectomy
- Type of operation: partial / radical, simple or with prostate, urethra, uterus or cervix.
- Inflate with formalin then bivalve coronally via urethral probe.
- Measure dimensions of all organs and Nõ., size, position and depth of any tumours.
- Is there macroscopic invasion of perivesical tissues (extravesical mass = pT3b) ?
- Blocks: ➤ tumour(s) – to see the factors described above [for biopsies] and completeness of excision; stage multiple tumours according to the most advanced and use the 'm' suffix e.g. pT2b(m)
  ➤ urethral and ureteric margins – to check for flat CIS
  ➤ bladder walls: dome, trigone, left, right, anterior, posterior
  ➤ any LN (defined according to TNM6 criteria) / accompanying organs (sample prostate well for synchronous prostate CA)

Prostate

Resections (radical prostatectomy)
- Weigh and ink left *vs.* right (*NB*: seminal vesicle on posterosuperior aspect helps orientation – see Figure 4.11).
- Shave (or cone) urethral margins from apex (inferior) and base (superior)
- Slice into transverse serial sections ± photo; use large blocks to embed whole sections (some local guidelines prefer to use standard-sized blocks concentrating on tumour and prostate capsule as these are easier to use for immuno, quicker to process and easier to get good thin diagnostic sections).
- Embed first slice above the apex and EITHER representative (if tumour can be seen going close to margins) and random blocks of peripheral margins OR embed the whole gland.
- Representative blocks of seminal vesicles (esp. proximally i.e. near the prostate)
- Accompanying lymphadenectomy specimens should be all embedded.
- Report: ➢ Gleason score
          ➢ is tumour organ-confined? (see criteria for extraprostatic extension in Chapter 16: Urological)
          ➢ circumferential margin, seminal vesicle and LN status .

T1 Prostate cancers (i.e. those diagnosed on TURP or core Bx)
- T1a involves ≤5% of the sample (by volume or area)
- T1b involves >5% of the sample (by volume or area)
- T1c if tumour is diagnosed on core Bx
- *NB*: these are *clinical* T stages that depend on histology – there is no pT1 category

> *NB:* the term 'minimal adenocarcinoma' is defined as CA involving <5% of the whole specimen (usu. applied to core Bx) and some 'experts' diagnose this on as few as 2–3 acini

TURP chips
- Protocol depends on attitude of local surgeons to T1 cancers re further management.
- In the following points 'AGE' is the age below which the patient will be considered for radical prostatectomy upon diagnosis of carcinoma (the UK National Dataset for 2000 suggests a value for AGE of 70 years. Some local practices use other values e.g. 65 years. However other factors may also contribute to the question of operability such as fitness, patient choice, etc.)
- In the following points, a filled cassette will contain about 2g of tissue.
- If known carcinoma, only process a small sample of 6g (3 cassettes) to compare grade.
- If not known carcinoma and:
  ☞ <AGE → embed all tissue
  ☞ >AGE and <12g total sample → embed all tissue
  ☞ >AGE and >12g → embed first 12g (6 cassettes) then 1 cassette per additional 5g
      (Some say embed the first 12g then the rest if no tumour detected in this first sample.)
- If high grade PIN is seen then more tissue should be embedded to detect carcinoma.
- Some local guidelines advise that:
      ① if initial sample shows high grade carcinoma → no further tissue embedded
      ② if initial sample shows low grade carcinoma → embed more tissue
- Needle core Bx: (cut multiple levels and spares for immuno)
      ① Bx from single nodule: confirm malignancy / grade
      ② sextant biopsies for ↑ PSA: detect carcinoma, grade and estimate extent of disease
          ➢ Nõ., site and size of cores and % involved by carcinoma (for each core).
          ➢ Whether carcinoma infiltrates adipose tissue, skeletal muscle or seminal vesicle.
          ➢ Report high grade PIN (if carcinoma is not present).
          ➢ Any other pathology that might account for ↑ PSA (e.g. active / chronic prostatitis).

Testicular Tumours

Aims: ➢ Distinguish spermatocytic seminoma *vs.* pure seminoma *vs.* tumours with NSGCT elements.
       ➢ Identify vascular invasion and invasion of any part of the cord or the *tunica vaginalis testis*.
Macro ➢ Note cysts / haemorrhage / necrosis and whether the tunica vaginalis slides freely on the testis.
       ➢ Blocks: cord (margin, mid, root); measure tumour(s) and take multiple blocks (≥1 per cm ∅), adjacent testis, uninvolved testis.
Micro ➢ List elements present and if there is ITGCNU; is there evidence of regression (scar + ITGCNU)
       ➢ Tumour size and invasion (vascular, rete, epididymal, cord, *tunica vaginalis testis*) – rete invasion includes invasion of the rete stroma i.e. tumour does not have to be seen in the rete tubule lumens
       ➢ Immuno: PLAP, AFP, hCG (also c-kit, CD30, NSE, EMA, CK).

Retroperitoneal LN
Assess: ① Margins

   ② Surviving tumour and types (esp. transformation to somatic malignancies)

   ③ Whether there is recognisable residual LN architecture. For detail, see p. 228.

Penis (Amputation)
- Insert a catheter (or Pasteur pipette) into urethra, fix (24 hours) and ink proximal margin of shaft and skin.
- Specify type (partial/full amputation or glansectomy), length of specimen and whether circumcised
- Describe tumour location, extent and type (exophytic or ulcerated)
- Bisect in sagittal plane (may use scissors to cut ventral urethra to skin first, then knife to complete)
- Sample to assess tumour depth (esp. if extending to urethra / corpora), ulceration, extent of shaft invasion, laterality and margins (skin and proximal shaft) – big blocks may be helpful.

Endometrial Cancer / Atypical Hyperplasia

Curettings:
- Presence of atypical hyperplasia or carcinoma (type, grade, background hyperplasia)

Hysterectomy
- Tumour type: endometrioid (FIGO grade) / others
- Invasion: myometrium, cervical stroma,[7] adnexa serosa, vessels, LN
- Peritoneal washings cytology (result alters FIGO and TNM sub-stage)
- Distinguish solid adenocarcinoma from squamous differentiation. Grade only on adeno part (For FIGO criteria for squamous differentiation, see p. 241)

Cervical Neoplasia

Biopsies
- Presence of CIN, CGIN, HPV and invasion
- If Bx large enough to include whole lesion: type, size and FIGO stage
- Completeness of excision (not if punch Bx)

Wertheim's Hysterectomy
- Tumour: size (max. dimension may be across blocks), type, grade, site, depth of invasion
- Margins: vaginal, soft tissue (anterior and posterior) and parametrial
- Sample full circumference of vaginal margin (because there may be microscopic lymphatic spread)
- Type: SCC (keratinising / non-keratinising), SmCC, basaloid, verrucous, glassy cell, adenosquamous

Vulval Bx and Vulvectomy
- Distinguish FIGO stage IA disease: ≤2cm max. ∅ and ≤1mm stromal invasion (depth measured from the level of the tip of an adjacent uninvolved dermal papilla)
- Background changes (VIN, HPV, dystrophies) – see p. 232 for the two types of SCC
- Type and differentiation of tumour (? no agreed guidance for Paget's disease)
- Minimum tumour-free margins (mm): skin, vaginal (urethral), anal, deep
- Vascular invasion
- LN status incl. extracapsular spread

Ovaries

Macro
- Measure ∅ of intact cyst (otherwise state it was collapsed).
- Sample ≥1 block per cm ∅ of solid (and non-smooth cystic) tumour. Upped to 2 blocks/cm for tumours >10cm in max. ∅. [These guidelines are to ensure that a borderline diagnosis is accurate – fewer blocks may be taken if the tumour is obviously malignant and homogeneous].
- Differentiate surgical puncture from tumoural perforation from tumour growing on the surface.
- State the size of the largest extra-ovarian tumour nodule (e.g. omental).

---

[7] Determines sub-stage of stage II disease: IIA = cx glandular involvement, IIB = cx stromal involvement

Micro

- Tumour type (or types if *mixed* – defined as minor component(s) comprising >10% of the tumour)
- Grade epithelial tumours and immature teratomas (grade 1° separately from deposits)
- State additional prognostic factors for non-epithelial tumours: mitotic count per 10 hpf (for sex cord / stromal tumours, dysgerminoma and FATWO); vasc. invasion (for dysgerminoma, FATWO and SCTAT); state if there is marked nuclear pleom. (for dysgerminoma, steroid cell tumour NOS and FATWO) and some tumour-specific features (heterologous elements in Sertoli/Leydig, sparse lympho-cytic infiltrate in dysgerminoma and stromal invasion in SCTAT)
- The result of any peritoneal washing cytology is included in the UK National Dataset report
- If the appendix is sent, embed it all and state the extent/site of any tumour (serosal, mucosal, intramural, etc.)

Breast Carcinoma

- Specify side, weight (except mastectomies) and type (core Bx, localisation Bx, segmental excision)
- Have you seen the specimen X-ray (one should be done for X-ray detected/localised lesions)? Is the radiographic abnormality present in the specimen? Sample such as to include it in the blocks [may need to X-ray your slices / blocks to confirm this and identify which blocks contain the lesion(s)].
- In axillary dissections aim to find ≥16 LN for accurate staging; identify the apical LN if possible
- Size of invasive tumour (max. dimension; combine macro and micro information as necessary):
  - ➤ this is the measurement used for TNM staging (not 'whole size' *vide infra*)
  - ➤ in multifocal tumours use the size of the largest focus (if they are discrete and separate)
  - ➤ if a single tumour mass is composed of ill-defined separate parts (i.e. not a well-defined main tumour with a well-defined small satellite) use the aggregate size of all the parts
- Whole size (= size of invasive tumour + overhanging DCIS) if there is an extensive DCIS component (defined as DCIS extending >1mm beyond the edge of the invasive tumour)
- Distance to nearest margin – for invasive tumour and separately for any extensive DCIS component
- Other factors: tumour type, grade and multifocality, peritumoural vasc. invasion, presence of Ca^{2+} (and whether assoc[d] with benign or malignant structures); any background disease.

Placenta

Indications

- Fetal abnormalities or neonatal diseases with possible intrauterine origin (incl. neurological signs)
- Premature rupture of membranes >36 hours
- Multiple gestation (to establish chorionicity ± other anomalies)
- Maternal illnesses that may affect the neonate (pyrexia / group B *Strep.*, HT/PET, CTD, DM (and other metabolic disease), thrombotic disorders, neoplasia, etc.)
- No examination is indicated for normal births of normal singleton infants regardless of whether there is placenta praevia, PPH or other maternal conditions such as HIV/ viral hepatitis, etc.)

Macro

- Clin.: maternal age, gestational age, birth weight, fetal presentation and mode of delivery, time of rupture of membranes, time of delivery, maternal PMHx, any complications
- Cord: length (<32cm is too short, >100cm is too long), insertion, knots (true and false), vessels, nõ. of twists (normally 1 per 5cm of length; sig. more – hypercoiling – may accompany hypoxia)
- Placental shape and if any succenturiate lobes
- Membranes: insertion, completeness, colour
- Maternal surface: completeness, thickness (average <2cm = abnormally thin), clots/craters/focal lesions (give position and % involvement)
- Twins/multiple: amount of placenta serving each fetus (keep cords and placental zones identifiable for each infant), vascular anastomoses (arteries lie superficial to the veins, veno-venous anastomoses are a worse prognostic than arterio-venous or arterio-arterial anastomoses). May need injection studies in the fresh placenta if ?twin-twin transfusion. Take 'T'-junction block to confirm chorionicity
- Measure the trimmed weight (membranes and cord removed) and state if fixed/fresh
- Blocks: cord (×2 ± funix), membrane roll, full-thickness placenta away from edge (×3).

Soft Tissue Sarcomas

- Type of operation, nature of specimen, anatomical landmarks
- Consider taking fresh tissue for cytogenetics esp. if young (e.g. <40) or a deep / large fatty tumour

- Tumour size and consistency (fleshy, gritty, and presence of bone, cartilage, haemorrhage, etc.)
- Presence and amount of necrosis (as a %): take 1 block per 2cm ∅ of tumour for this
- Margins

Bone Sarcomas
- Biopsies: make imprints (air-dried) for ALP-staining as an adjunct to histology; fix and decalcify the remainder
- Resections: ➤ description of whole specimen (operation, anatomy, attachments, etc.)
  - ➤ prepare a 5mm thick longitudinal slab in a plane through the max. ∅ of the tumour
  - ➤ X-ray the slab to see soft tissue extension and serve as block guide
  - ➤ many blocks (≥40) to assess % non-viable tumour (= chemoRx response), state of the excision margins and to confirm / exclude soft-tissue extension

Thyroid Tumours

Macro
- Weigh, ink, measure and specify left/right; lobectomy/thyroidectomy; total/'near-total'.
- Measure max. ∅ of main lesion (and search for others); sample any intrathyroid margins, parathyroids.
- Sample any LN and note site (contralateral / ipsilateral / central / level IV / other).
- MTC: block all specimen; PTC: sample tumour(s) + ≥2 blocks from uninvolved tissue of each lobe; follicular: sample capsule widely (≥10 blocks if not embedding the whole lesion).
- All tumours: samples to assess presence and extent of any extrathyroidal spread.

Micro
- Confirm max. ∅ if ≤20mm (*NB*: the UK RCPath Dataset advocates TNM5 i.e. pT1 is ≤10mm).
- In multifocal tumours, the largest tumour is used for the T part of the TNM classification.
- For mixed follicular *adenoma*/PTC the ∅ used for staging is that of the whole tumour (if there are multiple PTC foci in it) *or* the ∅ of the focus with recognisable PTC features (if it is the sole focus).
- Tumour: distance to margins, type(s) and differentiation by predominant area. If well-diff, state if minor foci of poorly diff carcinoma are present *but* if an undiff focus is seen, however small, the tumour is classified as anaplastic carcinoma.
- Distinguish follicular tumours with capsular invasion (only) from cases with vasc. invasion and state if the latter is extensive (e.g. >5 intracapsular or extratumoural vessels involved).

Parathyroid Carcinoma
- Macro: site, weight of gland(s), size, ?intact capsule (?breached during surgery); clin.: ?1°/recurence
- Micro: diagnosis, completeness of excision, state of LNs and any accompanying thyroid / parathyroids

Adrenal Tumours

Macro
- Site, weight, size, ?intact capsule, ?necrosis, ?invades surrounding tissues; clin: ?laparoscopic resect[n]
- Blocks: tumour (if <3cm ∅ block it all, else take 1 per cm ∅) + LN + uninvolved cortex (if cortical tumour) or medullary tail (if phaeochromocytoma) + any needed to give the micro information

Micro
- Tumour type, max. ∅, distance to margins, capsular/local invasion (?involves adjacent organs), mitotic count, vasc. invasion, background hyperplasia. [For features of ↑ risk of malignancy, see pp.275–276]
- A note on staging: There is no pTNM for phaeochromocytomas. A pathological staging' TNM for ACC in given in the 2006 RCPath National Dataset but this was designed as a per-operative clinical staging (done by the dissecting surgeon without microscopy). This explains the lack of any histological (micro) definition of local invasion in the literature:
  - ➤ T1 is defined by MacFarlane (1958) and Henley *et al.* (1983) as tumour ≤5cm ∅ and T2 as tumour >5cm ∅
  - ➤ T3 is defined by MacFarlane (1958) as 'infiltration locally reaching neighbouring organs' and refined by Henley *et al.* (1983) to 'tumour any size, locally invading to but not involving adjacent organs'
  - ➤ T4 is defined by MacFarlane (1958) as 'infiltration of neighbouring organs – kidney, veins, etc.' and by Henley *et al.* (1983) as 'tumour any size, locally invading adjacent organs'

Many sources speak of T3 as merely 'local invasion' but the originators of this staging system imply that the local invasion should reach upto (but not into) neighbouring organs. In the absence of a well-defined and standardised pTNM system, the application of this surgical TNM system by histopathologists is thus questionable.

Bibliography

Adachi, Y., Katsuata, T., Aramaki, M., *et al.* (1999) Proximal gastrectomy and gastric tube reconstruction for early cancer of the gastric cardia. *Digestive Surgery*, **16** (6), 468–470.

Albert, D. and Syed, N. (2001) Protocol for the examination of specimens from patients with uveal melanoma. A basis for checklists. *Archives of Pathology and Laboratory Medicine*, **125** (9), 1177–1182.

Anderson, J.R. (1997) Recommendations for the biopsy procedure and assessment of skeletal muscle biopsies. *Virchows Archiv*, **431** (4), 227–233.

Arnold, W.J., Laissue J.A., Friedmann, I., and Naumann, H.H. (1987) *Diseases of the Head and Neck*, Thieme Medical Publishers Inc., New York.

Barr, M.L. and Kiernan, J.A. (1988) *The Human Nervous System*. J.P. Lippincott Company, Philadelphia.

Carpenter, M.B. and Sutin, J. (1983) *Human Neuroanatomy*. Williams & Wilkins, Baltimore.

Catalona, W.J. (1988) Modified inguinal lymphadenectomy for carcinoma of the penis with preservation of saphenous veins: technique and preliminary results. *Journal of Urology*, **140** (2), 306–310.

Eichelberger, L.E. and Cheng, L. (2004) Does pT2b prostate carcinoma exist? Critical appraisal of the 2002 TNM classification of prostate carcinoma. *Cancer*, **100** (12), 2573–2576.

Ellison, D., Love, S., Chimelli, L., Harding, B.N., Lowe, J. and Vinters, H.V. (2004) *Neuropathology. A reference text of CNS pathology*. Mosby, Edinburgh.

Fasel, J.H.D., Gailloud, P., Terrier, F., Mentha, G. and Sprumont, P. (1996) Segmental anatomy of the liver: a review and proposal for an international working nomenclature. *European Radiology*, **6** (6), 834–837.

Fleming, S., Griffiths, D.F.R. (2005) Nephrectomy for renal tumour; dissection guide and dataset. *Journal of Clinical Pathology*, **58** (1), 7–14.

Ford, A.L., Mudhar, H.S., Farr, R. and Parsons, M.A. (2005) The ophthalmic pathology cut-up – Part 1: The enucleation and exenteration specimen, *Current Diagnostic Pathology*, **11** (4), 284–290.

Furness, P.N. (2000) Renal biopsy specimens, *Journal of Clinical Pathology*, **53** (6), 433–438.

Gibbs, A.R. and Attanoos, R.L. (2000) ACP Best Practice No.161: Examination of lung specimens. *Journal of Clinical Pathology*, **53** (7), 507–512.

Gosling, J.A, Harris P.F., Humpherson J.R., Whitmore I. and Willan P.L.T. (1985) *Atlas of Human Anatomy with Integrated Text*. Churchill Livingstone, Edinburgh.

Graadt van Roggen, J.F. (March 2001) The histopathological grading of soft tissue tumours: current concepts. *Current Diagnostic Pathology*, **7** (1), 1–7.

Hahn, H.P., Fletcher C.D.M. (Dec. 2005) The role of cytogenetics and molecular genetics in soft tissue tumour diagnosis – a realistic appraisal. *Current Diagnostic Pathology*, **11** (6), 361–370.

Hamoir, M., Desuter G., Grégoire V. *et al.* (2002) A proposal for refining the boundaries of level V in the neck. *Archives of Otolaryngology – Head and Neck Surgery*, **128** (12), 1381–1383.

Hargitai, B., Marton T. and Cox, P.M. (2004) Examination of the human placenta. *Journal of Clinical Pathology*, **57** (8), 785–792.

Harrist, T.J., Rigel, D.S., Day, C.L. *et al.* (1984) "Microscopic satellites" are more highly associated with regional lymph node metastases than is primary melanoma thickness. *Cancer*, **53** (3), 2183–2187.

Henley, D.J., van Heerden, J.A., Grant, C.S., Carney, J.A. and Carpenter, P.C. (1983) Adrenal cortical carcinoma — a continuing challenge. *Surgery*, **94** (6), 926–931.

Kim, K.W., Choi, B.I., Han, J.K. *et al.* (2002) Postoperative anatomic and pathologic findings at CT following gastrectomy. *RadioGraphics*, **22** (2), 323–336.

Jamieson, E.B. (1950) *A Companion to Manuals of Practical Anatomy*, Oxford University Press, London.

Junqueira, L.C., Carneiro, J. and Long J.A. (1986) *Basic Histology*, Appleton-Century-Crofts (Prentice-Hall), Norwalk, CT.

Lewis, W.H. (2000) *Gray's Anatomy*, Lea & Febiger, Philadelphia and Bartleby.com, New York. Available at www.bartleby.com/107 (accessed March 2007)

Lowe, D.G. and Jeffrey, I.M. (1990) *Macro Techniques in Diagnostic Histopathology*, Wolfe Medical Publications Ltd., London.

MacFarlane, D.A. (1958) Cancer of the adrenal cortex; the natural history, prognosis and treatment in a study of fifty-five cases. *Annals of the Royal College of Surgeons in England*, **23** (3), 155–186.

Mann, C.V. and Russell, R.C.G. (eds) (1992) *Bailey & Love's Short Practice of Surgery*, Chapman and Hall Medical, London.

McLatchie, G.R. (1990) *Oxford Handbook of Clinical Surgery*, Oxford Medical Publications Ltd., Oxford.

McMinn, R.M.H. and Hutchins, R.T. (1984) *A Colour Atlas of Human Anatomy*. Wolfe Medical Publications Ltd., London.

Poulos, C.K., Koch, M.O., Eble, J.N., Daggy, J.K. and Cheng, L. (2004) Bladder neck invasion is an independent predictor of prostate-specific antigen recurrence. *Cancer*, **101** (7), 1563–1568.

Pringle, J.A.S. (November 1996) Osteosarcoma: the experience of a specialist unit. *Current Diagnostic Pathology*, **3** (3), 127–136.

Quirke, P. (1998) The pathologist, the surgeon and colorectal cancer – get it right because it matters, in *Progress in Pathology*, vol. 4, (eds N. Kirkham, N.R. Lemoine), Churchill Livingstone, Edinburgh, pp. 201–213.

Shousha, S. (June 2000) Reporting breast biopsies. *Current Diagnostic Pathology*, **6** (2), 140–145.

Sobin, L.H. and Wittekind, Ch. (eds) (1997 – 5th edn; 2002 – 6th edn) *UICC TNM Classification of Malignant Tumours*, Wiley-Liss, New York.

Siewert, J.R. and Stein, H.J. (1998) Classification of adenocarcinoma of the oesophagogastric junction. *British Journal of Surgery*, **85** (11), 1457–1459.

Slootweg, P.J. (2005) ACP Best Practice No. 182: Complex head and neck dissections. How to handle them. *Journal of Clinical Pathology*, **58** (3), 243–248.

Snell, R.S. (1986) *Clinical Anatomy for Medical Students*, Little, Brown & Co. Inc., Boston.

Somner, J.E.A., Dixon, J.M.J. and Thomas, J.S.J. (2004) Node retrieval in axillary lymph node dissections: recommendations for minimum numbers to be confident about node negative status. *Journal of Clinical Pathology*, **57** (8), 845–848.

Sternberg, S.S. (ed) (1997) *Histology for Pathologists*, Lippincott Williams & Wilkins, Philadelphia.

Strasser, H., Klima, G., Poisel, S., Horninger, W. and Bartsch, G. (1996) Anatomy and innervation of the rhabdosphincter of the male urethra. *The Prostate*, **28** (1), 24–31.

Wainwright, H.C. (2006) My approach to performing a perinatal or neonatal autopsy. *Journal of Clinical Pathology*, **59** (7), 673–680.

Wilkins, B.S. (1997) Simplifying the spleen: a new look at splenic pathology, in *Progress in Pathology*, vol. 3, (eds N. Kirkham, N.R. Lemoine), Churchill Livingstone, New York, pp. 211–231.

Wittekind, Ch., Greene F.L., Henson D.E., Hutter R.V.P and Sobin L.H. (eds) (2003), *UICC TNM Supplement: A Commentary on Uniform Use*, Wiley-Less, New York.

Young, J.A. (1993) *Fine Needle Aspiration Cytopathology*, Blackwell Scientific Publications, Oxford.

Web sites

Papagiannis, G., Mlynarek, A., Massie, R., Chagnon, F. and Gesser, R. (2000–2004) *Discover the Larynx*, McGill University, Canada. www.sprojects.mmi.mcgill.ca/larynx/Default.htm (accessed March 2007)

Royal College of Pathologists. Standards and Datasets for Reporting Cancers. www.rcpath.org.uk (accessed March 2007)

5. Paediatric and Placental

Paediatric

Congenital / Malformative Anomalies
- Of the lung (see pp.82–83, p. 393 and *vide infra*)
- Of the heart (see p. 385, p. 386, p. 389 and p. 78)
- Of the urinary tract / testis (see pp. 212–213, incl. Potter's triad)
- Of skeletal muscle (see p. 191 and p. 184)

Alveolar capillary dysplasia
- Incompatible with recovery – ! so diagnosis results in termination of ventilatory support
- Alveolar walls are thickened, cellular and contain ↑numbers of prominent capillaries
- Capillaries not closely apposed to alveolar lining
- Misalignment of pulmonary veins: the small pulm. veins accompany the bronchi and pulm. arteries (*cf.* running separately in the interlobular septa) resulting in reduced septal vascularity
- d/dg peripheral lung injury due to ventilation, infection, etc. – look for the venous anomalies
- d/dg do not confuse pulmonary lymphangiectasia or interstitial emphysema for pulm. veins

Hirschprung's Disease (HD)
- Ultrashort segment (aganglionosis of distal rectum only)
- Short segment (upto the rectosigmoid junction)
- Long segment (beyond the rectosigmoid but not reaching the small bowel)
- Total colonic (includes variable amounts of small bowel)
- Easy to exclude HD (in a particular segment) by seeing the presence of ganglion cells
- Diagnosis based on neural morphology including acetylcholinesterase (AChE) staining:
  - ➤ absence of ganglion cells in the submucosa
  - ➤ hypertrophied nerve trunks and ↑ nerve fibres in the submucosa
  - ➤ ↑ density of AChE fibres in the lamina muscularis mucosae (all ages, pathognomonic)
  - ➤ ↑ density of AChE fibres in the lamina propria mucosae in older patients which are
    1. coarse
    2. extend to surface
    3. run parallel to surface
    4. not present in neonates with HD (! false −ve diagnosis if unaware of this)
  - ➤ ! false +ve if unaware of normal appearances, esp. close to the pectinate line i.e.
    - ☞ ↑ density of vessels (vessels are normally surrounded by AChE +ve fibres)
    - ☞ hypoganglionosis is normal 1–2 cm proximal to the pectinate line
    - ☞ occ. nerve trunks and fibres are normal in submucosa of right colon and rectum
    - ☞ d/dg ganglion cells *vs.* CMV inclusions of endothelium
  - ➤ ! false −ve if unaware that ganglion cells *look* different in neonates (small cells without prominent nucleoli – d/dg stromal cells)
- ∴ Must know age of patient, distance of Bx and examine ≥50 levels
- Some cases of total colonic HD may not show ↑ fibres in the muscularis mucosae → ! false −ve

Necrotising Enterocolitis
- Radiological pneumatosis in a premature baby ± pneumatosis macroscopically at cut-up
- Mural haemorrhage ± necrosis
- Pneumatosis (may show multinucleated GC around the spaces)
- ± signs of healing: granulation tissue, epithelial regenerative atypia, fibrosis (± stenosis)

CIBD in Children
- In UC, 1st presentation may be patchy with subtle/absent signs of chronicity and with rectal sparing
- In CD, upper GI involvement (usu. asymptomatic) is more common *cf.* adults

Infantile Respiratory Distress Syndrome (Hyaline Membrane Disease)
- Alveolar collapse
- Hyaline membranes in terminal and resp. bronchioles (*cf.* alveoli in adults)

Diagnostic Criteria Handbook in Histopathology: A Surgical Pathology Vade Mecum by Paul J. Tadrous
Copyright © 2007 by John Wiley & Sons, Ltd.

Cutaneous vascular lesions (according to the ISSVA Classification)
- Diagnosis depends on CPC: present at birth? progression/involution? results of flow studies, etc.

Neoplasms
- Congenital haemangioma (M=F, present at birth, subdivided by involution history into RICH/NICH)
    - ➢ RICH involutes from the centre with capillary lobules replaced by fibrosis, haemosiderin and thromboses ± Ca^{2+} leaving dilated abnormal channels with thick or thin walls; other features may overlap with infantile haemangioma but GLUT1 is −ve and capillaries may be thin-walled
    - ➢ NICH grows at the same rate as the child, features may overlap with RICH and infantile haemangioma but GLUT1 is −ve
- Infantile haemangioma (= 'juvenile / cellular haemangioma', *do not use* 'infantile haemangioendothelioma')
    - ➢ F≫M, *may* be present at birth, grows faster than the infant for a few months then involutes
    - ➢ proliferative phase: abundant lobules of small capillaries with diffusely GLUT1 +ve endothelium
    - ➢ endothelium is plump: lumena may not be evident (but you see packeted and tubular retic patterns)
    - ➢ involutional phase shows few capillary foci (GLUT1 +ve) with more stroma and prominent larger feeder vessels (have GLUT1 −ve endothelium by immuno) – see p. 318 for more
    - ➢ d/dg ! do not mis-diagnose involutional phase as AVM (which do not have GLUT1 +ve capillaries)
- Other (GLUT1 −ve): pyogenic granuloma, KS, HPC, Kaposiform haemangioendothelioma, tufted angioma (angioblastoma of Nakagawa), etc. For more information, see Chapter 21: Soft Tissues

Malformations
- Simple: one type of vessel (use D2-40 for lymph) ⎫ It is important to identify if there is an arterial
- Combined: >1 type e.g. lymphovenous or AVM ⎬ component (high flow malformations require
                                                                       ⎭ different Rx).
- d/dg involutional phase infantile haemangioma: malformations (esp. AVM) may show foci of proliferative immature vessels (+ve for Ki-67, αSMA and CD31 and may 'infiltrate' normal tissues) but these are GLUT-1 −ve

Spindle Cell Lesions of Childhood / Infancy
- *Fibrous hamartoma of infancy*   ① spindle cell fascicles (CD34 −ve) ⎫ For *mesenchymal hamartoma*
                                                                       ② fat as part of the lesion   ⎬ and other bone tumours, see
                                                                       ③ primitive mesenchymal cells ⎭ Chapter 22: Osteoarticular.
- *Digital fibroma of infancy*   ➢ affects fingers
                                                                       ➢ spindle cells with eosinophil inclusions (see p. 286)
- *Inflammatory myofibroblastic tumour:* systemic Sx, inflam^y cells, spindle cells, ALK1 +ve
- *Infantile fibromatosis:* single or multiple, 10% recur, Rx is local excision
- *Desmoid fibromatosis:* never regress, 80% recur, Rx is WLE (+ chemo/radioRx)
- *Infantile fibrosarcoma*: single lesion, may metastasise, 30% recur, Rx: chemoRx and WLE (good prog)
See also Chapter 21: Soft Tissues, for more on some of these entities and specialised textbooks.

Thymic Cyst
- A lymphoepithelial cyst usu. in the lateral neck. and present in <10 year olds
- d/dg branchial cyst:
    - ➢ thymic cysts present in young child, branchial in adults
    - ➢ thymic cyst contains thymic lymphoid tissue in the wall ± Hassall's corpuscles

Langerhans Cell Histiocytosis / Histiocytosis X (HX)
- Proliferation of Langerhans dendritic cell histiocytes:
    - ➢ abundant cytoplasm
    - ➢ elongated vesicular nucleus, may have a transverse 'fold' / 'belt'
    - ➢ immuno: +ve for CD1a, S100, HLA-DR (MHC class II). CD68 is weakly +ve
    - ➢ EM: 'tennis racket' Birbeck granules
- Usu. eosinophils also present, may be numerous

- Localised form ('eosinophil granuloma') has better prog. *cf.* systemic (Hand-Schüller-Christian and, worst of all, Letterrer-Siwe)
- d/dg ALCL (see p. 116 and p. 302); non-X histiocytoses (see p. 286); Gaucher's disease (see p. 123); Rosai-Dorfman (CD1a −ve, lymphocyte emperipolesis) and epithelioid granulomatous / eosinophilic inflam[n]

Ewing's, Peripheral Neuroectodermal Tumour (PNET) and Askin Tumour (of chest wall)
- Sheets of small glycogenated cells with scant, ill-defined cytoplasm   *Askin tumour* has features
- PNET (*cf.* Ewing's) it is more lobulated, more vascular ± occ. rosettes   intermediate between
- No fibrillar stroma or other neuroblastoma features   Ewing and PNET
- Cytogenetics: t(11;22)(q24;p12)(FLI1;EWS) – the same in Ewing's, PNET and Askin
- PNET and Ewing's immuno: vimentin +ve (dot-like), CD99 +ve (strong membranous[1]), CK −ve
- PNET selective immuno/stains: NSE, S100, Synaptophysin +ve (also, tends to be −ve for glycogen)

See pp.335–336 for more on Ewing's incl. EM, d/dg and prognostic factors.

Desmoplastic Small Round Cell Tumour (DSRCT)
- Multiple intra-abdominal masses in adolescent (M>F). Also reported in pleura, CNS and lymph node
- Low power: sharply outlined trabeculae of blue cells separated by desmoplastic stroma
- Central necrosis ± Ca^{2+}
- Uniform cells, scant cytoplasm, indistinct nucleoli, mitoses ++ (a variant has eosinophilic cytoplasm ++)
- t(11;22)(p13;q21) – said to be unique to DSRCT
- Immuno: co-expression of epithelial (CAM5.2, AE1/AE3), neural (vimentin, NSE) and muscle (dot-like desmin). CD99 +ve in 30%. C-terminal WT1 +ve (C19 Ab), MyoD1, myogenin and myoglobulin are −ve

Rhabdomyosarcoma (RMS)
- Occurs at sites of embryonic tissue fusion (head, neck and midline – the grey zone in the Figure 5.1)
- Classification by prognosis: ➢ best: botryoid and spindle cell
                                  ➢ intermediate: embryonal NOS
                                  ➢ poor: alveolar and pleomorphic
                                  ➢ unknown: RMS with rhabdoid features.

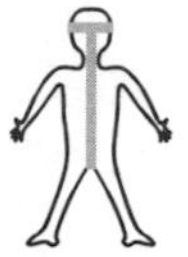

FIGURE 5.1
Sites of RMS

- Features of striated muscle differentiation: bright cytoplasmic eosinophilia ± cross striations
- Immuno: MyoD1 (nuclear), polyclonal desmin, MSA, myoglobulin, myogenin +ve; CD99 +ve in 15% (usu. weak granular cytoplasmic)
- d/dg: muscle infiltrative small blue round cells of regenerating muscle, see also Chapter 21: Soft tissues

Embryonal
- Variable cellularity with cambium layer (cellular condensation beneath mucosa) and pericellular retic
- Cells range from primitive stellate to elongated forms with bright eosinophilia ± cross striations
- Anaplastic cells may be present singly or as clonal clusters
- ± Myotube-like formations, ± 'smooth muscle-like' spindle forms with blunt nuclei, ± myxoid areas
- Variant: Botryoid – has polypoid nodules (usu. occurs in bladder and vagina)
- Variant: Spindle Cell – fascicles ± storiform, not anaplastic (usu. occurs in the paratesticular region)
- Cytogenetics: +8, +2, +11, rea.(12)(q13)

Alveolar
- Fibrous septa delineate cell aggregates with central dyscohesion. Reticulin is peri-aggregate
- Cells are rounded (! d/dg lymphoma) + focal striated muscle differentiation ± clear cells; myxoid is usu. absent
- Variant: solid – lacks the dyscohesion and fibrous septa but retic is not pericellular *cf.* embryonal RMS
- Variant: mixed alveolar / embryonal – consider this if there are spindle and myxoid areas
- Cytogenetics: t(2;13)(q35;q14) in 70% or t(1;13)(q36;q14)

Pleomorphic
- Whole tumour must be pleom. without foci of embryonal or alveolar variants; striations are rare
- Diagnosis requires at ≥ 1 striated muscle immuno plus H&E evidence of polygonal rhabdomyoblasts

---

[1] useful pattern to distinguish Ewing's/PNET from blastematous Wilms'

Teratoma (Non-gonadal)
- Commonest tumour in the neonate (i.e. within the first month of life)
- Usu. midline (sacrococcygeal, neck, palate, mediastinum, CNS), also: kidney, orbit, etc.
- Any tissue type may be present but if a well-formed axial skeleton is seen consider *fetus-in-fetu*
- Classification: benign, malignant, immature (degree of immaturity may $\propto$ aggressiveness)
- Immaturity assessed by discordance of tissue maturity with the age of the child (e.g. neuroblasts in a neonate are OK – but not in a 3-year-old)

For gonadal teratomas see pp.225- 226 and pp.251–252.

Pineoblastoma, Haemangioblastoma, Medulloblastoma and other CNS Tumours
See p. 184, p. 187 and p. 188.

Retinoblastoma
See p. 199 and p. 44.

Pleuropulmonary Blastoma
See p. 90.

Pancreatoblastoma
See p. 177 and p. 179 (under the d/dg of acinar cell tumour and NETs).

Neuroblastoma (NB) / Ganglioneuroblastoma / Ganglioneuroma
- Poorly diff NB: ➢ sheets of cells with hyperchromatic nuclei
  - ➢ lobular architecture with thin fibrous septa
  - ➢ fibrillar stroma (unmyelinated axons), S100 +ve cells in stroma
- Increasing differentiation
  - ➢ Homer-Wright pseudo-rosettes (no lumen, just fibrils) in 30% of cases
  - ➢ Some cells with more open nuclei, prom. nucleoli and more cytoplasm (i.e. obvious neuroblasts)
  - ➢ ganglion cells
  - ➢ more ganglion cells = ganglioneuroblastoma
  - ➢ all ganglion cells = ganglioneuroma
  - ➢ lots of trk expression (NGF receptor)
- Cytogenetics of NB: 1p del., N-myc amplification (dmin / HSR)
- Immuno of NB: CD99 −ve[2], NB84 +ve, CD57, NSE, CgA, PGP 9.5 +ve
- Favourable prognostic features in NB are: ganglion cells, tumour giant cells, low mitotic count (<10/10hpf) and focal calcification

Hepatoblastoma
- Large solitary variegated liver mass and ↑serum AFP (± hCG)
- ± Necrosis ++ (due to pre-op chemoRx in resected specimens, but not seen on 1° diagnostic core Bx)
- Stroma: fibrous septa, osteoid, primitive spindly mesenchyme (other elements are rare e.g. muscle)
- Epithelia (the first two are required for diagnosis):
  - ➢ embryonal liver: cords ± rosettes of small blue fusiform cells
  - ➢ fetal liver: small cells (vesicular nucleus, single nucleolus) in microtrabeculae ± bile plugs
  - ➢ ± macrotrabecular liver (adult HCC-like)
  - ➢ ± anaplastic small cell (SBRCT-like)
  - ➢ ± glandular elements (intestinal-like)
  - ➢ ± teratoid elements: ectopic epithelia (squamous, endocrine, etc.)
- Immuno: AFP, focal hCG, CAM5.2, CK7/19, CEA and S100 are all +ve in various elements

Nephroblastoma (Wilms' tumour)
- Classically triphasic (but biphasic / monophasic variants occur):
  - ① stroma (spindle cells)
  - ② blastema (dyscohesive small blue round cells) occurs in 3 organoid patterns (helps to distinguish monophasic blastematous subtype from d/dg lymphoma):

---

[2] CD99 +vity virtually excludes neuroblastoma. Wilms' is also CD99 −ve

> serpentine (anastomosing cords in myxoid stroma)
> nodular (rounded nests)
> basaloid (nests outlined by cuboidal / columnar cells)

③ epithelium (cells with elongated, moulded and wedge/carrot-shaped nuclei form glomeruloid and tubular structures – !d/dg entrapped renal parenchyma.
- Variant: predominantly cystic forms of Wilms' occur
- Stroma can be highly differentiated with 'heterologous elements': myxoid, fibroblastic, leiomyomatoid, adipose and chondroid (= 'teratoid Wilms' if prominent) and skeletal muscle or even rhabdomyoblastic elements (! d/dg RMS)
- Anaplasia (focal or diffuse) must have ALL of the following:
  > nuclear enlargement ≥ 3 fold *cf.* adjacent nuclei of same lineage
  > hyperchromasia of enlarged nuclei
  > enlarged or multipolar mitoses (each limb of an X or Y-shaped figure must be as large as a normal metaphase)
  So defined, it heralds poor prognosis and chemoresistance.
- Stage according to the NWTS system (I–V), simplified this is:
  I   confined to kidney, capsule intact, renal sinus[3] veins and lymphatics not involved
  II   spread beyond capsule / hilar plane but surgical margins clear
  III extends to surgical margins or residual local disease present
  IV   haematogenous mets
  V   bilateral renal tumours
- Cytogenetics: WT1 and WT2 on chromosome 11
- Immuno: epithelium (CK, WT1 +ve), blastema (desmin, WT1 +ve; vimentin, CK ±ve), CD99 −ve

Clear Cell Sarcoma of the Kidney
- Highly aggressive, resistant to Wilms' therapy, needs specific chemoRx
- Monotonous array of pale cells with nuclei having finely dispersed chromatin and small nucleoli
- Characteristic vasculature of parallel capillaries connected by transverse arcades
- Variant: sclerosing (may entrap nephrons and be confused for d/dg blastematous Wilms')

Placenta

Placental Growth (Weights) [4]

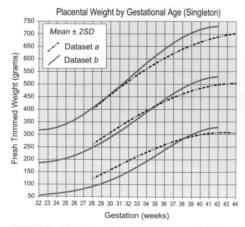

FIGURE 5.2 Placental weight by gestational age (Singleton)

- For twin placental mean weight multiply the mean 'Singleton Weight' by the 'Twin Factor' in the table (10th centile is ≈ 0.75 × the

TABLE 5.1

Gestation in weeks	Singleton Weight Mean (b) in g	Twin Factor	Fetus:Placenta Ratio
19	160 [synth]	1.33	-
20	165 [synth]	1.32	-
21	175 [synth]	1.32	-
22	186.11	1.35	-
23	189.37	1.46	-
24	195.52	1.57	2.9
25	204.56	1.67	3.1
26	216.44	1.76	3.3
27	231.05	1.82	3.5
28	248.22	1.87	4.9
29	267.73	1.9	5.1
30	289.3	1.91	5.3
31	312.58	1.92	5.4
32	337.2	1.91	5.6
33	362.7	1.89	5.8
34	388.58	1.87	6.0
35	414.27	1.84	6.2
36	439.15	1.82	6.4
37	462.55	1.79	6.5
38	483.75	1.76	6.6
39	501.94	1.73	6.7
40	516.29	1.7	6.8
41	525.9	1.68	7.0

---

[3] The renal sinus is that part of the pelvis lateral to the hilar plane
[4] The sources for datasets 'a' and 'b' in these charts and table are detailed in the Bibliography (*q.v.*)

twin mean and 90th centile is $\approx 1.25 \times$ the twin mean). [*NB*: The table entries marked 'synth' are not true singleton weights but were synthesised for the purpose of calculating twin weights]

- IUGR = birth weight below 2.5kg at term or below the 3rd centile for gestational age ['small for gestational age' = birth weight below the 10th centile]
- The normal fetal:placental weight ratio goes from 1:1 at 14/40 to $\approx$ 7:1 at 40–44/40

Large placenta (e.g. >90th centile)

- Maternal conditions (e.g. DM / anaemia)
- Fetal hypertrophy syndromes (e.g. Beckwith-Wiedemann syndrome)
- Congenital syphilis
- Fetal oedema (e.g. *hydrops fetalis*, less-severe anaemia, nephrotic syndrome)

Small placenta (e.g. <10th centile)

- IUGR (from various causes)
- PET
- ↑ Perivillous fibrin deposition
- Villitis of unknown aetiology
- Trisomies

Infarcts
- May occupy upto 3–5% of a term placenta without functional consequence (but >10–30% is sig.)
- Only diagnose on histology because the macro d/dg includes fibrin, MPVFD and chorangioma
- Early (red infarct):
  - ➤ ↑ maternal blood in intervillous space with central thrombus ⎫ Signs of
  - ➤ villous vessels congested and dilated ⎬ ischaemia
  - ➤ syncytial trophoblast necrosis and eosinophilia ⎭
- Later:
  - ➤ intervillous space collapses
  - ➤ perivillous fibrin deposition
  - ➤ villous vessels collapse → ghost-like villi
  - ➤ adjacent villi show ischaemia: ↑ syncytial knots, small terminal villi + big stem villi, empty intervillous space

Syncytial Knots
- Occur in 10–30% of villi in term placentae (! exclude d/dg thick section artefact)
- They are a sign of placental hyperplasia / maturity and are ↑ in:
  - ➤ maternal DM / HT / PET / anaemia
  - ➤ adjacent to infarcts
- They are uncommon <32 weeks but may be seen in mid-trimester abortions

Maternal HT incl. Pre-Eclamptic Toxaemia (PET) / Eclampsia
- Villous BM thickening
- Incomplete transformation of maternal vessels (i.e. they are lined by endothelium rather than tro-phoblast) esp. in the intra-myometrial portion of the arteries
- Maternal vessel acute atherosis (fibrinoid change/necrosis + intimal foamy lipid cells) ± thromboses
- Haematomas (placental / retroplacental)
- The resulting ischaemia / uteroplacental insufficiency → accelerated maturation (↑ vasculosyncytial membranes, ↑ knots, small villi, etc.) → small-for-dates baby (placental weight may be ↑ or ↓)

Maternal Diabetes
- Delayed maturation and big placenta (and baby)
- Fetal 'infarcts' (actually villous vessel thromboses *vide infra* under Villous Changes Following IUD)
- Villous BM thickening and ↑ knots
- ↑ Nucleated RBCs in villous vessels (i.e. nucleated RBCs easily found at term)

Maternal Antiphospholipid Antibody Syndrome (± SLE)
- Clin.: a cause of habitual abortion (= recurrent miscarriage = $\geq$3 consecutive pregnancy losses) incl. 1st trimester abortion; this is preventable by antithrombotic cover (see p. 351)
- In treated patients with uncomplicated live births the placenta usu. shows no specific abnormality

- Early POC may show incomplete vascular transformat^n (normal endothelium in endometrial vessels)
- Later fetal deaths may show MPVFD (but only in a minority of cases)
- One study showed decidual small vessel thromboses (non-inflam^y $\pm$ recanalisation) and infarcts $\rightarrow$ ischaemia (hypovascular/fibrotic villi and $\uparrow$ syncytial knots) but with $\downarrow$ vasculosyncytial membranes

Retroplacental Haematoma
- Clin.: may be the cause of fetal distress, sudden hypoxic death or pre-term labour
- Macro: haematomas are excavating (i.e. make a concave impression on the maternal surface) otherwise it is probably insignificant post-partum clot
- Overlying villi show signs of ischaemia (e.g. dilated congested vessels) or infarction

Intervillous Thrombus
- Intervillous space expanded by laminated fibrin and blood; it is largely devoid of villi
- There is no sig. infarction / ischaemia of the surrounding villi (unlike in d/dg haematoma)
- Situated near centre of cotyledon and not considered clinically important

Subchorial Thrombus
- Small: insignificant (= Langhans fibrinoid)
- Massive: assoc^d with fetal death, pre-term labour and 3rd trimester bleeding

Massive Perivillous Fibrin Deposition (MPVFD)
- Rare but assoc^d with IUGR and *recurrent* fetal loss ($\therefore$ important to recognise for future pregnancies)
- Extensive pallor *throughout* placenta (>80%, if concentrated in basal plate = maternal floor 'infarct', if with a reticular configuration = Gitter 'infarct')
- Fibrinoid is composed of fibrin + extracellular matrix proteins (e.g. laminin)
- Within abundant fibrinoid are *viable* villi (unlike d/dg infarction)
- Groups of intermediate trophoblast cells within the fibrinoid (called X-cell islands)
- d/dg infarction (see p. 61)
- d/dg minor perivillous fibrin (<20% is usu. functionally not sig.) $\approx$ focal perivillous fibrin deposition
- d/dg 'extensive perivillous fibrin deposition': 20–80% of the villi are surrounded by fibrin

Other Fetal Vascular Anomalies
- Chorionic vessel thrombosis
- Umbilical cord angioma / thrombosis
- Chorangiosis: affected villi are large and have $\uparrow$vessels centrally ($\geq$10 per villus). If diffuse (i.e. seen in $\geq$10 fields from $\geq$10 different blocks) it is assoc^d with fetal anomalies/mortality
- Chorangioma: macro: range from several cm $\varnothing$ to microscopic (d/dg focal chorangiosis); usu. subchorial and may be pale or red (d/dg thrombus/infarct). micro: capillary ($\pm$ larger vessel) haemangioma-like hamartoma $\pm$ infarct/thromboses/overlying hyperplastic trophoblast. $\pm$ fetal pathology: high output CCF +/ other haemangiomas

Avascular villi
- Fetal vessel thrombosis (maternal [e.g. DM, coagulopathy] and fetal causes)
- Hydatidiform mole and non-molar hydropic abortion
- Normal villi 1–2 weeks after IUD (d/dg infarct – these are ghost-like and have necrotic trophoblast)

Villous Changes Following IUD or Local Fetal Vessel Occlusion
- Microvascular contraction and vascular apoptoses / perivascular karyorrhexis (hours)
- Septation of large stem vessels by fibroblastic in-growth (from two days onwards)
- Fibrous avascular villi $\pm$ Ca^{2+} [with viable surface trophoblast and internal fibroblasts] ($\approx$ 1–2 weeks)

Sub-involution of the Placental Site Vessels
- Diagnosed as a cause of PPH *in the absence of other RPOC*
- Dilated tortuous vessels and fully involuted vessels co-exist
- Patent lumena / only partial occlusion by thrombus
- Hyaline replacement of normal vessel wall structure $\pm$ mural intermediate trophoblast
- Persistence of endovascular intermediate trophoblast (CAM5.2 +ve, hCG $-$ve)

Calcification
- Extravillous: normal finding in a mature placenta
- Intravillous: assoc[d] with IUD retained for >1 week

Meconium Staining of Membranes
- Full changes require >6 hours of exposure (though chorionic Mφ take up meconium after 3 hours) and are assoc[d] with fetal distress, fetal thrombotic vasculopathy, chorioamnionitis and Group B *Strep.* infection
- Pseudostratified, club-shaped vacuolated amniocytes ± pigment; later may slough off with necrosis of underlying decidua and peripheral layers of arterial smooth muscle in the umbilical cord after 24 hours
- Mφ containing green meconium pigment seen in the compact layer of the amnion after 12–24 hours

Villitis
- May be focal or extensive; basal or non-basal, acute or chronic (chronic is the default meaning)

Acute villitis
- Severe maternal infection ± prematurity or IUD

Chronic villitis
- Mixed infiltrate of lymphocytes, histiocytes (± specific changes in 2% – e.g. TORCH, listeria, syphilis)
- Associations: IUGR and may recur in successive pregnancy if extensive (?autoimmune aetiology)

Villous Oedema
- Normal if limited and focal
- Fetal infections: assoc[d] with ↑ nulceated RBCs in villous vessels (i.e. easily found at term)
- *Hydrops fetalis* (e.g. 2° to cardiac / thoracic anomalies, *erythroblastosis fetalis* [2° to the haemolysis of α-thalassaemia or, rarely, Rhesus incompatibility], IEM or idiopathic) ± ↑ nulceated RBCs
- Hydatidiform mole and non-molar hydropic abortion

Villous Fibrosis
- Result of long-standing IUD
- Stem vessel thrombosis / any cause of avascular villi or vascular insufficiency
- Infection (esp. CMV)
- Seen in IUGR

Squamous Metaplasia of the Amnion
- Stratification, hyperkeratosis ± granular layer
- No pathological significance

Amnion Nodosum
- Macro: smooth pale little mounds mostly on the fetal surface
- Micro: fragments of cells ± hair embedded in amorphous eosinophilic matrix (? vernix concretions)
- Signifies oligohydramnios and ∴ possible fetal anomalies

Twin Placentation
- Monochorionic excludes dizygosity but monozygotic can be anything (from two separate placentas to monoamniotic monochorionic)
- Death of one twin can cause abnormalities in the other – but only if they are monochorionic
- Normal (non-oedematous) amnion is upto 1/2 mm thick
- Normal histology of amnion and chorion and intertwin membrane is shown in the figure, below

Twin-Twin Transfusion Syndrome (TTTS)
- Is restricted to monozygotic twins
- Donor: large poorly vascularised villi   } but in both the villi may
- Recipient: smaller villi with dilated, engorged villous vessels } look normal

Complete Hydatidiform Mole (CM)

Mature / Late CM
- Generalised hydropic change with cisterns (! d/dg: do not confuse cisterns with an amnion-deficient gestational sac)

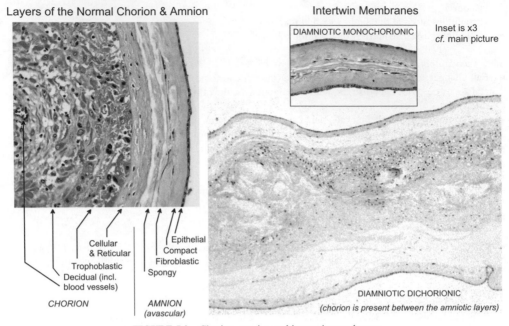

Layers of the Normal Chorion & Amnion

CHORION
- Cellular & Reticular
- Trophoblastic
- Decidual (incl. blood vessels)

AMNION (avascular)
- Epithelial
- Compact
- Fibroblastic
- Spongy

Intertwin Membranes

DIAMNIOTIC MONOCHORIONIC | Inset is x3 *cf.* main picture

DIAMNIOTIC DICHORIONIC
(chorion is present between the amniotic layers)

FIGURE 5.3 Chorion, amnion and intertwin membranes

- Avascular villi
- No fetal tissue ('fetal tissue' = nucleated RBCs, amnion or fetal parts)
- Circumferential proliferation of trophoblast (! d/dg: do not confuse with the abundant trophoblast seen in early gestations e.g. tubal ectopics or trophoblast proliferation 2° to perivillous fibrin deposition of any cause)

Earlier CM:
- Hydrops increases with gestational age, so at 11/40 only some villi are hydropic
- Hydropic change is due to MPS (not fibrosis as in partial mole) and stroma is hypercellular
- Villi may be polypoid ('budding' or 'fibroadenomatoid' – see Figure 5.4)
- Stromal cell karyorrhexis (not vessel) in well-preserved villi (i.e. not covered with necrotic trophoblast)
- Reticulin is perivascular (only)
- >90% of CM villi are vascularised before 11/40, dropping to 30% after 20/40
- Nucleated RBCs may be seen in some CM (an embryo begins to develop but does not progress)
- Trophoblast may strip off villous surface ∴ a) circumferential excess may not be seen, b) may see sheets of extravillous pleomorphic trophoblast (! d/dg: does not imply ChC)
- Molar implantation site: abundant interstitial trophoblast, no endovascular plugging, ± haemorrhage
- No dentate villi (*cf.* partial mole) and no rounded inclusions (may see larger irregular ovoid inclusions)
- Immuno: Ki67 LI is high and nuclear p57 (Kip2) is ↓/lost in the villous stroma and cytotrophoblast and intermediate trophoblasts of CM (use intervillous trophoblast islands and decidual cells as internal +ve controls for p57) – partial mole and HA have lower Ki67 and are p57 +ve
- CM are usu. diploid androgenones (95% monospermic XX, 5% dispermic XY)

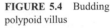

FIGURE 5.4 Budding polypoid villus

Partial Hydatidiform Mole
- Geographical / dentate / scalloped villi; may see a dual population of villi
- Excess circumferential trophoblast, often vacuolated / lacy and may strip off to appear multifocal
- Angiomatoid vessels (FVIIIRA +ve) [= 'Branching cisterns' esp. in late partial moles]
- Reticulin shows 'spider's web' pattern connecting one vessel to the another
- Fibrosis ↑ with gestational age
- Small rounded trophoblastic inclusions
- Extensive sampling may be needed to detect these features

- Partial moles are usu. triploid (2 of the 3 chromosome sets are from sperm) – can be useful in d/dg HA
- Fetal tissues are common and implantation site is normal
- ! d/dg mixed curettings from a twin gestation of CM and embryo (→ dual population of villi)
- d/dg stem villous hydrops (in PMD): no trophoblast hyperplasia, normal 3rd trimester fetus
- d/dg Beckwith-Wiedemann syndrome shows sig. hydrops of some villi without other molar features

Non-molar Hydropic Abortion (HA)
- Hydrops but of smooth round/ovoid contour and not large enough to be macroscopically visible
- Stroma is oedematous, fibrotic and often avascular – but hypocellular *cf.* moles
- Polar trophoblastic proliferation
- Invaginated trophoblast / rounded trophoblastic inclusions (see Figure 5.5)
- HA are usu. diploid (trisomies > monosomies) but non-molar fetal aneuploidy may show HA with some irregular-shaped villi and inclusions but no trophoblast proliferation (d/dg partial mole)

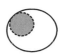

FIGURE 5.5   Rounded inclusion

Invasive Hydatidiform Mole
- Virtually all arise from CM but partial moles are monitored in case of possible diagnostic confusion
- Molar villi seen within myometrium/vessels (may embolise to other organs e.g. lung = *metastatic mole*)
- Residual trophoblast can be seen upto six months post ERPC ∴ !beware diagnosing choriocarcinoma in this period even if *no* villi are seen (i.e. sampled)

Morbidly Adherent Placentae
- Predisposed to by any cause of decidual deficiency e.g. PMHx of Caesarian section or laser ablation of the endometrium
- Paucity of decidua
- Villi and fibrinous basal plate (cytotrophoblast ++) penetrate to:
  - ➤ superficial myometrium   =   *placenta accreta*
  - ➤ deep myometrium   =   *placenta increta*
  - ➤ right through the myometrium   =   *placenta percreta*

Choriocarcinoma (ChC)
- Def^{n}: a tumour of villous trophoblast
- Clin.: can occur after any kind of gestation, monitored with hCG, cured with chemoRx. Suspect ChC if there is unexplained intracerebral haemorrhage or acute cor pulmonale
- LN mets are unusual (consider non-gestational 1° with trophoblastic differentiation – e.g. germ cell tumour – esp. if there is no evidence of gestational origin)
- Macro: haemorrhagic and bulky
- Micro: defined as an admixture of syncytiotrophoblast and cytotrophoblast (± intermediate trophoblast) that may grow in a laminar, plexiform, 'villous' or papillary architecture:
  - ➤ cytotrophoblast: usu. −ve for hCG, cells are polygonal, clear cytoplasm, well defined cell borders, central vesicular nucleus ± prominent nucleolus / chromocentres; architecture = cords / solid masses; ± weak staining for hPL
  - ➤ intermediate trophoblast: a mixture of mononuclear and multinucleated cells with more/stronger staining for hPL than hCG and +ve for CD146 (unlike other trophoblast)
  - ➤ syncytiotrophoblast: usu. +ve for hCG and inhibin-α, the syncytium contains smaller, denser nuclei within more basophilic cytoplasm (*cf.* cytotrophoblasts) that may be vacuolated
- No intrinsic tumour vasculature (but the tumour invades pre-existing vessels)
- No 2° or higher order chorionic villi – by definition (i.e. no villi containing stromal cores)
- Variant: cytotrophoblastic
  - ➤ (*cf.* d/dg PSTT) is predom. mononuclear, ↑ mitoses, intravascular *cf.* interstitial spread
  - ➤ (*cf.* usual type ChC) is more chemoresistant
- 'Choriocarcinoma *in situ*' = intraplacental ChC
- d/dg new pregnancy (or persistent trophoblast in CM). More likely to be ChC if abundant, very pleomorphic and found > 4 months after last known pregnancy.
- d/dg PSTT: more haemorrhagic, vascular mode of spread (*cf.* intramuscular in PSTT), laminar structure, cytotrophoblasts of ChC are less eosinophilic, more hCG +ve cells *cf.* hPL +ve

- d/dg carcinoma with trophoblastic differentiation: CA produces little hCG for its bulk, has a vascular stroma and is resistant to chemoRx. ChC contains paternal polymorphisms. Immuno unhelpful as ChC is +ve for CK, EMA and some CEA.
- d/dg invasive mole: moles have villi with stromal cores
- d/dg pleomorphic trophoblast without villi in curettage specimens (see sections on CM and 'Invasive Hydatidiform Mole' above) – do not diagnose ChC here without corroborating evidence

Placental Site Trophoblastic Tumour (PSTT)

- Def^n: a tumour of intermediate trophoblast (admixed mononuclear and multinucleate cells)
- Clin.: amenorrhoea / irregular bleeding months (>4) or years after some gestation
- Less metastatic but chemoresistant ∴ Rx is surgery, not chemoRx
- Eosinophilic pleomorphic cells (± cytoplasmic vacuoles / hyaline inclusions) infiltrating myometrium / decidua (occasional scattered foci of syncytiotrophoblast may be present)
- Hyaline and fibrin ++
- Much necrosis (not haemorrhage) → tumour cells survive only around vessels and may show endovascular growth (cling to or focally replace endothelium or are free in the lumen)
- ↑ Metastatic potential if mitoses > 5/10hpf
- Immuno: more hPL than hCG +ve cells (i.e. the converse of ChC); +ve for inhibin-α, AE1/AE3, CAM5.2 and CD146 (= Mel-CAM)
- d/dg exaggerated placental site reaction: mitoses, presentation > 4 months and large clusters of cells favour PSTT while villi, decidua vera and many multinucleate cells favour exaggerated placental site
- d/dg regressing placental site nodule: ↑↑ hyaline and central necrosis favour nodule
- d/dg non-gestational carcinoma: PSTT presents with gynae Sx. Immuno: hPL more useful than hCG

Bibliography

Al-Adnani, M., Williams, S., Rampling, D., Ashworth, M., Malone, M. and Sebire, N.J. (2006) Histopathological reporting of paediatric cutaneous vascular anomalies in relation to proposed multidisciplinary classification system. *Journal of Clinical Pathology*, **59** (12), 1278–1282.

Berenguer, B., Mulliken, J.B., Enjolras, O. *et al.* (2003) Rapidly involuting congenital hemangioma: clinical and histopathologic features. *Pediatric and Developmental Pathology*, **6** (6), 495–510.

Boyd, T., Gang, D., Lis, G., Juozokas, A. and Pfeuger, S. (2004) Appendix 2A in *Placental Pathology*, fascicle 3 in *Atlas of Non-Tumor Pathology* 1st series (eds F.T. Kraus, R.W. Redline, D.J. Gersell, D.M. Nelson and J.M. Dicke), AFIP, The American Registry of Pathology, Washington D.C.

Filipe, M.I. and Lake, B.D. (1990) *Histochemistry in Pathology*, 2nd edn, Churchill Livingstone, Edinburgh.

Fox, H. (1997) Trophoblastic disease, in *Progress in Pathology*, (eds N. Kirkham and N.R. Lemoine), Churchill Livingstone, NY, vol. 3, pp. 86–101.

Fox, H. (1997) *Pathology of the Placenta*, 2nd edn, W.B. Saunders Co. Ltd., London.

Fox, H. and Wells, M. (eds) (2002) *Haines & Taylor Obstetrical and gynaecological pathology*, 5th edn, Churchill Livingstone, London.

Glickman, J.N. (April 2005) Pathology of inflammatory bowel disease in children. *Current Diagnostic Pathology*, **11** (2), 117–124.

Gruenwald, P. and Minh, H.N.(1961) Evaluation of body and organ weights in perinatal pathology II. Weight of body and placenta in surviving and autopsied infants. *American Journal of Obstetrics and Gynecology*, **82** (2), 313–319.

Guillou, L., Coquet, M., Chaubert, P. and Coindre, J.M. (1998) Skeletal muscle regeneration mimicking rhabdomyosarcoma: a potential diagnostic pitfall. *Histopathology*, **33** (2), 136–144.

Hargitai, B., Marton, T. and Cox, P.M. (2004) Examination of the human placenta. *Journal of Clinical Pathology*, **57** (8), 785–792.

Lage, J.M., Minamiguchi, S. and Richardson, M.S. (Feb 2003) Gestational trophoblastic diseases: update on new immunohistochemical findings. *Current Diagnostic Pathology*, **9** (1),1–10.

Meijer-Jorna, L.B, van der Loos, C.M., de Boer, O.J., *et al.* (2007) Microvascular proliferation in congenital vascular malformations of skin and soft tissue. *Journal of Clinical Pathology*, **60** (7), 798–803.

Moore, I.E. and Baxendine-Jones, J. (2001) Diagnosis and molecular pathology of Hirschprung's disease, in *Recent Advances in Histopathology*, (eds D. Lowe, J.C.E. Underwood), Churchill Livingstone, Edinburgh, vol. 19, pp. 51–66.

Out, H.J., Kooijman, C.D., Bruinse, H.W. and Derksen, R.H. (1991) Histopathological findings in placentae from patients with intrauterine fetal death and anti-phospholipid antibodies. *European Journal of Obstetrics, Gynecology and Reproductive Biology*, **41** (3), 179–186.

Paradinas, F.J. (June 1998) The differential diagnosis of choriocarcinoma and placental site tumour. *Current Diagnostic Pathology*, **5** (2), 93–101.

Pinar, H., Sung, C.J., Oyer, C.E. and Singer, D.B. (1996) Reference values for singleton and twin placental weights. *Pediatric Pathology and Laboratory Medicine*, **16** (6), 901–907.

Sebire, N.J., Fox, H., Backos, M. *et al.* (2002) Defective endovascular trophoblast invasion in primary antiphospholipid antibody syndrome-associated early pregnancy failure. *Human Reproduction*, **17** (4), 1067–1071.

Sebire, N.J., Backos, M., Gaddal, S., *et al.* (2003) Placental pathology, antiphospholipid antibodies, and pregnancy outcome in recurrent miscarriage patients. *Obstetric Gynecology*, **101**, 258–263.

Sebire, N.J. and Rees, H. (2002) Diagnosis of gestational trophoblastic disease in early pregnancy. *Current Diagnostic Pathology*, **8** (6), 430–440.

Skordilias, K. and Howatson, A.G. (2003) The diagnostic challenge of paediatric small round cell tumours, in *Progress in Pathology*, (eds N. Kirkham, N.A. Shepherd), Greenwich Medical Media Ltd, London, vol. 6, pp. 1–27.

Smith, N.M and Keeling, J.W. (1997) Paediatric solid tumours, in *Recent Advances in Histopathology*, (eds P.P. Anthony, R.N.M. MacSween and D.G. Lowe), Churchill Livingstone, Edinburgh, vol. 17, pp. 191–218.

Wainwright, H.C. (2006) My approach to performing a perinatal or neonatal autopsy. *Journal of Clinical Pathology*, **59** (7), 673–680.

Wigglesworth, J. and Singer, D.B. (eds) (1991) *Perinatal Pathology*, 1st edn, Blackwell Medical Publishers Inc., Boston.

Wright, C. (June 2006) Congenital malformations of the lung. *Current Diagnostic Pathology*, **12** (3), 191–201.

Placental Weights Data Sources

Dataset 'a' for singleton placentas is based on the data for 1232 liveborn babies from Gruenwald and Minh (1961). (*NB*: Placental weights from the autopsied infants was found to be similar to the liveborn ones in this study). I fitted this data to a 3rd order linear polynomial for the purpose of plotting the chart. The fetoplacental weight ratios are also derived by fitting to data from this paper.

Dataset 'b' for singleton placentas is based on the data for liveborn babies as gathered by Boyd *et al.* (2004). I fitted this data to a 4th order linear polynomial for the purpose of plotting the chart.

The twin placenta factors are based on the twin placental weights of Pinar *et al.*, 1996.

6. Vascular

Normal and Age-Related Changes

- Elastic arteries are large Windkessel vessels (distend during systole to buffer the BP pulse) and have the outer $\frac{2}{3}$ of the wall supplied by *vasa vasorum* (e.g. aorta and main branches). Age → focal fibrosis and fragmentat^n of *medial* elastic with ↑MPS ± amyloid and some intimal fibrosis.
- Muscular arteries are the main distributors (e.g. coronaries). The wall muscle is disposed in a regular spiral helix angled ≈30° to the transverse plane of the vessel. Age → intimal and medial fibrosis, focal medial hyaline, IEL may show small breaks (± Ca^{2+}) and focal reduplication.
- Arterioles are defined as having: a lumen < 0.1–0.3 mm ⌀ +/ ≤ 6 concentric layers of medial muscle.
- Capillaries have no muscle, are the diameter of an RBC and have continuous, fenestrated or sinusoidal endothelium. Age → BM thickening.
- Post-capillary venules (PCVs) have 1–2 layers of muscle and no elastic.
- Veins are valved capacitance vessels with a lower wall-thickness:lumen-diameter ratio and poorly defined elastic laminae *cf.* arteries. The wall muscle is disposed in circular and longitudinal bundles in larger veins. Age → intimal fibrosis and medial hypertrophy.

Atherosclerosis

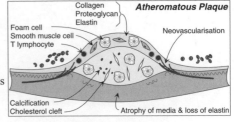

Time Course
- 10 years: | ➤ lipid streaks (subintimal foamy Mφ)
- | ➤ fibrofatty plaques ('atheromas')
- 40 years:↓ ➤ Calcification, Ulceration, Thrombosis
  - → clinical effects

FIGURE 6.1 Atheroma

Distribution
- Eccentric lumenal narrowing
- Sites of turbulence (bifurcations and ostia)
- Aorta (abdominal > thoracic), coronaries, circle of Willis, (kidney), lower limbs, small intestine
- Arterialised veins (such as occur in a CAVG)

Systemic Hypertension

Definitions
- HT should only be diagnosed on the average of ≥2 readings on ≥2 occasions
- *Borderline HT:* diastolic 90–95 mmHg systolic 140–160 mmHg
- *Established HT:* diastolic ≥ 95 or systolic ≥ 160 mmHg
- *Malignant HT:* rapidly increasing BP to > 130 mmHg diastolic (die in ≈2 years from RF if no Rx)

Benign HT (= Essential HT)
- Arteriosclerosis: ➤ medial hypertrophy and reduplication of the IEL
  - ➤ concentric intimal fibroplasia and patchy medial fibrosis
  - ➤ ↑MPS + fragmented elastic (i.e. myxoid degeneration)
  - ➤ d/dg: a) cystic medial necrosis (a matter of degree – see p. 73 under 'Aortic dissection')
    - b) Marfan's syndrome (≈ pre-mature ageing of the media, see p. 78)
    - c) age-related changes

- Hyaline arteriolosclerosis: ➤ hyaline change in the media, starts in the sub-intimal region
  - ➤ correlates with HT most in the kidney (least in the spleen)
  - ➤ diffuse, variable severity (→ granular contracted kidney at end-stage)
  - ➤ unusual in skeletal muscle, skin, brain (± Charcot-Bouchard microaneurysms), heart, GIT
  - ➤ d/dg: a) similar changes occur in the elderly & DM (without HT) and
    - b) radiation injury (*q.v.*)

Malignant HT:
- Hypertrophic arteriolosclerosis: concentric smooth muscle cell onion skin thickening of the intima
- Fibrinoid necrosis (necrotising arteriolitis) esp. kidney ('flea bite' haemorrhages and haematuria) – assoc[d] with more severe HT
- Microangiopathy → haemolytic anaemia, retinal haemorrhages, exudates and papilloedema
- The above changes are also seen in severe forms of TMA (see p. 207).
- d/dg athero/lipid emboli and the renal vascular changes of Alagille's syndrome (look for lipid)
- d/dg: PSS arteritis (*vide infra*)

Pulmonary HT

See Chapter 8: Respiratory and Mediastinum.

Vasculitides

Diagnostic Table
- In Table 6.1 √ means typically present and × typically absent – although exceptions occur. GN refers to the presence of glomerulonephritis (usu. necrotising FSGN or crescentic), not intra-renal arterial branch involvement. An important d/dg is TMA (see p. 207)
- d/dg of necrotising vasculitides includes radiation vasculopathy, severe HT changes and TMA (*q.v.*)

Giant Cell (Temporal) Arteritis
- Patients are usu. > 50 years old (a strong feature)
- Changes are focal and GC present in only 55% cases ∴ take multiple levels of long Bx (e.g. 4 cm)
- Early: medial necrosis and many PMN, smaller branch involvement.
- Later: granulomatous lesions in relation to fragments of the IEL (↑refractility but ↓staining)
- Non-specific transmural mononuclear cell infiltrate and scattered eos. ± PMN ± lumenal thrombus
- Healed phase: ➢ extensive fibrotic replacement of the IEL (e.g. $\frac{1}{4}$ circumference)
  - ➢ patchy lymphohistiocytic aggregates in media
  - ➢ patchy fibrosis of media ± neovascularisation
  - ➢ irregular intimal fibrosis.
- Steroids cause resolution of histology after 14 days continuous use
- d/dg normal age change (= elastic splitting, concentric intimal fibrosis, medial hyalinisation ± Ca^{2+})
- d/dg: Buerger's, Takayasu's, Bazin's/nodular vasculitis, Wegener's, Churg-Strauss

Takayasu's Disease (Takayashu's Disease, Pulseless Disease)
- < 50 years (strong feature), HT, arm claudication, BP difference >10mmHg between arms, visual Sx
- Early: granulomatous inflam[n] (± greater adventitial and intimal involvement *cf.* giant cell arteritis)
- Mixed chronic inflam[y] infiltrate (esp. adventitial) with elastic destruction
- ± Medial necrosis (proper)
- Intimal fibrosis ± proliferative endarteritis ± thrombosis
- d/dg giant cell arteritis, Syphilis, clinically other causes of 'pulseless disease' e.g. dissection

Polyarteritis Nodosa (PAN)
- Asthma and eosinophilia are strongly associated with the Churg-Strauss variant
- Main visceral arteries (no GN), cutaneous leukocytoclastic vasculitis may accompany PAN
- Patchy, transmural, fibrinoid necrosis with healing by fibrosis
- Leukocytes (PMN early, later mixed incl. variable eosinophils) are biased to the adventitia
- Acute, healing and healed stages usu. co-exist
- Segmental erosion → aneurysm/rupture/local inflam[n] → palpable nodule
- Consequences: ischaemic injury/infarcts/ulcers/thrombosis
- d/dg 2° arteritis (due to infarction, inflammation or infection)

Microscopic Polyarteritis
- Segmental fibrinoid necrosis ± leukocytoclasia (incl. venules)
- Necrotising GN and pulmonary capillaritis, also skin, muscle, GIT and mucosae
- All lesions tend to be of the same stage

TABLE 6.1   Diagnosing vasculitides

Vessel Type	Lung	GN	Skin	Diagnostic Antibodies/Comments
Large Elastic Arteries				
Giant cell arteritis	±	×	±	older patients & more restricted to media *cf.* Takayasu
Takayasu's disease	±	×	±	exclude Syphilis
Syphilitic aortitis				confirm with serology
CTD aortitis	±	±	±	usu. ascending only, sparing of major branches (*cf.* Takayasu) e.g. ankylosing spondylitis, RhA, SLE
Medium-sized Muscular Arteries				
Giant cell arteritis	±	×	±	±↑ESR, 50% have polymyalgia rheumatica (PMR)
Takayasu's disease	±	×	±	*vide supra* for d/dg with giant cell arteritis
PAN	√	×	√	HBV (40%), p-ANCA/c-ANCA (≤10%)
Buerger's disease	×	×	±	
Wegener's	√	√	√	c-ANCA (70%), p-ANCA (20%), neither (10%)
Churg-Strauss	√	√	√	p-ANCA (75%)
Kawasaki's disease				
Fungal	√			
CTD arteritis	±	±	±	Lupus can have dermo-renal involvement with non-proteinase-3 p-ANCA in 25%. RhA are seropositive for IgG rheumatoid factor
Arterioles +/ Capillaries				
Microscopic polyarteritis	√	√	√	c-ANCA (45%), p-ANCA (45%), neither (10%)
PAN	√	×	√	*vide supra.* Larger vessels also involved
Wegener's	√	√	√	c-ANCA (70%), p-ANCA (20%), neither (10%)
Churg-Strauss	√	√	√	
Rickettsial				
lymphocytic vasculitis	×	×	√	see Chapter 20: Skin
1° pauci-immune GN	×	√	×	p-ANCA (60%), c-ANCA (30%), neither (10%)
Goodpasture's	√	√	×	linear IgG + C3 in BMs. p-ANCA (25%).
leukocytoclastic vasculitis	±	±	√	HSP (± IgA ANCA), cryoglobulins (± HCV Ags) and serum-sickness can have dermo-renal involvement ± elastase p-ANCA. Drug reactions may have MPO/lactoferrin p-ANCA
Veins/Venules				
Buerger's disease	×	×	±	
Wegener's	√	√	√	c-ANCA (70%), p-ANCA (20%), neither (10%)
1° cutaneous granulomatous phlebitis	×	×	√	very rare
Trousseau's syndrome	×	×	√	migratory thrombophlebitis assoc[d] with metastatic adenocarcinoma. PMNs early, granulomas later
leukocytoclastic	±	±	√	
Lymphatics				
Crohn's/Sarcoid	±	±	√	Granulomatous vasculitis may be 2° to perivascular lymphatic involvement.

Wegener's Granulomatosis (WG)
For def[n] and lung and kidney features, see p. 87.
- Necrotising vasculitis away from necrotic areas (extensive fibrinoid change is unusual)
- Affects arteries, arterioles and veins
- Lymphocytes and plasma cells > giant cells and PMN, eos. are usu. sparse (except in the eosinophilic variant)
- Granulomatous inflammation may involve whole vessel wall and extend into lumen
- Arterioles, capillaries and veins may be involved (e.g. in alveolar septa) ± leukocytoclasia
- d/dg other granulomatous/PAN-like vasculitides (giant cell, Takayasu's, Churg-Strauss, etc.)

Churg-Strauss Vasculitis
- Eosinophilic PAN
- Eosinophilic microscopic polyarteritis
- Eosinophilic WG-like granulomatous vasculitis
- Eosinophilic phlebitis
- Eosinophilic leukocytoclastic vasculitis
- Necrotising FSGN (rarely)

For extravascular details and definition, see p. 87.

Buerger's Disease (Thromboangiitis Obliterans)
- Strong ($\approx$ dose-response) association with tobacco smoking
- Muscular arteries of the forelimbs, skip lesions early on, and involves adjacent veins
- Acute inflam^n (early) $\rightarrow$ chronic inflam^n $\rightarrow$ fibrosis affects whole vessel wall incl. adventitia and surrounding veins and nerves
- Inflamed, cellular thrombus
- $\pm$ Giant cells in/adjacent to thrombus (*cf.* in the media in other arteritides) ⎫ These are said to be
- $\pm$ Microabscesses in vessel wall ⎭ pathognomonic
- Separation of layers of the vessel wall by inflam^n/fibrosis
- Good preservation of the IEL (*cf.* giant cell/other arteritis or atheroma)
- d/dg atheroma: preserved IEL, early onset, upper limb involvement, vein involvement, inflam^y nature, small vessel involvement.
- d/dg giant cell arteritis: distribution, giant cell location, preservation of IEL, adventitial involvement, vein involvement.

Leukocytoclastic Vasculitis (LCV)
For morphology and further information, see p. 301. Example causes are given below.
- Most drug reaction vasculitides
- Henoch-Schönlein purpura (HSP)
- Cryoglobulinaemia (also results in membranoproliferative GN)
- Serum sickness (see p. 350)
- Behçet's disease (see p. 194 and p. 341)
- Some forms of paraneoplastic vasculitis
- *Neisseria* infections (e.g. *N. meningitidis*)

Urticarial Vasculitis and Lymphocytic Vasculitis
See Chapter 20: Skin.

Rheumatoid Vasculitis
- Nerves, skin and main visceral small arteries and capillaries, esp. hands and nail folds
- Transmural fibrinoid necrotising vasculitis
- Cutaneous lymphocytic vasculitis ⎫ These are said to be
- Cutaneous urticarial vasculitis ⎭ pathognomonic
- d/dg drug reaction

SLE Vasculitis
- Nerves, skin and main visceral small arteries and capillaries
- Transmural necrotising vasculitis (PAN-like with $\downarrow$overall inflam^n $\pm$ $\uparrow$PMN)
- Cutaneous urticarial vasculitis
- LN and spleen arteries may show 'onion skin' perivascular fibrosis
- For GN spectrum, see pp. 204–205; for further detail see pp. 297–298.
- d/dg lupus 'anticoagulant' thrombotic vasculopathy (fibrin thrombi in small vessels $\rightarrow$ *et seq.*) [also called antiphospholipid Ab syndrome: see p. 351 and pp. 61–62]

Progressive Systemic Sclerosis (PSS) Vasculitis
- Fibrinoid necrotising vasculitis of small arteries
- $\uparrow$ Mucopolysaccharide in intima
- Onion skinning of intima
- d/dg severe HT changes

Kawasaki's Disease
- Seen in children with the mucocutaneous LN syndrome (MCLNS)
- Transmural necrotising vasculitis with PMN predominating early on (PAN-like)
- Later → mixed mononuclear cell infiltrate (incl. intramural T-cells) and PMN
- Arterioles and venules may be involved in addition to muscular arteries
- d/dg: see p. 119, under 'Kikuchi-Fujimoto disease'

Miscellaneous

Radiation Angiopathy
- Muscular arteries, arterioles and capillaries. For veno-occlusive disease, see p. 169
- Early: ➢ endothelial atypia (nuclear hyperchromasia, swelling)
            ➢ fibrinoid necrosis
            ➢ RBC extravasation
            ➢ thrombosis
- Later: ➢ proliferative endarteritis and intimal fibroplasia
            ➢ foam cell accumulation and accelerated atherosclerosis
            ➢ small vessel telangiectasia
            ➢ adventitial fibrosis and distortion, fragmentation of the IEL $\pm$ inflam^n (d/dg vasculitis)
            ➢ hyaline arteriolosclerosis-like changes (*q.v.* – d/dg HT)

Congophilic (Amyloid) Angiopathy (CAA)
- Clin.: multifocal superficial cerebral haemorrhage/SAH ($\pm$ Alzheimer's)
- Hyaline eosinophilic material in meningeal +/ cerebral vessels   ⎫ These H&E features may
- $\pm$ Evidence of previous haemorrhage   ⎬ be subtle
- Immuno for A4 (β) amyloid is more sensitive *cf.* Congo red   ⎭

Aneurysms
Definition
- An abnormal localised dilatation of a vessel
- True – surrounded by a complete vessel wall (e.g. atheromatous, congenital, luetic, mycotic)
- False – extravascular haematoma communicating with the intravascular space (e.g. anastomotic leak, mycotic aneurysm)

Atherosclerotic:
- Usu. abdominal and below the renal arteries. Grow by deposition of thrombus (→ laminar structure)
- Atheromatous erosion (and ∴ weakening) of media
- Complications: ➢ rupture
                   ➢ occlusion of vessels/ostia by pressure or thrombus (e.g. renal/vertebral)
                   ➢ compress/erode adjacent structures (e.g. ureter/vertebrae)
                   ➢ embolism
                   ➢ infection ('mycotic aneurysm')
                   ➢ retroperitoneal fibrosis $\pm$ ureteric involvement

Luetic (syphilitic)
- Thoracic aorta (usu. the arch)
- Proliferative endarteritis of *vasa vasorum* → patchy necrosis (loss) of medial fibroelastic tissue
- Lymphoplasmacytic periarteritis of *vasa vasorum*
- Dense collagenous fibrous patches of intima with grooves ('tree bark' macro)
- Complications: ➢ rupture
                   ➢ occlude coronary ostia
                   ➢ compress/erode adjacent structures (→ respiratory difficulties/cough/pain)
                   ➢ annuloaortic ectasia *et seq.* → *cor bovinum*
- d/dg: aortitis of psoriasis, Reiter's or ankylosing spondylitis

Cirsoid aneurysms (Racemose aneurysms)
- These are dilated AVMs (congenital +/ traumatic)
- Occur in the scalp, leptomeninges and elsewhere

Venous aneurysms
- Rare and usu. 2° to trauma or abnormal infiltrates of the wall (*vide infra*)

Other conditions weakening the vessel wall
- Congenital (e.g. berry aneurysm)
- Inflammatory (e.g. PAN)
- Infective ('mycotic aneurysm')
- Infiltration by diffuse NF tissue in NF-1
- Trauma (as a result of stretching of the scar) e.g. cardiac, arteriovenous-fistula and caroticocavernous sinus aneurysms
- DM (capillary aneurysms e.g. retina)

Arterial Dissection (Dissecting 'Aneurysm')
- Tracking of blood between (usu.) the middle and outer thirds of the media. Commonest in the aorta
- Potentiating factors: HT and conditions with ↑ MPS deposition e.g. pregnancy/Marfan's
- Atheromatous plaques act as barriers to dissection

Aortic dissection:
- ± Intimal tear on ascending aorta (a distal tear → double barrel aorta → ↓risk of complications)
- ± 'Cystic medial necrosis' (disorganisat^n of the media, elastic fragmentat^n and pools of acid MPS forming pseudocystic [i.e. no lining] spaces – see also p. 78)
- Complications: ➢ rupture into a coelomic cavity → exanguination/cardiac tamponade
  - ➢ occlusion of ostia (e.g. carotid, coronary, renal, mesenteric)
  - ➢ impaired aortic valve function

Fibromuscular Dysplasia (Fibromuscular Arterial Hyperplasia)
- Muscular arteries; renal > carotid/other sites
- One or more of the following may be seen:
  - ➢ segmental medial hypertrophy alternates with medial thinning and attenuation of IEL
  - ➢ fibrous replacement of outer half of media
  - ➢ cellular concentric intimal fibroplasia
  - ➢ adventitial fibrous encasement
- Complications: stenosis, thrombosis, aneurysm (in thinned segments), dissection
- d/dg NF-1 assoc^d arterial dysplasia/vasculopathy (*vide infra*)

NF-1 Associated Vasculopathy (Vascular Neurofibromatosis)
- Veins and muscular arteries: → renovascular HT, aneurysm, fistulae, haemorrhage (! a per-operative risk)
- Veins (± arteries) may have their walls weakened by infiltration with diffuse NF spindle tissue
- Arteries show concentric cellular myointimal proliferation (MSA +ve cells) with MPS ++
- Nodules of smooth muscle spindle-cells may be seen in the arterial media and intima (S100 −ve)
- d/dg fibromuscular dysplasia (*vide supra*)

Thrombus and Thromboembolus (Features and Dating Criteria)
- d/dg embolus (e.g. PE)/thrombus *vs.* PM clot:
  - ➢ embolus is firmer (*cf.* 'chicken-fat' clot) and is *not* a cast of the vessel
  - ➢ clot does not have a laminar cross-section (lines of Zahn)
  - ➢ thrombus/embolus stands proud of the vessel wall when cut
- Dating thrombus:
  - ➢ sampling: take a block from the junction of thrombus and vessel wall
  - ➢ two days: endothelial bud proliferation begins
  - ➢ eight days to one year: haemosiderin deposits
  - ➢ age of fibrin (by the MSB method): early = yellow, medium = red, very old = blue

Ehlers Danlos Syndrome
- Excessive elastic tissue in small arteries

Thrombotic Microangiopathy (TMA) and DIC
See p. 207.

Transplant Rejection Angiopathy
See organ-specific chapters.

Tumours and Malformations
See Chapter 5: Paediatric and Placental, and Chapter 21: Soft Tissues.

Bibliography

Bellamy, C.O.C. (2004) Microangiopathies and malignant vascular injury in the kidney. *Current Diagnostic Pathology*, **10** (1), 36–51.

Cavallo, T. (1998) Pathologic approach to the diagnosis of vasculitis. *Current Diagnostic Pathology*, **5** (2), 70–81.

Cotran, R.S, Kumar, V. and Collins, T. (eds) (1999) *Robbins Pathologic Basis of Disease*, 6th edn, W.B. Saunders Co., Philadelphia.

Knight, B. (1983) *The Coroner's Autopsy*, 1st edn, Churchill Livingstone, Edinburgh.

Mooney, E.E. and Shea, C.R. (1997) Cutaneous vasculitis. *Current Diagnostic Pathology*, **4** (1), 1–9.

Ng, W-K. (2003) Radiation-associated changes in tissues and tumours. *Current Diagnostic Pathology*, **9** (2), 124–136.

Nopajaroonsri, C. and Lurie, A.A. (1996) Venous aneurysm, arterial dysplasia, and near-fatal hemorrhages in neurofibromatosis type 1. *Human Pathology*, **27** (9), 982–985.

Sheaff, M. and Baithun, S.I. (1997) Pathological effects of ionising radiation. *Current Diagnostic Pathology*, **4** (2), 106–115.

Sternberg, S.S. (ed) (1997) *Histology for Pathologists*, 2nd edn, Lippincott Williams & Wilkins, Philadelphia.

Symmers, W. St. C. (ed) (1976) *Systemic Pathology*, Vol. 1, 2nd edn, Churchill Livingstone, London.

Wheater, P.R., Burkitt, H.G. and Daniels, V.G. (1987) *Functional Histology: A text and colour atlas*, 2nd edn, Churchill Livingstone, Edinburgh.

7. Heart

Normal and Age-Related Changes

Valves
- Avascular except for microvessels at the root
- Three-layer sandwich of (from ventricular surface outwards):
    - ① *lamina ventricularis* lined by endothelium and containing most elastic fibres
    - ② *lamina spongiosa* (MPS-rich, containing muscle in the AV valves near the valve root)
    - ③ *lamina fibrosa* lined by endothelium, focally thickened at contact points (lines of closure)

Blood Supply
- LAD supplies: apex, anterior LV, anterior $\frac{2}{3}$ of the septum
- RMC supplies: RV free wall, posterior LV ($\rightarrow$ Posterior Descending if right dominant)
- LCirc supplies: lateral LV ($\rightarrow$ Posterior Descending if left dominant)
- Posterior descending supplies the posterior $\frac{1}{3}$ of the septum

Age-Related Changes
- Brown atrophy (lipofuscin) and basophil degeneration (glucan)
- Right shift and tortuosity of ascending aorta $\rightarrow$ HOCMoid sigmoid septum
- Aortic valve: calcinosis ($\pm$ stenosis)
- Mitral valve: bulging, atheromatoid changes, Ca^{2+}, Lambl's excrescences

Ischaemic Heart Disease

Angina
- May show myocardial scarring / infarction
- Sig. coronary disease may be absent in LVH or hyperthyroidism

MI (Regional)
- Usu. transmural and involving: LAD (50%), RMC (30%), LCirc (15%), LMC/combined (5%)
- Macro:
    - 8–10 hours   none, but NBT test may show focal lack of enzyme activity
    - 1–2 days   swelling, lack-lustre
    - 2–3 days   pale, soft, $\pm$ beginning of 'tigroid' haemorrhages
    - 3–7 days   yellow-grey, haemorrhages, softening ('*myomalacia cordis*')
    - 7–10days   sharp definition with vascular granulation tissue
    - 1–2 weeks   'gelatinous transformation' at the centre of the infarct
    - 3–12 weeks   scar tissue
- Micro:
    - 2–12 hours   blurring of striations, 'cloudy swelling' (= eosinophilia and granularity)
    - 1 day $\uparrow$eosinophilia, myocytes become angulated, wavey and 'pinched'
    - 2–7 days   PTAH shows striations undergoing granular disintegrat^n with clumping into 'contraction bands' (likened to Chinese writing), $\downarrow$nuclear staining, variable PMN infiltrate, beginning of granulation tissue by 1 week
    - 1st week   PMN are prominent
    - 2nd week   granulation tissue is prominent
    - 3rd week   collagenisation (scarring) begins
    - 6–12 weeks   fibrosis, $\downarrow$vascularity, myohypertrophy, chamber dilatation
    - months–years   fossilised infarct (an old MI containing a central area that looks like a recent MI)
- Complications:
    - immediate: arrhythmias and SCD
    - acute   ☞ rupture of ventricle, septum, pap. muscle
        - ☞ pericarditis
        - ☞ intracardiac thrombus (due to $\uparrow$thromboplastin and eddying)
        - ☞ LVF / CCF / cardiogenic shock

> chronic   ☞ aneurysm (15%) → LVF / emboli
>   ☞ angina (relief or production)
>   ☞ re-infarction (esp. smokers)
>   ☞ antimyocardial autoimmunity (→ Dressler's: fever, tachycardia, pleuroperi-carditis)

MI (Subendocardial)
- Severe coronary atheroma (except in aortic valve disease)
- Usu. whole LV circumference ± regional transmural infarct

Sudden Cardiac Death (SCD)
- May see an old infarct or angina changes
- Most do not have a fresh infarct

Inflammatory Heart Disease

Viral Myocarditis
- Coxsackie B (common in the UK) – diagnose by serology, pericardial fluid, throat swab / faeces
- Mixed mononuclear cell infiltrate
- ± Necrosis, ± granulomatous myocarditis

Systemic Diseases
- RhA: nodules
- SLE: fibrinoid, histiocytes, apoptoses, Libman-Sacks fibrin vegetations (not related to closure lines, present on the surface of the influx of blood, valve shows fibrinoid necrosis at site of attachment)
- Vasculitides: Wegener's, PAN, Kawasaki
- Sarcoid
- Whipple's disease: focal fibroses, valve deformities (d/dg rheumatic fever), DPAS +ve foamy Mφ
- Chagas' disease (of *Trypanosoma cruzi*): acute → fever, LNp, unilateral orbital oedema, rash, etc.; Chronic → megaoesophagus/colon/heart (cardiomegaly); see Chapter 23: Infection and Immunity

Granulomatous Myocarditis
- Idiopathic (not to be confused with idiopathic giant cell myocarditis)
- Sarcoid
- Infective: usu. TB or viral
- Rheumatic fever (Aschoff bodies)
- d/dg Mφ cytomyolysis which accompanies cerebral infarct, head injuries, etc.

Idiopathic Giant Cell Myocarditis
- Rapid clinical deterioration → death
- Serpiginous necrosis
- Giant cells at periphery

Floppy Mitral Valve
① focal destruction of the lamina fibrosa with replacement by . . .
② . . . accumulations of MPS

Acute Rheumatic Fever
- Pancarditis: pericarditis, myocarditis, endocarditis
- Aschoff bodies:
  > Aschoff cells: ☞ eosinophilic ragged cytoplasm
  >   ☞ nucleus has a clear zone around elongated nucleolus to give an 'owl's eye' or 'caterpillar' appearance
  > early: ☞ swelling, fragmentation and eosinophilic change of connective tissue
  >   ☞ interstitial basophilic material
  > later: granulomatous foci and fibrinoid change
  > located around small vessels

- Myocardial damage: ➢ lymphocyte predominant infiltrate
                      ➢ muscle necrosis, vacuolation and multinucleation
                      ➢ ± Aschoff bodies (esp. in septum)
- Vasculitis: ➢ affects vessels of any size
               ➢ may be PAN-like in larger vessels
               ➢ perivascular fibrin
               ➢ adventitial scarring
               ➢ medial oedema
               ➢ intimal and medial elastification with loss of distinction between intima and media
               ➢ thromboses and recanalisation
- Valve disease: ➢ seen along lines of closure
                  ➢ intimal ulceration
                  ➢ 'verrucae' of platelets and fibrin
                  ➢ ± Aschoff bodies

Chronic Rheumatic Fever Valve Disease
- Fibrosclerotic thickening
- Vascularisation of the valve
- ± Non-specific chronic inflammation

Cardiac Allograft (Transplant) Rejection
- Predominantly T-cell infiltrate
- ± Granulocytes (usu. eosinophils > PMN)
- ± Myocyte necrosis
- A mixed infiltrate (lymphocytes, plasma cells, histiocytes ± granulocytes) is said to be evidence *against* rejection
- Changes due to healing of a previous biopsy site:
    ➢ granulation tissue ± organising fibrin with local distortion of myocytes
    ➢ ± early lipofuscin ('ceroid') Mφ
    ➢ usu. seen on only one of the submitted fragments
- Ischaemia and reperfusion injury: foci of myocyte necrosis / vacuolisation / dropout ± a mild PMN infiltrate. No evidence of a rejection infiltrate (mononuclear cells ± eosinophils)
- Subendocardial thickening / fibrosis
- Subendocardial dense lymphocyte collections ('Quilty lesions') without (Type A) or with (Type B) infiltration of adjacent myocardium are of uncertain significance (? localised rejection)
- Mild Acute Rejection = sparse T-cells, no eosinophils or necrosis
- Moderate / Severe Acute Rejection = moderate multifocal infiltrate with eosinophils ± necrosis
- Chronic rejection:
    ➢ graft vasculopathy: concentric proliferative endarteritis with atheromatoid features
    ➢ myocardial cellular rejection
    ➢ myocyte vacuolisation / coagulative necrosis
    ➢ parenchymal fibrosis and atrophy
- Humoural rejection:
    ➢ = donor Ab-mediated vascular endothelial damage occurring during the acute and chronic rejection time periods (manifest as graft dysfunction not attributable to cellular rejection or ischaemia on endomyocardial biopsy)
    ➢ PMN/Mφ in capillaries, endothelial swelling, congest^n/haemorrhage, interstitial oedema
    ➢ immuno: C4d +vity in capillary endothelia (becomes negative as humoural rejection resolves)
- The presence of contraction band necrosis is said to be evidence *against* rejection if this is the only feature but within the context of a picture of acute rejection it is considered to be one form of 'myocyte damage' for grading purposes
- Opportunistic infection (if present, rejection cannot be reliably assessed):
    ➢ uncommon but important to exclude due to implications for immunosuppression Rx
    ➢ CMV: serology is best as inclusions tend to be cytoplasmic only and fragmented
    ➢ *Toxoplasma*: ! do not confuse intracellular granular Ca^{2+} for Toxoplasma (do von Kossa)
    ➢ a prominent PMN component should raise suspicion for infection
- Grading acute cellular rejection (Billingham *et al.*, 1990; Stewart *et al.*, 2005):

TABLE 7.1   Grading acute cellular rejection

2004 Revised Grade	ISHLT Grade	Myocyte Damage[a]	Large Lymphocytes	Granulocytes	Other Features
mild { 1R	1A	absent	multifocal (perivasc./interstitial)	absent	
1R	1B	absent	diffuse but sparse	absent	
1R	2	1 focus only	present	absent	
mod. 2R	3A	multifocal	multifocal	absent	
severe { 3R	3B	multifocal	more diffuse	present	
3R	4	present	diffuse	diffuse	oedema, vasculitis, haemorrhage

[a]myocyte damage includes myocytes with irregular border due to encroachment by inflam[y] cells, architectural dsturbance, partial replacement of myocytes or myocyte necrosis (incl. contraction band necrosis)

- For updates and illustrations see: University of Pittsburgh Transplant Internet Service (www.tpis.upmc.edu) and Slootweg & de Weger (1998).

Non-Inflammatory Heart Disease

Infiltrates / Deposits
- Amyloid
- Iron: haemochromatosis
- Calcium: calcinosis
- Oxalate: oxalosis
- Storage diseases (e.g. in rhabdomyomas or in glycogenosis Type 2 = Pompe's disease)

Hypertrophic Obstructive Cardiomyopathy (HOCM)
- All ages (even elderly, esp. if assoc[d] with myosin binding protein mutation). Macro may look normal
- Thickened endocardial patch with sharp lower border on the LV side of the septum is said to be pathognomonic (if present)
- 'Disarray' is the hallmark feature:
  ➢ present in ≥ 2 blocks (*away* from the insertion of the LV into the septum)
  ➢ fibre bundle disarray: loss of parallel arrangement and presence of fibroid-like whorls
  ➢ myocyte disarray: bizarre shapes and nuclear pleomorphism
  ➢ myofibrillar disarray: do a PTAH stain
- Interstitial fibrosis
- The RV is involved in $\approx \frac{1}{3}$ of cases

Arrythmogenic Right Ventricular Dysplasia (ARVD)
See Chapter 25: Autopsy.

Syndromic Conditions

The Marfan Syndrome / Cystic Medial Necrosis / Floppy Mitral Valve
- Aorta: ➢ disorganisation of the media
  ➢ disruption of medial elastic fibres
  ➢ pools of AB +ve MPS
- Valves: ➢ disruption of lamina fibrosa and elastica
  ➢ pools of acid MPS
  ➢ thickened and opaque cusp may develop 2° infective endocarditis

Pseudoxanthoma Elasticum
- Irregularly thickened and fragmented elastic fibres (in arteries and subendocardially)
- Fibrosis

Sudden Cardiac Death, Congential Heart Disease, Examination of the Heart

See Chapter 25: Autopsy.

Tumours

Cardiac Myxoma
- Usu. atrial wall
- Polypoid (smooth / fronded) ± stalk and attached atrial patch (= excision margin)
- Sparsely cellular myxoid matrix (hyaluronic acid) ± outer endothelial lining
- Stromal haemorrhage, Ca^{2+} ± Gamna-Gandy bodies (see Chapter 10: Lymphoreticular)
- Myxoma cells:
  - ➢ elongated / stellate / polygonal; may be single or multinucleated (syncytial giant cells)
  - ➢ finely vacuolated eosinophil cytoplasm with variably dense nuclei
  - ➢ distribution: perivascular, nested, dispersed
  - ➢ no mitoses
  - ➢ immuno: vimentin +ve
- Other cells: Mϕ, siderophages, myofibroblasts, smooth muscle, lymphocytes, plasma cells
- ± Mucous gland-like structures (+ve for CK, AB, DPAS)
- d/dg fibroelastoma (which is more likely if on a valve)
- d/dg myxoid MFH and myxoid liposarcoma

Rhabdomyoma
- Infant / child, nearly all have tuberose sclerosis
- Often multifocal, may be intracavitary
- Very swollen myocytes
- Glycogenic cytoplasmic clearing
- 'Spider cells' – central nucleus supported by strands of cytoplasm

Cardiac Fibroma
- Infant / child
- Interweaving bundles of collagen / elastic
- Haemopoietic islands
- Smooth muscle

Giant Lambl's Excrescence (Papillary Fibroelastoma)
- Adults
- Endocardial surfaces esp. aortic valve
- Filiform architecture with central dense collagenous cores covered by loose connective tissue
- Elastic ++

Malignant Tumours in the Heart
- 1°: angiosarcoma, RMS, mesothelioma, liposarcoma, MFH
- 2°: lung, breast, lymphoma, thyroid, tongue, stomach, pancreas, kidney, bladder, etc.

Bibliography

Becker, A.E. and Anderson, R.H. (1983) *Cardiac Pathology: An integrated text and color atlas*, 1st edn, Churchill Livingstone, Edinburgh.

Billingham, M.E., Cary, N.R., Hammond, M.E. *et al.* (1990) A working formulation for the standardization of nomenclature in the diagnosis of heart and lung rejection: heart rejection study group. *Journal of Heart Transplantation,* 9 (6), 587–93.

Burke, M.M. (1994) Complications of heart and lung transplantation and of cardiac surgery, in *Recent Advances in Histopathology*, (eds P.P. Anthony, R.N.M. MacSween and D.G. Lowe.), Churchill Livingstone, Edinburgh, vol.16, pp. 95–122.

Cotran, R.S., Kumar, V. and Collins, T. (eds) (1999) *Robbins Pathologic Basis of Disease*, 6th edn, W.B. Saunders Co., Philadelphia.

Crespo-Leiro, M., Veiga-Barreiro, A., Doménech, N. *et al.* (2005) Humoral heart rejection (severe allograft dysfunction with no signs of cellular rejection or ischaemia): Incidence, management, and the value of C4d for diagnosis. *American Journal of Transplantation*, 5 (10), 2560–2564.

Gallagher, P.J. (1994) The investigation of cardiac death, in *Recent Advances in Histopathology,* (eds P.P. Anthony, R.N.M. MacSween and D.G. Lowe), Churchill Livingstone, Edinburgh, vol. 16, pp. 123–146.

Knight, B. (1983) *The Coroner's Autopsy*, 1st edn, Churchill Livingstone, Edinburgh.

Pomerance, A. and Davies, M.J. (eds) (1975) *The Pathology of the Heart*, 1st edn, Blackwell Scientific Publications, Oxford.

Silver, M.D. (ed) (1983) *Cardiovascular Pathology*, 1st edn, Churchill Livingstone, NY.

Slootweg, P.J. and de Weger, R.A. (1998) Cardiac transplantation pathology: an update. *Current Diagnostic Pathology*, 5 (4), 198–203.

Snell, R.S. (1986) *Clinical Anatomy for Medical Students*, 3rd edn, Little, Brown & Co. Inc., Boston.

Stewart, S., Winters, G., Fishbein, M. *et al.* (2005) Revision of the 1990 Working formulation for the standardization of nomenclature in the diagnosis of heart rejection. *Journal of Heart and Lung Transplantation,* **24** (11), 1710–1720.

Symmers, W. St. C. (ed) (1976) *Systemic Pathology*, Vol. 1, 2nd edn, Churchill Livingstone, London.

Willis, R.A. (1952) *The Spread of Tumours in the Human Body*, Butterworth & Co. Ltd., London.

Web sites

University of Pittsburgh, Transplant Pathology Internet Service. www.tpis.upmc.edu (accessed April 2007).

8. Respiratory and Mediastinum

Upper Respiratory Tract

Rhinosporidiosis (Rhinosporidium seeberi)
- This PAS and mucicarmine +ve protofungus has its 200–300μ sporangia in the mucosa *and submucosa*
- d/dg vacuoles of cylindrical cell Schneiderian papilloma (mucosal only)
- d/dg myospherulosis: Grocott −ve encysted balls of swollen, pale RBC following oleic nasal packing. (A d/dg of myospherulosis is protothecosis which is Grocott +ve)
- Rx is excision ± antifungals

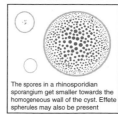

The spores in a rhinosporidian sporangium get smaller towards the homogeneous wall of the cyst. Effete spherules may also be present

FIGURE 8.1 Rhinosporidian sporangia

Rhinoscleroma (Klebsiella rhinoscleromatis)
- Gram −ve organisms (++ on silver stains) – d/dg non-tuberculoid leprosy
- Submucosal granulomas, plasma cells and clear foamy Mφ (Mikulicz cells)
- Rx is antibiotics (e.g. tetracyclines)

Inflammatory Nasal Polyps
- Uncommon before 20 years old, often bilateral ± Hx of asthma, aspirin sensitivity, etc.
- Mucofibrous stroma ± radiation-like atypical fibroblasts; (d/dg Microsporidiosis in the maxillary sinus)

Schneiderian ('Transitional Cell') Papillomas
- Usu. >30 years old, unilateral (± multifocal), tend to recur
- Variant: fungiform – often on nasal septum
- Variant: inverted – often on lateral wall and assoc^d with ↑risk of malignancy
- Variant: oncocytic (= cylindrical cell) – inverted, intraepithelial vacuoles contain inspissated mucus; d/dg Rhinosporidian sporangia (*vide supra*) or papillary variant of adenocarcinoma
- May have focal nuclear atypia or aggregates of atypical nuclei in lower $\frac{1}{3}$ of the mucosa
- PMN infiltration → inflammatory atypia
- Mitoses usu. few and parabasal but may be more extensive – never atypical
- d/dg papillary SCC (shows widespread severe atypia and & focal squamous nests), TCC

Nasopharyngeal Carcinoma (NPC)
- Keratinising SCC (usual histology)
- Non-keratinising SCC: cells have distinct cell borders and a 'paving stone' arch
- Undifferentiated NPC (lymphoepithelial carcinoma or lymphoepithelioma)
  - ➤ bimodal (children/teens–'50s), most radiosensitive of the group, best prognosis[1]
  - ➤ uniform epithelial cells with vesicular nuclei and indistinct cell borders (syncytial-like) arranged in solid patches (Regaud) or scattered small groups (Schmincke) in a lymphoid background
  - ➤ submucosal origin – may present with cervical LNs in which the LN metastasis may be misdiagnosed as lymphoma, esp. Hodgkin's if Schmincke type
  - ➤ tumour cells EBNA +ve and EBV serology +ve (if EBV −ve = 'lymphoepithelioma-*like* CA')
  - ➤ prognosis ∝ stage: I = confined, II = cervical LN +ve, III = into surrounding structures
  - ➤ pseudoepitheliomatous hyperplasia incited by T-cell lymphomas may cause misdiagnosis of lymphoepithelial carcinoma or mixed carcinoma / lymphoma
- d/dg *Sinonasal Undifferentiated Carcinoma*: this is organoid with necrosis, vasc. invasion, ↑ NCR and distinct cell borders but no squamous / glandular / neural diff^n (d/dg NB). CK and EMA +ve, NSE and S100 ±ve, CD99 and HMB45 −ve, NE granules on EM. It is insensitive to chemo/radioRx and survival is <1 year. d/dg NSE +ve high grade olfactory neuroblastoma, but NB has focal / weak / −ve CK and EMA staining

---

[1] ∴ it is important to distinguish this from *Sinonasal Undifferentiated Carcinoma* (see d/dg)

Other Sinonasal Lesions
- Vascular: angiofibroma ($\approx$ erectile tissue), HPC-like tumour, glomus tumour
- Neural/endocrine: paraganglioma, olfactory neuroblastoma (see Chapter 13: Central Nervous System and Skeletal Muscle), SmCC
- Soft tissue: RMS, leiomyoma / leiomyosarcoma, angioma / angiosarcoma, nerve sheath tumours
- Lymphoid: lymphomas (esp. angiocentric TCL and lymphomatoid granulomatosis), florid lymphoid hyperplasia, plasmacytoma (d/dg plasma cell granuloma)
- Inflammatory pseudotumour (= plasma cell granuloma)
  - ➤ unlike d/dg plasmacytoma, this has: ——— other cell types / a range of plasma cell differentiation / prominent Russell bodies.

Larynx

Lesions in the d/dg of SCC
- Squamous papilloma: *juvenile* ones are prepubertal, multiple, due to HPV, non-keratinising, show koilo-cytosis but no dysplasia and are benign but may be obstructive / recurrent; *adult* ones are keratinising, may show dysplasia and may be the tip of a verrucous carcinoma or assoc^d with SCC
- PEH (see Chapter 11: Alimentary Tract, under 'Mouth and Oropharynx' and Chapter 20: Skin) e.g. associated with a granular cell tumour
- CIS/severe dysplasia: desmoplasia, single cell invasion and stromal reaction to keratin favour early invasion
- Soft tissue lesions (e.g. plasma cell granuloma) *vs.* spindle cell SCC
- FS for margins: ! do not confuse radiation atypia (in spindle stromal cells or epithelium) for SCC

Laryngeal Nodule / Singer's Node in Reinke's Space
- Vascular type: dilated thin vessels with intra and extravascular fibrinoid $\pm$ granulation tissue – d/dg haemangioma (but these are supraglottic and have thicker-walled vessels)
- Myxoid type: myxohyaline stroma, fewer vessels – d/dg amyloid (Congo red +ve), myxoma (has stellate and mast cells)

Contact Granuloma (Contact Ulcer) of the True Cord
- Florid granulation tissue radiating to the surface $\pm$ ulceration; d/dg pyogenic granuloma (is lobular not radiating)

Cystic Lesions
- Laryngocoele (of the saccule): usu. acquired (forced blowing), stratified ciliated lining $\pm$ focal lymphocytic aggregates
- Laryngeal cyst: retention (respiratory-type lining) or congenital (squamous lining) $\pm$ lymphocytes
- Laryngeal duct cyst with papillary hyperplasia ('adenoma' / 'cystadenoma'): tall cells, often oncocytic, line tubules, acini and papillae $\pm$ goblet cells; usu. occurs in the saccule and is rare
- Cystic lesions / neoplasms of minor salivary glands (see pp.133–134)

Malformative/Congenital Anomalies

Congenital Cystic Adenomatoid Malformation (CCAM / CAM / CPAM)
- Stocker Classification (Stocker, 2002):

Type 0: = *acinar dysplasia*: widespread and bilateral, small cysts (5mm $\varnothing$), respiratory epithelial lining, cartilage (i.e. bronchial structures) but no normal alveoli (macro: lungs are small and solid)

Type I: localised mass, large cysts (2–10cm $\varnothing$), resp. epithelium, mucus cell rows, polypoidal infolds, intervening fibromuscular tissue, presents at all ages, risk of malig. transformation (to BAC / sarcoma)

Type II: usu. confined to 1 lobe (d/dg sequestration), medium cysts (0.5–2.0cm $\varnothing$, back-to-back), simple columnar cells, interspersed alveolar ducts $\pm$ striated muscle $\pm$ renal anomalies (= *rhabdomyomatous dysplasia* if widespread $\pm$ CVS anomalies)

Type III: solid/small cysts with simple cuboidal lining (mimics late fetal lung), may involve upto whole lung

Type IV: peripheral location, mesenchymal cysts with alveolar lining, no resp. epithelium / cartilage, risk of blastematous transformation if stromal hypercellularity. d/dg pleuropulmonary blastoma

- Except for type II, CCAM presents in neonates. Types II and IV have a good prog. (others poor)
- d/dg CCAM I *vs.* simple foregut cyst: CCAM has polypoidal infolds and rows of pure mucus cells
- d/dg CCAM I *vs.* bronchogenic cyst: CCAM lacks cartilage and mural mucus glands
- d/dg CCAM IV *vs.* grade I pleuropulmonary blastoma: may be histologically identical – use CPC
- d/dg CCAM *vs.* cystic mesenchymal hamartoma: CCAM lacks a mesenchymal cambium layer
- d/dg CCAM *vs.* sequestration: CCAM has a pulmonary arterial supply, communication with bronchial tree and presence of normal alveoli (usu. at the periphery of the lesions) except type 0

Sequestration
- Lower lobe regions affected in $\frac{2}{3}$ of cases
- Common to all: arterial supply is systemic and 'airways' do not communicate with rest of the lungs
- *Intralobar* (i.e. within the visceral pleura): adults, has a pulmonary venous drainage, *usu.* acquired
- *Extralobar*: infants, systemic venous drainage, developmental, like CCAM II ± lymphangiectasia
- Poorly developed lung with columnar / cuboidal epithelium lining dilated spaces ± cartilage
- Normal alveoli are not usu. present though there may be collapsed / consolidated alveolar tissue

Cystic Mesenchymal Hamartoma
- Multilocular cyst; bland simple cuboidal/columnar lining
- (Endometrial stroma-like) mesenchyme with a cambium layer (see CCAM d/dg), mitoses are rare
- d/dg endometrial stromal sarcoma (metastatic) or pleuropulmonary blastoma (*vide infra*)

Chronic Bronchitis, Emphysema and Bronchiectasis

Chronic Bronchitis
- Def^n: phlegmatic cough on most days for ≥ 3 months for ≥ 2 consecutive years
- Goblet cell hyperplasia
- ↑Bronchial gland volume – can be estimated by the Reid Index (= thickness of mucosal glandular layer [superficial surface of glandular layer to superficial perichondrium] divided by the total mucosal thickness [surface epithelial BM to superficial perichondrium]) using main or lobar bronchi where the epithelium is parallel to the cartilage. Reid's original mean values: healthy ≈ 0.25 (upper limit 0.36), bronchitic ≈ 0.6 (lower limit 0.4) – but other studies showed sig. overlap

Pulmonary Emphysema
- Def^n: airway dilatation and destruction distal to the terminal bronchioles
- Centrilobular: ➤ respiratory bronchioles worst affected
                   ➤ occurs in smokers / coal workers
                   ➤ severe effects due to shunting ++ ('blue bloater' hypercapnoeic respiratory failure, pulm. HT, cor pulmonale)
- Panacinar: ➤ alveolar ducts and alveoli worst affected
                   ➤ focal form is very common in elderly, diffuse form occurs in α_1 AT deficiency
                   ➤ milder effects, compensatable by ↑ventilation ('pink puffer')
- Localised forms: paraseptal, paracicatricial, unilateral (McLeod's syndrome), etc.

Bronchiectasis
- Def^n: airway dilatation and destruction proximal to the terminal bronchioles
- Due to scarring 2° to bronchopneumonia, pertussis, measles, CF, bronchiolitis, narcotics, etc.
- Cavities accumulate infected fluid → ulceration, haemoptysis, metastatic abscesses, amyloid, inflammatory atypical squames on cytology

Interstitial Lung Disease

Non-Specific / Insignificant Changes (d/dg Lung Disease)
- Non-specific inflam^n, fibrosis ± honeycombing may occur in the extreme tips of the lobes (esp. the lingula and right middle lobe) without implying specific disease
- Sub-pleural fibrosis, non-specific chronic inflam^n and larger alveoli may occur in the lung apices
- Scarring (any cause) may have adjacent type II pneumocyte hyperplasia: d/dg BAC (p. 92)
- Scarring (any cause e.g. smoking/city dwellers) may have adjacent pulm. artery endarteritic changes (incl. intimal fibrosis and medial hypertrophy) without pulmonary HT

Lung Transplant Pathology
- Rejection and infect[n] may be asymptomatic and are more common in the lungs *cf.* heart in combined Tx
- Acute rejection: perivenular mononuclear cell infiltration (d/dg infection – can be difficult)
- Intermediate: diffuse and patchy peribronchial and peribronchiolar mixed mononuclear infiltration with exocytosis (into the respiratory epithelium) ± granulation tissue but no collagen fibrosis
- Chronic rejection: patchy obliterative bronchiolitis (*q.v.*) → vanishing bronchiole syndrome

Cryptogenic Fibrosing Alveolitis (CFA / IPF) Showing Usual Interstitial Pneumonia (UIP)
- Chronic, terminal (median survival 3–5 year) condition requiring strong immunosuppression
- Dry cough, bibasal creps, restrictive pattern ± characteristic HRCT, non-organ-specific auto-Abs
- Hamman-Rich acute terminal deterioration (ARDS-like) may occur (= AIP)
- BAL show lymphocytes and granulocytes
- Bronchial Bx can exclude bronchocentric disease (sarcoid, EAA, RBILD) but *cannot* diagnose CFA
- Only diagnose CFA on open lung Bx or PM and then only if specific features present (else = NSIP)
- Periph. (sub-pleural) disease with central sparing. Basal lower lobes worst affected (± honeycomb)
- Distal acinar involvement with central sparing (else rethink the diagnosis)
- Temporal heterogeneity is the hallmark (fibroblastic foci *and* mature collagenised areas)
- Variegate pathology (normal septa to gross thickening and distortion in the same section)
- Lymphoplasmacytic infiltrate in septa (and granulocytes in alveoli) ± giant cells with blue bodies
- Fibroblastic foci (re-epithelialised Masson bodies) ± marked Type II pneumocyte atypia
- Alveolar lining varies from normal to columnar with ciliated / mucus metaplasia
- Stromal smooth muscle and arterial thickening with intimal proliferation
- DIP is no longer considered part of CFA as it has a distinct, more benign course
- d/dg of UIP:
    - CTD: pleural thickening/inflam[n] suggests a CTD, look for other signs (vasculitis, nodules, etc.)
    - nitrofurantoin (can look identical to CFA), NSIP, LIP
    - EAA, BOOP, chronic eosinophilic pneumonia, sarcoid, radiation, HX
    - infection, pneumoconioses, lymphangitis carcinomatosa, Goodpasture's
    - pulmonary alveolar proteinosis

Desquamative Interstitial Pneumonia (DIP)
- Diffuse distribution of lightly haemosiderotic Mφ in alveoli
- Mild interstitial inflam[n] / light fibrosis – no temporal heterogeneity
- d/dg of DIP:
    - smoking (RBILD): patchy (bronchocentric), brown Mφ ('smoker's Mφ')
    - amiodarone / other drugs
    - 2° to proximal airway obstruction
    - EAA, chronic eosinophilic pneumonia, pulmonary alveolar proteinosis, HX

Honeycomb Lung (Causes)
- CFA, sarcoidosis, asbestosis, HX, EAA and non-specific

Non-Specific Interstitial Pneumonia (NSIP)
- Grade 1 = cellular (d/dg LIP – but NSIP does not expand septa like LIP)
- Grade 2/3 = fibrotic: spatially and temporally uniform without fibroblastic foci (*cf.* CFA)
- Exclude causes: drugs, hypersensitivity, etc.

Giant Cell Interstitial Pneumonia (GIP)
- Peribronchiolar DIP with multinucleated alveolar Mφ ± eos. (! ≠ measles epithelial GC pneumonia)
- Multinucleated cells may show emperipolesis / phagocytosis of other inflammatory cells
- Usu. Hx of hard metal exposure (e.g. tungsten, cobalt, titanium and their alloys)

Diffuse Alveolar Damage (DAD)
- Fibroblastic expansion of the interstitium with variable inflammation
- Hyperplasia of atypical type 2 pneumocytes
- Hyaline membranes ($\propto$ disease phase)

- Thrombi in small pulmonary arteries
- Megas in capillaries (d/dg viral/malig. cells) – also seen in sepsis without DAD and in normal lungs
- See 'Shock lung' (ARDS) on p. 383 and d/dg OP (*vide infra*).

Bronchiolitis Obliterans (Organising Pneumonia [OP], COP and BOOP)
- Plugs of cellular myxoid tissue (Masson bodies) in bronchiole lumens and peribronchiolar alveoli
- Inflam^y cells and proteinaceous exudate may be prominent in early lesions
- Alveolar reaction to terminal obstructions: ① type 2 pneumocyte hyperplasia, ② intra-alveolar foamy (lipoid) Mϕ, ③ cellular debris ± cholesterol clefts
- 1°: COP (= idiopathic BOOP) – BAL shows a mixed cell content
- 2°: infection, WG, EAA, HX, eosinophilic pneumonia, allergies, some gases
- Granulomas, vasculitis, PMN, necrosis, and BAL showing single cell type predominance are all features which may help identify the underlying aetiology in any given case of OP
- d/dg DAD, AIP and NSIP: in OP, the changes are patchy and restricted to peribronchiolar tissue; also there are no hyaline membranes

Obliterative Bronchiolitis / Bronchitis
- Fibrosis within and around bronchial / bronchiolar wall (*cf.* lumenal in OP), epithelial sloughing
- Bronchovascular bundles with missing bronchi are the end result and a good diagnostic clue
- Distally the air spaces may accumulate foamy Mϕ
- Seen 2° to BMTx, lung Tx, RhA and drugs (esp. gold / penicillamine), viruses, mycoplasma, gases

Extrinsic Allergic Alveolitis (EAA)
- Peribronchiolar and centriacinar (*cf.* CFA which is distal acinar)
- Spatially heterogeneous (i.e. patchy) but temporally uniform (unlike CFA)
- Inflam^n: lymphocytes (T8) and plasma cells > PMN; eos. are sparse; ± intra and extra-alveolar foam cells
- Lymphocyte-rich BOOP-like areas
- Bronchiolar muscle hypertrophy
- Most cases have poorly formed granulomas ± giant cells containing cholesterol clefts
- ± DIP-like pattern

Pneumoconioses
Coal worker's pneumoconiosis
- Upper $\frac{2}{3}$ of the lung worst affected
- **Simple**: 2–5mm stellate macules of anthracotic Mϕ in immobile alveoli (centrilobular) and sub-pleurally (may follow lymphatics). Nodules (<1cm ∅) are well-circumscribed and palpable due to ↑collagen (a reaction to coal with higher mineral:carbon ratio)
- **Complicated** (= progressive massive fibrosis): ≥1cm ∅ (Caplan nodules are excluded from PMF), compensatable, haphazard collagen with pigment, well-circumscribed, ± central breakdown and TB
- Caplan's syndrome (in RhA): upto 5cm ∅, necrobiotic collagen with *concentric bands* of dust (*cf.* randomly intermingled dust) and palisaded Mϕ
- **Grade** the amount of dust present from i. to v. thus:
- State if dust foci are soft or palpable

i.	dust-free
ii.	slight diffuse pigmentation
iii.	sparse dust foci (≥1cm apart)
iv.	moderate dust foci (>1 per cm)
v.	numerous dust foci

Silicosis
- Whorled laminar collagen with birefringent silicates[2] and peripheral plasma cells

Asbestosis
- This is a clinicopathological diagnosis; histological confirmation, when needed, requires: ① diffuse interstitial fibrosis of the asbestotic type and ② evidence of asbestos as the cause (asbestos bodies)
- The interstitial fibrosis should be EITHER of at least grade 3 (*vide infra*) OR, if lower grades, the distribution and clinical should be typical (i.e. not elderly smokers with mainly upper lobe disease)
- Typical pattern: symmetric, lower lobes worst affected with sub-pleural accentuation but broad areas of fibrosis (i.e. obliterating architecture), not lace-like (preserved arch.) as in CFA.

---

[2] silicates are co-inhaled with the silica but it is the silica which causes the fibrosis

- Asbestos bodies:
  - ➤ only visible when ferruginated →golden [unstained] / Prussian blue [stained] coat
  - ➤ found in the walls of the RB +/ assoc^d with intra-alveolar Mϕ
  - ➤ >1 asbestos body in 1 or several 5μ thick Perls-stained tissue section(s) from 1 or several blocks is usu. considered significant. Normal (non-asbestotic) controls may show, on average, 1 asbestos body per 100 sections, each section being 2cm^2 in area.[3] However, in some populations the norm is higher (e.g. in Finland, $\approx \frac{1}{3}$ of people unlikely to have been exposed to asbestos had an average of 1 body per section)
  - ➤ asbestos body concentrat^n can vary 10-fold depending on site (for sampling, see p. 48)
  - ➤ use of 30μ thick unstained sections greatly reduces the time it takes to find asbestos bodies
  - ➤ asbestos bodies may also be quantified by EM or in BAL fluid (for sample acceptability criteria and reference ranges see De Vuyst et al., 1998)
  - ➤ asbestos (and erionite) bodies have a long and (usu.) straight core (0.5μ thick) that is clear (not yellow) and transparent (not black). The Fe-protein coating may be uniform or segmented and it stifles birefringence (∴ they are usu. not birefringent)
  - ➤ d/dg other ferruginous bodies: sheet silicates (e.g. talc, kaolinite) are broader/scrolled with a yellow clear core. Black-cored bodies are usu. carbon (not birefringent, many shapes incl. long and thin) or titanium oxide rutile (birefringent).
  - ➤ ! mixed dust inhalation occurs incl. asbestos with other types so:
    1. finding other fibre types does not exclude asbestosis, and
    2. finding a heavily ferruginated body in a patient with a PMHx of asbestos exposure should not be assumed to be an asbestos body if the core is obscured
- Asbestos-related pleural plaques (may have nodular macro and 'basket weave' collagen micro) are common and are not compensatable
- Compensation is given for asbestosis, diffuse pleural fibrosis, or asbestos-related neoplasia
- Asbestos-related neoplasms are mesothelioma and any histotype of lung carcinoma[4]
- d/dg of asbestos-related diffuse pleural fibrosis: sarcomatoid mesothelioma, TB, CTD, adenoCA

Grading the severity of fibrosis (esp. w.r.t. asbestosis)

⓪ No fibrosis around respiratory bronchioles (RB)

① Mild peribronchiolar fibrosis ± non-linking septa (involving the immediate layer of adjacent alveoli)

② As for 1 but septa involve ≥2 adjacent layers of alveoli or alveolar ducts

③ As for 2 but with at least focal bridging (no non-fibrotic alveolar septa between two bronchioles)

④ As for 2 but with new spaces forming (> alveolar size – upto 1cm ∅) – 'honeycomb lung'

Grading the extent of RB fibrosis (esp. w.r.t. asbestosis)

A. An occasional RB only (affected by any grade of fibrosis) ⎫ Latterly, the term 'occasional' has
B. More than occasional but <50%   ⎬ been interpreted to mean <25% of
C. 50% of all RB involved   ⎭ the lung tissue.

Immunological / Autoimmune / Connective Tissue Diseases

Relapsing Polychondritis
- Death is usu. due to resp. cartilage involvement (esp. tracheal)
- Perichondrium is the original site of inflam^n → invasion of cartilage with ↓basophilia and ↑PAS +vity
- Changes over time: PMN → plasma cells → lymphocytes → fibrosis and cartilage atrophy in late stages
- Systemic CTD with vasculitis may develop later or be concurrent

Asthma and Status Asthmaticus
See p. 382, under 'Anaphylaxis'.

Necrotising Sarcoid Angiitis (NSA) / Necrotising Sarcoid Granulomatosis / Necrotising Sarcoidosis
- Peribronchiolar (obliterated), confluent, sarcoidal granulomatous areas
- Irregular areas of necrosis (non-caseating) that are *not* intimately assoc^d with the granulomas

---

[3] Roggli and Pratt, 1983
[4] Asbestos is probably *not* a cause of laryngeal carcinoma (related to alcohol and tobacco – which were confounding factors in earlier studies that suggested an asbestos link).

- More typical sarcoid granulomas elsewhere [i.e. tight, non-necrotising, naked, ± Schaumann or asteroid bodies]
- Pulmonary arteritis of the giant cell type or wall infiltrated by sarcoidal granulomas
- d/dg WG: WG may have a few sarcoid-like granulomas but not as many as NSA
- d/dg infective granulomas – must be excluded
- d/dg berylliosis (a classical mimic of sarcoid)

Eosinophilic Pneumonia
- This is a clinical term for patients with radiological pulm. infiltrates and PB eosinophilia
- Histologically: eosinophils in alveoli and alveolar septa +/ granulomatous inflammation
- Later ± →organising pneumonia with diminished eosinophils
- Main causes :
  - ① Churg-Strauss syndrome (for more details on the vasculitis see pp. 69–71)
    - ➢ clinically: fever, asthma, blood eosinophilia
    - ➢ histologically (esp. skin, kidney, lung):
      1. tissue eosinophilia
      2. vasculitis (PAN-like, WG-like)   } All three need not be present in the same
      3. granulomas: ☞ eosinophilic granulomas / abscesses } tissue.
                      ☞ necrobiotic palisaded granulomas
    - ➢ d/dg eosinophilic variant of WG
  - ② Asthma (esp. if there is mucus plugging or allergic bronchopulmonary aspergillosis)
  - ③ Drugs / toxins (e.g. penicillin, smoke, some metals)
  - ④ Reaction to infection: e.g. fungi, helminthes (e.g. tropical eosinophilia due to filariasis)
  - ⑤ Simple pulmonary eosinophilia (Loeffler's syndrome):
    - ➢ *transient* eosinophilic pneumonia (changes last 1 month to 1 year)
    - ➢ retrospective diagnosis
    - ➢ due to toxocariasis, drugs or intestinal ascaris in some cases
    - ➢ 'Loeffler's syndrome' may also refer to endomyocardial fibrosis with eosinophilia.

Wegener's Granulomatosis (WG)
- Clin: URT/LRT mucosal ulceration (esp. nasal septum) and c-ANCA +vity are good clinical pointers
- WG is currently defined by: ① necrotising extravascular granulomas in the URT and LRT
                                 ② generalised vasculitis
                                 ③ GN (necrotising FSGN / crescentic, pauci-immune)

Pulmonary histology
- Vasculitis (for the features, see p. 70) – essential for a confident histodiagnosis
- Serpiginous / geographic necrosis with nuclear debris ++ ('dirty' necrosis)
- Necrosis is surrounded by loose / palisaded granulomatous inflam^n ± giant cells
- Multifocal ulceration of airways
- The (lung) limited form (± skin) has a better prognosis (but may heal with fibrosis ++)
- Limited WG may develop into classic WG with renal / other organs involved years later
- Variants: eosinophilic, bronchocentric, BOOP-like
- d/dg lymphomatoid granulomatosis (has atypical lymphocytes, *vide infra*)
- d/dg Wegener's cavitating lung granulomas may resemble TB
- d/dg necrotising sarcoid angiitis (has many more sarcoid-like granulomas *cf.* Wegener's)
- d/dg invasive (necrotising) pulmonary Aspergillosis

Pulmonary Haemorrhagic Syndromes

Wegener's Granulomatosis (vide supra)

Idiopathic Pulmonary Haemosiderosis
- Recent and old intra-alveolar haemorrhage (do Perls – intra-alveolar RBC may be due to Bx artefact)
- Minimal / no inflammation or fibrosis
- Diagnosis of exclusion

Goodpasture's Syndrome
- Recent and old intra-alveolar haemorrhage (do Perls – intra-alveolar RBC may be due to Bx artefact)

- ± Leukocytoclastic vasculitis
- Necrotising FSGN
- Immunofluorescence: linear IgG and C3 on BM of alveolar septa and capillaries
- 25% are p-ANCA +ve

Pulmonary Hypertension

Normal Histology
- Pulm. arterial pressure is 25 (at rest) to 30 mmHg (during exercise)
- Arteries travel with bronchi, have distinct internal and external elastic laminae and muscle wall thickness is upto 7% of vessel external ∅
- Veins travel in interlobular septa and have indistinct muscle and elastic
- Arterioles and venules lack muscle and have a single elastic lamina
- Supernumerary arterioles branch directly from larger arteries into the respiratory parenchyma (these branch points are the typical site of plexiform and dilatation lesions – see Figure 8.2)

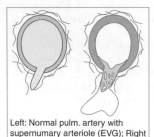

Left: Normal pulm. artery with supernumary arteriole (EVG); Right plexiform lesion with distal dilatation lesion & medial hypertrophy (H&E)

FIGURE 8.2   Pulmonary arteries

Progression of Lesions in Congenital / 1° Arterial Pulmonary HT
1. Muscularisation of arterioles (esp. in children and hypoxic adults)
2. Medial hypertrophy (thickness >15% of ∅ is definitely abnormal)
3. Concentric cellular intimal thickening (d/dg acellular hyaline venous sclerosis of the aged)
4. Concentric laminar fibroelastosis   ⎫ These four
5. Dilatation lesions (may occur as clusters = angiomatoid lesions) ⎪ are
6. Necrotising arteritis (fibrinoid necrosis) ⎬ irreversible
7. Plexiform lesions (usu. <300µ and focal ∴ may need serials to detect) ⎭ changes.

1° Arterial Pulmonary HT
- Associations: youth, female, CTD, liver disease, HIV, miscellaneous (toxic oil, aminorex, eosinophilia myalgia syndrome, schistosomiasis)
- Plexiform lesions: VEGF-1 +ve cellular recanalisation-like plugs but with proximal local cellular intimal thickening, distal dilatation lesions and occur at supernumerary arterioles; d/dg thrombotic or embolic recanalisation sites which usu. affect larger vessels and don't show dilatation lesions.
- Thrombotic (small distal arteries ∴ normal angiogram or distal pruning)
- Medial and intimal thickening (changes 2. and 3. above) may be the only anomalies seen

1° Venous Pulmonary HT (Pulmonary Veno-Occlusive Disease)
- Associations: BMTx and chemoRx; arterial pulm. HT occurs secondarily but no plexiform lesions
- Thrombosed and recanalised septal veins with local congestion and loose-textured intimal fibrosis
- Septal fibrosis, capillary haemangiomatosis ± granulomatous reaction to Fe/Ca^{2+} deposits in elastic
- Larger veins are normal

2° Venous Pulmonary HT
- Associations: acquired heart disease (LVF, myxoma), mediastinal disease, sarcoid
- Venous medial hypertrophy and arteriolisation (i.e. inner and outer elastic laminae become distinct)
- Haemosiderosis, ↑ lymphatics, septal oedema and fibrosis, osteoliths, ↑ in arterial adventitia and media

2° Arterial Pulmonary HT
- Thromboembolic: ➢ radiol: arterial filling defects and ventilation-perfusion mismatches
                    ➢ recanalisation in larger elastic arteries
- Thrombotic: ➢ smaller muscular arteries show eccentric fibrosis or multilumenal recanalisation
                ➢ 2° to low flow (pulm. stenosis), haematological conditions and emboli (talc / tumour)
- Interstitial lung disease and chronic hypoxia: changes 1. 2. and 3., above. Hypoxia may also result in longitudinal smooth muscle cells / bundles on the intimal side of the IEL

Drugs and Toxins

Cocaine and 'Crack Lung'
- Alveolar haemorrhage, DAD, organising pneumonia
- Interstitial and intra-alveolar inflammatory cell infiltration (eosinophils ++)
- Bullous emphysema (fragmentat[n] of elastic fibres) → may present with pneumothorax/mediastinum
- Vascular: medial hypertrophy, 2° pulm HT (± extrapulmonary eosinophilic angiitis)
- Immuno: deposition of IgE in both lymphocytes and alveolar macrophages

Cannabinoids (e.g. marijuana)
- Changes similar to tobacco smokers: squamous metaplasia, chronic bronchitis, RBILD, ↑ CA risk
- ↑ Incidence of allergic bronchopulmonary aspergillosis and other fungi (from mouldy marijuana)
- ± Surgical emphysema, pneumothorax and bullae (due to forced deep inhalation practices)

Narcotics (e.g. heroin)
- Exacerbations of pre-existing asthma
- Pulmonary oedema ± subsequent bronchiectasis
- Aspiration pneumonitis risk (due to impaired consciousness during use)

Intravenous (any drug)
- Emboli of foreign substances → thromboses, pulm. HT, granulomatous reactions, PMF
- Talc-induced panacinar emphysema
- Particles may be clear, black, basophilic (d/dg 'bacteria'), eosinophilic, PAS +ve, carminophilic, birefringent, etc. For further details on identification, see Tomashefski and Felo, 2004

Paraquat Lung
- Found in weed-killers (trademarked as Gramoxone®, Weedol®, Pathclear®, etc.)
- Lowest fatal dose for adults is 17mg/kg (liver, kidney, brain and other organs are also affected)
- Pneumocytes actively uptake paraquat → oxidative damage (DAD)
- Early: intense vascular congestion, pulm. oedema and alveolar haemorrhage
- Late (few days): hyaline membranes and intra-alveolar obliterative fibrosis (elastic / Masson bodies)

Pleural Tumours

Mesothelioma
Aetiology
- Asbestos, heredity, erionite, radiation, chronic inflam[n], SV40 virus (controversial)
Subtypes
- Epithelioid: tubulopapillary, solid, glandular, small cell, clear cell, deciduoid (PLAP −ve), signet ring, lymphohistiocytic (d/dg lymphoma), pleomorphic, myxoid
- Sarcomatoid: desmoplastic[5], metaplastic (cartilage/bone), fibrosarcoma-like, MFH-like, lymphoid-rich
- General points: mitoses are scant in epithelioid; sarcomatoid may be αSMA and desmin +ve; biphasic must be differentiated from d/dg thymic carcinoma, carcinosarcoma, biphasic sarcoma and pulmonary blastoma
Mesothelioma *vs.* carcinoma
- +ve in meso: AB (hyaluronidase sensitive), CK5/6, calretinin (nuclear), thrombomodulin, WT1, D2-40
- +ve in CA: DPAS (strong, big globule), MNF, TTF-1, pCEA, Ber-EP4, CD15, B72.3, BG8, MOC-31
- AMAD-2 is +ve in most mesotheliomas but is rare in adenocarcinomas
- MUC4 was expressed by 94% of lung adeno CA but not meso (i.e. 100% specific for adenoCA)[6]
- Mesothelioma may show characteristic cytogenetic changes
- Ber-EP4 may be +ve in mesothelioma but never diffuse and strong (<50% of cells and usu. <25%). It is esp. good at discriminating mesothelioma from adenocarcinoma of pulmonary origin
- CK +vity in the deepest parts of the tumour is better evidence of malignant mesothelioma (*cf.* superficial +vity). CK5/6 is +ve in most SCC of lung, −ve in most adenocarcinomas
- −ve CEA is strong evidence *against* adenocarcinoma

---

[5] if > 50% of tumour is hypocellular
[6] Llinares *et al.*, 2004

Mesothelioma *vs.* reactive mesothelial hyperplasia
- Papillary, solid and even minimally invasive forms of hyperplasia exist
- Hx of prior (esp. recurrent) irritat^n, effusion or disease of underlying viscus favours reactive
- Radiology helps: presence of mass lesion or mesothelioma-like pattern
- Necrosis in hyperplastic looking lesion = strong evidence of mesothelioma
- Invasion with desmoplasia and lack of inflam^n (sub-mesothelial cells disrupted, tumour goes into lung etc.). True invasion is haphazard and perpendicular to the mesothelial surface (*cf.* parallel entrapment)
- Cytology of fluid may help (see pp.359–360) as it samples the whole mesothelial surface *cf.* Bx
- ↑ Cytological atypia, mitoses and papillary arch. favour (but are not diagnostic of) mesothelioma
- p53 +ve (diffuse and strong) in mesothelioma
- Reaction pattern with EMA (see Figure 8.3):
- Desmin +vity favours reactive mesothelial hyperplasia over malignant mesothelioma

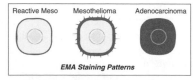

FIGURE 8.3   Mesothelial immuno

Desmoplastic mesothelioma *vs.* reactive fibrous pleurisy
- Generous sampling / block all tissue
- Meso: invasion, collagen necrosis, atypical mitoses, organised collagen patterns (storiform, etc.)
- Pleurisy: more cellular, inflam^y, 'maturation' of spindle cells towards the surface, vertical capillaries

Sarcomatoid mesothelioma *vs.* other tumours
- Diagnostic criteria for meso: ① chest wall/lung invasion, ② bland necrosis and ③ sarcomatoid areas
- Calretinin is only +ve in ≈ 50% and other mesothelial markers less so; CK and vimentin are most reliably +ve
- ! But some sarcomas are CK +ve (e.g. synovial sarcoma) ∴ use other markers, cytogenetics, clin./radiol.
- Proliferating non-neoplastic sub-mesothelial cells (≈ fibroblasts) acquire CK +vity as they migrate towards the surface, ∴ CK +ve spindle cells do *not* imply sarcomatoid mesothelioma. In this situation you need: ① Unequivocal invasion (e.g. into lung parenchyma) *and*
        ② Cytological evidence of malignancy
- d/dg spindle sarcomas or malignant SFT (*vide infra*)
- d/dg: calcifying fibrous pseudotumour, radiation, sarcomatoid carcinoma, melanoma, RCC

Epithelioid mesothelioma *vs.* papillary serous carcinoma of the peritoneum / ovary
- PLAP is −ve in mesothelioma but +ve in 50% of papillary serous carcinoma
- S100 is −ve in (most but not all) mesothelioma but +ve in 25% of papillary serous carcinoma
- CK5/6 is −ve in peritoneal CA, +ve in 25% ovarian carcinoma and +ve in 50% of mesothelioma

Pleuropulmonary Blastoma of Infancy
- Solid component: may be undiff or contain multiple sarcomas (leiomyosarcoma/RMS/chondro/osteosarcoma)
- Cystic component: lined by bland (?entrapped benign) epithelium ∴ probably not truly biphasic
- d/dg pulmonary blastoma: adults, biphasic (has an immature epithelial component), see p. 92

Other Tumours
- Solitary fibrous tumour (see SFT on p. 94 and pp. 324–325)
- Multicystic mesothelial proliferation of the pleura (see peritoneal type in Chapter 11: Alimentary Tract)
- Adenomatoid tumour, pseudomesotheliomatous angiosarcoma, synovial sarcoma, lymphoma, *etc.*

Pulmonary Lymphoid Lesions

Reactive
- LIP: mainly T-cells with aggregated B-cells (d/dg MALT which has mainly B-cells), expanding the septa (MALToma destroys them and NSIP doesn't expand them). Must exclude EAA. Idiopathic LIP is *very rare* ∴ look for a cause (HIV, CTD, etc.)
- Follicular Bronchiolitis: Like LIP, this occurs in three settings: CTD, immunosuppression, idiopathic
- Nodular lymphoid hyperplasia (= those few 'pseudolymphomas' that don't fulfil the criteria for MALToma)

Angiocentric Lymphoid Proliferations
- Grade 1: BLAG is composed of small mature lymphocytes and has the lowest Ki-67 LI of the three
- Grade 2: Lymphomatoid granulomatosis (usu. an angioinvasive and angiodestructive EBV-related T-cell-rich DLBCL + geographic necrosis ± granulomas but occ. TCL/NK tumours show this histol.)
- Grade 3: Angiocentric T-cell lymphoma

MALT Lymphomas and 'Pseudolymphoma'
- Reactive MALT is induced by smoking, autoimmune disease and CFA. LIP also has ↑risk of lymphoma
- Low grade (see also pp.110–112):
  - ➢ clin./radiol.: age >30 years, air bronchograms
  - ➢ arch: destructive masses with surrounding perilymphatic and bronchovascular bundle extension (sparing vessels), septal and subpleural infiltration
  - ➢ ± non-necrotising transmural infiltrates of large vessels
  - ➢ other: hyaline sclerosis, giant lamellar bodies, LEL ++ (in the lung the lymphocytes may not look monocytoid), granulomas (not caseous), amyloid
- The term *pseudolymphoma* was used for what we now consider to be true low grade MALToma and it should no longer be used. (The same goes for gastric – but not cutaneous – 'pseudolymphoma']
- High grade (= DLBCL): symptomatic, destructive growth, necrosis (see p. 113)

Other Types and d/dg of Pulmonary Lymphoma
- 1° intravascular lymphoma: high grade B-cell, poor prognosis, d/dg *lymphangitis carcinomatosa*
- 1° effusion lymphoma (PEL): a DLBCL but B markers are usu. −ve (positive for CD138, EMA, CD30, HHV8 and clonal EBV). Assoc[d] with AIDS and KS
- Pleural lymphoma: usu. DLBCL, assoc[d] with chronic inflammation / TB (i.e. PAL, usu. −ve for CD30, HHV8 and EBV)
- d/dg: SmCC, lymphoepithelioma-like CA, lymphohistiocytic / lymphocyte-rich mesothelioma, thymoma, Askin

Other Tumours

Mucinous Cystic Tumours
- Benign cystadenoma: very rare, purely mucus-cell lining, no atypical features
- Borderline: periph.; mucinous lining with folds, stratificat[n], cytol. atypia ± microglandular solid foci
- d/dg cystadenocarcinoma has obviously malignant cytology +/ frank invasion
- d/dg mucinous adenocarcinoma (this is like colloid carcinoma in other organs)
- d/dg bronchogenic cyst has cartilage and bronchial glands in wall
- d/dg CCAM has cells other than mucinous in its lining and usu. presents in younger patients
- d/dg mucus cell adenoma of bronchial glands: macro: more solid, proximal and protrudes into lumen; micro: bland-lined mucus cysts (= dilated bronchial glands) ± papillary foci but ≈ no mitoses

Atypical Adenomatous Hyperplasia (= Bronchioalveolar Adenoma)
- ≤5mm diameter (if larger it is diagnosed as BAC – *vide infra*)
- Assoc[d] with adenocarcinoma / SCC and metastases
- Consists in Type II pneumocytes / Clara cells (but no ciliated / mucus cells)

Adenocarcinoma
- WHO def[n]: 'a malignant epithelial tumour with tubular, acinar, or papillary growth patterns, and/or mucus production by the tumour cells.'
- Subtypes: acinar (= mostly glandular structures ± pap / solid areas), papillary, BAC, mucinous (colloid carcinoma) and solid (solid type must have demonstrable mucin in 'many' tumour cells – some define 'many' as ≥5 cells per hpf must stain for mucin in ≥2 hpf)
- Grading: degree of solidity *vs.* gland formation, degree of mucin production, cytol. atypia and mitoses
Bronchioalveolar Carcinoma (BAC):
- Def[n]: >5mm in maximum dimension, lepidic growth pattern, no well-formed glands, no invasion[7]
- Types: Mucinous (columnar, little atypia), Non-mucinous (hobnail, more atypia), mixed
- Multicentric has a worse prognosis than unicentric (28% *vs.* 78% 5YS)

---

[7] no invasion (incl. lymph / blood vascular invasion) is a 1999 WHO criterion but is controversial

- Mucinous worse than non-mucinous (more likely to be multicentric)
- Invasive worse than non-invasive (invasive tumours = 'adenocarcinoma with a BAC growth pattern')
- d/dg alveolar adenoma: rare, well circ., <3cmØ, serum-filled cysts lined by bland flat-cuboidal pneumocytes ± hobnailing. ! Do not misdiagnose as d/dg lymphangioma
- d/dg atypical Type II pneumocytes in ARDS / chemoRx (Type II pneumocyte hyperplasia has an indistinct boundary, lacks tufts, has variable cytological atypia and has a background of interstitial lung disease)
- d/dg Lambertosis (local extension of bronchial ciliated cells to line alveolar septa)

Endometrioid adenocarcinoma (Pulmonary endodermal tumour resembling fetal lung, 'Monophasic blastoma')
- Low grade endometrioid features with glycogen-rich cytoplasm; bland spindle stroma
- Squamous morules showing focal NE differentiation and biotinylated nuclei
- d/dg pulmonary blastoma: these are biphasic tumours of adults with complex / cribriform gland formations (with elongated hyperchromatic cells as well as endometrioid clear cells ± morulae) and a cellular mitotic mesenchymal stroma ± divergent differentiation (d/dg pleuropulmonary blastoma)

Squamous Cell Carcinoma (SCC)
- Def^n: a tumour with at least one of the following: ← ① Keratin production
- Variants: ➢ spindle cell   ② Squamous pearls
  - ➢ lymphoepithelioma-like   ③ Intercellular bridges
  - ➢ basaloid carcinoma: well-defined solid islands with peripheral palisading, mitoses ++ and absence of NE features (unlike d/dg SmCC); worse prognosis *cf.* usual SCC
- Grading ∝ amount of squamous differentiation, cytological atypia, mitoses and necrosis (comedonecrosis is usu. seen in high grade – d/dg large cell NEC)
- d/dg reactive or atypical squamous metaplasias (e.g. necrotising sialometaplasia-like lesions)

Adenosquamous Carcinoma (ASC)
- Each component should comprise ≥10% of a single tumour mass (by WHO – others accept ≥5%)
- Each component should fulfil the criteria for adenoCA or SCC; they are *usually* intimately admixed
- d/dg MEC: ASC has well-developed adenocarcinoma (often with high grade nuclei) and SCC (± frank keratinisation); ASC may be peripheral (as well as central) and have CIS

Mucoepidermoid Carcinoma (MEC)
- Usu. a central, endobronchial and exophytic tumour (for histology, see p. 132)
- Low grade MEC: many bland mucus cells (! d/dg bronchial gland adenoma doesn't have 3 cell types)
- MEC is favoured in a poorly diff tumour if there are areas of lower grade MEC differentiation
- d/dg ASC: *vide supra* (but in some cases it may be impossible)

Undifferentiated Large Cell Carcinoma
- WHO def^n: 'a malig. epithelial tumour with large nuclei, prom. nucleoli, abundant cytoplasm and usu. well-defined cell borders, without the characteristic features of SCC, SmCC or adenocarcinomas.'
- Central necrosis may cause confusion with d/dg Large Cell NE Tumour (*q.v.*)
- Variant: giant cell CA – has dyscohesive pleom. cells incl. multinucleated giant forms; poor prognosis

Carcinosarcoma / Sarcomatoid Carcinoma / Pleomorphic Carcinoma
- Well-demarcated areas of spindle and epithelioid differentiation with CK +vity in both
- Sarcomatoid carcinoma (= spindle cell carcinoma) has no epithelioid areas
- Pleomorphic carcinoma has spindle +/ giant cells with no SCC / adenocarcinoma differentiation

Lymphangiomyomatosis (LAM, Lymphangioleiomyomatosis)
- F≫M ± haemoptysis; complications (due to muscle constricting effects): pneumothorax, chylous effusions; LAM is progressive unless Rx is given (e.g. progestagens) or menopause starts
- Lung involvement is unusual (*cf.* major lymphatic ducts or deep LNs) and is a poor prognostic
- Spindle cellular masses in the walls of endothelial-lined cystic spaces (lymphatic)
- ± Siderophages
- Immuno of cellular masses: αSMA +ve, HMB45 +ve (PEComa), S100 −ve
- Immuno of cystic spaces lining: endothelial markers +ve

- Associations: female hormones (regress post menopause), tuberose sclerosis, endocrinopathies
- d/dg smooth muscle proliferations in CFA
- d/dg benign metastasising leiomyoma or leiomyosarcoma (immuno for endothelial cells may help, also non-PEComa smooth muscle tumours are usu. HMB45 −ve)
- d/dg HX (immuno may help)

Pulmonary Neuroendocrine Proliferations
WHO Classification of NE tumours
- NE tumours are classified as described in the subheadings below
- Any SCC or adenoCA with only focal NE differentiation = the appropriate type 'with NE features' unless the NE differentiation is in the form of SmCC in which case it is called 'combined SmCC'
NE Cell Hyperplasia
- 'Lentiginous' proliferation within the airway's BM
- May be more florid with nesting but still confined by the bronchial BM (else = tumourlet/carcinoid)
Tumourlets
- Nodular prolif^n assoc^d with airways (*cf.* d/dg meningothelioid nodules – assoc^d with septal veins)
- Called 'carcinoid' if ≥ 5mm ⌀ (or if there is evidence of malig. behaviour e.g. LN mets)
- If multiple, may be a cause of obstructive airways disease due to fibrogenetic cytokines
- Assoc^d with bronchiectasis, carcinoid and carcinomas
Well diff NE tumours (Carcinoids)
- Commoner in children and least assoc^d with smoking
- Typical arch: central tumours are trabecular (macro dumbbell), peripheral ones insular (may spindle)
- Variants: some have an adenopapillary arch. and many others are biphasic with S100 +ve sustentacular cells (= paraganglioid because the tumour cells are CK +ve, unlike true paragangliomas)
- Other changes: oncocytic, melanin and mucin (small amounts); stromal cartilage / bone / APUDamyloid
- Nuclei: finely granular ± slight clumping with small / inconspicuous nucleoli
- Vessels: thin-walled and variably dilated
- Paraneoplasia: carcinoid syndrome (affects left sided heart valves), Cushing's, acromegaly, etc.
- d/dg paraganglioma, adenoCA, clear cell sugar tumour, glomus tumour (esp. solid/infiltrating types)
- d/dg SmCC (overdiagnosing SmCC is a potential pitfall in crushed bronchial biopsies)
    - carcinoids may show crush artefact and dot-like CK – but not the Azzopardi phenomenon
    - chromatin texture, Ki-67 LI (if <20% it is unlikely to be SmCC, if >50% it is unlikely to be carcinoid) and stromal vessel features all help in the d/dg
    - strong staining for CgA / synaptophysin, weak or −ve TTF-1 and peripheral location favour carcinoid
Moderately diff NE tumours (Atypical carcinoids)
- Clin.: lack SmCC chemosensitivty, 70% metastasise, more associated with smoking, 60% 5YS
- Def^n: contain mitoses (at a rate of 2–10/10 hpf) +/ necrosis
- A non-WHO system requires ≥2 of: ≥5/10hpf mitoses, focal necrosis, some pleom., focal arch. loss
- Nuclei: more coarsely granular / vesicular (*cf.* carcinoid) and has variable nucleoli
- Ki-67 LI is 10–48% (i.e. intermediate between carcinoid and SmCC)
- Peripheral tumours with SmCC-like cytology are likely to be atypical carcinoid (i.e. have insular / trabecular arch.) and should be excised
- d/dg SmCC: see above under carcinoid d/dg
Poorly diff NE tumours (SmCC and Large cell NE carcinoma)
- Small cell carcinoma (SmCC):
    - clin.: elderly, smokers, central location (rarely peripheral)
    - close-packed (nuclear moulding), small to medium-sized cells in sheets, strands or single cells
    - Azzopardi phenomenon (DNA encrustation of vessels) and smudging: these are not sufficient for diagnosis
    - overlying epithelium may show atypical squamous metaplasia or Pagetoid infiltration
    - nuclei: dark, fine and evenly dispersed chromatin, inconspicuous/absent nucleoli, mitoses ++, occ. giant nuclei
    - vessels: some glomeruloid prloliferations / thick-walled vascular channels in cords
    - 'combined' group have distinct SmCC and non-SmCC components (and ? worse prog.)
    - immuno: CgA can be −ve (ISH is usu. +ve); +ve for CAM5.2 (paranuclear dot), CD56, NSE, Ki-67 LI typcially >50%

➢ EM: NE dense core granules (50–200nm ∅) [squamous/mucinous features may be seen at EM, but this does not change the diagnosis]
➢ d/dg lymphoma / inflam^n / PNET – all may show Azzopardi (do CD45, CD99)
➢ d/dg Merkel cell CA: Merkel is CK20 +ve, CK7 −ve, SmCC of the lung is CK20 −ve, CK7 +ve
➢ d/dg non-SmCC (go by nuclear features – not cell size – see also carcinoid d/dg above)
➢ d/dg basaloid carcinoma (*vide supra*)
• Large Cell NE carcinoma
➢ non-SmCC nuclei (i.e. peripherally clumped chromatin with prom. nucleoli), mod. cytoplasm
➢ arch.: well-defined large groups that typically have periph. palisading and central necrosis
➢ atypical carcinoids with ≥11 mitoses per 10hpf (2mm^2) are classified as large cell NEC.

Meningothelioid (Arachnoid) Nodules (old term = Minute Pulmonary Chemodectomas)
• Interstitial nests of epithelioid cells (≈ meningiomas) assoc^d with septal veins (*cf.* d/dg tumourlets)
• Immuno: EMA and vimentin +ve (i.e. *not* a paraganglial phenotype)
• EM: shows features of arachnoid granulations
• d/dg 1° meningioma is a well-defined tumour usu. ≫3mm ∅ ± foamy Mφ +/ bone
• d/dg glomus tumour (see Chapter 20: Skin) or paraganglioma (see Chapter 19: Endocrine)

Solitary Fibrous Tumour (Localised Fibrous Tumour / SFT)
• Patternless pattern and 'ropey' collagen and stromal degenerations (see pp. 324–325)
• Triad of positivity: CD34, Bcl-2, CD99; CK is −ve; CD34 is often −ve in high grade tumours/foci
• Signs of malignancy: mitoses ≥4/10 hpf, ↑cellularity and pleom.; (p53 is usu. +ve in ≫1% of cells)
• d/dg mesothelioma (important because Rx is different): SFT is localised, mesothelioma is diffuse; SFT is CD34+ve, CK−ve, mesothelioma is converse: ! exceptions occur; use CPC; EM may help
• d/dg: synovial sarcoma or pulmonary adenofibroma (because entrapped mesothelial cells / type II pneumocytes→ CK +ve cysts / clefts to give a biphasic or fibroadenomatoid appearance in SFT)
See Chapter 21: Soft Tissues, for more d/dg and for the Calcifying Fibrous Pseudotumour variant.

Histiocytosis X (HX, Langerhans Cell Histiocytosis, Eosinophil Granuloma)
• Progressive cough / dyspnoea (± pneumothorax esp. in acute / active disease); assoc^d with smoking
• Peribronchiolar (± perivascular) cellular masses, may be stellate, may ulcerate
• Cystic spaces ± siderophages
• Highly active lesion: Langerhans cells ++, ± DIP reaction
• Subsiding activity: siderophages replace the Langerhans cells.
• Healed lesion: stellate scar with siderophages ± eosinophils
• May result in honeycomb lung
• Immuno: CD1a +ve, S100 +ve (see also pp.57–58)
• d/dg LAM (because they share: cellular masses, cystic spaces and siderophages)
• d/dg UIP / DIP
• d/dg Erdheim-Chester disease: in this the scarring follows the lymphatics, ± foamy Mφ or Touton GC and the Mφ are CD68 and S100 +ve but CD1a −ve, + other anomalies in the bones, pituitary, skin, etc.

Sclerosing Pneumocytoma (Sclerosing Haemangioma)
• Asian, F>M, middle-age
• Small (≈ 5cm ∅), well-circumscribed intraparenchymal (unrelated to bronchus)
• Papillary, angiomatous and solid growth patterns
• Bland round / polygonal cells without nucleoli
• No mitoses or necrosis
• Foamy Mφ, fibrosis, angiomatous areas
• Immuno: +ve for surfactant, vimentin, EMA, ± CK, ± NE markers

Epithelioid Haemangioendothelioma (See also p. 321)
- Typically multifocal/bilateral tumours with myxohyaline centres (d/dg amyloid tumour)
- The periphery of the nodules are cellular and show a lobular/polypoidal intra-alveolar arch.
- d/dg epithelioid mesothelioma (*q.v.*) – esp. if there is diffuse intrapleural growth – but this is rare

Clear Cell Tumour (Sugar Tumour)
- Clear cells with inconspicuous nucleoli (no mitoses, necrosis or atypia)
- Gaping vessels, little stroma
- PEComa (HMB45 +ve, PAS +ve, DPAS −ve)

Intrapulmonary Thymoma
- CK strong +ve (unlike d/dg most sarcomas)
- No NE differentiation (unlike d/dg carcinoids)   } See 'Mediastinal Pathology', below,
- Lack atypia (unlike d/dg spindle cell carcinomas)   } for more on thymomas.
- d/dg lymphoma: the epithelial component and phenotype of the lymphocytes in thymoma help

Other Tumours
- Minor salivary gland-like tumours (see Chapter 11: Alimentary Tract)
- Kaposi sarcoma: nodular or diffuse (see Chapter 21: Soft Tissues)
- Squamous papilloma, Type II pneumocyte papillary adenoma (well-circ.), adenofibroma, 1° melanoma, etc.
- Pulmonary hyalinising granuloma: inflammatory pseudotumour in which hyaline collagen bundles predominate in a trabecular pattern (see p. 310)

Frozen Section Diagnoses
- d/dg adenoCA *vs.* carcinoid (with acini or endocrine-type atypia) and type II pneumocyte hyperplasia
- d/dg SCC *vs.* squamous (or necrotising sialo-like) metaplasia in regenerative parenchyma
- d/dg carcinoma *vs.* organising pneumonia (due to the fibroblastic prolif[n] and reactive pneumocytes mimicking desmoplasia and malignant epithelium respectively)
- Necrotic lesions are usu. infective (e.g. TB, fungi, VZV), infarctive (e.g. Wegener's) or neoplastic

Mediastinal Pathology

Sclerosing Mediastinitis (Causes)
- *Histoplasma*, TB, autoimmune, trauma, drugs
- Idiopathic (see p. 311)
- d/dg sclerosing DLBCL

Thymoma
- 1917 Bell defined thymoma as a thymic epithelial tumour that may be benign or malignant and is typified by the presence of elements of the thymic epithelial reticulum and lymphocytes
- 1962 Bernatz and Lattes (B&L) classified them by the predominant cell type (spindle = good prog):
  Predominantly: lymphoid / epithelial / mixed / spindle
- 1976 Rosai and Levine used *invasiveness* and '*metastatic potential*' to classify thymomas:
  Probably benign: encapsulated, non-invasive / bland spindle
  Invasive   ➢ Category I: minimal invasion ± mild cytological atypia
               ➢ Category II: cytologically malignant (usu. widely invasive)
- 1989 Müller-Hermelink (M-H) used the *organoid histology of the thymus* and noted that aggressiveness ∝ cortical differentiation:

Medullary	= WHO Type A
Composite	= WHO Type AB
Predominantly cortical (organoid)	= WHO Type B1
Cortical	= WHO Type B2
Well-diff Thymic Carcinoma	= WHO Type B3

- 1999 WHO essentially follows M-H but does away with the names (because it is uncertain whether thymoma differentiation truly resembles normal thymic histology and because the term 'well-diff thymic carcinoma' (WDTC) is inappropriate for a thymoma because usual-type thymic carcinomas are very aggressive and some series have lumped WDTC with other thymic carcinomas thereby muddying the results)

- Common features for thymomas:
  - ➢ organoid growth pattern (even invasive foci are organoid)
  - ➢ fibrous septa
  - ➢ EMA +ve microcysts
  - ➢ CD20 +ve epithelial cells (CD20 may be −ve in type A/B), also +ve for CK (e.g. MNF116)
  - ➢ scattered CD20 +ve B-cells
  - ➢ perivascular serum lakes (increase in prominence from medullary to cortical differentiation)
  - ➢ follicular hyperplasia and MG are assoc[d] with cortical differentiation
  - ➢ red cell aplasia and hypogammaglobulinaemia are assoc[d] with medullary differentiation
- Medullary thymoma (Type A)
  - ➢ non-invasive
  - ➢ pericellular reticulin is present (*cf.* type B3)
  - ➢ few lymphocytes (these are of mature phenotype: −ve for Tdt, CD99 and CD1a)
  - ➢ no Hassall's corpuscles (HC) and no foci of epidermoid differentiation.
  - ➢ differs from B&L 'predom. spindle' in that the latter also includes spindle cell WDTC
- Composite (Type A/B)
  - ➢ two distinct components:
    1. medullary (may form cellular 'septa' dividing up the cortical areas)
    2. lymphocyte rich areas with 'starry sky' and stellate epithelial cells with open nuclei
  - ➢ the cortical component has immature T-cells (+ve for CD2, CD3, Tdt, CD99 and CD1a)
  - ➢ no HC and no foci of epidermoid differentiation.
- Predominantly Cortical – Organoid Thymoma (Type B1)
  - ➢ large tumours which typically show local invasion
  - ➢ full range of differentiation of normal thymus incl. medullary islands containing HC
  - ➢ well-formed lobules, thin septa, lymphocyte rich (immature T-cells)
  - ➢ epithelial cells (and nucleoli) are smaller than in cortical thymoma
- Cortical (Type B2)
  - ➢ invasion is the rule
  - ➢ lobular architecture, medullary differentiation much less obvious
  - ➢ large epithelial cells with prominent eosinophilic nucleoli
  - ➢ epidermoid differentiation at periphery of lobules
  - ➢ immature lymphocytes (fewer than B1) and lymphoid follicles (esp. with MG)
- WDTC (Type B3)
  - ➢ sheets of large epithelial cells with a squamous quality (± keratin) and mitoses and mild atypia
  - ➢ sclerosis is prominent
  - ➢ palisading along septa and around perivascular serum lakes
  - ➢ small numbers of immature T-cells
  - ➢ spindle cell variants can mimic medullary but cells are large with mild cytological atypia
  - ➢ lack pericellular reticulin (*cf.* type A)

Invasive thymoma
- Lobular organoid infiltration into fat / surrounding tissue
- 'Naked' lobules (lack a surrounding fibrous mantle)

Thymic Carcinoma
- Cytological atypia
- CD5 +ve epithelial cells occur in 60–80% of cases
- C-kit +ve epithelial cells (membranous) in 86% (−ve in d/dg thymoma)
- Usual type is SCC: ➢ lacks immature thymic lymphocytes
  - ➢ has prominent intercellular bridges
  - ➢ shows a desmoplastic response when invading
  - ➢ has an infiltrative (*cf.* pushing) invasive margin
  - ➢ tumour cell islands separated by fibrous septa (i.e. some organoid features)
- d/dg WDTC – see points above
- d/dg 2° SCC: has more tendency to necrosis, less organoid, CD5 −ve, clinical Hx
- d/dg borderline thymic epithelial tumour (atypical thymoma) – features in between thymic carcinoma and thymoma (rare)
- Other types include: lymphoepithelioma-like, sarcomatoid / carcinosarcoma, basaloid, clear cell, mu-coepidermoid, etc.

Other Mediastinal / Thymic Mass Lesions

- Lymphomas: Hodgkin's (esp. NSHL), T-ALL, DLBCL (sclerosing)
- Castleman's disease
- Carcinoid (often atypical ± Cushing's syndrome)
- Germ cell tumours (teratoma, seminoma, YST)
- Thymolipoma
- Thymic hyperplasia
- Cysts, incl. congenital ± PEH (! d/dg thymoma/carcinoma/carcinoid arising in the wall)

Bibliography

Arnold, W.J., Laissue, J.A., Friedmann, I. and Naumann, H.H. (eds) (1987) *Diseases of the Head and Neck: An atlas of histopathology*, 1st edn, Thieme Medical Publishers Inc., NY.

Attanoos, R. (2005) Pitfalls in pulmonary pathology. *Current Diagnostic Pathology*, **11** (1), 45–51.

Attanoos, R. L., Galateau-Salle, F., Gibbs, A. R., *et al.* (2002) Primary thymic epithelial tumours of the pleura mimicking malignant mesothelioma. *Histopathology*, **41** (1), 42–49.

Attanoos, R.L. and Gibbs, A.R. (2003) Asbestos-related neoplasia, in *Recent Advances in Histopathology*, vol. 20 (eds. D. Lowe and J.C.E. Underwood), Royal Society of Medicine Press Ltd, London, pp.73–87.

Attanoos, R.L. and Gibbs, R.A. (1997) Pathology of mesothelioma. *Histopathology*, **30**, 403–418.

Bacon, C.M., Du, M-Q. and Dogan, A. (2007) Mucosa-associated lymphoid tissue (MALT) lymphoma: a practical guide for pathologists. *Journal of Clinical Pathology*, **60** (4), 361–372.

Burke, A. and Virmani, R. (1996) Evaluation of pulmonary hypertension in biopsies of the lung. *Current Diagnostic Pathology*, **3** (1), 14–26.

Butnor, K.J. (2006) My approach to the diagnosis of mesothelial lesions. *Journal of Clinical Pathology*, **59** (6), 564–574.

Corrin, B. (1997) Neuroendocrine neoplasms of the lung. *Current Diagnostic Pathology*, **4** (4), 239–250.

Corrin, B. (1996) Unusual tumours and tumour-like conditions of the lung. *Current Diagnostic Pathology*, **3** (1), 1–13.

Corrin, B. and Nicholson, A. (2006) *Pathology of the Lungs*, 2nd edn, Churchill Livingstone, NY.

Craighead, J.E., Abraham, J.L., Churg, A. *et al.* (1982) The pathology of asbestos-associated diseases of the lung and pleural cavities: diagnostic criteria and proposed grading schema. *Archives of Pathology and Laboratory Medicine*, **106** (11), 544–596.

Crouch, E., Churg, A. (1984) Ferruginous bodies and the histologic evaluation of dust exposure. *American Journal of Surgical Pathology*, **8** (2), 109–116.

De Vuyst, P., Karjalainen, A., Dumortier, P. *et al.* (1998) Guidelines for mineral fibre analyses in biological samples. Report of the ERS Working Group. *European Respiratory Journal*, **11** (6), 1416–1426.

Dunhill, M.S. (1987) *Pulmonary Pathology*, 2nd edn, Churchill Livingstone, Edinburgh.

Flieder, D.B. (2004) Recent advances in the diagnosis of adenocarcinoma: the impact of lung cancer screening on histopathologists. *Current Diagnostic Pathology*, **10** (4), 269–278.

Forrester, J., Steele, A., Waldron, J. and Parsons, P. (1990) Crack lung: an acute pulmonary syndrome with a spectrum of clinical and histopathologic findings. *American Review of Respiratory Disease*, **142** (2), 462–467.

Gosney, J.R. (1994) Endocrine pathology of the lung, in *Recent Advances in Histopathology*, vol. 16 (eds. P.P Anthony, R.N.M. MacSween and D.G. Lowe), Churchill Livingstone, Edinburgh, pp.147–166.

Hasleton, P.S. (1998) Current developments in lung cancer, in *Progress in Pathology*, vol. 4 (eds. N. Kirkham and N.R. Lemoine), Churchill Livingstone, Edinburgh, pp.165–177.

Hasleton, P.S. (2001) New WHO classification of lung tumours, in *Recent Advances in Histopathology*, vol. 19 (eds. D. Lowe and J.C.E. Underwood), Churchill Livingstone, Edinburgh, pp.115–129.

Hasleton, P.S. and Roberts, T.E. (1999) Adult respiratory distress syndrome – an update. *Histopathology*, **34**, 285–294.

Henderson, D.W., Shilkin, K.B. and Whitaker, D. (1998) Reactive mesothelial hyperplasia *vs.* mesothelioma, including mesothelioma in situ. *American Journal of Clinical Pathology*, **110** (3), 397–404.

Karjalainen, A., Nurminen, M., Vanhala, E., Vainio, H. and Anttila, S. (1996) Pulmonary asbestos bodies and asbestos fibers as indicators of exposure. *Scandinavian Journal of Work, Environment & Health*, **22** (1), 34–38.

Katzenstein, A-L. and Myers, J.L. (1998) Idiopathic pulmonary fibrosis – clinical relevance of pathologic classification. *American Journal of Respiratory Critical Care Medicine*, **157** (4, part one), 1301–1315.

Knight, B. (1983) *The Coroner's Autopsy*, 1st edn, Churchill Livingstone, Edinburgh.

Kon, O.M., Redhead, J.B.G., Gillen. D. *et al.* (1996) "Crack lung" caused by an impure preparation. *Thorax*, **51** (9), 959–960.

Llinaris, K., Escande, F., Aubert, S. *et al.* (2004) Diagnostic value of MUC4 immunostaining in distinguishing epithelial mesothelioma and lung adenocarcinoma. *Modern Pathology*, **17** (2), 150–157.

MacSweeney, F., Papagiannopoulos, K., Goldstraw *et al.* (2003) An assessment of the expanded classification of congenital cystic adenomatoid malformation and their relationship to malignant transformation. *American Journal of Surgical Pathology*, **27** (8), 1139–1146.

McCaughy, W.T.E., Kannerstein, M. and Churg, J. (1983) Tumors and pseudotumors of the serous membranes. *Atlas of Tumor Pathology Fascicle No. 20*, 2nd edn, Armed Forces Institute of Pathology, Washington DC.

Miettinen, M. and Sarlomo-Rikala, M. (2003) Expression of calretinin, thrombomodulin, Keratin 5, and mesothelin in lung carcinomas of different types. *American Journal of Surgical Pathology*, **27** (2), 150–158.

Mooi, W.J. and Grünberg, K. (2006) Histopathology of pulmonary hypertensive diseases. *Current Diagnostic Pathology*, **12** (6), 409–450.

Müller-Hermelink, H.K., Marx, A. and Kirchner, Th. (1994) Advances in the diagnosis and classification of thymic epithelial tumours, in *Recent Advances in Histopathology*, vol. 16 (eds. P.P. Anthony, R.N.M. MacSween and D.G Lowe), Churchill Livingstone, Edinburgh, pp. 49–72.

Nicholson, A.G. (2000) Pulmonary lymphoproliferative disorders. *Current Diagnostic Pathology*, **6** (2), 130–139.

Nicholson, A.G. and Corrin, B. (1997) Pulmonary lymphoproliferative disorders, in *Recent Advances in Histopathology*, vol. 17 (eds. P.P. Anthony, R.N.M. MacSween and D.G. Lowe), Churchill Livingstone, Edinburgh, pp. 47–68.

Ordóñez, N.G. (1999) Role of immunohistochemistry in differentiating epithelial mesothelioma from adenocarcinoma. *American Journal of Clinical Pathology*, **112**, (1), 75–89.

Pan, C-C., Chen, P.C-H. and Chian, H. (2004) KIT (CD117) is frequently overexpressed in thymic carcinomas but is absent in thymomas. *Journal of Pathology*, **202** (3), 375–381.

Pelosi, G., Rodriguez, J., Viale, G. and Rosai, J. (2005) Typical and atypical pulmonary carcinoid tumor overdiagnosed as small-cell carcinoma on biopsy specimens. *American Journal of Surgical Pathology*, **29** (2), 179–187.

Rice, A.J., Wells, A.U. and Nicholson, A.G. (2003) The classification of interstitial pneumonias, in *Progress in Pathology*, vol. 6 (eds N. Kirkham and N. Shepherd), Greenwich Medical Media Ltd, London, pp. 51–77.

Roggli, V.L., Pratt, P.C. (1983) Numbers of asbestos bodies on iron-stained tissue sections in relation to asbestos body counts in lung tissue digests. *Human Pathology*, **14** (4), 355–361.

Sheppard, M.N. and Nicholson, A. (1995) The role of trans-bronchial and open lung biopsies in non-neoplastic lung disease, in *Progress in Pathology*, vol. 2 (eds N. Kirkham and N. Lemoine), Churchill Livingstone, Edinburgh, pp. 13–30.

Stocker, J.T. (2002) Congenital pulmonary airway malformation – a new name for and an expanded classification of congenital cystic adenomatoid malformation of the lung. *Histopathology*, **41** (Suppl), 424–431.

Symmers, W. St. C. (ed) (1976) *Systemic Pathology*, Vol. 1, 2nd edn, Churchill Livingstone, London.

Tomashefski Jr., J.F. and Felo, J.A. (2004) The pulmonary pathology of illicit drug and substance abuse. *Current Diagnostic Pathology*, **10** (5), 413–426.

Travis, W.D., Colby, T.V., Shimosato, Y. and Brambilla, E. (1999) *Histological Typing of Lung and Pleural Tumours (WHO: International Histological Classification of Tumours)*, 3rd edn, Springer-Verlag, Berlin.

Underwood, J.C.E. (1981) *Introduction to Biopsy Interpretation and Surgical Pathology*, 1st edn, Springer-Verlag, Berlin.

Wallace, W.A.H. and Lamb, D. (1996) Cryptogenic fibrosing alveolitis: a clinico-pathological entity. *Current Diagnostic Pathology*, **3** (1), 27–34.

Wick, M.R. and Ritter, J.H. (2002) Neuroendocrine neoplasms: evolving concepts and terminology. *Current Diagnostic Pathology*, **8** (2), 102–112.

Wright, C. (2006) Congenital malformations of the lung. *Current Diagnostic Pathology*, **12** (3), 191–201.

Yaziji, H., Battifora, H., Barry, T.S. *et al.* (2006) Evaluation of 12 antibodies for distinguishing epithelioid mesothelioma from adenocarcinoma: identification of a three-antibody immunohistochemical panel with maximal sensitivity and specificity. *Modern Pathology*, **19** (4), 514–523.

9. Bone Marrow

Normal Ranges for Trephines

Cellularity

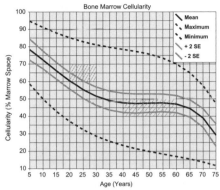

FIGURE 9.1 Bone marrow cellularity

- The curves are a 4th order polynomial regression fit to data from Hartsock *et al.*, 1965 (177 cases).
- This was an autopsy study of sudden death victims and used large chunks of bone from the anterior iliac crest – not trephines.
- They estimated % marrow space occupied by cellular marrow using point-counting volumetry using only 4 points per ×430 field (≈ ×40 objective), and measured many hundreds of fields per case
- They noted much variation from field to field (! this has implications for applying these ranges to trephine cores).
- The shaded boxes show the normal ranges for 2 age groups from more recent data collated by Thiele *et al.*, 2005.

Reticulin

TABLE 9.1 Grading bone marrow reticulin

Grade	Features
0	no staining
N	an occasional fine individual fibre
1	focal fine fibre network (in <50% of section)
2	fine fibre network (in >50% of section); coarse fibres are absent
3	diffuse network, occasional coarse fibres; mature collagen is absent
4	diffuse network, many coarse fibres and mature collagen present

- Based on Bauermeister, 1971 (121 cases)
- This study used mostly Gomori-stained paraffin-embedded bone fragments recovered from *aspirates* – not trephine. Hence the area of tissue is much smaller than a trephine (! this has implications for interpreting terms such as 'diffuse' and 'focal' coverage and 'covering most of the section' i.e. >50%)
- The normal range is grade 0–2; grading should only be done in cellular, haematopoietic areas
- Grade 3 (= 'reticulin fibrosis') may not be obvious on H&E whereas grade 4 usu. is obvious and may show ectatic sinusoids and streaming of haemopoietic cells

- Definition of 'mature collagen' is:
  - ➢ stainable with Masson's trichrome
  - ➢ shows birefringence with polarised light
  - ➢ thick, wavy fibres (obvious on H&E)
- Pitfalls:
  - ➢ thick coarse fibres are normal around bone spicules and vessels (even mature collagen around vessels is normal)
  - ➢ reactive grade 4 fibrosis can be seen at the site of a previous Bx.
  - ➢ falsely low scores may be obtained from fatty (non-cellular) or oedematous areas
- Causes of marrow fibrosis ± new bone formation usu. fall into:
  - ➢ abnormal infiltrates: haematological (MPD, MDS – esp. if 2° to alkylating agents, lymphomas – esp. HL, leukaemias – esp. AML M7), mastocytosis, HX, carcinomas, etc.
  - ➢ inflam[y] / reactive: post chemo/radioRx, infection, GVHD, granulomatous inflam[n], PSS, SLE etc.
  - ➢ metabolic diseases e.g. ↑PTH, ↓vitamin D, Gaucher's disease

Iron
- Iron is lost from a trephine Bx during decalcification so should be assessed (and graded) on the aspirate.
- Perls' on a separate (non-decalcified) clot may give useful information.
- Perls' on trephines are useful where the aspirate is inadequate for iron assessment (i.e. < 7 particles).
- The result of Perls' on a trephine cannot be graded – state if iron is present / appears increased (you should not state that iron is absent, only that Perls' is negative).

Diagnostic Criteria Handbook in Histopathology: A Surgical Pathology Vade Mecum by Paul J. Tadrous
Copyright © 2007 by John Wiley & Sons, Ltd.

Mast Cell Immunocytochemistry / Enzyme Histochemistry
- +ve for: CD43, CD45, CD68, CD117 (c-kit), CD138 (= Syndecan-1, B-B4)
- +ve for: mast cell tryptase (is the most specific), lysozyme, α_1AT and α_1ACT
- +ve for: vimentin and S100
- CAE +ve (but PMN myelocytes are also +ve, so do MPO as well)
- TRAP +ve in 67% of mastocytosis cases
- +ve for: CD2 and CD25 in mastocytosis (but not normal mast cells — as shown by flow cytometry)
- −ve for: MPO, MUM1, CD14, CD15, CD3, CD20

> *NB*: Enzyme histochemical stains like CAE may not work in decalcified tissue.

Plasma Cell Immunocytochemistry
- Usu. −ve: LCA (CD45), CD20, PAX5
- Variably +ve: CD79a
- Usu. +ve: Syndecan-1 (CD138, B-B4), CD38, p63 (vs38c[1]), cytoplasmic Ig
- Benign: CD19 +ve, CD56 −ve, CD58 −ve
- Malignant: CD19 −ve, CD56 +ve, CD58 +ve; also ±ve for c-kit (CD117), CD20 and CD28
- CD20 +ve myeloma may be PAX5 +ve; plasma cell leukaemia may be CD56 −ve
- CD30 and EMA positivity are more common in benign plasma cells *cf.* myeloma
- cyclin D1 (PRAD1, Bcl-1) nuclear +vity occurs in myeloma with t(11;14)[2]
- CD45RO (UCHL1) +ve myeloma have a worse prognosis

Megaloblastic Anaemia
- Hypercellularity – may be marked with loss of fat spaces → AML-like 'packed marrow'
- Marked erythroid hyperplasia with predominance of early blasts (!d/dg AML) and megaloblasts[3]
- Megakaryocytes (hypersegmented) may be present in normal or reduced numbers
- Giant metamyelocytes are esp. helpful when megaloblastic change is inconspicuous due to Fe deficiency
- d/dg AML: in megaloblastic anaemia the cells are erythroid[4], there is preserved arch. and giant metamyelocytes; the blood film[5] and aspirate may also help.
- Islands of early erythroblasts → d/dg carcinoma / ALIPs (an ALIP is a cluster of usu. ≥4 myeloid precursors in a central location away from the trabeculae) – do immuno to confirm erythroid nature

HIV
- Cellularity ↑/↓
- Serous atrophy of fat (gelatinous transformation)
- Reticulin fibrosis ('streaming' of cells)
- Lineages:
  - erythroid: large, poorly-formed islands ± megaloblasts
  - myeloid: ± infection response (↑granulocytes and left shift) } ! d/dg MDS
  - megakaryocytes: ↑numbers, bare nuclei, clustering, dysplasia
  - (a *cluster* of megakaryocytes is usu. defined as ≥4 megas in contact)
- Opportunistic infections
  - granulomas: TB, *Histoplasma, Leishmania, Cryptococcus, Toxoplasma*
  - focal necrosis → think *Cryptococcus*
  - Gaucher-like cells → think MAI
  - epithelioid angiomatosis → think bacillary angiomatosis
  - *Pneumocystis*
- Lymphoid proliferations
  - polymorphous lymphocytic aggregates incl. eos. (! d/dg T-cell lymphoma)
  - reactive plasmacytosis / myeloma
  - malignancies: HL, DLBCL, Burkitt lymphoma, KS
  - Castleman's disease
- d/dg MDS or MPD (*q.v.*)

---

[1] vs38c recognises the endoplasmic reticulum-assoc[d] p63 antigen which is not the same as the basal cell nuclear marker which is also called p63.

[2] 60% of myeloma patients have translocations of the Ig heavy chain gene at 14q; t(11;14) is the commonest.

[3] megaloblasts are cells with cytoplasmic maturation (haemoglobinisation) and nuclear immaturity.

[4] AML M6 can be a problem ∴ rely on the other features described.

[5] but a film may show leukoerythroblastic reaction due to infection, etc. so raise suspicion of AML.

Spindle Cells in Fibrotic Bone Marrow
- Any cause of severe fibrosis will cause a spindly effect or 'streaming' of cells
- Systemic mastocytosis shows paratrabecular spindled cells (c-kit and mast cell tryptase +ve)
- Myeloma, lymphomas, carcinomas (esp. RCC)
- MPD tending towards myelofibrosis
- HIV marrow with fibrosis

Reactive Lymphoid Follicles / Infiltrates
- Reactive aggregates (! which are common after Rx for lymphoma) are suggested by:
  - sharp circumscription (stellate borders or loose arrangement with cells streaming off into the interstitium favour a malignant infiltrate). Stellate borders are typical of splenic MZL mets – which may also show germinal centres
  - non-paratrabecular location (and esp. if perivascular)
  - mixture of cells (Mϕ, plasma cells, eos.) with B-cells (predom. small and mature) and admixed T-cells ++
  - presence of a central arteriole / germinal centre (but ! d/dg mets from a splenic MZL – some pathologists say the presence of a germinal centre should prompt suspicion of lymphoma)
  - assoc[d] with lipid granulomas and reactive plasmacytosis
- Reactive dispersed lymphocytes are usu. in a ≥4:1 ratio of T-cells:B-cells
- Associat[ns]: ↑age, infection, inflam[n]/autoimmunity (RhA, SLE, thyroid), Castleman's, post BMTx
- Extensive / florid in AIDS or phenytoin reaction
- Rarer causes:
  - thymoma: interstitial and nodular *T-cell* infiltrate
  - persistent polyclonal B-cell lymphocytosis (of middle-aged female smokers, RhA, Gaucher's or hyposplenics): interstitial and intravascular infiltrate ± binucleate lymphocytes; (! some may be Bcl-2 and FMC7 +ve with t(14;18)); −ve for CD23, CD5 and CD43

Histiocytosis (Reactive)
- Any condition assoc[d] with marrow hyperplasia or ineffective haemopoiesis
- Any condition assoc[d] with granulomas
- Any condition assoc[d] with haemophagocytosis (± granulomas, ± haemophagocytic syndrome)
- Post GM-CSF Rx (e.g. molgramostim) or at presentation of ALL

Granulomas
- Lipid granulomas are common and of no clinical significance *per se* but the vacuoles may be so small so as to mimic sarcoid / other epithelioid granulomas from which they must be distinguished
- Ring (doughnut) granulomas: empty space surrounded by PMN, lymphocytes, histiocytes and fibrinoid seen in Q fever – also HL, IM, typhoid (and CMV in immunosuppressed patients)
- Drug-induced granulomas: usu. poorly formed lymphohistiocytic-type with eos. ± vasculitis
- Foamy Mϕ containing: MAI, typhoid, Leprosy
- Other bugs include: TB (± necrotising), Brucella, Histoplasma (small ± necrotising), Cryptococcus, Leishmania, Toxoplasma (for more on morphology, see Chapter 23: Infection and Immunity)
- Malignancies: myeloma (involved marrow), lymphomas (also uninvolved marrow), carcinomas
- Foreign bodies: talc, silicosis, berylliosis, anthracosis

Haemophagocytic Syndrome
- Clin: peripheral cytopenias, hepatosplenomegaly and fever
- Malignant histiocytosis: sheets of mitotic Mϕ, ± monocytes}mild haemophagocytosis
- Reactive: infections, malignancies (incl. lymphoid, esp. T), familial}marked haemophagocytosis
- Erythrophagocytosis (only) may be due to anti-RBC Abs

Mast Cell Infiltrates and Systemic Mastocytosis
- See p100 for mast cell staining properties (see p.229 for cutaneous mastocytoses)
- Assoc[d] with fibroplasia of any cause e.g. fracture callus, MPD, MDS and also AML/CGL
- Mast cells ↑ in infection, renal failure, lymphoproliferations and aplastic anaemia
- Bony trabeculae may be wide and irregular or thinned with ↑ osteoclasts
- distribution of mast cell aggregates: paratrabecular, perivascular, interstitial ('pseudogranulomas')

- The mast cells are assoc[d] with eosinophils, lymphocytes, plasma cells and MPD-like hyperplasias (e.g. granulocytic)
- d/dg MPD, CGL, LPL[6], AITCL, hairy cell leukaemia[7], granulomas, HL
- *Systemic mastocytosis* (prog. $\propto$ cellularity) defined as EITHER 1 major + 1 minor OR 3 minor criteria:
  - ➢ major criterion: multiple aggregates (of ≥ 15 mast cells per aggregate) in marrow +/ other non-skin sites [mast cells must be confirmed by special stains]
  - ➢ minor criteria:
    - ☞ >25% of all mast cells are atypical (spindled / immature / hypogranular / epithelioid with irregular nuclei – ! d/dg Mϕ)
    - ☞ a specific KIT point mutation is present
    - ☞ mast cells co-express CD117 with CD2 +/ CD25
    - ☞ serum total tryptase is >20 ng/ml (in the absence of a clonal myeloid disorder)
- Variants: many are defined by the WHO using clinicopathological criteria; the histological components are:
  1. % marrow infiltration (esp. if >30%)
  2. presence of non-mast cell myeloproliferation not amounting to a neoplasm by WHO criteria
  3. presence of a non-mast cell MDS, MPD, lymphoma, AML, other haemolymph neoplasm
  4. mast cell cytology grade (high/low) ⎫ e.g. *Mast Cell Sarcoma* is defined as a solitary, high grade
  5. destructive growth pattern ⎬ destructive lesion without systemic / cutaneous mastocytosis.
- Types of mastocytic marrow infiltration (Horny, Parwaresch & Lennert, 1985):
  - I focal infiltrate with normal background marrow ($\approx$ 'benign systemic mastocytosis', usu. with urticaria pigmentosa)
  - II focal with fat loss and either granulocytic hyperplasia or ↑ blasts ($\approx$ 'malignant mastocytosis')
  - III diffuse replacement with fat loss and haemopoietic hypoplasia ($\approx$ 'mast cell leukaemia' – has PB changes)

Chronic Idiopathic Myelofibrosis in the Cellular Phase
- Hyperplasia of all three cell lineages
- Retic only mildly ↑
- Megas: large and hyperlobated

Grading Myelofibrosis (Thiele *et al.*, 2005)
MF0 – sparse linear fibres, none crossing, no collagen
MF1 – loose mesh with many crossovers, no collagen
MF2 – dense mesh, minor foci of collagen ± osteosclerosis
MF3 – dense mesh, significant collagen + osteosclerosis

Myelodysplasia (MDS)
- Histologically (*cf.* cytology and cytogenetics) this is a diagnosis of exclusion
- Hypercellular (usu.) or hypocellular marrow with peripheral cytopenias, Pelger-Huet anomaly, etc.
- Deranged architecture:
  - ➢ erythroid islands poorly formed / very large   ① round nucleoli on Giemsa
  - ➢ myeloid ALIP – distinguished from erythroid by[8] ⇐ ② glycophorin C / spectrin −ve
  - ➢ megas: clustering / paratrabecular   ③ CD68 / MPO / PMN elastase +ve
- Deranged cytology
  - ➢ erythroid: megaloblastic / multinucleated / mulberry nuclear budding / ringed sideroblasts
  - ➢ myeloid: hypogranular PMN, acquired Pelger-Huet anomaly / Auer rods
  - ➢ megas: hypolobated megas and micromegakaryocytes (esp. useful if $< 30\mu$ $\varnothing$)
- Apoptoses ++
- Reticulin fibrosis   ➢ more common in 2° MDS / CMML
                        ➢ correlates with   ① megakaryocyte numbers and atypia
                                            ② poor prognosis and cytogenetics
- Reactive changes: lymphoid follicles, siderophages post transfusion, etc.
- d/dg hypocellular MDS *vs.* aplastic anaemia or hypoplastic AML
- d/dg HIV (*q.v.*) or the effects of drugs (e.g. methotrexate or arsenic)

Polycythaemia Rubra Vera (PRV)
- ↑(Hb, RBC, PMN, platelets), hepatosplenomegaly; → myelofibrosis +/ AML
- Marked ↑cellularity ($\geq 90\%$)

---

[6] LPL often has an accompanying reactive mast cell infiltrate which may be mis-called 'mastocytosis'.
[7] esp. when the mastocytosis cells are evenly-spaced, not spindly and +ve for TRAP and CD25.
[8] *NB:* Glycophorin C is recognised by the antibody ret40f.

- Hyperplastic erythropoiesis with normal morphology (granulopoiesis also ↑)
- Pleomorphic megas (large polylobated to micromegas), clustering, emperipolesis
- Mild retic ↑ in early stages which may progress to myelofibrosis
- Increased numbers of sinusoids and dilated sinusoids

Secondary Polycythaemia
- No hepatosplenomegaly
- Only moderate ↑cellularity
- Normal megas, retic and sinusoids

Essential Thrombocythaemia
- Sustained ↑platelets to >600 × 10^9/l; normal to moderately ↑cellularity
- Megas: ↑ nõ., ↑ size, well-spaced nuclear lobes ('staghorn nucleus') loose clustering, paratrabecular (not pleomorphic with micromegakaryocytes as in PRV)

Idiopathic (Immune) Thrombocytopenic Purpura (ITP)
- Bone marrow Bx indicated prior to steroid Rx to rule out underlying lymphoma (esp. ALL)
- Normocellular with ↑numbers of megas
- Megas are of ↓size overall with some giant forms. No abnormal architecture

Marrow Eosinophilia with Maturation
- May be due to infection, allergy, drugs, CML[9], Hodgkin/T-cell lymphoma
- May be due to aberrant T-cell clone[10] with no morphological evidence of lymphoma
- May be idiopathic – a proportion later present with AML M2-Eo / CML ∴ F/U required

Acute Myeloid Leukaemia (AML)
- Replacement of marrow and fat by blasts (≥20%) ± necrosis
- May show signs of maturation (e.g. Charcot-Leyden crystals and eosinophil granules in AML M2-Eo)
- FAB classification:
  - ➤ M0 minimally diff (MPO −ve, some myeloid Ag +ve)
  - ➤ M1 without maturation (minority MPO +ve, myeloid Ag +ve)
  - ➤ M2 with maturation (incl. M2-Baso and M2-Eo subtypes)
  - ➤ M3 promyelocytic (hyper or hypogranular variants)
  - ➤ M4 myelomonocytic (PB monocytes, marrow looks like M2)
  - ➤ M5 monocytic (M5a PB promonocytes / monoblasts, M5b PB monocytes)
  - ➤ M6 erythroleukaemia
  - ➤ M7 megakaryocytic (± myelofibrosis)

> *NB*: Monoblasts are −ve for MPO but NSEst +ve. Megakaryoblasts and lymphoblasts are MPO −ve.

- WHO Classification:
  - ➤ AML with recurrent cytogenetic anomalies
  - ➤ AML with multilineage dysplasia (± preceding MDS, MPD)
  - ➤ AML related to Rx
  - ➤ AML NOS (includes most of the FAB groups plus acute panmyelosis with myelosclerosis)

Post-Treatment Effects (The Recovering Marrow)

Toxic myelopathy (post chemoRx / radioRx)
- ↑ Fe in stromal cells and ↑ siderophages – fading with time
- Granular proteinaceous degeneration of the stroma and transient ↑reticulin (lasting ≈ 2 months)
- Dissolution of adipose with multiloculated adipocytes and foamy Mφ
- Bone necrosis, woven bone and reactive granulomas
- Haemopoietic hypocellularity

Haemopoietic recovery
- Occurs first at ≈ 1 week and in areas of stromal (esp. adipose) recovery
- Cellularity increases non-linearly (≈ power law) to normal by 1 month
- First to appear are the erythroid (tight colonies) +/ myeloid (loose colonies) as immature blasts in a linear formation. Mixed colonies appear later. There may be dysmorphic features due to Rx
- Megas are usu. the last to regenerate (as scattered islands) though some may be found earlier

---

[9] CML must be excluded by blood cytogenetics.
[10] Detectable by T-cell cytogenetics.

Residual disease

- AML:
    - ➤ !do not misdiagnose erythroid blasts as recurrent AML (do spectrin/glycophorin)
    - ➤ numerous MPO +ve blasts in the first week is indicative of recurrent disease
    - ➤ regenerating promyelocytes have regular smooth oval nucleoli (do MPO to ensure you are looking at myeloid cells and not erythroid)
    - ➤ lymphomas: use immuno to detect non-haemopoietic lineages e.g. Tdt, CD30, etc. for lymphomas and ! do not misdiagnose CD10 +ve stromal cells as recurrent ALL
- Distinguish MDS *vs.* chemo/radioRx atypia: persistence of changes beyond 1 month favour MDS
- Distinguish CML / MPD *vs.* regenerative hyperplasia

Plasmacytosis (Reactive)

- 10–20% of nucleated cells (rarely upto 50%) with small aggregates but no monotypic nodules
- Polytypic: κ:λ = 2.5:1 (which, incidentally, is same ratio of κ to λ myelomas)
- Pericapillary and peri-Mφ distribution
- Inclusions (Russell, Mott, thesaurocytes, flaming), binucleate, sparsely nucleolated forms, Dutcher [11]
- Assoc^d changes: lymphoid aggregates, granulocytic hyperplasia, ↑Mφ (incl. haemophagocytic)
- Assoc^d conditions: HIV, infections, chronic inflam^n e.g. RhA, DM, cirrhosis, malignancies[12]
- PB plasmacytosis is unusual and often light
- d/dg myeloma: κ:λ > 10:1 or λ:κ > 5:1 suggests a neoplastic infiltrate

Plasma Cell Myeloma (incl. Multiple Myeloma, Plasmacytoma and Plasma Cell Leukaemia)

- WHO def^n: *EITHER* 1 major + 1 minor criterion *OR* the first 2 + 1 other minor criteria:
  Major: A) Bx-proven plasmacytoma, B) >30% plasma cells (on aspirate), C) very high paraprotein[13]
  Minor: ① >10% plasma cells, ② high paraprotein, ③ bone lesions, ④ ↓ normal serum Ig to <50%
- *Indolent myeloma* = as above but with ① no infections ② ≤ 3 lytic bone lesions and no compression fractures, ③ normal serum [Ca^{2+}] and renal funct^n and ④ paraprotein at lower end of myeloma ranges
- Outcome: *refractory myeloma* ± leukaemia, DLBCL[14], 2° MDS / AML. Death is usu. by infection
- Homogeneous nodules of monotypic plasma cells, paratrabecular infiltrates and cytological atypia favour myeloma
- Atypia incl. plasmablasts[15], multinucleation ++, multinucleolation ++, inclusions (either Dutcher bodies or cytoplasmic inclusions e.g. crystals, Mott cells, Russell bodies)
- Amyloid: vascular / interstitial
- Immuno: see separate section on plasma cell immuno above
- Prognosis ∝   ① Stage (pattern and extent of infiltration)
  ② Grade (% plasma blasts)
  and is worse if there is ↑vascularity +/↑ osteoclastic activity +/ t(4;14)(p16;q32)

TABLE 9.2 Myeloma stage & grade

Stage	Grade
interstitial	1 (<10%)
nodular	2
packed	3 (>50%)

- d/dg ALCL / anaplastic carcinoma *vs.* anaplastic myeloma: use CPC and a broad immuno-panel as all three may be CD138, CD30 and EMA +ve:
    - ➤ ALCL : CD45, CD20 / T-cell, ALK +ve and *cytoplasmic* Ig −ve (occ. CK +ve)
    - ➤ carcinoma: CK +ve, vs38c −ve, κλ −ve
- d/dg spindle cell myeloma *vs.* other spindle cell infiltrates: do immuno for plasma cells (*vide supra*)
- d/dg myeloma *vs.* LPL / other NHL with plasmacytic differentiation: these will show a range of cytological differentiation to include small lymphocytes, but myeloma has >90% plasma cell purity (by morphology or CD138)
- d/dg Hodgkin lymphoma (*vide infra*)
- d/dg reactive: need CPC / κλ immuno as some reactive (e.g. HIV) have sheets of plasma cells
- d/dg MGUS has a minimal reactive-like infiltrate, κ:λ ratio is usu. <16 either way (myeloma is >16 and usu. >100) – see also the WHO clinicopathological definition of MGUS, below

---

[11] Dutcher bodies are more characteristic of neoplastic infiltrates but are not exclusive to neoplasia.

[12] In HL you can get nodules of plasma cells with fibrosis suggestive of myeloma.

[13] The definitions of 'very high' and 'high' for blood and urine paraprotein (also called M-protein) are specified by the WHO (*q.v.*). *NB:* upto 4% of myelomas are non-secretory (have no M-protein).

[14] Immunoblastic type.

[15] Plasmablasts have mature plasma cell cytoplasm with immature nucleus (i.e. nucleoli ± diffuse chromatin).

Monoclonal Gammopathy of Undetermined Significance (MGUS) and Smouldering Myeloma
- MGUS: No lytic bone lesions or myeloma Sx, paraprotein < myeloma levels, <10% plasma cells on aspirate
- *Smouldering myeloma*: as MGUS but paraprotein in myeloma range and plasma cells are 10–30% on aspirate
- Minimal focal infiltration (≈ reactive), κ:λ ratio usu. <16 either way
- Many patients go on to develop myeloma, NHL or 1° (AL) amyloid over 30 years

Lymphomatous / Leukaemic Infiltrates

Adequacy of Bx for assessment
- ≥ 5 well-preserved marrow spaces (but depends on focality of expected disease)

Hairy cell leukaemia (HCL)
- Heavy infiltrate: packed marrow, usu. diffuse (nodules may occur with fibrosis)
- Fine reticulin pattern ('chicken-wire mesh') until late when fibrosis may occur
- Evenly-spaced small lymphocytes with round or bean-shaped nuclei and clear cytoplasm/halos
- Immuno/stains: CD20/79a, TRAP, CD25, DBA44 and cyclin D1 +ve; mitoses are rare
- d/dg mastocytosis (esp. when it is diffuse, non-spindled and TRAP / CD25 +ve) or aplastic anaemia (because HCL can suppress the background marrow and the infiltrate may be light & focal)

ALCL
- Mild dispersed infiltrate or extensive; d/dg IM (EBV and CD30 +ve, ALK −ve)

Follicular lymphoma (FCL)
- Paratrabecular infiltrates 'coat' the trabeculae (but not always and may be fibrotic / hypocellular)
- ! CD10 may be −ve in the marrow
- d/dg: other lymphomas may show this mixed with other patterns; *very rarely* SLE and some infections

Marginal zone lymphoma (incl. Splenic MZL)
- Loose interstitial nodules, intrasinusoidal cords (revealed by CD20: typical, but not specific, for splenic MZL)
- May have stellate shape or germinal centres (nodules are more common after splenectomy in splenic MZL)
- d/dg hepatosplenic γδ TCL can also show a subtle intrasinusoidal pattern with medium-sized lymphocytes

ALL
- Interstitial, monotonous, diffuse
- Immuno: usu. +ve for T/B-cell, CD34, Tdt and CALLA (CD10) [! stromal cells are also CD10 +ve]
- Crenated nuclear envelope, small nucleoli, chromatin more open than mature lymphocytes

CLL
- Interstitial, monotonous nodular (± proliferation centres) and diffuse component
- Richter's transformation: immunoblasts and RS-like large cells ± residual small cell component. At any site, Richter's is a typical DLBCL (solid / sheet-like growth) arising in CLL *cf.* paraimmunoblastic or prolymphocytic transformations of CLL which show a scattered increase in paraimmunoblasts or prolymphocytes (these transformations also have a more aggressive course)

LPL
- Interstitial, monotonous nodules and diffuse component, plasmacytoid differentiation
- Mast cells ++

DLBCL
- Usu. not subtle but subtle infiltrates take the form of intrasinusoidal / intravascular lymphoma cells
- Marrow infiltrate may be of lower grade (e.g. show the features of follicular lymphoma)
- d/dg: dysplastic megas, melanoma, carcinoma, early leukaemia, proliferation centres in CLL

Hodgkin lymphoma (HL)
- Low power recognised as an area of paucicellular fibrosis or dense cellular nodules
- Cellular nodules may be comprised predominantly of plasma cells
- d/dg myeloma – use CPC and look for:
  - admixed cells of other types and other nodules of a more classic mixed cellularity type
  - H/RS cells – these are necessary to diagnose marrow involvement by HL but may need many levels to find. If not found then 'infiltrate suggestive of HL' may be stated.

See also p117.

Bibliography

Anagnostou, D. (2005) Pitfalls in the pattern of bone marrow infiltration in lymphoproliferative disorders. *Current Diagnostic Pathology*, **11** (3), 170–179.

Bain, B.J., Clark, D.M., Lampert, I.A. and Wilkins, B.S. (2001) *Bone Marrow Pathology*, 3rd edn, Blackwell Science Ltd., Oxford.

Bauermeister, D.E. (1971) Quantitation of bone marrow reticulin – a normal range. *American Journal of Clinical Pathology*, **56** (1), 24–31.

Chetty, R., Echezarreta, G., Comley, M. and Gatter, K. (1995) Immunohistochemistry in apparently normal bone marrow trephine specimens from patients with nodal follicular lymphoma. *Journal of Clinical Pathology*, **48** (11), 1035–1038.

Cotran, R.S., Kumar, V. and Collins, T. (eds.) (1999) *Robbins Pathologic Basis of Disease*, 6th edn, W.B. Saunders Co., Philadelphia.

Escribano, L., Beatriz, D.A., Bravo, P. *et al.* (1999) Immunophenotype of bone marrow mast cells in indolent systemic mast cell disease in adults. *Leukaemia Lymphoma*, **35** (3–4), 227–35.

Frisch, B. and Bartl, R. (1997) Fibrosis in the bone marrow: histology and pathogenesis. *Current Diagnostic Pathology*, **4** (1), 36–44.

Hartsock, R.J., Smith, E.B. and Petty, C.S. (1965) Normal variations with aging of the amount of haematopoietic tissue in bone marrow from the anterior iliac crest. *American Journal of Clinical Pathology*, **43** (4), 326–331.

Horny, H.P., Parwaresch, M.R. and Lennert, K. (1985) Bone marrow findings in systemic mastocytosis. *Human Pathology*, **16** (8), 808–814.

Hurwitz, N. (1997) Bone marrow trephine biopsy changes following chemotherapy and/or bone marrow transplantation. *Current Diagnostic Pathology*, **4** (4), 196–202.

Jaffe, E.S., Harris, N.L., Stein, H. and Vardiman, J.W. (eds.) (2001) *WHO Classification of Tumours: Pathology and Genetics Tumours of Haematopoietic and Lymphoid Tissue*, 1st edn, IARC Press, Lyon.

Joshi, A. and Aquel, N.M. (2003) Hodgkin's disease of bone marrow masquerading as a heavy plasma cell infiltration and fibrosis. *British Journal of Haematology*, **122** (3), 343.

Keats, J.J., Reiman, T., Maxwell, C.A., *et al.* (2003) In multiple myeloma t(4;14)(p16;q32) is an adverse prognostic factor irrespective of FGFR3 expression. *Blood*, **101** (4), 1520–1529.

Kroft, S.H. and McKenna, R.W. (1997) Histiocytic disorders involving bone marrow. *Current Diagnostic Pathology*, **4** (4), 203–209.

Müller-Hermelink, H.K., Zettl, A., Pfeifer, W. and Ott, G. (2001) Pathology of lymphoma progression. *Histopathology*, **38** (4), 285–306.

Schmid, C. and Isaacson, P.G. (1992) Bone marrow trephine biopsy in lymphoproliferative disease. *Journal of Clinical Pathology*, **45** (9), 745–750.

Stuart-Smith, S.E., Hughes, D.A and Bain, B.J. (2005) Are routine iron stains on bone marrow trephine biopsy specimens necessary? *Journal of Clinical Pathology*, **58** (3), 269–272.

Thiele, J., Kvasnicka, H.M., Faccetti, F., Franco, V., van der Waalt, J. and Orazi, A. (2005) European consensus on grading bone marrow fibrosis and assessment of cellularity. *Haematologica*, **90** (8), 1128–1132.

Thomas, J. St J. (2004) The diagnosis of lymphoid infiltrates in the bone marrow trephine. *Current Diagnostic Pathology*, **10** (3), 236–245.

Wilkins, B.S. (1995) The bone marrow trephine biopsy: recent progress and current issues, in *Progress in Pathology*, vol. 1 (eds. N. Kirkham, and P.A. Hall), Churchill Livingstone, Edinburgh, pp. 77–97.

Wilkins, B.S. (1997) Simplifying the spleen: a new look at splenic pathology, in *Progress in Pathology*, vol. 3 (eds. N. Kirkham and N.R. Lemoine), Churchill Livingstone, NY, pp. 211–231.

Wilkins, B.S. and Clark, D. (2003) Recent advances in bone marrow pathology, in *Recent Advances in Histopathology*, vol. 20 (eds. D. Lowe and J.C.E. Underwood), Royal Society of Medicine Press Ltd, London, pp. 145–166

10. Lymphoreticular

Normal Ranges in Peripheral Blood

- Total WCC 4–11 $\times 10^9$/l ($\uparrow$ in children upto 18×10^9/l in infants)
- Lymphocytes are 1–4 $\times 10^9$/l (20–45% in the differential count)
- PMN are 40–75% in the differential count
- Eosinophils should not be $>1.5 \times 10^9$/l or persistently $>0.35 \times 10^9$/l

Some Useful Antigens, Stains and Staining Patterns

α_1AT   PMN, mast cells and monocytes / Mϕ

α_1ACT   mast cells and Mϕ

ALK-1   = CD246: ALCL, RMS, NB, DLBCL with full length ALK, inflammatory myofibroblastic tumour

Bcl-1   = PRAD1, Cyclin D1: nuclear stain. +ve in MCL, myeloma and HCL

Bcl-2   memory cells (incl. mantle B-cells and many T-cells), FCL and most large cell (blastic) lymphomas; −ve in normal B-blasts / germinal centre B-cells, spindle cell lipoma, SFT, synovial sarcoma, some epithelia

Bcl-6   nuclear stain for normal and neoplastic germinal centre cells (FCL and a DLBCL subset)

Bcl-10   nuclear +/ cytoplasmic stain for MZL (+ve in ≈45%) esp. gastric & lung MALToma. Also cytoplasmic +vity in normal follicle centre cells (esp. Cb); nuclear +vity in 55% of LPL

CAE   Chloroacetate Esterase (Leder's stain): a histochemical stain for myeloid granules (and mast cell granules but does not stain lymphoid, Mϕ, monocyte or erythroid lineages)

CD1a   Langerhans cells, immature (thymic) T-cells and a poor prognostic subset of T-ALL

CD2, 3, T-cells, CD7 often lost in later stages of mycosis fungoides. Cytotoxic T-cells are +ve for CD8
4, 7, 8 and TIA-1 +/ granzyme B (the latter two are −ve in T-suppressor). CD2 is +ve in abnormal mast cells

CD5   T-cells, some B-cell lymphomas (CLL, MCL), +ve in thymic carcinoma epithelial cells

CD6   germinal centre B cells, a subset of DLBCL

CD10   = CALLA: normal and neoplastic follicle centre B-cells, ALL, Burkitt's, AITCL[1], some DLBCL, PMN, stromal cells (bone marrow and endometrium), myoepithelia, bile canaliculi, non-chromophobe RCC (and an aggressive subset of chromophobe), −ve in AML

CD11a   HCL (NB: CD11a is LFA-1α and it marks all normal leukocytes by flow cytometry)

CD14   Mϕ (see also CD68); −ve in mast cells

CD15   H/RS cells, granulocytic / monocytic, adenocarcinomas (vs. mesothelioma); −ve in mast cells

CD16   NK cells (see also CD56)

CD19   B-cells.

CD20   B-cells and medullary thymoma epithelial cells, usu. −ve in plasma cells and immature B-cells and can fail to stain B-cells in patients who received anti-CD20 Ab Rx (e.g. rituximab). CD20 stains reactive nucleoli / chromocentres in any tissue or tumour (as a cross-reaction)

CD21   FDC

CD22   B-cells and HCL (which may respond to anti-CD22 Rx)

CD23   CLL, normal mantle cells, FDC

CD24   IDC (interdigitating dendritic cells)

CD25   hairy cell leukaemia and HTLV-1 lymphoma

CD30   = Ki-1: activated lymphocytes (T/B), H/RS cells, ALCL, myeloma, some DLBCL, embryonal carcinoma, a poor prognosis subset of mycosis fungoides, LyP, mesothelioma, myeloid sarcoma

CD31   (PECAM-1) linear membranous in endothelia, granular membranous in Mϕ / monocytes

---

[1] most peripheral TCL are CD10 −ve

Diagnostic Criteria Handbook in Histopathology: A Surgical Pathology Vade Mecum by Paul J. Tadrous
Copyright © 2007 by John Wiley & Sons, Ltd.

CD33	myeloid incl. AML (but some ALL and myeloma also +ve), histiocytes +ve; RS-cells −ve
CD34	endothelia (crisp membranous staining), myeloblasts and lymphoblasts (membranous and granular cytoplasmic staining), KS, interstitial dendritic cells of soft tissue (SFT, spindle cell lipoma)
CD35	C3b-receptor: FDC, mantle cell lymphocytes
CD36	dermal dendrocyte subset (dermal dendrocytes are also +ve for FXIIIa)
CD38	plasma cells (see also CD30, CD56, CD138 and vs38c/p63)
CD42b	megakaryocytes, platelets and some precursors / stem cells
CD43	mast cells, most T-cells, CLL, MCL, some LPL but not FCL / MZL (MALToma may be +ve), AML (may be useful in trephines)
CD44	various isoforms said to be useful as markers for various tumours (? significance)
CD45	(CD45RA) = LCA: −ve in H/RS cells in all HL except LPHL. Mast cells are +ve
CD45	(CD45RO) = UCHL1: old marker for T-cells but not specific and no longer widely used
CD56	= NCAM: NK cells, NE differentiation (e.g. small cell / Merkel cell), bile ductules, malignant plasma cells
CD57	= HNK-1, Leu-7: NK cells and some CNS tumours e.g. oligo. Other evidence of NK differentiation is lack of B & T-cell markers (although CD2 may be +ve) and +ve perforin, granzyme B and TIA-1, CD57 is not as specific as CD56 for NE differentiation
CD61	megakaryocytes (= platelet glycoprotein IIIa)
CD63	= NKI-C3: melanoma of reduced metastasis risk, cellular neurothekeoma, monocytes, endothelium
CD68	PGM1 is +ve in Mφ ; KP1 is common to mast cells, Mφ , monocyte, granulocytes, AML, some carcinomas, megakaryocytes, osteoclasts, melanomas and myofibroblasts (e.g. nodular fasciitis)
CD79a	B-cells including early pre-B and plasma cells
CD99	immature (thymic) T-cells, ALL, Ewing's, synovial sarcoma, 50% of Merkel, some osteosarcoma, etc. See also p.16.
CD103	HCL (which is also +ve for CD11c, CD22, CD25, DBA44 and Bcl-1)
CD105	newly formed microvessels (in embryos, tumours and granulation tissue) not mature vessel endothelium
CD117	= c-kit: mast cells, GIST, germ cells and much more (for a list, see p.16)
CD138	= B-B4, syndecan-1: plasma cells, osteoblasts, some epithelia, some large cell NHL
CD146	= Mel-CAM: +ve in intermediate trophoblasts and their tumours
CD171	= L1, N-CAM: related to CD56, this is +ve in 75% of GISTs and some PNST but −ve in smooth muscle tumours and desmoids
CD236	= ret40f, glycophorin C: erythroid precursors (incl. earlier forms *cf.* spectrin)
CD246	(see ALK-1 above)
DBA44	HCL (see also CD103)
EMA	T-cells, some TCL, some myelomas, LPHL (−ve in H/RS cells of classical HL), ALCL, PEL
FMC7	flow cytometric +vity in some B-cell neoplasms (e.g. prolymphocytic leukaemia, HCL) but −ve in CLL
FOX-P1	+ve in the activated peripheral B-cell type of DLBCL (more aggressive)
Granzyme B	marker of cytotoxic function (as are perforin, TIA-1)
Ig Heavy Chains	= IgM/A/D/G/E: characterising some lymphomas (e.g. LPL, IPSID, MZL)
Ig Light Chains	= κ and λ: to assess clonality (both are absent in IPSID)
J-chain	+ve in LPHL
Ki-67	(e.g. using the MIB1 Ab): a nuclear stain for cells in cycle. Detected at all stages of the cell cycle except G0 – not just the division stages. A lymphoma 'progression' marker
LMP	for EBV, a granular cytoplasmic and membranous stain
Lysozyme	PMN, mast cells and monocyte / Mφ
MALT1	variable cytoplasmic +vity in MALTomas, Positive in normal follicle centre cells esp. Cb
MBP	= Eosinophil Major Basic Protein: +ve in eosinophils
MPO	myeloid lineage/PMN and monocyte/Mφ (but not monoblasts, lymphoblasts or megakaryoblasts)

MUM1	= IRF4: melanoma and most lymphomas (B-cell, T-cell, ALCL, classical RS cells, plasma cells / myeloma, activated B subtype of DLBCL), −ve in Burkitt's, mast cell and histiocytic lesions
NP57	= Neutrophil Elastase: myeloid lineage / PMN
NSEst	= non-specific esterase: diffuse cytoplasmic +vity in monoblasts (spotty/Golgi in lymphoblasts)
p24	= an HIV nucleocapsid protein: stains HIV-infected FDC
p53	nuclear stain 'progression marker' in lymphomas
p63	= vs38c: endoplasmic reticulum protein, stains the cytoplasm / membrane of plasma cells, naevocytes and some melanoma cells. ! Do not confuse with the p53-related protein (also called p63) which stains nuclei of basal cells of various epithelia
PAX5	nuclear +vity in pre-B to mature B-cells (incl. lymphomas −ve for CD45, CD20 & CD79a) but may be −ve in plasma cells and CD20 −ve myelomas; −ve in most non-lymphoid neoplasia (except a minority of Merkel and TCC)
perforin	marker of cytotoxic function (see also granzyme B, TIA-1, CD57)
S100	Langerhans cells, IDC, mast cells (for a longer list, see Chapter 2: Histological Techniques)
Tdt	a nuclear stain (cytoplasmic staining should be discounted) for pre-T or pre-B cells
TIA-1	T-cell Intracellular Ag 1: marker of cytotoxic function (see also granzyme B, perforin, CD57)
TRAP	HCL and some mast cells
vs38c	see p63 above (plasma cells, naevocytes, melanoma cells)
Zap-70	+ve in CLL with un-mutated Ig genes (more aggressive than mutated CLL)

Interdigitating Reticulum Cells (= Interdigitating Dendritic Cells, IDC)
- Paracortical histiocytoid cells related to Langerhans cells
- Immuno: +ve for S100, CD24, HLA-DR; −ve for CD1a,3,20,21,30,35,79a
- EM: no desmosomes (unlike FDC) or Birbeck granules

Lymphomas Positive for the Triad–CD30, EMA, CD138
① ALCL, ② anaplastic myeloma, ③ primary effusion lymphoma (PEL)

B-Cell Reactions

Follicular Hyperplasia
- d/dg FCL see under 'Follicular Lymphoma'
- d/dg Hodgkin lymphoma (*vide infra*)
- d/dg progressive transformation of the germinal centres (*vide infra*)
- d/dg RhA (also Felty syndrome) which may show:
  - ➤ florid follicular hyperplasia – may seem to be present throughout the LN – d/dg FCL
  - ➤ ↑ plasma cells in medulla and paracortex
  - ➤ assoc^d with splenic B-cell hyperplasia
- d/dg adult Still's disease (also shows a paracortical T-cell reaction)
- d/dg SLE or other CTD
- d/dg HIV (*vide infra*)
- d/dg toxoplasmosis (for a full list of features, see Chapter 23: Infection and Immunity)
- d/dg leishmaniasis (Leishman-Donovan bodies in epithelioid Mφ – see pp.348–349)
- d/dg drainage of inflammatory sites (CIBD, peptic ulcer, etc.)
- d/dg 1° and 2° syphilis, but these also show:
  - ➤ 1° shows capsulitis with ↑ vascularity and plasma cells
  - ➤ 2° shows fibrotic thickening of capsule and septa
  - ➤ 1° and 2° show ↑ plasma cells and paracortical epithelioid Mφ aggregates
  - ➤ perivascular spirochaetes demonstrable in tissue (!serology may be −ve if HIV co-infection)

Sinus Lymphocytosis (Sinus B-Cell Reaction)
- B-cells (often monocytoid) predominate in sinuses
- Occurs in: prolonged reactive states, toxoplasmosis, HIV, EBV, early stages of some lymphomas
- d/dg CLL or nodal MZL
- d/dg sinus histiocytosis (esp. if monocytoid B-cells)

B-Cell Lymphomas

Small Cell B-cell Lymphomas – Immuno and General Points

TABLE 10.1   Small cell B-cell lymphomas

	CD5	CD10	CD23	Other positive findings
FCL	−	+	−	Bcl-2, Bcl-6, CD21 & CD23 [FDC network], t(14;18)
CLL	+	−	+	± proliferation centres, CD43 +ve
MCL	+	−	−	Bcl-1, t(11;14), crinkly cells, epithelioid Mφ
LPL*	−	−	−	cytoplasmic IgM (not D), epithelioid Mφ , elderly, high stage
MZL	−	−	−	translocations ± Bcl-10, MALT1 & IgM, Bcl-2 ±ve, Bcl-6 −ve
Splenic MZL	−	−	−	IgD may be +ve (unlike other MZL variants)
IPSID	−	−	−	IgA (α heavy chain only – no κ or λ light chains)
HCL	−	−	−	+ve for CD25, DBA44, TRAP (& Bcl-1 in 50–85%)
rare cases . . .	+	+	depends	. . . of otherwise typical FCL, MCL, CLL, B-ALL, DLBCL

*Lymphoplasmacytic lymphoma is a diagnosis of exclusion: exclude CLL, FCL, MZL

- MCL are CD43 +ve and upto 20% of MCL are Bcl-1 −ve
- Some MCL are CD5 −ve, Bcl-1 +ve; these have typical morphology and most have a t(11;14)
- FCL are CD43 −ve and upto 40% of FCL are CD10 −ve. Bcl-2 may be −ve in cases without t(14;18)
- MCL *vs.* CLL: ➤ CLL can be CD38 +ve (upto 40% – represent a good prognosis subgroup)
  - ➤ MCL are CD38 −ve and do not have paraimmunoblasts / proliferation centres
  - ➤ MCL have a 'two-tone' positivity for CD5 (T-cells stain strongly, MCL cells weakly)
  - ➤ CLL have strong diffuse staining for CD5
  - ➤ Ki-67 +vity may be clustered on CLL but is diffuse in MCL
- MCL has classical, blastic, pleomorphic, small cell and other morphological variants
- CLL transformations: Richter's, paraimmunoblastic and prolymphocytoid – see p.105
- LPL *vs.* CLL: ① lack of CD5 in LPL ② strong cytoplasmic Ig (heavy chains) in LPL
- Nodal MZL = 'monocytoid B-cell lymphoma'

Cutaneous B-cell Lymphomas
- Diagnosis requires CPC, best left to a specialist pathologist as these break many of the rules of nodal lymphomas. See Cerroni (2006), Slater (2003) and Goodlad and Hollowood (2001) in the Bibliography for details.
- 1° MZL: ➤ follicles with germinal centres and expanded mantle zone
  - ➤ sheets of small B-cells in between the follicles (may be vaguely nodular / perivascular)
  - ➤ LEL may be absent and the neoplastic B-cells may be CD43 +ve
  - ➤ combination of cell types: monocytoid, plasma cells / plasmacytoid, centrocyte-like
  - ➤ colonisation of germinal centres: shown as CD10 and Bcl-6 −ve cells in follicle centres with surrounding condensation of FDC (+ve for CD21 and CD23). (Also, the germinal centre looses its 'starry sky' appearance on H&E as the tingible body Mφ are replaced)
  - ➤ locally recurrent but tends not to spread to other organs / systems
- 1° FCL: ➤ follicles with attenuated / absent mantles
  - ➤ CD10 and Bcl-6 +ve cells outside follicles as well as inside
  - ➤ CD21 +ve FDC network visible
  - ➤ Bcl-2 and t(14;18) often negative: if +ve, you should consider skin involvement by systemic spread of nodal FCL
- 1° DLBCL incl. intravascular lymphoma (see p.113) – may not require toxic systemic chemoRx if it is a solitary lesion confined to the skin
- MCL: this is rarely a 1° skin tumour – look for nodal / GI disease, etc.
- CLL: ➤ diffuse pattern superficially
  - ➤ ± heavy perivascular pattern deeper
- Lymphomatoid granulomatosis: see p.91
- d/dg B-cell cutaneous lymphoid hyperplasia: if follicular, there are well-formed mantles with a mixed interfollicular infiltrate (B:T-cell ratio <3:1); no sheets of plasma cells; B-cells are CD43 −ve; adnexa are not destroyed; infiltrate is top-heavy (a weak feature); a stimulus is seen (e.g. tattoo pigment) or discovered from the history (for a list, see p.302 under 'B-Cell and Other Lymphomas')

Signet Ring Lymphomas
- FCL or myeloma variant (due to immunoglobulin cytoplasmic globules)
- Some T-cell lymphomas may also show this pattern
- d/dg signet ring carcinoma

Follicular Lymphoma (FCL)
- Commonest adult lymphoma in UK, rare in people <30 years old
- FDC are present – their presence, esp. in a nodular configuration, is supportive evidence for FCL *vs.* other lymphomas and is a useful feature for core Bx diagnosis of FCL
- 'Early' FCL is confined to the follicles with normal small lymphocytes in interfollicular areas
- Progression to higher grades is accompanied by infiltration of interfollicular areas by FCL cells with consequent blurring of follicular definition, merging of follicles and ↑ mitotic rate
- 'Follicles' throughout the node (! but this may also be seen in florid reactive nodes e.g. RhA)
- Extension into perinodal (not hilar) fat *as nodules* or *mindless sheets*
- Reticulin: ➤ 'early': reticulin-free[2] follicles with condensation of interfollicular areas
                ➤ 'later': destruction of interfollicular reticulin as follicles merge
                ➤ generally: loss of sinus architecture
- 'Signet ring' FCL contains cells with large cytoplasmic globules of immunoglobulin
- Grading FCL depends on the centroblast (Cb) count as follows:
    1. 0–5 / 1 hpf   ⎫ a hpf is 0.45 mm diameter (0.159 mm² area) and the count
    2. 6–15 / 1 hpf   ⎬ should be adjusted for other field diameters (e.g. by counting
    3. >15 / 1 hpf   ⎭ <10 fields for microscopes with larger diameter hpf)
        3a. centrocytes (Cc) still present
        3b. sheets of Cb without Cc (d/dg DLBCL – FCL 3b is still nodular but it often lacks t(14;18) and is Bcl-2 −ve)
    ➤ must count in 10 *representative* neoplastic follicles (not those with most Cb) – 10hpf in each
    ➤ must distinguish Cb from large centrocytes and FDC nuclei
    ➤ variation in grade between regions of the LN should be noted (e.g. 'predom. G1 with focal G3a')
- If <75% follicular architecture state proportion of diffuse (DLBCL) component
- If <25% follicular this is considered a focally follicular DLBCL
- Diffuse variant of FCL: see 'Diffuse Large B-Cell Lymphoma', p.113, for definition and d/dg
- d/dg follicular hyperplasia (see Table 10.2)

Progressive Transformation of Germinal Centres
- The follicles are larger, more centrally placed within the node and ill-defined
- Residual tingible body Mφ may be seen
- More reactive T-cells and ↑ marginal zone *cf.* ordinary follicles
- Peripheral 'collections' of epithelioid Mφ
- May be an isolated reactive feature or assoc[d] with lymphoma e.g. LPHL (d/dg FCL)

Regressed Follicle
- Smaller
- Absence of transformed lymphocytes
- No mantle
- Mφ and PAS +ve hyalinised vessels prominent (≈ Castleman's disease)

MALT Lymphoma (MALToma, Extranodal MZL)
- In the GIT these are usu. localised and amenable to surgery (but can be disseminated e.g. IPSID)
- Lymphoepithelial lesions (LEL) show epithelial damage / destruction (swelling, eosinophilia and loss – use CAM5.2 to demonstrate LEL if not obvious) by *clusters* of ≥3 B-lymphocytes per cluster – not just interposition of lymphocytes in between epithelial cells
- Cytol. of neoplastic lymphocytes: small non-descript / centrocyte-like / monocytoid (abundant clear cytoplasm) / plasma cell / scattered blasts (≤10%). Reactive plasma and T-cells admixed

---

[2] except immediately around blood vessels

TABLE 10.2   Follicular lymphoma or follicular hyperplasia? Table reprinted (with modifications and additions) from *Lymph Node Biopsy Interpretation*, Stansfeld AG, d'Ardenne AJ (Eds.), Ch. 9 'Low grade B-cell lymphomas', p.253, Copyright (1992), with permission from Elsevier Ltd.

Feature	Follicular Hyperplasia	Follicular Lymphoma
Architecture	preserved	lost (unless partial LN involvement)
Distribution of follicles	predom. cortical	spread throughout the node
Extracapsular spread	absent / limited	present as nodules & 'mindless sheets'
Size of follicles	variable with large ones	uniform in any given case[†]
Shape of follicles	may be irregular	usu. regular and rounded
Definition of follicles	usu. sharp, no cracks	sharp (± cracks[‡]) / poorly defined
Mantle zone	present (unless the germinal centre is very large)	usu. absent or narrow
Reticulin	(see text)	(see text)
Bcl-2 positivty in B-cells[X]	absent	present (except cutaneous FCL)
Polarity/Ki-67 zonation	present	absent
Acetyl cholinesterase activity	present	absent
AED[**] in follicles	often present	occ. present
Mitoses in follicles	numerous, typical	fewer, ± atypical forms
Tingible body Mϕ	frequent	occ. present but usu. absent
centrocytes	confined to follicles	not confined unless 'early' FCL
maturing plasma cells and other inflam[y] cells in interfollicular areas	often numerous	scant / absent

[†] Cases with large ('giant') follicles correspond to the original Brill-Symmers disease; [‡] these are artefactual cracks between the follicle edge and surrounding lymphoid tissue; [X] it is usu. the centrocytes that stain best with Bcl-2 (*cf.* centroblasts): [**] AED = acidophilic extracellular deposits.

- Dense diffuse infiltrates of B-cells between reactive follicles and interstitially between mucosal glands
- Colonisation of germinal centres ($\rightarrow$ loss of 'starry sky' admixture of tingible body Mϕ):
  - invasion of the germinal centre by CD10 and Bcl-6 −ve neoplastic cells (! but may be Bcl-2 +ve)
  - displacement and peripheral condensation of FDC (CD21 and CD23 +ve)
- Immuno: CD20 +ve, CD43 +vity in B-cells is helpful if present (but T-cells are also +ve), light chain restricted and heavy chain +ve (usu. IgM) but IgD −ve; −ve for CD5, CD10, Bcl-1 and Bcl-6
- Transformation to DLBCL (do not use 'high grade MALT lymphoma') is diagnosed when there are solid sheets of transformed blasts; some accept clusters (of usu. >20) blasts but ! d/dg germinal centres
- Some translocations are seen in the various MALTomas, the following three are mutually exclusive:
  - t(11;18)   ☞ rare in nodal or splenic MZL; usu. does not have any other chromosomal anomaly
    - ☞ indicates: ① resistance to response to anti-helicobacter Rx ⎱ in gastric
      ② resistance to (i.e. protection against) ⎰ MALToma
      transformat[n]
    - ☞ immuno: moderate nuclear +vity for Bcl-10, weak cytoplasmic +vity for MALT1
  - t(1;14)   ☞ occurs in a small proportion of gastric and pulmonary MALTomas
    - ☞ immuno: strong nuclear +vity for Bcl-10, weak cytoplasmic +vity for MALT1
  - t(14;18)   ☞ found in extraintestinal MALToma (salivary gland, eye, liver, etc.)
    - ☞ it is different to the t(14;18) seen in FCL
    - ☞ immuno: strong cytoplasmic +vity for both Bcl-10 and MALT1
- Other MALTomas have none of the above translocations and these usu. show weak cytoplasmic +vity for both Bcl-10 and MALT1
- Nuclear Bcl-10 +vity in ocular MALTomas may confer a worse prognosis

Intestinal Lymphomas (other than MALToma)

FCL
- Usu. 2° so diagnose 1° only if limited to gut wall and local draining LN
- Well-defined nodules based on an FDC network
- Frequently produce IgA (not IgG as in 1° nodal FCL)
- t(14;18) frequent (unlike intestinal MALToma)
- Do not show plasma cell differentiation (MALTomas often do)

MCL
- CD43 +ve unlike FCC (but CLL and some MALTomas are CD43 +ve)
- Plasma cell differentiation is not seen
- LEL are sparse or absent
- d/dg DLBCL *vs.* blastoid variant of MCL

Lymphomas in chronic inflammatory bowel disease
- Related to immunosuppression
- Usu. EBV +ve
- Includes extranodal HL with   ① polyclonal H/RS cells
                                 ② possible regression upon stopping immunosuppression

EATL/ETTL (see p.115)

Extra-Intestinal MALT Lymphoma of Salivary Gland
- Arises on a background of LESA (also known as MESA) – see pp.132–133
- The earliest lymphomatous change is the presence of a pale zone of clear monocytoid centrocyte-like (Cc-like) cells around a duct or epimyoepithelial island
- These Cc-like cells loose their mantle B-cell phenotype (IgD +ve, IgM +ve) to display a marginal zone phenotype (IgD −ve, IgM +ve) and show light chain restriction
- Later Cc-like cell zones coalesce to form sheets that destroy the epimyoepithelial islands and displace/colonise and replace the follicles
- ± Sclerosis
- ± Granulomas
- Transformation to DLBCL may occur (defined as the presence of solid sheets of blasts)

Diffuse Large B-Cell Lymphoma (DLBCL)
- 'Large' is defined as ≥ twice the size of a normal lymphocyte
- Centroblastic, immunoblastic[3], plasmablastic (oral, HIV, EBV), anaplastic (unrelated to ALCL)
- Need >90% immunoblasts to classify as immunoblastic DLBCL
- LN involvement may be partial, interfollicular or sinusoidal
- Variants: ➤ T-cell-rich   ⎤ a 'rich' variant is defined as a tumour where
             ➤ histiocyte-rich ⎦ <10% of the cells are neoplastic
             ➤ sclerosing 1° mediastinal / thymic: CD45 +ve (unlike d/dg classical HL), CD30 +ve and CD10 −ve. Also CD23 +ve unlike most other DLBCL
             ➤ PEL (1° effusion lymphoma – see p.362)
             ➤ PAL (pyothorax-assoc[d] lymphoma – see p.362)
             ➤ 1° CNS
             ➤ intravascular (cyclin D1 and CD23 −ve)
             ➤ DLBCL with full length ALK (see under d/dg of ALCL on p116)
- Immuno: pan-B +ve, CD5 ±ve, CD10 (+ve in 50%), CD30 +ve (esp. in anaplastic)
- Adverse prognostic variant: 'Activated' B-cell phenotype: high Ki-67 LI, p53 +ve in >50% of the cells, Bcl-2 strongly +ve, FOX-P1 +ve, Bcl-6 −ve, CD10 −ve, often immunoblastic morphology
- Good prognostic variant: 'Germinal Centre' B-cell phenotype: centroblastic, Bcl-6 +ve, CD10 +ve
- d/dg blastoid MCL: DLBCL is Bcl-1 −ve
- d/dg mediastinal grey zone lymphoma = clinical, morphological and immuno features in between NSHL and 1° mediastinal DLBCL; M>F; some treat as for DLBCL not HL but more data needed.
- d/dg diffuse FCL: ➤ diffuse FCL *must* ① have centroblasts as the minority of the neoplastic cells
                                            ② be grade 1 or 2 at most (if grade 3 then = DLBCL)
                                            ③ have no follicular areas
                     ➤ presence / absence of a CD21 +ve FDC network is not useful

Burkitt's Lymphoma
- Children, extra-nodal (jaws, gonads, breast, intestines), EBV-assoc[d]
- Medium-sized B-cells with squared-off cytoplasm
- Round nuclei with multiple small central nucleoli
- Monotonous population

---

[3] an immunoblastoid variant expressing cytoplasmic IgA is ALK +ve, t(2;5) −ve and highly aggressive

- ++ Mitoses, apoptoses and tingible body Mφ ('starry sky')
- Immuno: +ve for: lipid, surface IgM, CD10, Bcl-6, pan-B; −ve for: CD5, Tdt, Bcl-2, CD23
- Immuno: Ki-67 LI ≈ 100%

Atypical Burkitt's Lymphoma (Burkitt-like Lymphoma)
- Adults, nodal
- CD10 −ve Burkittoid lymphocytes
- Less monotonous – half way between classical Burkitt and DLBCL
- Cells have more prominent (but fewer) nucleoli *cf.* classical Burkitt
- Ki-67 LI of ≈ 100% is required for diagnosis

Microlymphoma (HHV8-Associated)
- Usu. occurs in the context of multicentric Castleman's disease in LN or spleen
- Defined by small confluent aggregates of HHV8 +ve plasmablasts, often impinging on germinal centres
- There is light chain restriction by immuno but may be polyclonal or monoclonal (by genetics)

Post Transplant Lymphoproliferative Disorders (PTLD)
- Plasmacytic hyperplasia: nodal, normal architecture, ! may be adjacent to a worse grade PTLD
- PTLD IM-Like: nodal and Waldeyer's ring, normal architecture, blasts prominent
- PTLD Plasma Cell Rich: nodal and extranodal; equivalent to plasmacytoma
- PTLD Polymorphic: invasive and destructive, oligoclonal
- PTLD Monomorphic: immunoblasts or follicle centre cells, monoclonal, less likely to respond to a reduction in immunosuppression, N-ras / p53 mutations common
- PTLD Multiple Myeloma-like: monoclonal, N-ras, not likely to respond to ↓immunosuppression
- PTLD T-cell Type: Not EBV-related (unlike most of the others), aggressive, poor prognosis
- PTLD Hodgkin's-Like: Few cases, must fulfil criteria for HL (because RS-like cells occur in other PTLD)
- PTLD Composite: two distinct types must be present – not a gradation
- PTLD NOS
- EBV-unrelated PTLD: ➤ may be related to HHV8
  ➤ occur later
  ➤ may respond to ↓immunosuppression
  ➤ most are conventional lymphomas

T-Cell/NK Lymphomas and Reactions

Abbreviated List of T-Cell / NK Lymphomas
- **T**-ALL/CLL
- **H**epatosplenic (γδ type) – see p.124 and p.105
- **ETTL**[4] (= EATL)
- **PTCL-U** (peripheral TCL – unspecified)
- **S**ubcutaneous panniculitis-like TCL (αβ type) and mucocutaneous γδ lymphoma
- **A**ngiocentric/Angioimmunoblastic/Adult TCL (HTLV-1)/Anaplastic
- **L**arge granular lymphocyte lymphoma
- **M**ycosis Fungoides and variants (e.g. Pagetoid Reticulosis)

Subcutaneous Panniculitis-like TCL (+ve for CD8 and αβ; −ve for CD56 and EBV)
- Restricted to the adipose (unlike γδ); is one cause of *cytophagic histiocytic panniculitis* (CHP)
- Rimming of adipocytes by variably-sized Ki-67 +ve lymphocytes, clear cytoplasm, ±necrosis ++
- In CHP cytophagocytotic histiocytes from 'bean bag' cells full of RBC ±WBC ±debris
- d/dg: other causes of CHP (EBV, nasal-type NK/TCL), subcutaneous MF, γδ TCL

T-CLL
- Like B-CLL but no proliferation centres
- LN infiltrate accompanied by high endothelial venules
- Immuno: pan-T +ve (incl. CD4 and CD7), Tdt −ve

---

[4] WHO terminology = Enteropathy *Type* TCL (*cf. Associated* – because there may not be enteropathy)

Enteropathy Type / Associated TCL (EATL / ETTL)
- In un-complicated coeliac disease the IELs are CD8 +ve
- In *refractory coeliac disease* (± *ulcerative jejunitis*) the IELs loose CD8 and become monoclonal (= *intraepithelial EATL*)
- The subsequent invasive EATL (infiltration of mucosa and submucosa) may be dominated by medium to large lymphocytes of the same clone as for refractory coeliac
- An ulcerated mass next to atrophic small intestinal mucosa is the typical macro
- ! The stromal inflammatory component (incl. eosinophils and histiocytes) may obscure the lymphoma
- Immuno: CD8 ±ve, CD4 −ve (an unusual phenotype for a T-cell lymphoma)

Angioimmunoblastic TCL (AITCL)
- Elderly, generalised LNp, systemic Sx, d/dg drug reaction (antibiotic / phenytoin, etc.)
- Effacement of architecture but preserved subcapsular sinus and regressed follicles
- Arborising proliferation of high endothelial venules
- Proliferation of CD21 +ve FDC-like cells *outside* follicles around vessels → fascicles / whorls of plump spindle cells
- Small–medium T-cells incl. clear cell clusters and sheets → 'mottled' look at medium power
- Immunoblast clusters (may be intravascular)
- Background: rich in plasma cells ± eosinophils ± epithelioid Mɸ clusters
- ± RS-like cells (CD15 +ve, CD30 +ve, EBV ±ve, CD20 ±ve)
- Grading: no numerical score but disease progression ∝ amount of immunoblasts
- Immuno: mainly T4 cells, CD10 +ve (most periph. TCL are −ve), interspersed B-cells also present
- d/dg:
  - ➢ T-cell-rich DLBCL: but atypical cells are T and B-cells are polytypic (κ and λ)
  - ➢ PTCL-U, but AITCL has: ⟵ distinctive clinical
  - ➢ AILD (*vide infra*)   arborising high endothelial venules
  - ➢ Classical HL   plasma cell-rich background
                                extrafollicular FDC proliferation

Angioimmunoblastic Lymphadenopathy with Dysproteinaemia (AILD)
- Similar clinical features to AITCL with polyclonal hypergammaglobulinaemia
- Similar arch., arborising high endothelial venules and extrafollicular FDC prolif^n to AITCL
- Overall hypocellular
- Lack clear cells or immunoblasts in clusters / islands / sheets
- No cytological atypia

Angioimmunoblastic Lymph Node Reaction / Immunoblastic Reaction
- Preservation of architecture and follicles
- Otherwise like AILD
- Specific causes include:
  - ➢ drugs
  - ➢ infections: EBV / other viral infection, brucellosis
  - ➢ adult Still's disease

Angiocentric TCL (WHO: Extranodal NK/TCL, Nasal Type)
- Nose ('*lethal midline granuloma*'), pharynx, skin, testis
- Diffuse angiocentric and angiodestructive infiltrate
- Coagulative necrosis, apoptoses (and ulceration at mucosal sites ± PEH)
- Cell size varies from case to case (small to anaplastic)
- Nucleoli inconspicuous or small, even in large cell types
- Mitoses ++, even in small cell types
- ± Heavy mixed inflammatory cell infiltrate (hence old name: *polymorphic reticulosis*)
- Immuno: +ve for CD2, EBV, CD56, TIA-1 and granzyme B; −ve for CD3

HTLV-1 Adult T-cell Leukaemia / Lymphoma
- Hypercalcaemia and lytic bone lesions (d/dg myeloma), multi-organ involvement
- CD25 +ve CD3 +ve cells infiltrating skin esp. at dermoepidermal junction
- Cerebriform atypical cells (medium-sized)

- Assoc^d with hyperinfection with *Strongyloides stercoralis* (see p.350)
- d/dg MF
- Immuno: ➢ positive for CD3,CD25,CD30($\pm$ve)
  ➢ negative for ALK, CD7, TIA-1, granzyme B

Anaplastic Large Cell Lymphoma (T/Null/NK Type) – Nodal (for Cutaneous, see p.302)
- 1° (nodal/cutaneous/soft tissues/bone/lung) or 2° (transformation of nodal TCL / MF / LyP / HL)
- Sinusoidal, diffuse or interfollicular growth pattern (d/dg HL)
- Anaplastic cells, horseshoe / wreath nuclei surrounding central eosinophilic blob, multiple nucleoli
- Variants: ➢ lymphohistiocytic   } more typical ALCL large neoplastic cells tend
  ➢ small cell   } to cluster around vessels in these variants
- Immuno: ☞ $\pm$ve for CD30 (Golgi blob), EMA, CD25, CD45, LMW CK
  ☞ ALK ① nucleus and cytoplasm (nucleophosmin-ALK translocation)
  ② granular cytoplasmic (clathrin-ALK translocation)
  ③ diffuse cytoplasmic (other ALK translocations)
- Criteria for assigning T-cell differentiation:
  ➢ any of CD2,3,4,8 +ve (CD3 and CD8 are often −ve)
- Criteria for null-cell differentiation:
  ➢ CD2,3,4,8 all negative
  ➢ B-cell markers all negative
- Criteria for NK-cell differentiation (whether T or Null):
  ➢ CD56, TIA-1, granzyme B, perforin
- Prognostics: ➢ ALK −vity is a bad prognostic unless 1° cutaneous form
  ➢ many NK-type T-cells are a bad prognostic
- d/dg systemic *vs.* 1° cutaneous ALCL:
  ➢ 1° cutaneous is usu. −ve for EMA, −ve for ALK t(2;5) translocation and is rare in children
  ➢ systemic/1°LN ALCL are assoc^d with aberrant clusterin expression
- d/dg other ALK +ve tumours:
  ➢ RMS and neuroblastoma
  ➢ inflammatory myofibroblastic tumour
  ➢ the rare immunoblastic 'DLBCL with full length ALK' (are t(2;5) −ve, CD30 −ve, IgA +ve)
- d/dg classical HL: ➢ CD15 rarely expressed in ALCL and then only focal sparse cells
  ➢ ALCL are EBV −ve

Hodgkin Lymphoma (HL, older term = Hodgkin's Disease)

Classical Reed-Sternberg (at least two nuclear lobes / nuclei) and Hodgkin (mononuclear) cells
- Rounded nuclei
- Accentuated nuclear membrane
- Large eosinophilic nucleoli (*cf.* smaller bluer nucleoli of florid reactive immunoblasts)
- Pale chromatin
- Abundant amphophil cytoplasm
- $\pm$ Mummified forms: pyknosing nuclei and condensed eosinophilic cytoplasm
- Variants:
  ① L&H: has a multilobated nucleus with small nucleoli (nucleus looks like a *popcorn*)
  ② lacunar: see 'Nodular Sclerosis HL (NSHL)', below
  ③ pleomorphic
  ④ small cell
- Immuno: there are two immunophenotypes
  ① the L&H cell phenotype seen only in NLPHL (*q.v.*)
  ② the phenotype of all other H/RS cells in all other variants of HL (see 'Lymphocyte-rich classical HL (LRCHL)', below)
  ➢ CD15, CD30 (and EMA in NLPHL) typically show membranous accentuation with a Golgi dot
- d/dg RS-like cells in AITCL have variable intensity CD30 staining (uniform in HL)
- d/dg reactive blasts show diffuse cytoplasmic (or membrane + dot) CD30, are −ve for CD15 and +ve for T/B markers

Diagnosing HL Recurrence or Occurrence Outside LN (e.g. Bone Marrow, Effusions, etc.)
- Must have either Hodgkin or RS cells (CD15 +ve and/or CD30 +ve) in an appropriate background
- Seeing an appropriate (e.g. mixed cellularity) background without H/RS cells is not sufficient to confirm HL but may suggest it
- Plasma cell nodules or broad areas of fibrosis in a bone marrow trephine should suggest the possibility of HL and search for H/RS cells instigated if clinically consistent
- Epithelioid granulomas may be found together with HL or in LN without HL draining sites affected by HL

Mixed Cellularity
- Diffuse, vaguely nodular or interfollicular growth pattern
- LN capsule not thickened and no bands of fibrosis / sclerosis (else = NSHL)
- Classical H/RS cells
- Background of lymphocytes, plasma cells, eosinophils, neutrophils, Mφ ± granulomas

Nodular Lymphocyte Predominant HL (NLPHL, Nodular Paragranuloma)
- Adult, M≫F, low stage, good prog., assoc[d] with progressive transformation of the germinal centres
- L&H popcorn cells rosetted by CD57 +ve T-cells in a background of mantle B-cells (but may resemble more classical Hodgkin cells morphologically)
- L&H cells lie predominantly *centrally* in the nodule of mantle B-cells
- the nodules contain an expanded FDC network (seen with CD21) but not tight rounded clusters of FDC representing remnants of ordinary follicles overrun by lymphoma as seen in LRCHL
- Eosinophils and neutrophils are absent in both nodular and diffuse regions
- Immuno of L&H cells: BOB-1, OCT2, J-chain, Bcl-6, EMA, CD20, CD45 +ve; CD30 ±ve; CD15 −ve; EBV −ve (this is important, if EBV is +ve reconsider diagnosis – e.g. LRCHL)
- d/dg: T-cell-rich DLBCL:
  - ➤ just one nodule typical of NLPHL in an otherwise diffuse pattern is sufficient to diagnose NLPHL
  - ➤ the background small lymphocytes are predominantly *B-cell* (in the nodular areas) of NLPHL *cf.* T-cell in DLBCL
- d/dg Lymphocyte-rich classical HL: *vide infra*

Lymphocyte-Rich Classical HL (LRCHL)
- Usu. nodular with attenuated T-zone (but rarely it is diffuse with a mainly T-cell background)
- Classical H/RS cells (although some may resemble L&H cells)
- CD57 +ve T-cells are present but not rosetting H/RS cells
- Eosinophils and neutrophils are sparse / absent
- H/RS cells appear to lie *eccentrically* within the follicles with germinal centre to one side. They lie in the expanded mantle of the follicle and not in the germinal centre
- Immuno: CD15 +ve, CD30 +ve, EBV ±ve, EMA −ve[5], −ve for J-chain, CD45, BOB-1 and OCT2, CD20 is *usu.* −ve but not in all cases
- d/dg NLPHD (*q.v.*): ! this is a common mis-diagnosis amongst general pathologists

Nodular Sclerosis HL (NSHL)
- Nodular growth, fibrous bands and thickened capsule
- RS cells have multiple small lobes with multiple small nucleoli and retraction artefact ('lacunar cells') – this artefact is not seen on frozen section.
- Lacunar cells may form aggregates (= *syncytial variant* if this is pronounced)
- Necrosis may be present
- Variable background: mixed cellularity to hypocellular
- Grading (BNLI method):
  - I ≥75% of the nodules have scattered RS cells with a non-neoplastic cell-rich background (lymphocytes, mixed cellularity or fibrohistiocytic)
  - II ≥25% have at least 1 × 40 field filled with RS cells. (These are also usu. associated with lymphocyte depletion but it is the abundance of RS cells that make it a grade II)

---

[5] but upto 20% of cases may be focally +ve for EMA

Lymphocyte Depleted HL (LDHL)
- Rarest type, extranodal sites or retroperitoneal LN preferred
- Predominance of classical H/RS (or pleomorphic variant) cells to background lymphocytes
- *Diffuse fibrosis* subtype: low cellularity, H/RS cells rare, fine fibrosis with proteinaceous material
- *Reticular* subtype: numerous H/RS with bizarre forms (= '*Hodgkin's sarcoma*')
- d/dg NSHL: if there is nodular sclerosing fibrosis don't call it LDHL (it is NSHL, probably grade II)
- d/dg ALCL: LDHL should have CD15 +ve H/RS cells and the diagnostic features of ALCL are absent

Interfollicular HL
- A name given to HL (of various subtypes) that occurs in the interfollicular regions of a LN
- It is accompanied by follicular hyperplasia so may be mis-diagnosed as reactive

Sentinel Node Pathology

Melanoma
- Most mets are in the subcapsular sinus and ≈ all are S100 +ve
- Benign naevus cells are co-present in >10% cases and are usu. HMB45 −ve but will give a +ve tyrosinase test on PCR (hence limitations of non-histological methods for SN assessment)
- '*Enhanced histopathology*' (multiple levels and immuno) of SN is predictive of local LN field mets
- Lymphadenectomy of SN +ve cases only: spares unnecessary morbidity
- Lymphadenectomy of SN +ve cases only: may be therapeutic (but ? survival advantage)
- ≈ 20% of SN show mets by enhanced histopathology (∝ Breslow thickness and Clark level)
- ≈ $\frac{1}{3}$ of these also have +ve LN other than the SN

Breast
- Similar clinical points and +vity stats as for melanoma (SN immuno for CK is esp. sensitive in ILC)
- Good for local control by selective axillary clearance or radioRx for SN +ve cases
- It can also identify internal mammary LN +ve cases (worse prognosis)
- Per-operative assessment by imprint cytology (= 'dabs') or FS is becoming popular

Colorectal
- High level of false −ves in literature (>10%) mean that routine sampling of SN for enhanced histopathology is not justified outside research
- SN mapping may be useful to guide surgery by identifying unexpected lymphatic drainage routes

Other Lesions and Reactions of Lymph Nodes

Benign LN Inclusions
- ! A source of overdiagnosis of malignancy on FS
- Epithelial:
  - ➤ peri/intra-parotid / submaxillary LN – salivary duct inclusions
  - ➤ axillary LN – breast epithelium, usu. cystic +/ squamous / apocrine change
  - ➤ periaortic LN – Müllerian metaplastic epithelium
  - ➤ mesenteric LN – colonic glands
  - ➤ pelvic / inguinal LN – tubal-type epithelium without stroma, usu. women
- Mesothelial:
  - ➤ mediastinal LN
  - ➤ epithelioid cells in sinuses
  - ➤ bland nuclei, low NCR, well-defined cell borders ± windowing
  - ➤ immuno: mesothelial (see p.89 and p.360)
- Naeval:
  - ➤ usu. intracapsular / intraseptal in axillary LN (!d/dg single file ILC cells)
  - ➤ inguinal / neck LN – sinus naevocytes drained from congenital naevi[6]
- Decidual: ! do not mistake for metastatic SCC
- Haemopoietic: megakaryocytes are AE1/AE3 −ve (d/dg carcinoma)

---

[6] the original skin naevus may show intravascular naevocytes

Necrotising Histiocytic Lymphadenitis (Kikuchi-Fujimoto Disease)
- Clin.: systemic Sx (*NB*: Kikuchi may be a *forme fruste* of SLE)
- Cortical / paracortical foci of necrosis
- Histiocytes of phagocytic (not epithelioid) type
- PMN are absent
- ± Marked immunoblastic reaction
- 'Banana' nuclear fragments (apoptotic crescents)
- d/dg non-reactive TB (do ZN and Wade-Fite for atypical mycobacteria)
- d/dg lupus lymphadenitis (look for vasculitis, advise serology)
- d/dg adult Still's disease (also has follicular hyperplasia and paracortical T-cell reaction)
- d/dg *Yersinia*/cat scratch (*Bartonella* [*Rochalimaea*] *henselae*)/LGV (*Chlamydia trachomatis* serotypes L1, L2, L3): show serpiginous / bifurcating palisaded granulomas around central PMN / necrosis
- d/dg tularaemia (*Francisella tularensis*): histologically like *Yersinia*, TB (or sarcoid)
- d/dg Kawasaki's disease: look for vasculitis, PMN and geographic (*cf.* focal) necrosis

HIV Lymphadenopathy
- 'Explosive' follicular hyperplasia with depleted mantles ('naked follicles')
- Germinal centres may fuse to give irregular giant germinal centres
- Mantle cells encroach into germinal centres → 'folliculolysis'
- Plasmacytosis, immunoblasts, vascularity of interfollicular areas
- Monocytoid sinus B-cell reaction
- Warthin-Finkeldey multinucleate FDC and IDC
- Late changes: regression and disappearance of follicles, lymphocyte depletion, nodal fibrosis
- Assoc^d changes: MAI, focal nodal KS, mycobacterial pseudotumour, etc.

Spindle Cell Tumours and Tumour-like Lesions in LN
- Metastatic carcinoma (SCC, RCC, medullary thyroid, etc.)
- Melanoma
- Synovial sarcoma
- Kaposi sarcoma
- Mycobacterial pseudotumour
- Palisaded myofibroblastoma
- Ectopic thymoma
- Vascular transformation of LN sinuses (see p.319)
- IDC tumour / sarcoma
- FDC tumour / sarcoma
- LAM (for details, see pp.92–93)

Castleman's Disease (Angiofollicular Lymph Node Hyperplasia)

Localised – hyaline vascular type
- Large node (single rounded mass), local effects but no systemic Sx
- Loss of sinus architecture
- Large mantle zone of concentric ('onion skin') lymphocytes
- Central regressed germinal centre with FDC and hyaline vessels
- 'Lollipop' sign of interfollicular vessel traversing to centre of follicle
- Interfollicular zone contains lymphocytes, lots of vessels and few reactive cells (plasma cells, immunoblasts, eos.)
- d/dg regressed follicle – lacks expanded onion skin mantle
- d/dg Castleman-like reactive LN: common at some sites (e.g. mesenteric), does not form a large mass and is probably of no clinical significance
- d/dg HL (because an occ. FDC may be pleomorphic simulating Hodgkin cells)
- d/dg MCL
- d/dg Castleman's disease-like FCL
- d/dg Castleman's disease-like HIV lymphadenopathy:
    - ➤ small / absent mantle
    - ➤ more florid interfollicular plasmacytosis
    - ➤ less vascular interfollicular zone

> ➢ preserved sinus architecture
> ➢ other features of HIV LNp / infection / focal KS

Localised – plasma cell type
- Matted group of large nodes, systemic Sx
- Obliteration of sinuses
- Follicular hyperplasia ± scattered regressed follicles (hyaline vascular follicles are rare)
- Mantle zone surrounded by sheets of plasma cells (polyclonal or monotypic)
- Diagnosis of exclusion: d/dg: CTD (e.g. RhA), syphilis, HL, plasmacytoma, HIV

Systemic (multicentric) type
- Rare, multiple peripheral LN / systemic (liver, kidney, skin, bone marrow, CNS, etc.)
- Preserved sinuses with 'inspissated' lymph
- Mixture of regressed and hyperplastic follicles ± hyaline vascular follicles
- Perifollicular sheets of plasma cells
- HHV8 +ve plasmablasts in the mantle zone (may form aggregates of microlymphoma)
- ± Interfollicular vascular proliferation
- Associations: HHV8 (even if HIV −ve), KS / plasmablastic lymphoma, osteosclerotic myeloma (Crow-Fukase POEMS syndrome), other neoplasms (e.g. chordoid meningioma)
- d/dg: exclude Castleman-like lymphomas, HIV, CTD, nodal KS, HL

Dermatopathic Lymphadenopathy
- Skin lesions may or may not be present
- Mottled expansion of the paracortex by histiocytes, plasma cells, immunoblasts ± Cc-like cells
- Pigment (melanin / haemosiderin) may be sparse to abundant ± cholesterol
- Langerhans cells and eosinophils are usu. present in the infiltrate
- d/dg HX, HL, monocytoid leukaemia
- d/dg nodal involvement by MF (this requires partial effacement of architecture by MF cells)

EBV Lymphadenopathy (Infectious Mononucleosis)
- Florid paracortical angioimmunoblastic reaction ± sheets of immunoblasts
- Sinus B-cell reaction with transformed cells
- Destruction of B-cell areas (esp. in advanced cases, this mimics loss of architecture)
- Mitoses ++
- Bi-/multi-nucleated immunoblasts (nucleoli usu. smaller and more haematoxyphilic *cf.* H/RS cells)
- Immuno: immunoblasts show CD20, CD30 (Ki-1), CD43, LMP +ve
- d/dg lymphoma (esp. ALCL / HL) but preserved architecture, characteristic IM clinical, serology and PB atypical T-cells and −vity for ALK all help

Eosinophil Granuloma (HX)
- Langerhans cell infiltrate is sinus-centric *cf.* paracorticocentric as in dermatopathic LNp
- See also: pp.57–58, p.94 and p.333.

Follicular Dendritic Cell Sarcoma (= Dendritic Reticulum Cell Sarcoma, FDC Sarcoma)
- Clin.: usu. one nodal site, may locally recur but mets / death are rare
- Arch: storiform, fascicles, sheets, meningothelioid whorls (± nuclear pseudoinclusions), ± cysts
- Cytology: spindle cells with bland, oval, vesicular nuclei
- Other: sharp demarcation from uninvolved areas, intratumoural and perivascular lymphocytes (B and T) ± follicles
- Immuno: +ve for EMA, CD21,23,35; ±ve for S100, MSA, CD20,45,68; −ve for CD1a,3,34,79a, CK, desmin, HMB45
- EM: desmosomes are present (unlike d/dg IDC sarcoma) but no Birbeck granules or melanosomes
- d/dg: see list in 'Spindle Cell Tumours in LN' section; also inflammatory myofibroblastic tumour / inflammatory pseudotumour (esp. if extranodal)

Interdigitating Dendritic Cell Sarcoma (= Interdigitating Reticulum Cell Sarcoma, IDC Sarcoma)
- Clin.: usu. one nodal site initially ± B symptoms; mets / death are common (upto 50% of cases)
- Arch: tumour is centred in the paracortex (if LN is not completely replaced), necrosis is usu. absent

- Cytology: spindle cells with spindle to round / convoluted nuclei of variable grade; epithelioid cells with ill-defined cytoplasm (may be pleomorphic); sheets of round cells may also be seen
- Other: intratumoural T-cells (hardly any B-cells)
- Immuno: +ve for S100, vimentin; ±ve for CD45,68; −ve for EMA, CD1a, 3, 20, 21, 25, 30, 34, 35,79a, CK (see also p.109)
- EM: desmosomes are absent (unlike d/dg FDC sarcoma) and no Birbeck granules or melanosomes
- d/dg: see list under 'Spindle Cell Tumours in LN', above; also histiocytoses / histiocytic sarcoma, ALCL

The Spleen

Normal (see Fig. 10.1)
- Capsule and septa, white pulp (PALS and follicles) and red pulp (cords of Billroth and sinusoids)
- Marginal zone (MZ) is for carbohydrate responses (e.g. pneumococcal vaccine / HS)

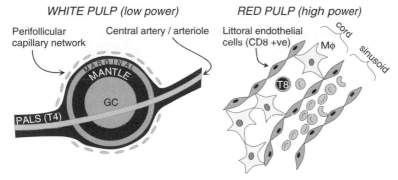

FIGURE 10.1   Normal spleen

Causes of a Small Spleen
- Old age
- Intestinal malabsorption e.g. coeliac disease
- Sickle cell anaemia
- HIV
- Congenital hypoplasia

Trauma
- ↑ White pulp
- ↑ Prominence of perifollicular capillary network (= 'perifollicular flare')

Reactive Patterns
- White pulp:
  - ➢ germinal centre formation
  - ➢ ↑ MZ ± perifollicular flare (seen esp. in post vaccination [pneumococcal] spleen)
  - ➢ ↑ PALS (incl. more blasts)[7]
- Red pulp: congestion, plasmacytosis, T8 lymphocytosis, cord fibrosis

SLE
- Periarteriolar concentric fibrosis (also occurs in sarcoidosis)
- Plasmacytosis
- Reactive white pulp (*vide supra*)

---

[7] analogous to LN paracortical reaction and seen esp. with viral infections / ITP

Red Cell and Platelet Sequestration Disorders
In Table 10.3 ↑ indicates reactive hyperplasia and ↓ represents atrophy.

TABLE 10.3   Differential features in sequestrations

	Red Pulp	White Pulp
HS	RBC loose in cords & empty sinusoids	↑(esp. MZ)
ITP	platelets in cord Mφ ('Gaucher-like')	↑/↓ (± NHL)
AIHA	RBC in sinus Mφ	↑/↓ (± NHL)

Sickle Cell Disease
- Early: drepanocyte (sickle cell) expansion of the cords with sinus compression
- Later: multiple infarcts
- Later: siderotic calcific fibrous foci (Gamna-Gandy bodies[8]) – which may contain vessels and in which some of the encrusted collagen fibres have a hyaline greenish appearance and may branch
- Eventually: spleen replaced by a small siderotic fibrous nodule ('autosplenectomy')

EBV Spleen (Infectious Mononucleosis)
- Florid CD30+ve immunoblastic reaction in red pulp
- Infiltration of trabecular vein intima by immunoblasts
- ± Haemophagocytosis (histiocytes ++)
- ± Granulomas (may be necrotising)
- d/dg leukaemia / ALCL: use CPC; EBV shows mixed T + B-cell immuno and lacks a macro tumour

HIV
- Early: splenomegaly
- Secondary: infection / KS / lymphoma / ITP-like pattern but with ↑T8 cells
- Late: atrophy

Granulomatous Splenitis
- Infective:
  - ➤ miliary TB, EBV, syphilis, *Brucella*, toxoplasmosis (white pulp features similar to LN)
  - ➤ histoplasmosis (granulomas aggregate, encapsulate and ultimately calcify); 'infantile' form shows diffuse red pulp histiocytosis with parasitised Mφ – d/dg leishmaniasis
- Paraneoplastic: (e.g. accompanying lymphoma – does not imply lymphoma in spleen)
- Other: sarcoidosis (± onion skin periarteriolar fibrosis), lipogranulomas, foreign body, granulomatous vasculitides (e.g. WG)

Histiocytic and Histiocytoid Infiltrates
- ITP (*q.v.*)
- Histiocyte-rich B-cell lymphoma
- Haemophagocytic syndromes (incl. T-cell lymphomas, viral infection and MDS)
- Granulomatous splenitis (*vide supra*)
- 'Infantile' form of histoplasmosis (disseminated red pulp parasitised Mφ) d/dg leishmaniasis
- Visceral leishmaniasis (also get plasmacytosis) d/dg infantile histoplasmosis
- Malaria (slate colour macro; red pulp Mφ with pigment)
- Lipidoses (e.g. hypertriglyceridaemia / cholesterolaemia which may be 2° e.g. to DM) and storage diseases e.g. Gaucher's disease (*q.v.*)
- HX (*q.v.*) – the Hand-Schüller-Christian variant has lipidised Mφ
- FDC sarcoma and true histiocyte neoplasms (very rare)

Systemic Mastocytosis
- Red pulp mast cells with tendency to aggregate
- Paratrabecular / subcapsular predilection
- Assoc[d] fibrosis
- d/dg HCL but HCL is diffuse and has different immuno (for more detail, see Chapter 9: Bone Marrow)

---

[8] also seen in other conditions e.g. congestion 2° to portal HT and may be the result of intrafollicular haemorrhage

Gaucher's Disease (Gaucher-Schlagenhaufer Cerebroside Kerasinosis)
- Autosomal recessive defect of glucocerebrosidase $\longrightarrow$ accumulation of 'Gaucher cells':
  - ➤ bloated Mϕ with small eccentric nucleus and abundant 'tissue paper' cytoplasmic folds
  - ➤ DPAS +ve, TRAP +ve
- Spleen: stuffed cords with sparing of white pulp (unlike d/dg malignancy) $\pm$ infarcts
- Liver: stuffed sinusoids $\pm$ portal tract aggregates
- Bone marrow: interstitial aggregates
- LN: paracortical aggregates
- Other: fever, anaemia, skin pigmentation, ocular conjunctival melanosis and pingueculae

MDS
- Erythrophagocytosis
- Plasmacytosis
- EMH
- $\pm$ CMML infiltration of red pulp
- $\pm$ Transformation foci (of AML blasts)

Extramedullary Haemopoiesis (EMH)
- Physiological EMH: ➤ small foci
  - ➤ megakaryocytes normal (not clustered)
  - ➤ other organs have similar foci
- Pathological EMH: ➤ peliosis
  - ➤ megakaryocytes large, hyperlobated and clustered
  - ➤ occurs in chronic myeloprolifcrative diseases (as a form of metastasis)

CML
- Diffuse infiltration of red pulp (cords and sinuses)
- Over-running and obliteration of white pulp
- Myeloid cells maturing to granulocytes
- MPO and CAE +ve
- d/dg granulocytic hyperplasia 2$°$ to G-CSF Rx (e.g. filgrastim or lenograstim)

Myelofibrosis
- A cause of massive splenomegaly (upto 7Kg)
- Red pulp expansion by pathological EMH ++ with small dysplastic megas ($\pm$ large clusters)
- White pulp atrophy
- Infarcts common
- $\pm$ Capsular +/ red pulp fibrosis
- Features of pre-existing MPD (e.g. PRV / CML / ET)

Hairy Cell Leukaemia (HCL)
- Weight may range from upper end of normal to $\geq$1–2 Kg
- Diffuse infiltration of red pulp (evenly spaced-out cells without prominent nucleoli)
- Limited white pulp involvement / atrophy
- Paracortical involvement of LNs and sinusoidal involvement of liver (see p.105 for bone marrow)
- d/dg splenic MZL (but MZL has a nodular infiltrate in bone marrow)
- d/dg B-prolymphocytic leukaemia
- d/dg mastocytosis but HCL is diffuse, lacks mast cell-assoc[d] fibrosis and has different immuno
- Immuno / other features: see p.105

Lymphomas

Macro:
> *General*: Splenic size is not important. Sample any hilar LN
> *Specific:*   ➤ low grade B-cell: FCL, MCL, MZL $\rightarrow$ miliary nodularity (also seen in reactive)
>   ➤ high grade B-cell: large white nodules
>   ➤ HL: discrete nodules

Micro:

    General: most low grade lymphomas have a 'follicular' pattern – not just FCL

      Specific: ➤ FCL: Cb and Cc, no red pulp extension

                ➤ MCL: monotonous, Cc-like[9] cells and red pulp satellite nodules

                ➤ MZL: ☞ ↑ MZ (immunoblastoid) → 'reversal of follicles'

                           ☞ satellite nodules in the red pulp

                           ☞ granulomas, ± circulating villous lymphocytes (SLVL)

                ➤ CLL: ☞ para-immunoblasts and proliferation centres

                           ☞ involves white pulp and extends into the red ± invades vessel walls

                           ☞ ± plasmacytoid cells (also seen in LPL)

                ➤ Hepatosplenic γδ TCL: An aggressive lymphoma of young adults (M>F); no peripheral LNp; diffuse red pulp involvement and sparing / atrophy of the white pulp. CD3, TIA-1 and TCRδ1 +ve, CD56 ±ve, rearranged TCRγ, [i(7q)] +ve

Immuno:

- For specific conditions see previous sections in this chapter and see Chapter 9: Bone Marrow
- CD21 for FDC, shows: ➤ expansion of germinal centres by FCL
                                ➤ colonisation of germinal centres by MZL
                                ➤ destruction of germinal centres by MCL.

Bibliography

Anagnostou, D. (2005) Pitfalls in the pattern of bone marrow infiltration in lymphoproliferative disorders. *Current Diagnostic Pathology*, **11** (3), 170–179.

Arno, J. (1980) *Atlas of Lymph Node Pathology*, 1st edn, MTP Press Ltd, Lancaster.

Bain, B.J., Clark, D.M., Lampert, I.A. and Wilkins, B.S. (2001) *Bone Marrow Pathology*, 3rd edn, Blackwell Science Ltd, Oxford.

Bacon, C.M., Du, M-Q. and Dogan, A. (2007) Mucosa-associated lymphoid tissue (MALT) lymphoma: a practical guide for pathologists. *Journal of Clinical Pathology*, **60** (4), 361–372.

Cerroni, L. (2006) Lymphoproliferative lesions of the skin. *Journal of Clinical Pathology*, **59** (8), 813–826.

Cerroni, L. and Kerl, H. (2001) The clinicopathological spectrum of cutaneous B-cell lymphomas, in *Progress in Pathology*, vol. 5 (eds N. Kirkham and N.R. Lemoine), Greenwich Medical Media Ltd, London, pp. 1–16.

Chan, J.K.C., Banks, P.M., Cleary, M.L. *et al.* (1994) A proposal for classification of lymphoid neoplasms (by the International Lymphoma Study Group) *Histopathology*, **25** (6), 512–536.

Cochran, A.J. (2001) Sentinel node pathology, in *Progress in Pathology*, vol. 5 (eds N. Kirkham and N.R. Lemoine), Greenwich Medical Media Ltd, London, pp. 45–56.

Cotran, R.S., Kumar, V. and Collins, T. (eds) (1999) *Robbins Pathologic Basis of Disease*, 6th edn, W.B. Saunders Co., Philadelphia.

Cserni, G. (2003) Nodal staging of colorectal carcinomas and sentinel nodes. *Journal Clinical Pathology*, **56** (5), 327–335.

Cserni, G., Bianchi, S., Vezzosi, V. *et al.* (2006) The role of cytokeratin immunohistochemistry in the evaluation of axillary sentinel lymph nodes in patients with lobular breast carcinoma. *Journal of Clinical Pathology*, **59** (5), 518–522.

Dong, H.Y. (2003) B-cell lymphomas with coexpression of CD5 and CD10. *American Journal of Clinical Pathology*, **119** (2), 218–230.

Dupin, D., Diss, T.L., Kellam, P. *et al.* (2000) HHV-8 is associated with a plasmablastic variant of Castleman disease that is linked to HHV-8-positive plasmablastic lymphoma. *Blood*, **95** (4), 1406–1412.

Franco, R., Camacho, F.I., Caleo, A. *et al.* (2006) Nuclear bcl10 expression characterizes a group of ocular adnexa MALT lymphomas with shorter failure-free survival. *Modern Pathology*, **19** (8),1055–1067.

Goodlad, J.R. and Hollowood, K. (2001) Primary cutaneous B-cell lymphoma. *Current Diagnostic Pathology*, **7** (1), 33–44.

Isaacson, P.G. and Norton, A.J. (eds) (1994) *Extranodal Lymphomas*, 1st edn, Churchill Livingstone, London.

Jaffe, E.S., Harris, N.L., Diebold, J. and Müller-Hermelink, H-K. (1994) World Health Organisation classification of neoplastic diseases of the hematopoietic and lymphoid tissues – a progress report. *American Journal of Clinical Pathology*, **111** (Suppl.1), S8–S12.

Jaffe, E.S., Harris, N.L., Stein, H. and Vardiman, J.W. (eds) (2001) *WHO Classification of Tumours: Pathology & Genetics Tumours of Haematopoietic and Lymphoid Tissue*, 1st edn, IARC Press, Lyon.

Jensen, K.C., Higgins, K.P.T., Montgomery, K. *et al.* (2007). The utility of PAX5 immunohistochemistry in the diagnosis of undifferentiated malignant neoplasms. *Modern Pathology* **20** (8), 871–877.

Junqueira, L.C., Carneiro, J. and Long, J.A. (1986) *Basic Histology*. 5th edn, Appleton-Century-Crofts (Prentice-Hall), Norwalk, CT.

Kaifi, J.T., Strelow, A., Schurr, P.G *et al.* (2006) L1 (CD171) is highly expressed in gastrointestinal stromal tumors. *Modern Pathology*, **19** (3), 399–406.

Lee, F.D. (1994) Unusual sites and types of lymphoma, in *Recent Advances in Histopathology*, vol. 16 (eds P.P. Anthony, R.N.M. MacSween and D.G. Lowe), Churchill Livingstone, Edinburgh, pp. 73–93.

Lin, P., Mahdavy, M., Zhan, F. *et al.* (2004) Expression of PAX5 in CD20-positive multiple myeloma assessed by immunohistochemistry and oligonucleotide microarray. *Modern Pathology*, **17** (10), 1217–1222.

Liu, Z., Dong, H.Y., Gorczyca, W. *et al.* (2002) CD5-Mantle cell lymphoma. *American Journal Clinical Pathology*, **118** (2), 216–214.

---

[9] here Cc-like just means 'like centrocytes' and does not imply the Cc-like cells of MALToma / MZL

MacLennan, K.A, and Diebold, J. (1998) Anaplastic large cell lymphoma. *Current Diagnostic Pathology*, **5** (4), 165–173.

McKenney, J.K., Weiss, S.W. and Folpe, A.L. (2001) CD31 Expression in Intratumoral Macrophages: a potential diagnostic pitfall. *American Journal of Surgical Pathology*, **25** (9), 1167–1173.

Merzianu, M., Jiang, L., Lin, P., *et al.* (2006) Nuclear BCL-10 expression is common in lymphoplasmacytic lymphoma/Waldenström macroglobuli-naemia and does not correlate with p65 NF-κB activation. *Modern Pathology*, **19** (7), 891–898.

Murray, C.A., Leong, W.L., McCready, D.R. and Ghazarian, D.M. (2004) Histopathological patterns of melanoma metastasis in sentinel lymph nodes. *Journal of Clinical Pathology*, **57** (1), 64–57.

Robb-Smith, A.H.T. and Taylor, C.R. (1981) *Lymph Node Biopsy: A Diagnostic Atlas*, 1st edn, Miller Heyden Ltd, London.

Schraders, M., de Jong, D., Kluin, P. *et al.* (2005) Lack of Bcl-2 expression in follicular lymphoma may be caused by mutations in the BCL2 gene or by absence of the t(14;18) translocation. *Journal of Pathology*, **205** (3), 329–335.

Smellie, W.S.A., Forth, J., Smart, S.R.S. *et al.* (2007) Best practice in primary care pathology: review 7. *Journal of Clinical Pathology*, **60** (5), 458–465.

Slater, D.N. (2003) Diagnosis and classification of cutaneous lymphoproliferative disease, in *Recent Advances in Histopathology*, vol. 20 (eds D.Lowe and J.C.E. Underwood), Royal Society of Medicine Press Ltd, London, pp. 53–72.

Simpson, R.H.W. and Sarsfield, P.T.L. (1997) Benign and malignant lymphoid lesions of the salivary glands. *Current Diagnostic Pathology*, **4** (2), 91–99.

Stansfeld, A.G. and d'Ardenne, A.J. (eds) (1992) *Lymph Node Biopsy Interpretation*, 2nd edn, Churchill Livingstone, London.

Stevenson, F.K. and Wright, D.H. (1998) Hodgkin's disease and immunoglobulin genetics, in *Progress in Pathology*, vol. 4 (eds. N. Kirkham and N.R Lemoine), Churchill Livingstone, Edinburgh, pp. 99–111.

Swerdlow, S.H. (1997) Post-transplant lymphoproliferative disorders: a working classification. *Current Diagnostic Pathology*, **4** (1), 28–35.

Symmers, W. St. C. (ed) (1976) *Systemic Pathology*. vol. 2, 2nd edn, Churchill Livingstone, London.

Taylor, C. and Cote, R.J. (2006) *Immunomicroscopy. A Diagnostic Tool for the Surgical Pathologist.*, 3rd edn, Saunders Elsevier, London.

Warnke, R.A., Weiss, L.M., Chan, J.K.C., Cleary, M.L. and Dorfman, R.F. (1995) Tumors of the lymph nodes and spleen, fascicle 14 in *Atlas of Tumor Pathology* 3rd series, AFIP, Washington D.C.

Wheater, P.R., Burkitt, H.G. and Daniels, V.G. (1987) *Functional Histology: A text and colour atlas*, 2nd ed., Churchill Livingstone, Edinburgh.

Wilkins, B.S. (1997) Simplifying the spleen: a new look at splenic pathology, in *Progress in Pathology*, vol. 3 (eds N. Kirkham, N.R. Lemoine), Churchill Livingstone, NY, pp. 211–231.

Ye, H., Gong, L., Liu, H. *et al.* (2005) MALT lymphoma with t(14;18)(q32;q31)/IGH-MALT1 is characterised by strong cytoplasmic MALT1 and BCL10 expression. *Journal of Pathology*, **205** (3), 293–301.

Web sites

Royal College of Pathologists (2002) *Standards and minimum datasets for reporting cancers: Minimum dataset for the histopathological reporting of lymphoma*. Available online at: www.rcpath.org.uk (accessed May 2005).

11. Alimentary Tract

Normal

Mucins
- Gastric: neutral mucin ($\pm$ acid mucin in some foveolar cells but not in goblet form)
- Small intestinal goblets: both neutral and acid mucin (sialomucin i.e. carboxylated)
- Colonic goblets: both neutral and acid mucin (sulphomucin i.e. sulphated)

Oesophagus
- l.p. papillae should rise to $\leq 1/2$ the squamous epithelial thickness
- Basal layer is usu. <3 cells thick or 15% of the squamous epithelial thickness
- IELs: an occasional squiggle cell is normal (T8)

Stomach
- Lymphoid tissue:
  - ➢ superficial l.p. should have none or only an occ. lymphocyte +/ plasma cell[1]
  - ➢ deep l.p. should have no diffuse lymphocytes or plasma cells
  - ➢ an occ. 1° lymphoid aggregate may be seen just superficial to the m.m.
  - ➢ IELs (T8): <25/100 epithelial cells, and usu. <3/100
- Cardiac mucosa:
  - ➢ spaced-out and irregularly distributed mucinous glands (simple & compound) with foamy mucin (Brunner's gland-like) and some cystically dilated
  - ➢ smooth muscle slips may rise to separate glandular lobules
  - ➢ light lymphoplasmacytic infiltrate is probably normal
  - ➢ $\pm$ some oxyntic (parietal / acid-producing) cells
- Pyloric mucosa: glands gradually change to duodenal type $\therefore$ do not diagnose intestinal metaplasia here

Duodenum
- Lymphoid tissue:
  - ➢ l.p.: many lymphocytes, IgA plasma cells, few eos; mast cells (<8 per hpf); no PMN
  - ➢ l.p. lymphocyte gradient: most are in the deeper l.p. & fewest at villus tip
  - ➢ 2° follicles are normal and more numerous in the distal SI
  - ➢ IELs (T8): <20 per 100 epithelial cells (gradient: fewest at villus tip)
- Villus height is $\geq 2 \times$ crypt length (and often $3 \times$ to $5 \times$) away from Brunner's / lymphoid follicles
- Vertical smooth muscle slips extend up into normal villi
- *Pseudomelanosis duodeni*: iron-containing pigment in l.p. Mϕ

Colon
- l.p. lymphoplasmacytic gradient: the infiltrate is most intense superficially and least deep
- Caecal and right colon may have some plasma cells in the deepest l.p. at the crypt bases
- More distal colon should have no plasma cells at crypt base
- 'Herniation' of crypts into superficial submucosal lymphoid follicles may occur (lymphoglandular complex)
- Paneth cell gradient: most in caecum and decrease to zero by the mid-right colon
- Endocrine cells: most in rectum, decreasing to transverse; second peak in caecum, decreasing to transverse
- IELs (T8): <20 per 100 epithelial cells – in fact, 'normal' colon averages 4 per 100

Erosion, Ulceration and Aphthae

- Loss of surface epithelium may be artefactual $\therefore$ need evidence of pathology (e.g. fibrin)
- *Erosion* is ulceration that does not extend beyond the *lamina muscularis mucosae*
- *Ulcers* involve the full-thickness of the mucosa and extend (at least) into the submucosa

---

[1] the one exception being the cardia where a light infiltrate is considered normal

---

Diagnostic Criteria Handbook in Histopathology: A Surgical Pathology Vade Mecum by Paul J. Tadrous
Copyright © 2007 by John Wiley & Sons, Ltd.

- *Aphthae* are a clinical diagnosis in which histology usu. shows a circumscribed superficial erosion with a mixed chronic inflam^y infiltrate at the base and may overlie mucosal lymphoid aggregates. In the colon in Crohn's they have a characteristic structure that may help in diagnosis (*vide infra*)

Grading (General Criteria for Alimentary Tract Carcinomas)

- This general 'system' from the UICC applies to many carcinomas (not just GI) as part of TNM6 but see specific tumour types for detailed guidance and variant methods
- Applies to: oesophagus, upper & lower GI, anus, pancreas, gallbladder, extrahepatic biliary tree
- GX: grade cannot be assessed
- G1-4: well diff, moderately well diff, poorly diff, undifferentiated

Dysplasia (General Criteria for Glandular Dysplasia) and Carcinoma

- Criteria are modified depending on site and circumstance (see specific examples e.g. DALM in UC)
- Cytological: ➢ nuclear enlargement, hyperchromasia, pleomorphism, stratification
                 ➢ mitotic activity (increased, abnormal, beyond usual proliferative compartment)
- Architectural ➢ gland crowding, branching, budding, cribriformity, papillarity, surface villosity[2]
                 ➢ lack of maturation (abnormalities continue to the surface)
                 ➢ abrupt transition to non-neoplastic glands
- Vienna classification of GI neoplasia (an attempt to unify Western and Japanese reporting):

Category 1:   negative for dysplasia
Category 2:   indefinite for dysplasia (see 'Oesophagus' pp. 135–136 and 'Flat Dysplasia in Chronic idiopathic Inflammatory Bowel Disease (CIBD)', p. 150)
Category 3:   non-invasive low grade neoplasia (= low grade dysplasia / adenoma)
Category 4:   non-invasive high grade neoplasia
        4.1: high grade dysplasia / adenoma
        4.2: non-invasive carcinoma (= CIS)
        4.3: suspicion of invasion (incl. suspicion of invasion into the l.p.)
Category 5:   invasive carcinoma (see criteria below)
        5.1: intramucosal (incl. l.p./m.m.): l.p. invasion is insufficient for *colorectal* CA in the UK
        5.2: submucosal and beyond: this required for a diagnosis of *colorectal* CA in the UK

- Carcinoma: ➢ cribriform formations (a criterion accepted by some Eastern pathologists)
               ➢ solid cell islands   ⎱ at least one of these (together with
               ➢ single cell invasion   ⎰ dysplastic glands) is required by
               ➢ desmoplastic reaction   ⎰ most Western pathologists
               ➢ *NB*: desmoplasia is not always seen in early invasion and atypical architectures (e.g. cribriform) are more suggestive of invasion if expansile and disrupting other normal structures
- d/dg Isaacson lesions (reactive changes seen beneath ulcers):
Type I (epithelial): crowded acini with cytological atypia in a fibrinoid matrix: mitoses are scant / absent and the acini merge with benign reactive glands at the periphery
Type II (stromal): spindle / bizarre cells ± macronucleoli, cytoplasm may show granularity: homogenous chromatin, mitoses scant / absent. Many of these are endothelial.
- d/dg chemoRx/radioRx atypia: see 'Dysplasia (Flat / Non-Polypoid)' on p. 138 and see p. 148.

Mouth and Oropharynx

Classification of Odontogenic / Facial Cysts
A)   Developmental   ① dentigerous cyst
                     ② odontogenic keratocyst (may be a benign neoplasm *cf.* developmental)
B)   Inflammatory   ① radicular cyst   ⎱ both arise from a
                     ② paradental cyst   ⎰ periapical granuloma

---

[2] villosity is also seen in normal small bowel mucosa / metaplasia & UC inflammation without dysplasia

Dentigerous Cyst
- Assoc^d with an unerupted tooth (usu. 3rd molar 'wisdom' in adults / canine in a child)
- Can be very large; cyst is attached to the crown of the tooth
- Cyst *envelops the crown* of the tooth ∴ important to check X-ray
- Inflammation only in traumatised areas – otherwise uninflammatory
- Thin and regular squamous lining (gets thicker with age)
- *Focal* keratinisation in 10% of cases

Odontogenic Keratocyst
- Large soap bubble scalloped lucency which erodes bone but spares nerve
- If multiple consider Gorlin-Goltz (basal cell naevus) syndrome
- Inflammation only in traumatised areas – otherwise uninflammatory
- Cyst has hairpin bends and 'satellite cysts' (see Figure 11.1)
- Prominent basal layer with reversed polarity (d/dg cystic ameloblastoma)
- Thin squamous lining (8–12 cell layers) with corrugated surface and without rete pegs
- Most (85%) are parakeratotic but some (15%) are orthokeratotic
- Progresses, recurs and enlarges ∴ → radical surgery with jaw prosthesis

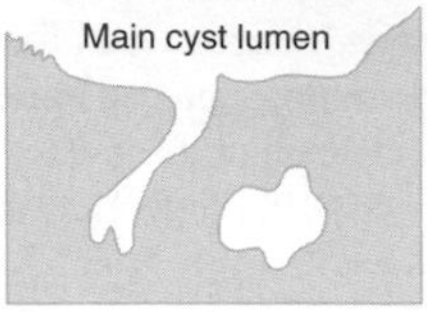

Main cyst lumen

FIGURE 11.1 Odontogenic keratocyst

Radicular (Dental) Cyst
- Assoc^d with a carous non-vital tooth (or PMHx thereof) – this is necessary for diagnosis
- Stratified squamous epithelium
- Epithelium has an arcade-like / reticular configuration at first (becomes attenuated with age)
- Inflammation (in wall) and cholesterol clefts (in wall and contents) ± foam cells
- Mucinous metaplasia (40%, ± respiratory epithelium in maxillary cysts)
- Hyaline laminated crescents (Rushton bodies – only seen in 5% but specific) ± PMN

Apical Granuloma
- This is a sequel to pulpitis in a carous tooth; may progress to form a radicular cyst
- Chronic inflammatory granulation tissue
- Squamous epithelium (as nests or a lacy network) permeates the lesion

Paradental Cyst
- Similar to apical granuloma but assoc^d with a partially impacted 3rd molar ('wisdom' tooth)

Ameloblastoma
- Adults, uni/multicystic ('soap bubble' lucency on X-ray)
- Biphasic: ① palisaded columnar / cuboidal epithelium with reversed polarity
            ② stellate reticulum
- No hard tissue formed except in some desmoplastic types that can have bone (if hard tissues are present consider d/dg craniopharyngioma)
- The stellate reticulum may show squamoid (± keratin) +/ granular cell change
- Epithelium may show focal squamous metaplasia in cystic areas
- Bland cytology and no mitoses (if more than a few mitoses consider malignant ameloblastoma)
- Variants: follicular, plexiform (interconnecting strands), desmoplastic, papilliferous and basaloid
- d/dg ameloblastic hyperplasia in the wall of a dentigerous cyst
- Malignant change: ➢ mitoses
                      ➢ clear cell areas (= low grade malignancy if otherwise benign ameloblastoma)
                      ➢ cytological atypia and cell crowding ± necrosis
                      ➢ NOT invasive margins (non-metastasising tumours may show invasion)

Ameloblastic Fibroma
- Child / adolescent
- Branching mushrooms of ameloblastoma-like epithelium in loose cellular fibrous stroma
- Cell-free zone in stroma around epithelium
- Mitoses uncommon

- Multiple sections to exclude dentine (otherwise = ameloblastic fibro-dentinoma or ameloblastic fibro-odontome if enamel has formed over the dentine)
- d/dg – !do not call this ameloblastoma – because unnecessarily radical surgery will result

Squamous Odontogenic Tumour
- Islands / strands of bland squamous epithelium with no peripheral palisading
- ± Keratin, ± cystic areas, ± dystrophic Ca^{2+} (but no amyloid)
- d/dg SCC: bland cytology
- d/dg ameloblastoma: no palisading
- d/dg Pindborg tumour: no amyloid / round masses of calcium / anisonucleosis

Calcifying Epithelial Odontogenic Tumour (Pindborg)
- Sheets / cribriform structures / nests of squamoid epithelium ± intercellular bridges
- Anisonucleosis with even chromatin
- Mitoses uncommon
- Hyaline amyloid amongst the epithelium (rounded masses, may calcify)

Clear Cell Odontogenic Tumour
- Elderly, aggressive tumour
- Cords and nests of clear cells and basaloid cells
- Mitoses ++
- No amyloid, calcium or mucus but glycogen is present
- d/dg clear cell tumours of salivary gland / clear cell ameloblastoma / Pindborg tumour

Primary Intraosseous Carcinoma
- Usu. in mandible and usu. SCC
- d/dg odontogenic tumours
- d/dg metastasis esp. RCC
- d/dg ameloblastoma / adamantinoma (*q.v.*)

Fibro-osseous Lesions
- Cementoblastoma: osteoblastoma at root of tooth (well-circumscribed, see p. 335)
- Ossifying fibroma: clearly defined margin on X-ray, well-circumscribed
- Fibrous dysplasia: poorly defined margin on X-ray (for features, see p. 334)
- Periapical cemental dysplasia

Oral Fibrous Polyps
- Fibroma of the lip: uninflamed un-orientated collagen bundles (i.e. they go in all directions)
- Fibrous epulis: inflamed vertically oriented collagen bundles continuous with underlying corium
- Pyogenic granuloma: inflamed lobular capillary growth ± ulceration
- Denture-assoc^d hyperplasia: simple lobulated hyperplastic polyp around denture edges
- Giant cell fibroma: large stellate stromal myofibroblasts ± multinucleation
- Ca^{2+} and ossification may occur in the stroma of any of these

Dysplasia in Squamous Oral Mucosa
- Grading is based on less-severe changes *cf.* CIN in the cervix (particularly for mild dysplasia)
- Rete peg elongation alone is not an arch. feature of dysplasia (*cf.* bulbous / 'drop'-shaped rete pegs)
- Mild: ➤ basal cell crowding with bulbous rete pegs and mild atypia (no need for ↑mitoses)
- Moderate: ➤ bulbous rete ± lateral projections (i.e. 2° nodules of basal cells extending laterally)
  - ➤ mild to moderate cytological atypia, suprabasal mitoses
  - ➤ changes extend to the middle $\frac{1}{3}$ (but do not completely fill the basal and spinous layers)
- Severe: ➤ atypia fills the basal and spinous layers (but need not extend to the surface, else = CIS)
  - ➤ cytological atypia is worse than in moderate dysplasia ± atypical mitoses
  - ➤ changes extend to upper $\frac{1}{3}$ (but surface cell nuclei may be normal)
- d/dg chronic candidiasis (incl. median rhomboid glossitis): see 'Pseudoepitheliomatous Hyperplasia (PEH) in the Oral Cavity', p. 133
- d/dg lichen planus: if dysplasia is present with LP call it 'dysplasia with a lichenoid reaction' not LP
- d/dg koilocytic atypia (HPV) occurs (esp. with HIV) but is not considered dysplasia in the mouth

SCC of Oral Mucosa
- 'Microinvasive' is not defined in terms of a depth measurement but as invasion to only the most superficial regions beneath the BM
- Verrucous carcinoma: criteria are as for skin (see p. 285)
- d/dg: PEH ± granular cell tumour (a deeper Bx may be needed to reveal this) / other cause
- d/dg: papillary hyperplasia of the palate: this shows nodular fibroplasia and irregular cross-sections of deep broad rete pegs with parakeratosis ± PEH with pseudo-'pearls' (! do not call it SCC)
- d/dg necrotising sialometaplasia (*vide infra*): SCC rarely occurs on the hard palate
- d/dg: lichenoid reactions (drugs, LP, discoid LE) cause irregularity of the basal layers and inflam^n
- SCC rarely arises on the dorsum of the tongue (unlike d/dg chronic Candida / granular cell tumour)

Salivary Glands

Pleomorphic Salivary Adenoma (PSAd)

Pathognomonic features   ① Chondromyxoid stroma (± adipose / bone)
                          ② Plasmacytoid myoepithelial cells (also seen in myoepithelioma)
                          ③ 'Streaming' pattern of myoepithelial cells (like a 'swarm of bees')
                          ④ Thick, fluffy elastic bands (centrally – shown well by EVG)
Prognostic features
- Margins
- The more the matrix the more the recurrence risk
- The more the cells the more the malignancy risk
Immuno
- Epithelium: CEA, PSA, EMA +ve
- Myoepithelium: calponin (for other myoepithelial cell markers, see p. 18)
- Low Ki-67 LI (1.6% *cf.* >20% for d/dg AdCC)
Malignancy and pleomorphic salivary adenoma
- Metastatic PSAd is a complication of surgery
- Carcinoma *ex* PSAd: ➤ any salivary CA that doesn't fit a standard type think CA *ex* PSAd (do EVG)
                         ➤ any type (except acinic cell) may occur
                         ➤ prognosis depends on whether the tumour is:
  ① *In situ* (↑/abnormal mitoses, coagulative necrosis, expansile nodule, widespread atypia [3]) or
  ② Invasive (distance of invasion from the PSAd capsule [some quote 8mm, others 5 to 6mm as the threshold for prognostic change], grade and type are all important features to assess)

Myoepithelioma of Salivary Gland (and Myoepithelial Carcinoma)
- Well-circumscribed
- Solid, myxoid and reticular architectures
- Myoepithelial cells may be: **s**pindled, **p**lasmacytoid, **e**pithelioid or **c**lear (rare)
- Spindle morphology is commonest in parotid with plasmacytoid in minor glands
- ± Small ducts (<10% of tumour)
- Immuno: S100, GFAP & CK14 +ve (and other myoepithelial markers – see p. 18)
- Malignancy (= *myoepithelial carcinoma*): ➤ invasion
                                            ➤ ↑ proliferation: ☞ mitotic count >7/10 hpf
                                                               ☞ Ki-67 LI >10%

Basal Cell Adenoma (and Basal Cell Adenocarcinoma)
- Major salivary glands; two subtypes (membranous and non-membranous)
- Two cell types: ① small dark with scant cytoplasm, ② larger with amphophil cytoplasm
- Cell nests surrounded by PAS +ve BM material (± peripheral palisading)
- Variant: Non-membranous:
  ➤ M=F, rarely recur or become malignant
  ➤ well-circumscribed, nests/trabeculae
  ➤ cells are admixed with dark ones tending to the periphery of the nests

---

[3] if atypia is mild then it is called 'atypical PSAd' rather than 'carcinoma *ex* PSAd'

> $\pm$ ducts and whorled eddies of epithelial cells
> variably cellular stroma contains S100 +ve spindle cells
- Variant: Membranous:
  > M$\gg$F, multicentric, $\frac{1}{4}$ recur locally, $\frac{1}{3}$ become malignant
  > unencapsulated, multinodular jigsaw pattern architecture
  > the PAS +ve BM material around islands and blood vessels is thick and hyaline
  > 50% assoc^d with dermal cylindroma / spiradenoma / other skin adnexal tumours
- Malignancy: invasiveness (= *basal cell adenocarcinoma*)
- d/dg adenoid cystic carcinoma: AdCC has more cytological atypia and mitoses and does not have epithelial whorled eddies and is not palisaded

Canalicular Adenoma
- Small
- Interconnecting strands of bilayered small, dark epithelial cells
- Loose vascular stroma
- No pleomorphism, mitoses or invasion (! but multifocality can mimic invasion)
- Immuno: strongly and diffusely S100 +ve
- d/dg adenoid cystic carcinoma: AdCC has true invasion and only focal or weak S100 +ve

Oncocytoma / Oncocytosis / Multinodular Oncocytic Hyperplasia (MNOH)
- PMHx of radioRx
- Round *central* nuclei with distinct nucleoli   } *cf.* d/dg acinic cell carcinoma
- Granular cytoplasm: DPAS −ve, PTAH +ve
- Prone to infarction → squamous metaplasia with 'reparative' nuclear atypia (!d/dg SCC)
- Malignancy: > invasiveness
              > coagulative tumour cell necrosis (not infarction)
              > abnormal mitotic figures
              > (atypia beyond the reparative type expected)

Adenoid Cystic Carcinoma (AdCC)
- Minor > major glands esp. palate, breast, bronchial glands (d/dg spread from salivary gland)
- Invasion (esp. perineural invasion)
- Cylindroma-like BM thickening around islands of basaloid cells with cribriform cystic spaces (acini)
- Basaloid acini are 'inverted' i.e. contain acid mucin (often with a central neutral mucin blob)
- Basaloid cells have angular hyperchromatic nuclei with a degree of pleomorphism
- True epithelial tubules are also admixed with central neutral mucin
- Immuno: +ve for c-kit (membranous), p63 (nuclear), S100 (focal, weak)
- Solid variant: > focally jagged islands of basaloid cells (not palisaded)
                 > $\pm$ small ducts within the basaloid islands
                 > $\pm$ coagulative tumour cell necrosis
                 > d/dg basal cell adenoma: (*vide supra*)

Salivary Duct Carcinoma
- Usu. major gland in middle aged
- Like high grade ductal carcinoma of the breast with comedo DCIS. In salivary glands this comedocarcinoma is considered to be an invasive component (unlike in the breast)
- Immuno: +ve for EMA, PSA, CEA, GCDFP15, $\pm$ PgR; −ve for ER and myoepithelial components
- d/dg metastatic carcinoma: breast 1° must be excluded clinically
- d/dg high grade MEC: esp. if more than sparse mucin is present

Polymorphous Low Grade Adenocarcinoma (PLGA, Terminal Duct Carcinoma)
- Usu. minor salivary glands
- Cells are rounded / oval; nuclei are uniform with finely speckled chromatin $\pm$ PTC-like vacuoles
- 'Architectural diversity' (ducts, cribriform, ILC-like, diffuse infiltration)
- Capsular, vascular and perineural invasion (the latter may be 'targetoid')
- Immuno: triad of EMA, S100, vimentin +ve
- Papillary variants are more aggressive
- d/dg AdCC: > cytology (AdCC has angular, hyperchromatic nuclei with pleomorphism)
             > proliferation fraction by MIB1: <10% for PLGA, >10% for adenoid cystic CA

Acinic Cell Carcinoma
- May be bilateral
- Microcystic / thyroid follicular / solid arch. with regimented *marginal* nuclei } *cf.* oncocytic
- Granular cytoplasm: DPAS +ve, PTAH −ve } tumours
- Stromal lymphoid follicles
- Good prognosis subtype: ➢ well-circumscribed
                            ➢ microcystic } throughout
                            ➢ lymphoid follicles

Mucoepidermoid Carcinoma (MEC)
- Any age, major/minor salivary gland, tracheobronchial tree, jaw bones
- Macro: solid ± cystic areas
- Micro: infiltrative as irregular islands (solid ± cystic with mucin) and variable stromal fibrosis and inflammation (? due to a reaction to extravasated mucin)
- Three cell types: ① epidermoid (intercellular bridges but keratin rare), ② intermediate, ③ mucus cells
- Low grade: ➢ well-developed mucus cells and cysts make up a large proportion of the tumour (intracystic spaces account for >10% of tumour area by Evans' criteria [not counting stroma and areas occupied by extravasated mucin])
              ➢ squamoid features not well developed (bridges hard to demonstrate, no keratin)
              ➢ fibroinflammatory stroma prominent
- High grade: ➢ mostly solid
               ➢ squamoid features well developed ± minor keratinisation (full keratinisation and pearls still rare)
               ➢ mucus cells (necessary for diagnosis) – may need DPAS/mucicarmine to show them
               ➢ aggressive invasion pattern plus at least one of the following
               ➢ 'other high grade features': high grade cytological atypia, ↑ mitoses (>4 per 10 hpf), tumour necrosis, perineural / vascular / bony invasion
- Intermediate Grade: *EITHER* a) some minor cystic areas and well-developed mucus cells *OR* b) predom. composed of intermediate cells with aggressive invasion but no 'other high grade features'
- Variant: Sclerosing MEC has paucicellular keloidal central scarring with inflammatory aggregates mixed with tumour islands at periphery (!d/dg benign inflammatory lesion)
- d/dg poorly diff adenocarcinoma, SCC or ASC: see p. 92
- d/dg Warthin or PSAd with squamous differentiation
- d/dg salivary cystadenoma / cystadenocarcinoma
- d/dg mucocoele (*vs.* low grade MEC)
- d/dg salivary duct carcinoma with mucus cells (*vs.* high grade MEC)

Mucus Clear Cell Tumours of Salivary Glands
- MEC
- Variants of salivary duct carcinoma

Non-mucus Clear Cell Tumours of Salivary Glands
- Monomorphic: 1. Epithelial: Hyalinising Clear Cell Carcinoma
                2. Myoepithelial: Myoepithelioma / carcinoma
- Dimorphic: *Epithelial myoepithelial carcinoma* ➢ well-circ., lobules, organoid, low grade
                                                   ➢ clear cells glycogen +ve
                                                   ➢ epithelial (eosinophilic) cells DPAS +ve
- Metastatic: RCC, thyroid, melanoma, SCC with clear cell change
- Clear cell variants of: *Acinic* (DPAS +ve, PTAH −ve) or *Oncocytic* (DPAS −ve, PTAH +ve) tumours

Myoepithelial Sialadenitis = Lymphoepithelial Sialadenitis (MESA / LESA) = Autoimmune Sialadenitis
- Old name = *benign lymphoepithelial lesion*; assoc[d] with autoimmune / CTD
- Early: ➢ duct dilates
          ➢ light / focal infiltrate of duct epithelium by B-cells with centrocyte-like morphology (Cc-like cells) that merge with the mantle zones of the surrounding follicles
          ➢ duct surrounded by lymphoid tissue with follicles and germinal centres
          ➢ plasma cells also present (esp. around the ducts)

- Later: ducts condense with obliteration of the lumen to leave solid nests of epithelial, myoepithelial and B-cells (epimyoepithelial islands) – highlighted by CK immuno
- The earliest change of transformation to MALToma (MZL) is the presence of a pale zone of clear Cc-like cells around the duct or epimyoepithelial island. These cells loose there mantle B-cell phenotype (IgD +ve, IgM +ve) to display a marginal zone phenotype (IgD −ve, IgM +ve).

Non-Autoimmune Sialadenitis (e.g. due to duct obstruction)
- Lymphocytic infiltration of the ducts is mild and there are scarce/no LEL (*cf.* d/dg LESA)
- Ducts may contain PMN, calculus +/ squamous metaplasia
- Main inflammation is in the acini
- Late changes = acinar atrophy, stromal fibrosis ± heavy chronic inflammation ± germinal centres. These can cause a hard palpable gland (= *Küttner's tumour* in the submandibular gland)
- Some forms of Küttner's tumour may have IgG4 +ve plasma cells (see multifocal fibrosclerosis)

Necrotising Sialometaplasia
- Usu. minor glands, ischaemic aetiology (post radiation / FNA or adjacent to infarction, *etc.*)
- Lobular architecture is preserved
- Extensive squamous metaplasia of both ducts and acini
- Inflammation ± granulation tissue / residual infarction
- PEH of overlying squamous epithelium (e.g. in palatal lesions)
- d/dg SCC: retained lobular architecture goes against SCC, and metaplastic ducts may retain lumena

Oral Hairy Leukoplakia
- Due to EBV; seen in immunosuppression regardless of HIV status
- Hyperkeratosis and acanthosis with minimal / no underlying inflammation
- Ballooning degeneration of keratinocytes ± intranuclear ground glass inclusions / beaded nuclei
- ± Koilocytic atypia (may also be due to d/dg HPV)
- d/dg chronic biting, Candida, maceration, white sponge naevus

Pseudoepitheliomatous Hyperplasia (PEH) in the Oral Cavity
- Chronic hyperplastic candidosis incl. median rhomboid glossitis: more usually this gives broad-based enlargement of the rete with atrophy over the connective tissue papillae but PEH may occur: look for PMN ± microabscesses and fungal hyphae on PAS
- Granular cell tumour (esp. tongue)
- Necrotising sialometaplasia (esp. palate, looks like a 'malignant ulcer' clinically) – *vide supra*
- Papillary hyperplasia of the palate (usu. due to poorly fitting or continuously worn dentures) – *vide supra*
- d/dg SCC: SCC is rare on the dorsum of the tongue and hard palate and shows abrupt squamous differentiation / keratinisation (not maturation from a basal layer like PEH) – see also p. 285

Cystic Lesions of Salivary Glands
- Warthin's tumour:
  - bilayer of oncocytic epithelium (inner columnar often with nuclei towards lumen, outer cuboidal)
  - ± squamous (! d/dg atypical squamous metaplasia is not SCC), mucous, ciliated metaplasia
  - stroma may be lymphoid rich or poor (esp. in the elderly)
  - malignancy in epithelium: SCC / poorly diff carcinoma / MEC
  - malignancy in stroma: any lymphoma that affects LNs
- Benign lymphoepithelial cyst (= 'simple cyst'):
  - lining is branchial-type (squamous +/ respiratory +/ columnar +/ cuboidal)
  - wall contains reactive lymphoid tissue ± follicles
  - no epimyoepithelial islands
- Cystic LESA:
  - instead of contracting to form epimyoepithelial islands, some ducts dilate → multicystic
- Cystic lymphoid hyperplasia of HIV:
  - LESA variant with Cc-like B-cells infiltrating cyst lining ± epimyoepithelial islands
  - multiple cysts lined by squamous epithelium (or cuboidal / columnar / respiratory)
  - undulating appearance to the epithelial lining

> florid HIV-type lymphoid reaction in the wall:
  - ☞ follicular hyperplasia (± 'naked follicles' i.e. without mantles)
  - ☞ folliculolysis, plasmacytosis, *etc.* (for more details, see p. 119)

- Cystic MALToma: can develop in cystic LESA
- Cystic MEC:
  > d/dg benign lymphoepithelial cyst (see box):
  > d/dg mucocoele: *vide infra*, also mucocoeles are very rare in major salivary glands

MEC has more mucous cells *cf.* squames
MEC shows solid areas
MEC has a mixture of cell types
MEC is infiltrative

- Cystic metastatic carcinoma: d/dg cystic SCC *vs.* benign lymphoepithelial cyst *vs.* keratocystoma
- Keratocystoma: multiple benign squamous cysts usu. in a major gland and without mucous cells, lobular arch. or skin adnexa (*cf.* d/dg trichoadenoma / dermoid / SCC / necrotising sialometaplasia)
- Papillary cystic acinic cell carcinoma: (see 'Acinic Cell Carcinoma', above)
- Cystadenoma (papillary cystadenoma):
  > major / minor glands, slow growing and painless
  > single / multicystic
  > dense fibrotic stroma
  > cysts lined by attenuated ductal epithelium ± papillary projections
  > bland nuclei, mitoses scant / absent
  > ± metaplasias (mucous, oncocytic, squamous)
  > d/dg salivary duct ectasia
  > d/dg cystic MEC (solid areas, infiltrative, mixed cell types)
  > d/dg cystadenocarcinoma (invasion)
- Cystadenocarcinoma (papillary cystadenocarcinoma):
  > major and minor glands, asymptomatic, low grade malignancy
  > single / multicystic with great variation in cyst size within any given tumour
  > fibrotic / sclerotic / desmoplastic stroma
  > single layer to pseudostratified cuboidal / columnar cells
  > prominent nucleoli and mild to moderate atypia
  > invasion into surrounding parenchyma is the diagnostic feature
  > d/dg papillary cystic acinic cell carcinoma and salivary cystadenoma (*q.v.*)
- Polycystic disease of the parotid (dysgenetic disease):
  > retained lobular architecture
  > honeycomb multicystic dilatation of lobules
  > cysts contain flocculant material
- Sclerosing polycystic adenosis: > lobular architecture retained
  > variably-sized cysts
  > adjacent cellular areas resembling sclerosing adenosis of the breast
- Retention mucocoele: (usu. in minor salivary glands) has an intact epithelial lining
- Extravasation mucocoele: (usu. in minor salivary glands)
  > small ones may collapse to a muciphagic granuloma otherwise you see. . .
  > a pool of mucin with peripheral foamy Mϕ,
  > ± lined by granulation tissue / fibrosis
  > large cysts may have a rim of compressed Mϕ (! do not confuse for an epithelial lining)
  > sublingual gland extravasation mucocoeles lying to one side of the frenulum can be large and are known as *ranula*. They may dissect the deep soft tissues of the head and neck ($\rightarrow$ plunging / dissecting ranula) and excision of sublingual gland is required for cure

Oesophagus

Reflux Oesophagitis (part of Gastro-Oesophageal Reflux Disease – GORD)
- Basal layer hyperplasia (alone this may be normal / physiological)
- Oedema / spongiosis
- ↑ IELs, eosinophils, PMN
- ↑ Height of papillae into upper $\frac{1}{2}$ of epithelium
- Superficial engorged capillaries

- ± Peptic ulceration
- d/dg: pemphigus, *etc.*: in systemic skin disease the changes are usu. in mid to upper oesophagus
- d/dg: HSV, candidal or CMV oesophagitis
- d/dg ! beware local reflux changes adjacent to carcinoma (∴ do levels if clinically ? CA)
- d/dg adult eosinophilic oesophagitis is favoured by dysphagia (*cf.* heartburn), M>F, age <45, rings & lack of hiatus hernia on endoscopy, l.p. fibrosis & eos., many intraepithelial eos. (≥20–25 in 1 hpf or ≥15 in ≥2 hpf), eos. abscesses; (important because Rx is allergen exclusion rather than antacids)

Progressive Systemic Sclerosis (PSS) ± CREST Syndrome
- Intimal thickening and elastosis of arteries
- Submucosal fibrosis and atrophy of smooth muscle
- GORD

Achalasia of the Cardia
- May be 1° (idiopathic ?autoimmune) or 2° (e.g. to neoplasia, sarcoid, vagotomy, MEN 2b, etc.)
- Distal constrict^n: loss of myenteric plexus neurons ± patchy fibrosis, lymphocytic & eos. inflam^n ± Lewy bodies
- Proximal dilatation: fibrosis, muscularis propria hypertrophy ± severe GORD ± ulceration
- Other 2° changes incl.: BO, haemorrhage, Candida, SCC
- d/dg Chagas' disease: *T. cruzi* amastigotes (≈ *Leishmania*) in intracellular 'cysts' seen in early stages

Barrett's Oesophagus (BO)

Def^n: *Classical BO*:   > 3cm from GOJ shows any of: cardiac mucosa / atrophic fundic mucosa / intestinal metaplasia — this is a combined endoscopic and histological diagnosis

Short-segment BO: < 3cm but only i.m. is allowed

Ultra-short-segment BO = i.m. within the SCJ

Classical and short: ➢ assoc^d with reflux (gastro-oesophageal acid, SI contents and bile)
                 ➢ CagA +ve *H. Pylori* may be protective
Ultrashort   ➢ not necessarily assoc^d with reflux or classical BO
            ➢ assoc^d with *H. Pylori* gastritis (may be a form of carditis)

Histodiagnosis of BO[4]:

- *Definite*: native oesophageal structures[5] juxtaposed to metaplastic glandular mucosa[6]
- *Conditional*:   ➢ inflammation in disorganised gastric mucosa
  (on endoscopy)   ➢ intestinal metaplasia (only the presence of i.m. is a definite cancer risk)
- *Other features*: a reduplicated m.m. (new component superficial to old) ± hyperplastic polyps

Soft Tissue Tumours
- Carcinosarcoma (d/dg inflammatory pseudotumour – see Chapter 21: Soft Tissues)
- Inflammatory fibroid polyp (*vide infra*)
- Granular cell tumour (± PEH – don't mis-diagnose as SCC)
- Leiomyoma (d/dg GIST).   ➢ arise from muscularis propria / m.m. / vessels
                        ➢ <5cm and unencapsulated (1–2mm ones are 'seedling leiomyomas')
                        ➢ histology as for leiomyoma elsewhere
                        ➢ d/dg very rare leiomyosarcoma: >5cm, necrosis, mitoses >5/10 hpf
                        ➢ d/dg diffuse leiomyomatosis: adolescents, hereditary associat^{n}s

Glandular Dysplasia
- No universally agreed criteria to distinguish low grade from high grade (see also p. 127)
- Cytology alone cannot distinguish dysplasia from invasive carcinoma (∴ need histology)
- High grade should be corroborated by an 'expert' (at least double reporting) or 2nd Bx

---

[4] the term 'Barrett's epithelium' refers to simple tall columnar mucinous epithelium (± goblet cells) with thin and irreg. (partially beaded) apical mucin that may occur in BO – this term is best avoided given the current clinicopathological definitions of BO and given that some people use the terms 'Barrett's epithelium / metaplasia / oesophagus' interchangeably in the literature
[5] i.e. oesophageal ducts (with a stratified squamoid lining) and submucosal glands (≈ minor salivary glands)
[6] not necessarily intestinal metaplasia

- Low grade:
    - ➤ cytology equivalent to mild / moderate dysplastic colonic adenoma
    - ➤ nuclei ovoid or pencil-like and usu. stratified (but often mild or not full-thickness)
    - ➤ architectural abnormalities are usu. mild
- High grade: (some require these changes to be present in > 1 or 2 crypts to qualify as high grade)
    - ➤ *EITHER* cytology ≈ severely dysplastic colonic adenoma *AND/OR* severe arch. abnormalities
    - ➤ rounded nuclei with open chromatin and prominent nucleoli which may be irregular
    - ➤ the nuclear arrangement is more disorganised than just stratified
    - ➤ more severe arch. changes (budding, complexity, etc.)
    - ➤ 50% have co-existent invasive carcinoma, esp. if there is a nodule or ulcer on endoscopy
- BCDA: has *both* arch. complexity and dysplasia-type cytological atypia but with surface maturation
- Immuno: AMACAR +vity may suggest neoplasia (–vity means nothing), p53 is controversial
- Features causing problems in diagnosis: (usu. false positive)
    - ➤ ↑ size of proliferative zone
    - ➤ variable position of proliferative zone in different types of metaplasia (gastric *vs.* intestinal)
    - ➤ change to intestinal-type epithelium (esp. a patch of intestinal metaplasia in an otherwise gastric area)
    - ➤ inflammation esp. acute (→ 'indefinite for dysplasia') or reactive (chemical) gastritis-type
    - ➤ surface re-epithelialisation with squamous mucosa: may mask the underlying dysplastic glands (difficult because there is no glandular surface to help assess loss of maturation)
    - ➤ artefacts e.g. cross-cutting, variable thickness or staining, etc. (consider 'indefinite for dysplasia')
    - ➤ d/dg Isaacson lesions (esp. Type II *vs.* SCC) – see p. 127
- Management: ➤ *Indefinite* → early (3 month) re-endoscopy after Rx for inflammation
    - ➤ *Low grade* → close F/U with endoscopies
    - ➤ *High grade* → laser/photodynamic/submucosal resection/surgery[7]

Squamous Dysplasia
- Same criteria as squamous dysplasia elsewhere (except oral cavity)
- Low grade if <1/2 the epithelial thickness involved, high grade if >1/2
- d/dg ! exclude inflammatory atypia ⎫ these have vesicular nuclei with nucleoli (may be irregular
- d/dg ! exclude regenerative atypia ⎬ or elongated) and normal mitoses. Dysplasia has ↑ NCR, hyperchromasia, mitoses ++ (that may be abnormal) ⎭ and disturbed cytoarchitecture

Oesophageal Carcinoma
- Main 1° types: SCC, adenoCA, SmCC, ASC: grade by worst area (well/mod./poorly diff./undiff)
- Invasion of submucosal lymphatics results in 'skip' lesions away from any macroscopic main lesion
- d/dg SCC *vs.* PEH (esp. when 2° to granular cell tumour)

Neoadjuvant Rx (Pre-op ChemoRx ± RadioRx)
- Mucin pools, keratinous nodules and effects of chemoRx/radioRx on benign tissues may be seen
- Only viable tumour epithelial cells allow diagnosis of residual tumour for staging purposes (apoptotic cells or mucin/keratin alone do not count) – multiple levels and CK immuno may be used to detect viable epithelial cells. (See also 'Neoadjuvant Rx (Pre-op RadioRx ± ChemoRx)' in 'Colorectal Carcinoma')

Other Nodular / Mass Lesions and Cysts
- Squamous papilloma: filiform arch., hyperplastic non-dysplastic squamous epithelium ± HPV changes
- Adenoma (see 'Adenomatous Polyp (Gastric Adenoma)', p. 138) – may occur as part of Barrett's dysplasia
- Minor salivary gland-type tumours arising from oesophageal glands
- 2° tumours: melanoma, breast carcinoma, testicular tumours, etc.
- Glycogenic acanthosis
- Fibrovascular polyp: usu. lined by squamous epithelium but not filiform (*cf.* papilloma)
- Cysts: duplication, bronchogenic, pseudodiverticular, etc.

---

[7] ? a role for F/U endoscopy i.e. conservative – always check local Mx protocols with clinicians

Stomach

Chronic Gastritis (Usual Types)
A) atrophic: body, PA, ECL-cell hyperplasia / tumourlets. Assoc[d] with i.m., adenoma, adenocarcinoma
B) bacterial (HLO): mention presence and severity of chronic inflam[n], activity (= *intraepithelial* PMN), i.m., atrophy, lymphoid follicles, HLOs, dysplasia and malignancy. HLOs are assoc[d] with activity, 2° lymphoid follicles, i.m. & MALToma.; intestinal metaplasia is associated with adenocarcinoma
C) chemical / reactive (due to alcohol, bile reflux, NSAID, etc.): foveolar hyperplasia, fibrosis, oedema, vertical smooth muscle in l.p., superficial vascular ectasia and sparse chronic inflam[n]. GAVE = florid type C gastritis

Lymphocytic Gastritis and Collagenous Gastritis
- ↑ T-cells in both l.p. and epithelium (≥ 25 per 100 epithelial cells)
- Small mature T-cells with pericellular clear halo
- ± Aphthae
- 'collagenous gastritis' if there is a subepithelial collagen band (>10μ thick)
- Assoc[d] with: coeliac, Crohn's, *H. Pylori*, lymphoma, adenocarcinoma, HIV and idiopathic

Eosinophilic Gastritis
- Eosinophils predominate throughout the l.p.
- l.p. fibrosis
- Assoc[d] with allergies, parasites, CTD, Crohn's and idiopathic

Granulomatous Gastritis
- Infective: H. pylori, TB, fungi, Whipple's, syphilis, etc.
- Sarcoidosis
- Crohn's (also has patchy acute inflam[n] ± fissures / ulcerat[n] ± eos. ± submucosal lymphoid aggregates ± focal destruction of glands by T-cells [= *focally enhanced gastritis* ≈ focal lymphocytic gastritis])
- Foreign body-type (assoc[d] with erosions or peptic ulcer)
- Idiopathic (= 'isolated') or rarer specific causes

Alcoholic Gastropathy (Haemorrhagic Gastropathy, Portal HT Gastropathy)
- 'Snakeskin' appearance at endoscopy may be seen (vascular changes) – fundal predominance
- Superficial mucosal haemorrhages ± haemosiderin
- Adjacent oedema
- Usu. lacks inflammation
- d/dg Erosive 'Gastritis': this is similar and is commonly seen in very ill patients (stress-related)

Intestinal Metaplasia (i.m.)
- Assoc[d] with ↑ risk of carcinoma – esp. in incomplete types and esp. in type III.
- Goblet cells contain both neutral and acid (either sialo or sulpho) mucin
- Complete i.m. (type I): goblet cells surrounded by intestinal absorptive cells (± Paneth / NE cells)
- Incomplete i.m. (types II and III): goblet cells surrounded by altered columnar mucinous cells (altered such as to have acid mucin and in smaller amounts *cf.* normal gastric mucin cells).
- Subtyping is based on the columnar (not goblet) cell acid mucin: sialo = type II, sulpho = type III (also known as type IIa and IIb respectively)

Ménétrier's Disease
- Protein-loosing hypertrophic gastric body fold disease. Progressive in adults / self limiting in a child
- Massive body / fundus foveolar hyperplasia with cystic glands deeper
- Mucus plugs in glands
- Atrophy of chief and parietal cells (∴ ↓ gastric acid unlike ZE syndrome)
- d/dg infection (esp. CMV)
- d/dg ZE Syndrome: ECL-cell hyperplasia, parietal cell hyperplasia and pancreatic / duodenal gastrinoma → hypergastrinaemia (unlike Ménétrier)
- d/dg hypertrophic hypersecretory gastropathy (very rare)

Fundic Gland Polyp
- Usu. fundal mucosa and average size <5mm
- Cystically dilated fundic glands
- Bland, often attenuated epithelium in cysts
- Assoc^d with: idiopathic, long term gastric acid suppression, FAP (dysplasia common)

Inflammatory Fibroid Polyp
- Macro: smooth submucosal mass that may ulcerate, usu. <5cm, occurs in upper & lower GIT
- Submucosal vascular granulation tissue with variable inflammatory infiltrate
- Perivascular hypocellular zones
- Variable nõ. of eosinophils (but not peripheral eosinophilia)
- ± Leiomyoma / Schwannoma-like areas with nuclear palisading
- Immuno: CD34 +ve, >95% are −ve for c-kit

Peutz-Jeghers Polyp – See p. 149

Hyperplastic Polyp (Regenerative Polyp)
- Usu. junctional mucosa and average size 1cm (if >2cm have ↑ risk of dysplasia / carcinoma)
- Cystic ± branching foveolar hyperplasia and 'onion skin' concentric arrangement of glands
- Stromal oedema ++, ± inflam^n, smooth muscle fibres extend up around gland aggregates
- Bland epithelium ± inflam^y atypia / ulceration (! d/dg focal dysplasia / CA which may also occur)

Dysplasia (Flat / Non-Polypoid)
- Usual features of dysplasia extending to the surface in the absence of complicating factors
- Low grade: cytological features not marked, mitoses normal, architecture minimally disturbed
- High grade: marked cytological +/ arch. atypia, abnormal mitoses
- May occur within i.m. (goblets may loose polarity) or apart from i.m. but is often assoc^d with i.m.
- Immuno: p53 nuclear +vity and Ki-67 extending to the surface epithelium favour dysplasia
- d/dg (complicating factors): sig. PMN infiltrate, foveolar hyperplasia, granulation tissue, ulcer slough
- d/dg chemoRx / radioRx atypia shows surface maturation, preserved polarity, cytoplasmic eosinophilia/vacuoles, microcystic arch. in deeper glands, normal mitoses present in normal distribution (also p53 −ve & Ki-67 restricted to usual proliferative zones), no i.m. nearby

Adenomatous Polyp (Gastric Adenoma)
- Usu. sessile, solitary and antral and may be large (few cm) ± nearby intestinal metaplasia
- Arch.: tubular, villous and TV ± underlying non-dysplastic cystic gastric glands
- Cytology: mild / moderate / severe dysplasia (criteria are as for colonic adenomas)
- ± intestinal differentiation (absorptive, goblet, NE and Paneth cells) which may predominate
- Invasive foci: single cell infiltration / solid areas / back-to-back cribriform areas
- Must assess completeness of excision
- d/dg hyperplastic / other polyps: presence of dysplasia and intestinal differentiation in adenomas

Gastric Carcinoma: Classification, Grading and Typing
- Laurén's classification of gastric carcinoma:
  - intestinal (tubules/papillae ± solid foci, cuboidal / columnar cytoplasm, basal nuclei)
  - diffuse (infiltrative polygonal cells, often signet ring). Signet ring cells usu. have acid mucin *cf.* the neutral mucin of benign gastric epithelium hence the use of an ABDPAS for screening gastric biopsies (! but some signet ring carcinomas have purely neutral mucin).
  - mixed / unclassified (Carneiro's classification is similar but subdivides the unclassified group into solid [cords and islands] and mixed [diffuse plus intestinal / solid – the smallest component being ≥5% of the tumour] subtypes)
- Ming's classification of gastric carcinoma:
  - expansile margin with discrete nodules (better prog. unless early gastric cancer)
  - infiltrative (worse prognosis unless early gastric cancer)
- Mucin-based (intra and extracellular) classifications (e.g. intracellular mucin with Goseki):
  - mucin poor: better prog. (Goseki group 1 – well-formed tubules, 3 – poorly-formed tubules)
  - mucin-rich: poorer prog. (Goseki group 2 – well-formed tubules, 4 – poorly-formed tubules)
- WHO classification:
  - by predominant pattern: papillary, tubular, mucinous, signet ring, special types (*vide infra*)
  - widely believed to be prognostically useless

- Grading: UK National Dataset method is based on the most poorly diff. area as:
  - ➢ poorly diff: i.e. diffuse / signet ring / non-cohesive tumours
  - ➢ other: usu. intestinal type / cohesive growth pattern
- Grading: WHO method is based on the proportion of tumour composed of glands:
  - ➢ well diff: >95%
  - ➢ moderately diff: 50–95%
  - ➢ poorly diff: <50%
- Types of gastric carcinoma other than typical intestinal-type adenocarcinoma:
  - ➢ signet ring carcinoma (WHO def^n requires >50% signet ring type)
  - ➢ mucinous carcinoma (WHO def^n requires >50% mucinous type)
  - ➢ SCC, ASC, SmCC, ChC, carcinosarcoma and spindle cell carcinoma
  - ➢ medullary carcinoma (>50% is poorly diff, lymphoid stroma, lack of fibrous tissue)
  - ➢ anaplastic carcinoma with extensive PMN infiltration
  - ➢ malignant rhabdoid tumour (vimentin +ve)
  - ➢ hepatoid (bile canaliculi & AFP +ve, typical adenocarcinoma foci elsewhere)
  - ➢ metastatic (very rare, may be multiple, usu. submucosal centric and arise by lymphatic or blood spread from: melanoma, breast, thyroid, testis, lung, oesophagus and elsewhere)

Differential Diagnosis of Signet Ring Carcinoma of Stomach (esp. on Frozen Section)
- ILC of the breast
- Signet ring carcinoma from other 1° sites: e.g. prostate, bladder, cholangiocarcinoma, etc.
- Malakoplakia (variant with non-mineralised PAS +ve bodies), muciphages or xanthelasma
- Signet ring lymphoma / mesothelioma / melanoma / ovarian stromal tumour / uterine leiomyoma/sarcoma / amphicrine MTC, signet ring morphology in CNS tumours (oligodendroglioma and ependymoma)

Neuroendocrine Pathology of the GIT
- The following criteria and terms relate to the upper GIT but some apply them in the colon also
- Hindgut (rectosigmoid) carcinoids are different. They arise in the submucosa, are usu. trabecular and poor prognostics are: invasion of muscularis propria, size >1 cm (add esp. if >2 cm), lymph/blood vasc. invasion, tumour ulceration, mitotic count.
- d/dg includes glomus tumour, paraganglioma and adenocarcinoma

NE cell hyperplasia
- Def^n: ↑ numbers of NE cells *within* a pre-existing gland / crypt:
- Confined to the mucosa (by definition)
- May be linear or nodular with nodules no wider than the width of a normal gland / crypt (sometimes called 'micronodules' hence 'micronodular hyperplasia')
- Each nodule surrounded by BM
- Adenomatoid hyperplasia = ≥5 micronodules close to each other with interposed BM

NE Cell Dysplasia (= pre-carcinoid)
- Fusion of micronodules with loss of intervening BM
- Micronodules enlarge beyond the size of a normal gland / crypt
- Total size >0.15 mm but <0.5 mm in max. ∅
- ± Cytological atypia
- ± Microinvasion of the lamina propria

Microcarcinoid (= Tumourlet)
- Def^n: NE-proliferation >0.5mm ∅, the upper measurement limit is not defined but it must be confined to the mucosa and not macroscopically (clinically / endoscopically) visible

Carcinoid
- Def^n: a well diff. NE-proliferation >0.5mm ∅ which either:
  - ① invades the muscularis mucosae or
  - ② is large enough to be macroscopically visible (clinically / endoscopically).
- The following is a guide to aggressiveness but the terms 'benign', 'borderline' and 'malignant' are best avoided since all carcinoids are potentially malignant
- 'Benign': <1cm ∅, no angioinvasion, tumour limited to mucosa / submucosa
- 'Borderline': either ① <1cm with angioinvasion but limited to mucosa / submucosa or
                        ② 1–2cm, no angioinvasion, limited to mucosa / submucosa

- Mucinous carcinoid / goblet cell carcinoid: more aggressive *cf.* other carcinoids and is probably a form of argyrophil adenocarcinoma (for details, see 'Appendix', p. 152)
- *Atypical carcinoid*: any of the following: ① necrosis (usu. punctate, not extensive)

  ② mitoses >2/10 hpf

  ③ cytological atypia (e.g. prominent nucleoli)
- 'Malignant': any of the following: ➢ functioning tumour (NE peptide effects)
  - ➢ 1–2cm with angioinvasion
  - ➢ >2cm without angioinvasion
  - ➢ invades the muscularis propria or beyond

Types of upper GI / gastric carcinoid

- Any type of carcinoid may have a sub-population of cells expressing any other NE peptide
- The four main types of NE cell (and tumours) in the stomach / upper GI are:

① ECL-cell (histamine, 5-HT or no product in carcinoids):
  - ➢ proliferate in response to hypergastrinaemia (any cause)
  - ➢ d/dg EC-cell: ECL-cell is +ve for VMAT-2, CgA, Grimelius; −ve for serotonin and argentaffin
  - ➢ gastric ECL-cell carcinoids occur usu. in the proximal stomach and are typed as:

Type I: assoc^d with ↑gastrinaemia 2° to chronic atrophic gastritis ⎤ usu. multiple, small & arise on a
Type II: assoc^d with ↑gastrinaemia without atrophy e.g. MEN 1/ZE ⎦ background of ECL-cell hyperplasia
Type III: sporadic and more likely to be solitary & show features of malignancy / atypia (*vide supra*)

② EC-cell (serotonin) tumours occur in the distal duodenum, acinar pattern

③ G-cell (gastrin)   proximal duodenum, trabecular, may cause ZE syndrome, ± MEN-1

④ D-cell (somatostatin) → somatostatinoma (50% have NF-1):
  - ➢ periampullary, glandular/acinar pattern, psammoma bodies
  - ➢ immuno/stains: somatostatin +ve, ! CgA / Grimelius may often be negative
  - ➢ d/dg: well diff adenocarcinoma (! esp. on FS) but somatostatinoma has low grade NE nuclei, low/absent mitoses & somatostatin +ve immuno

Gastrointestinal Stromal Tumour (GIST)
- Occur in any part of GI tract (and 7% are extra GI: mesenteric ones have worse prog. *cf.* omental)
- Spindle cell type:
  - ➢ variable cellularity
  - ➢ interlacing bundles / whorls of uniform spindle cells with blunt nuclei
  - ➢ ± paranuclear vacuole
  - ➢ ± multinucleated 'wreath' cells
  - ➢ ± prominent vascularity
  - ➢ ± neural features (e.g. palisaded nuclei)
  - ➢ ± skeinoid fibres (extracellular globoid / curvilinear collagen aggregates)
  - ➢ stroma may be hyaline or myxoid
  - ➢ ± foci of liposarcoma / chondrosarcoma / RMS
- Epithelioid type:
  - ➢ sheets / nests
  - ➢ rounded / vacuolated / clear / epithelioid / plasmacytoid cells
  - ➢ variable nuclear atypia to (*very rarely*) frank pleomorphism with large nucleoli
  - ➢ ± multinucleated tumour cells
  - ➢ thought to have worse prognosis *cf.* spindle type but is indolent if part of Carney triad[8]
- Gastrointestinal autonomic nerve tumour (GANT):
  - ➢ a non-myogenic GIST of either spindle / epithelioid type
  - ➢ diagnosis depends on ultrastructural features (processes, synapses, vesicles, etc.)
  - ➢ often has peritumoural lymphoid infiltrates (similar to some deep Schwannomas)
  - ➢ possibly worse prog. *cf.* other GISTs but no longer necessary to separate out this sub-type
- Immuno +ve: c-kit (membrane accentuation), DOG-1 (useful for CD117 −ve GIST – some of these also respond to Glivec®), CD34, CD171 (in 75%); nestin, (± neural +/ smooth muscle markers), PDGFRα (as for DOG-1 but also +ve in 25% of desmoids)

---

[8] Carney triad = ① epithelioid GIST, ② pulmonary chondroma and ③ non-adrenal paraganglioma

- d/dg (c-kit [CD117] is +ve in many things – see also p. 16 – do not use Ag retrieval):
  - leiomyoma / sarcoma: c-kit −ve, CD171 −ve, desmin +ve, ER may be +ve (−ve in GIST)
  - cellular Schwannoma of the GIT[9] / MPNST: c-kit −ve, S100 +ve; nestin & CD171 rarely +ve
  - fibromatosis: c-kit +ve (but with cytoplasmic blob [myofibroblast] pattern not membranous), PDGFRα ±ve, CD171 & CD34 −ve; (! don't mis-call a post-op desmoid 'recurrent GIST')
  - inflammatory fibroid polyp: CD34 +ve (like GIST), eosinophils (see p. 138)
  - SFT: triad of CD99, Bcl-2, CD34 +ve; some are also c-kit +ve (see p. 324)
  - spindle cell carcinoma and mesothelioma: CK +ve (rare in GISTs) and −ve for c-kit and CD34
  - glomus tumour (vs. epithelioid GIST) – see pp. 285–286
- Prognosis (NB: it is good practice never to report a GIST as 'benign'):
  - good prognostics are: ☞ spindle type with only smooth muscle markers
                             ☞ any type with only neural markers
                             ☞ <1 cm and incidental finding (these may be truly benign)
                             ☞ gastric or omental site
  - bad prognostics are: ☞ frank invasion (= malignant, whatever the mitotic count / size)
                             ☞ recurrence after Rx: abdominal cavity and liver commonest sites
  - pleomorphism is irrelevant to prognosis in epithelioid tumours
  - grading ∝ size and mitotic count but SI GISTs may be more aggressive for any given size
                             ☞ any tumour >10cm or with >10/50 hpf mitoses is high risk (see Figure 11.2)
                             ☞ if it has >20–50 mitoses / 50 hpf it is considered very high grade

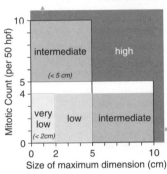

FIGURE 11.2 GIST risk groups. Based on Fletcher et al. 2002 and Wong et al. 2003.

Lymphoma
See also Chapter 10: Lymphoreticular.
- A solid swathe of lymphocytes covering the whole Bx suggests lymphoma (but it may be more subtle)
- MALToma: low grade is assoc[d] with *H. pylori* and may respond to antibiotics (high grade = DLBCL)
- An LEL is defined as a group of ≥3 IELs with destruction of epithelium (CK immuno may help e.g. CAM5.2; also T & B to demonstrate B-cells [unlike the T-cells of focally enhanced gastritis])
- True LEL may also be seen in severe chronic gastritis not just MALToma
- CD20 immuno may fail (false −ve) if patient previously Rx with anti-CD20 Ab ∴ use CD79a

- If a post-Rx Bx shows dense diffuse or nodular infiltrates or *H. pylori* then further Rx is indicated
- d/dg includes glomus tumour in the stomach (see pp. 285–286)

Small Intestine

Causes of Malabsorption
- **F**lora: blind loops / diverticula
- **I**ntestinal: ➤ sprues (incl. coeliac disease)
                    ➤ radiation
                    ➤ infection ————————
                    ➤ lymphoma / amyloid (e.g. Waldenström)
                    ➤ drugs including chemoRx

    ⟨ bacterial (MAI, *Tropheryma whippelii*)
      viral
      protozoal (*Giardia lamblia*)
      helminthic (*Diphylobothrium latum*)

- **D**igestion: pancreatic, gastric and biliary diseases
- **L**ymphatic obstruction: lymphangiectasis and LN pathology
- **E**ndocrine disorders: Addison's pernicious anaemia (PA), thyroid, DM
- **S**hort gut syndromes: resections, fistulous short circuit
- **B**iochemical: IEM (e.g. disaccharidase deficiencies and abetalipoproteinaemia)
- **V**ascular insufficiency of the gut
- *NB*: to diagnose crypt atrophy one should see ≥ 4 villi in a row (this gives assurance of proper orientation) and to exclude patchy disease (e.g. some cases of Coeliac) you need ≥ 3–5 Bx

---

[9] not encapsulated like other Schwannomas and may have peritumoural lymphoid infiltrates / follicles

Villous Atrophy of the Crypt Hyperplastic Type

Coeliac disease
- Clin: +ve serology for anti tTG Abs is more specific *cf.* anti gliadin (both are unreliable if <2 years old)
- Some cases show nearly normal villous architecture, however these have a greater concentration of IELs near the tip of the villi *cf.* the base (i.e. loss or reverse of the normal gradient of IELs)
- IELs are usu. > 30-40 / 100 villous (not crypt) enterocytes in established coeliac disease
- ↑ l.p. chronic inflam[y] cells (esp. plasma cells); ↓ height of enterocytes and brush border ± vacuolation
- d/dg acute (HLO-assoc[d] or peptic) duodenitis: ↑PMN, gastric metaplasia[10] ++, HLO (hard to identify in small bowel because they are fewer and more coccoid)
- d/dg refractory coeliac disease – see p. 115; for other d/dg *vide infra*

Other causes
- Tropical sprue: also affects the TI villi (unlike coeliac disease) in the later stages of the condition
- HIV enteritis (also has ↑ crypt apoptoses)
- Iatrogenic: drugs (e.g. mefenamic acid, NSAID), radioRx, post surgical blind loops, etc.
- ↑ IELs in other immune diseases (CVID, SLE, allergies, GVHD, CIBD), infections, ischaemia, etc.

Villous Atrophy of the Crypt Atrophic Type
- Chemo/radioRx (chemoRx causes ↑crypt apoptoses, radiation-induced villous atrophy is a transient event) – see p. 148 for other morphological features of chemo/radioRx
- Folate & vitamin B12 deficiency
- Prolonged TPN
- Drugs e.g. progestagens, NSAID
- HIV enteritis (also has ↑ crypt apoptoses)

Whipple's Disease
- M ≫ F; middle-age; usu. diffuse but can be patchy and submucosal after antibiotics
- l.p. packed with Mφ with intensely DPAS +ve *coarse* granules (but may be Gaucher-like after Rx)
- Villi show large lipid vacuoles in the l.p. (dilated lacteals)
- Stains: EM +/ immuno for *T. whippelii*; ZN −ve (d/dg MAI has ZN +ve fine rods)

Drug Reactions (incl. NSAID)
- **Vacuolation** of villous tip enterocytes (d/dg coeliac / infections)
- **Atrophy** of villi (crypt hyperplastic or atrophic) and apoptoses in crypts (with chemoRx)
- **Chronic** inflam[n] (incl. eosinophils)
- **Ulceration** which may be transverse peptic-like, pseudomembranes (if extensive), ± perforation
- *Diaphragm disease*: the diaphragms contain submucosa but not muscularis propria and they have mucosal prolapse changes [± ulcerat[n]] and submucosal fibrosis at the diaphragm aperture

Common Variable Immunodeficiency (CVID)
- Lack of plasma cells in l.p., ± villous atrophy, ± *Giardia*, CMV, *Candida*, etc., ± MALToma
- Nodular lymphoid hyperplasia ± granulomas

For more details, see p. 351.

Brunner's Gland Hyperplasia, Nodule(s) and Adenoma
- ↑Amount of normal lobulated Brunner's gland tissue with intervening slips of smooth muscle
- The difference between these entities is an arbitrary matter of size/amount of glands

Lymphoma
See also Chapter 10: Lymphoreticular.
- Small intestinal MALToma:
  - ➤ LEL are less prominent & DLBCL transformation more common (*cf.* gastric)
  - ➤ multifocality and stage are important prognostics
  - ➤ solid sheets of blasts = DLBCL (Bcl-2 & p53 may be prognostic)
- Others: EATL, IPSID, EBV-assoc[d] high grade B-cell (HIV / PTLD), Burkitt's, FCL

---

[10] in general, anywhere in the alimentary tract, *heterotopias* are distinguished from *metaplasias* by the presence of gastric parietal or chief cells or pancreatic acinar cells or adrenocortical cells

Post-Colectomy Ileitis (= Pre-stomal ileitis or Neoterminal ileitis)
- Occurs months to years post colonic surgery (for UC, colonic carcinoma or other causes), F≫M
- Wall thickening ± stricture
- Patchy variable acute and chronic inflam^n ± ulcerat^n, fissures and TLA but no granulomas or bugs
- d/dg Crohn's disease: but in post-colectomy ileitis there is a history of colectomy, CPC and review of past specimens confirms UC or show no evidence of Crohn's, granulomas are absent and TLA are limited to areas of deep mucosal fissuring/activity

CIBD
- Duodenum: focal aggregates of PMN in the l.p. and epithelium may be the only sign in Crohn's
- TI: patchy active inflam^n and UACL are typical of Crohn's and strongly favour Crohn's over UC
- TI: the 'backwash ileitis' of UC occurs with right-sided UC and shows diffuse superficial activity (no erosions or deep ulcers and no UACL) – it is not a contraindication to the formation of a pouch.

Lower GI

Infective Colitis

General bacterial colitis
- Oedema
- Mild to moderate inflammation, PMN dominant
- Inflammation tends to be more superficial in the mucosa and surface epithelium
- Cryptitis with preserved architecture (except amoebic colitis)
- Beaded crypt absceses ('string of pearls' sign)
- Crypt withering (also seen in radioRx effect and ischaemia)
- Microgranulomas (≥ 5 Mϕ) away from inflamed crypts – esp. in *Salmonella / Campylobacter*
- Haemorrhage
- Tufting of surface epithelium (may be antibiotic-related)
- Resolution (i.e. it goes away on F/U)

Entamoeba Histolytica
- Crypt distortion
- 'Flask-shaped' ulcers (have overhanging edges)
- Amoebae have pale-staining spherical nuclei (unlike Mϕ nuclei that are darker and bean-shaped)
- Amoebae have engulfed RBC (unlike non-pathogenic *Entamoeba coli*)
- Amoebae stain magenta with DPAS – sensitive method to detect them – and are CD68 –ve
- d/dg carcinoma (macro / radiology) and UC (histology)

Clostridium difficile[11] (Pseudomembranous Colitis)
- Multiple discrete foci of disrupted crypts
- Affected crypts are dilated superficially
- A 'volcanic spray'-like exudate forms a 'mushroom cloud' pseudomembrane of cellular debris, fibrin, mucus and inflam^y cells (! similar exudate can occur in SRUS – need to see underlying mucosa)
- Intervening mucosa is normal
- d/dg ischaemic colitis, severe CIBD / defunctioned UC, CMV, *Shigella*, *E. coli*, (rarely) acute CC
- d/dg PMC may also be caused by drugs, e.g. gold, not just antibiotic-assoc^d *C. difficile* infection

Chronic idiopathic Inflammatory Bowel Disease (CIBD)

Common pitfalls in diagnosis
- Pericryptal cells (pseudogranulomas)
- Muciphage collections (pseudogranulomas)
- Cryptolytic lesions (foreign-body-type granuloma adjacent to a crypt that has spilled its mucin) seen in: UC, diversion colitis, pouchitis, diverticular disease-assoc^d colitis, etc.; usu. in superficial l.p.
- Isolated crypt abscesses (can be seen adjacent to focal lesions / other situations)
- Branching crypts (seen at normal innominate grooves and in any situation of regeneration / growth)
- Normal chronic 'inflam^n' and NE cells of the caecum; normal rectal NE cells (*vs.* NE cell hyperplasia)
- 'Atrophy' at the anorectal margin (normal histology)
- Infective colitis (esp. amoebic / CMV)

---

[11] *NB: difficile* is a Latin word of four syllables (di-fi-chi-lay) – not French

- Ischaemic colitis
- Behçet's, peritumoural and diverticular disease-associated colitis (esp. d/dg Crohn's disease)
- Post-colectomy ileitis (!do not call it Crohn's disease in a patient with established UC) – see p. 143
- Diversion reaction / colitis
- Ileoanal pouch changes
- Drug-induced colitis e.g. bowel prep colitis (esp. d/dg Crohn's) or cholestyramine / polystyrene colitis
- Failure to correlate clinical information and macroscopic appearances / distribution with histology

Per-operative diagnosis of CIBD (incl. FS)

- Used during some ileoanal pouch-forming procedures because Crohn's disease is a contra-indication
- Determine: Crohn's disease / UC / don't know (*not* 'indeterminate colitis' *q.v.*)
- Macro appearances at surgery helps (see macro features of Crohn's disease and UC, below)
- FS from: ➢ the largest LN – granulomas? (be wary of pitfalls and acceptable criteria)
  - ➢ full-thickness lesional bowel – characteristic features present?
  - ➢ full-thickness 'normal' interlesional bowel – is disease truly patchy?

Ulcerative Colitis (UC)

- Macro: ➢ diffuse involvement of diseased colon from distal to proximal ($\pm$ backwash ileitis)
  - ➢ specific skip lesions can occur (appendix & caecal patch) $\pm$ rectal sparing if treated
- Micro (mucosal):
  - ➢ crypt distortion (!beware of nearby causes e.g. ulcers, lymphoid aggregates, innominate grooves)
  - ➢ surface villosity
  - ➢ chronic inflam^n: diffuse throughout the full thickness of the mucosa and length of the Bx and continuous throughout the involved segment (except with the UC skip lesions *vide supra*); tends to be worse distally
  - ➢ acute activity (PMN in the l.p [esp. if >100 per mm] / cryptitis / crypt abscesses): this is diffuse but patchiness can occur ① at the junction of involved and uninvolved bowel and ② in cases of treated UC
  - ➢ mucin depletion (associated with activity, weak feature)
  - ➢ cryptolytic granulomas and muciphage collections may be seen in UC
  - ➢ quiescent UC: ☞ the lamina propria may be hypocellular
    - ☞ distortion and atrophy (crypt bases do not reach the m.m.)
    - ☞ NE cell hyperplasia and Paneth cell metaplasia
  - ➢ patchiness of disease *severity* is OK for UC (as opposed to patchiness of disease *presence* in Crohn's) as not all sites may be at the same degree of severity of inflam^n. Finding quiescent UC in between two active biopsies is OK. Finding completely normal bowel in between two diseased biopsies is not (consider Crohn's or other d/dg, however, fulminant UC may be patchy with rectal sparing)
  - ➢ the rectal mucosa in UC may return to histological normality esp. after Rx ∴ a normal rectal Bx does not exclude UC
- Micro (transmural / resection): *diffuse* inflammation can occur *transmurally* at sites of ulceration

Crohn's disease

- Macro: ➢ SI involvement $\pm$ colon favours Crohn's (but isolated Crohn's colitis is possible)
  - ➢ fat-wrapping, serosal exudate, thickening of bowel wall, strictures, fistulae
  - ➢ skip lesions, fissures, snail-track ulcers, cobblestone mucosa, etc.
  - ➢ Abnormalities are worst on the mesenteric aspect
- Micro (mucosal Bx $\pm$ submucosa):
  - ➢ there is less crypt distortion and less mucin depletion (*cf.* UC)
  - ➢ patchiness of inflam^n – both acute and chronic, both within and between biopsies, esp. single crypt abscesses flanked by normal crypts. Completely normal intervening biopsies in a series
  - ➢ epithelioid granulomas, esp. when multiple, small (<200μ), between crypts and abutting the muscularis mucosae (d/dg infective microgranulomas, cryptolytic lesions, pseudogranulomas)
  - ➢ patchy lamina propria fibrosis and oedema (d/dg ischaemia which is favoured by mucosal capillary telangiectasia and siderophages – but these are not always seen)
  - ➢ disproportionate submucosal inflam^n (not assoc^d with an ulcer)
  - ➢ the typical Crohn's aphtha begins at the crypt base as a triangular ('mountain-top') ulcer pointing upwards sending a stream of PMN up the crypt and often overlying a lymphoid

aggregate (see Figure 11.3). Fissures develop as continuations of the angles at the base of the ulcer. The adjacent mucosa is normal. It is useful in d/dg UC but is not specific for Crohn's.

- Micro (transmural / resection):
  - ➤ inflam[n] is transmural with patchy discrete lymphoid aggregates, seen esp. running along serosa
  - ➤ granulomas (following lymphatics) are found in two-thirds of cases; ± granulomatous lymphovasculitis
  - ➤ fibrosis and oedema (± submucosal lymphangiectasia & neuronal hyperplasia – not seen in UC – ± perineural chronic inflam[n])
  - ➤ deep fissures (esp. if narrow, lined by inflam[n] and arising from the base of Crohn's-like aphthae)
  - ➤ well-formed, sarcoid-like epithelioid granulomas in draining lymph nodes help establish the diagnosis esp. in peroperative frozen section

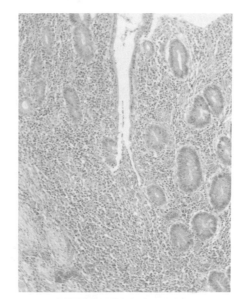

FIGURE 11.3   Crohn's aphtha

- d/dg TB is favoured by confluent granulomas, caseous necrosis or ≥10 granulomas per Bx
- d/dg Crohn's-like reaction (macro & micro) limited to a DD segment or peritumoural
- d/dg *idiopathic granulomatous appendicitis*: only the appendix is affected, no other signs of Crohn's
- d/dg Behçet's colitis: deep/perforating ileocaecal ulcers or colitis histologically identical to Crohn's
- d/dg focal inflam[n] may occur in inflam[y] polyps or anastomotic lines and does not favour Crohn's

Indeterminate Colitis (IC)
- Only diagnose when small bowel disease has been excluded clinically and whole colon sampling is available (colectomy or multiple biopsies)
- Using CPC and Bx findings try to qualify IC with a probable aetiology: UC, Crohn's (subserosal lymphoid aggregates unrelated to ulcers or gross skip lesions), other (e.g. infective / obstructive), unknown
- IC should be considered a temporary diagnosis pending F/U whenever possible

Acute type IC
- A confident pre-op Bx diagnosis of UC should not be overruled by indeterminate resection findings
- Macro: ➤ usu. acute severe segmental colitis affecting the middle 1/3 of the colon
  - ➤ ulceration ± extensive denudation ± toxic megacolon
  - ➤ ± transverse fissures
- Micro:
  - ➤ non-cryptolytic/non-foreign-body granulomas exclude IC (esp. if beyond the mucosa)
  - ➤ undermining ulcers with adjacent mucosa showing normal / minimal architectural or inflammatory response (pronounced and diffuse architectural distortion favours UC)
  - ➤ fissures may be transmural but are 'V'-shaped (*cf.* thinner in Crohn's disease) and show minimal adjacent inflam[n] (more prominent in Crohn's)
  - ➤ myocytolysis with capillary engorgement in parafissural muscularis propria
  - ➤ transmural inflam[n] is diffuse (*cf.* aggregates in Crohn's) and restricted to areas of severe ulceration

Non-acute type IC
- A confident endoscopic / pre-op Bx diagnosis should not be overruled by subsequent IC findings
- Micro (if normal colonoscopy): abnormalities not sufficient for diagnosis of microscopic colitis
- Micro (if abnormal colonoscopy): features not diagnostic of a specific colitis e.g. UC, Crohn's, drugs, ischaemia, infection, diverticular disease-assoc[d] colitis, etc.
- d/dg non-specific colitis (*vide infra*)

Non-Specific Colitis and Focal Active Colitis
- Only diagnose non-specific chronic colitis if:
  - ➢ you can't suggest even a probable aetiology and
  - ➢ features similar to IC (Non-Acute) but IC is not diagnosable due to limited sampling
- Diagnosis should come with a recommendation for F/U or further investigation
- Focal active inflam^n with no other abnormality (= focal active colitis), incl. no evidence of chronicity (unlike non-specific colitis) is also non-specific and may be due to infection, drugs, ischaemia, etc.

Microscopic Colitis (Lymphocytic Colitis [LC] / Collagenous Colitis [CC])
- Prolonged watery diarrhoea with (nearly) normal endoscopy. Assoc^d with coeliac disease
- Transverse colon (*cf.* sigmoid) may be the most sensitive Bx site for diagnostic features
- Lymphoplasmacytic infiltrate of the lamina propria
- Epithelial damage (flattening, detachment, ↑lymphocytes ($\geq$20 per 100 enterocytes in LC)
- Collagen band (strands parallel to the lumen, 7–90μ thick, may contain vessels) – in CC only (! may also get collagen band in other things e.g. metaplastic polyps – so use multiple criteria, as usual)
- PMN may be seen in LC / CC (some say that mild crypt distortion is also allowed)
- d/dg PMC *vs.* severe acute CC (quite rare, use CPC)
- d/dg amyloidosis *vs.* CC: surface epithelial damage in CC; CR +vity & CPC in amyloid

Diverticular Disease-Associated Colitis
- Four main types occur (possibly together):
① lumenal narrowing → *obstructive colitis* proximal to the diverticular disease (DD) segment
② impacted stools → localised ischaemia (= *crescentic fold colitis*)
③ more diffuse inflam^n affects the whole DD segment – *segmental colitis*
④ redundant fold prolapse → *inflammatory myoglandular polyp*-like change (≈ '*cap polyp*')
- Mild forms of crescentic fold and segmental colitis show: ➢ mild diffuse chronic inflammation
                                                                                              ➢ surface pus / erosions
                                                                                              ➢ normal architecture
- Severe forms can mimic CIBD with gland distortion, crypt abscesses, TLA, etc.
- d/dg CIBD:
  - ➢ DD colitis *tends* to be around the mouths of the diverticula, sparing the intervening mucosa
  - ➢ UC or Crohn's affecting *only* the sigmoid is unusual
  - ➢ TLA in DD colitis tend to radiate out from an affected diverticulum unlike Crohn's

Obstructive Colitis
- Varies from mild superficial ulceration to severe (resembling indeterminate colitis)
- Haemorrhage and congestion in adjacent mucosa
- The 2–3cm of mucosa immediately proximal to the obstruction is spared

Ischaemia
- Acute changes include ulceration and haemorrhagic necrosis starting with the most superficial layers of the mucosa (earliest changes) to deeper (with more prolonged / severe ischaemia)
- Long term ischaemia: stromal haemosiderosis and changes similar to d/dg chronic radiation enteritis (*q.v.*) but without the atypical stromal fibroblasts and vessel wall damage

Amyloid
- Usu. 2° (to Crohn's, RhA, etc.)
- d/dg collagenous colitis (*vide supra*): lack of surface epithelial cell damage goes against CC
- d/dg collagen in systemic sclerosis / myopathies in the muscularis propria (do CR / SAP immuno)

Endometriosis
- Endometrial glands *and stroma* (do CD10 if necessary) – *unlike d/dg colonic carcinoma*
- May infiltrate all layers the bowel wall
- May give radiological and clinical features suggestive of malignancy
- ! d/dg carcinoma – overcalling endometriosis as carcinoma is the main danger
- d/dg SRUS
- d/dg *colitis cystica profunda* (but endometrial glands are not mucinous)

- d/dg Crohn's (clinically, due to adhesions, deformity and fibrosis with PR bleeding of endometriosis)
- d/dg ischaemia (due to intermittent bleeding and pain and fibrosis with haemosiderin on histology)

Diversion Proctocolitis
- Lymphoid hyperplasia and diffuse chronic inflammation = *diversion reaction*
- + Aphthae and acute inflammation   = *diversion colitis*
- Lumenal narrowing and thickening of the submucosa and muscularis propria } do *not* imply
- ± Occ. well-formed mucosal epithelioid granulomas (controversial)   } Crohn's
- Microcarcinoids
- Involution (if severe may preclude re-anastomosis):
    - ➢ excessive adipose infiltration of submucosa and muscularis propria
    - ➢ mucosal atrophy
- Normal architecture unless prior CIBD
- UC / indeterminate colitis: ➢ transmural lymphoid aggregates   ∴ a diagnosis of Crohn's must not
  (get worse after diversion)   ➢ fissures   be based solely on the histology
                               ➢ granulomas (incl. in LN)   of the defunctioned rectum
                               ➢ pseudomembranous colitis (PMC)
- Crohn's disease: ➢ ↑ fibrosis
  (gets better)   ➢ granulomas hyalinase (± Schaumann bodies)

Ileal Reservoirs and Pouchitis (= Chronic Relapsing Acute Pouchitis)
- ↑Chronic inflam^n & a degree of crypt hyperplastic villous atrophy is normal but
- Subtotal villous atrophy (colonization[17] = Type C mucosa) is a minor risk factor for dysplasia → F/U
- Active pouchitis clinical: diarrhoea, blood, pain, contact bleeding on endoscopy
- Active pouchitis histol.: acute inflammation, surface erosion and focal superficial ulceration – UC-like
- d/dg exclude: infection, prolapse, ischaemia (i.e. ischaemia as a 1° cause of the pathology [e.g. due to surgical complications])
- d/dg Crohn's disease:
    - ➢ any single feature of Crohn's may be present in the pouch without Crohn's being the cause of it:
        - ☞ granulomas (esp. in lymphoid follicles) – but granulomas in SI beyond the pouch favour Crohn's
        - ☞ vertical fissures (usu. seen in relation to ruptured deep crypt abscesses / anastomoses)
        - ☞ fistulae (e.g. colovesical)
    - ➢ ∴ a first diagnosis of Crohn's should never be made on pouch histology alone
- St Mark's pouchitis score (score acute and chronic features separately) – based on Shepherd *et al.* (1987) – see table 11.1:

TABLE 11.1 St Mark's pouchitis score

Acute: (add PMN and ulceration scores to get a total score out of 6)

Score	PMN Infiltrate	Ulceration
0	absent	absent
1 (mild)	restricted to surface epithelium and focal*	superficial
2 (moderate)	+ crypt abscesses (occasional)	
3 (severe)	+ crypt abscesses (numerous)	widespread & deeper

Chronic: (add chronic inflammatory cell and atrophy scores to get a total score out of 6)

Score	Cellular Infiltrate	Villous Atrophy
0	normal	normal architecture
1 (mild)	focal	minor anomalies
2 (moderate)		partial
3 (severe)	more extensive	subtotal

*'restricted to surface epithelium' includes cryptitis

Melanosis Coli (Pseudomelanosis)
- Lipofuscin 2° to chronic apoptosis
- Anthraquinones, NSAID, etc.
- d/dg haemosiderosis (ischaemia) and *brown bowel syndrome* (muscle)

---

[12] 'colonization' (colonic phenotypic change) also connotes a change in mucin type to colonic

Drug Reactions (incl. NSAID)
- **P**MC or acute self limiting colitis (e.g. with antibiotics)
- **U**lceration ± superficial PMN infiltrates
- **M**elanosis / Microscopic colitis
- **I**schaemia (incl. stricture & diaphragm disease)
- **C**rypt apoptoses
- **E**osinophil infiltrates
- Specifics:
  - ➢ *Bowel Prep Colitis*: focal proximal active colitis (d/dg Crohn's)
  - ➢ *Cholestyramine or Polystyrene sulphonate*: can mimic CIBD (ZN +ve crystals)
  - ➢ *Barium Granuloma*: blue-grey / light green 'foamy' Mφ with birefringent crystals (stain red with rhodizonate – as does Pb, Zn, Sr and Hg)

Chemotherapy / Radiation
- *NB*: vitamin B12 / folate deficiency show similar cytological atypia to chemoRx changes

Early changes
- Ulceration and mucosal necrosis
- Apoptoses
- Epithelial cells may show a syncytial-like appearance
- Marked cell enlargement with nuclear atypia d/dg dysplasia / carcinoma:
  - ➢ gland architecture is preserved
  - ➢ nuclear abnormalities too bizarre for neoplasia forming such good glands
  - ➢ NCR not markedly increased (esp. given degree of nuclear atypia)
  - ➢ cytological atypia also present in surrounding endothelial and stromal cells
  - ➢ no mitoses (except in normal numbers and in their normal locations)
  - ➢ no infiltrative growth

Later changes
- Chronic ulceration
- Fibrosis / stricture / adhesions   } d/dg Crohn's disease (! in this regard note that there have
- ± Chronic inflamⁿ in lamina propria } been case reports of radiation-assocᵈ granulomas)
- Hyaline fibrosis of the lamina propria
- Crypt loss (and 'withering') with single large dark crypts standing out (regenerative hyperplasia)
- Radiation fibroblasts (plump, vesicular nuclei, binucleate forms, etc.)
- *Colitis cystica profunda* is also assocᵈ with radioRx
- Vascular changes: ectatic capillaries, endarteritis obliterans, foamy Mφ accumulation with hyaline change in vessel walls

Squamous Metaplasia in the Rectum (causes)
- Upgrowth from the anus 2° to distal rectal ulceration
- Repeated self-induced trauma by insertion of foreign objects
- Radiation-induced
- Persistent chronic inflammation (e.g. in UC)

Common Variable Immunodeficiency (CVID)
- Lack of plasma cells in l.p., ± Cryptosporidia, etc., ± MALToma
- ± Nodular lymphoid hyperplasia ± granulomas. See p. 351 for more detail.

Graft vs. Host Disease (GVHD)
- In the first 3 weeks post BMTx it is impossible to differentiate from pre-BMTx chemoRx changes
- Apoptoses in basal enterocytes, chronic inflammatory cells are few
- ± More extensive necrosis and ulceration and PMN
- Crypt loss with NE gravestones and regenerative crypt distortion
- Fibrosis of lamina propria (helps to distinguish from d/dg UC) ± transmural fibrosis
- d/dg: ↑apoptoses of crypts is also seen in HIV, CMV, drugs / viruses, chemoRx, radioRx

Angiodysplasia (of Upper or Lower GIT)
- Ectatic veins in the submucosa (may extend through to subserosa and become conglomerated)
- Communicate with ectatic capillaries in l.p. (not always seen but diagnose with caution if not seen)
- Arterial component seen if severe (but diagnosis should not be made in those with angiomas)
- Bleeds are assocᵈ with age, true diverticula (those with all muscle coats), aortic stenosis, etc.

Solitary Rectal Ulcer Syndrome (SRUS) / Mucosal Prolapse Syndrome
- Proctoscopy shows a pale area with erythematous base, may be multiple, usu. anterior
- Fibromuscular obliteration of the lamina propria
- Vertical smooth muscle in the lamina propria
- Telangiectasia / engorgement of superficial lamina propria capillaries
- Mild hyperplasia of crypts $\pm$ 'diamond-shaped' cross sections
- $\pm$ Submucosal vessels thickened and hyalinised
- $\pm$ Surface erosion

Mucosal Prolapse and Inflammatory Myoglandular Polyp / Cap Polyp
- Elongated, tortuous glands $\pm$ florid hyperplasia (matures to surface goblet cells, unlike dysplasia)
- Proliferated smooth muscle in stroma irregularly surrounds glands (unlike d/dg P-J polyps)
- A 'cap' of granulation tissuc is seen in cap polyps
- Often sited on the crest of a fold and multiple
- d/dg CIBD (due to arch. distortion and inflam^n) / dysplasia (due to hyperplasia and arch.)

Inflammatory Cloacogenic Polyp
- Polypoidal mucosal prolapse near anorectal junction (see SRUS and Mucosal Prolapse, above)
- Arch.: tubular deep ($\pm$ focal *colitis cystica profunda*), villiform superficial
- Partly covered by transitional epithelium
- d/dg villous adenoma (macro)/ dysplasia (micro – incl. high gradc duc to hyperplasia and arch.)

Inflammatory Polyp
- Macro: finger-like, irregular, fused and on a background of UC / Crohn's disease / ischaemic colitis
- Cystic glands
- Inflammatory and granulation tissue stroma
- d/dg juvenile polyp

Pseudolipomatosis Coli
- $2°$ to pneumatosis, insufflation, H_2O_2 on endoscope, etc.

Peutz-Jeghers Polyp (P-J Polyp)
- Upper and lower GI tract
- Arborising smooth muscle (of muscularis mucosae)
- Normal mucosa (appropriate to that part of the GI tract the polyp is in)

Juvenile Polyp
- Macro: rounded, on thin stalk – may tort
- Cystic glands lined by normal colorectal epithelium
- Stromal overgrowth (without muscularis mucosae)
- $\pm$ Cartilage / bone
- $\pm$ Surface ulceration
- $\pm$ purulent inflammation in lamina propria
- d/dg inflammatory polyp ('pseudopolyp')

Lymphomas
For details, see Chapter 10: Lymphoreticular.
- MALToma (extranodal MZL)
- MCL (= *lymphomatous polyposis coli*) has fewer LEL *cf.* MALToma

Dysplasia in Sporadic Adenomas (Polypoidal, Serrated and Flat)
- Generally: the degree of dysplasia is called according to the worst focus *not* the predominant grade
- Mild:
  (Low grade)
  - ➢ nuclear elongation and crowding, polarity essentially preserved, ↑mitoses
  - ➢ ↓ mucin in cells but both goblet cells and columnar cells are still present
  - ➢ cytoplasm becomes darker and more amphophilic
- Moderate:
  (Low grade)
  - ➢ nuclei elongate further, loss of polarity

- goblet cells transformed into cells with apical vacuoles or simple columnar cells
- ± architectural disturbance (branching / budding)
- Severe: ➢ roundening and vesiculation of nuclei with prominent nucleoli
  (High grade)   ➢ no mucin secretion
                             ➢ more architectural disturbance ± cribriform/gland-in-gland morphology
- Tubular, Tubulovillous (TV) and Villous Adenoma:
    - if >80% of one architecture call it that, else = tubulovillous
    - tubular types have closely compacted tubules that may branch
- Serrated Pathway Polyps (combined and transitional forms occur and all may coexist in *serrated adenomatous polyposis*):
    - *hyperplastic polyp* (*metaplastic polyp*): bottom half has straight hyperplastic non-serrated crypts with little or no mucin ± focally increased eosinophilic endocrine cells; top half has 'metaplasia' (serration with pink cell change ± collagen band). No dysplasia.
    - *serrated adenoma*:   ☞ serrated architecture in ≥ 50% of the lesion (otherwise = adenoma with serrated areas)
                            ☞ arch. is like hyperplastic polyp +/ sessile serrated polyp but must see dysplastic change extending to the surface at least focally. They often have less mucin with irregularly distributed goblet cells.
                            ☞ the serrated arch. may result in over-grading the dysplasia (if it is mis-diagnosed as an ordinary adenoma)
    - *sessile serrated polyp* (also called *'sessile serrated adenoma'*). These have a pre-malig. association and are rarely pedunculated.
        - ☞ lack of a subepithelial collagen band and lack of eosinophilic endocrine cells
        - ☞ focal mucin depletion (to little apical vacuoles) with cytoplasmic eosinophilia
        - ☞ persistence of mucinous cells and serration at all levels incl. deep in the crypt
        - ☞ other deep crypt arch. anomalies close to the m.m.: dilated crypts (± papillaroid serrated tufting +/ mucin distension), horizontal crypt orientation, L-shaped crypts, branching, etc.
        - ☞ mitoses high in crypts
        - ☞ non-stratified nuclei: may show irregularity, enlargement, vesiculation and prom. nucleoli but these do not extend to the surface (else = serrated adenoma)
- Flat adenoma:
    - wedge-shaped region of dysplasia (with central point of wedge deepest in mucosa)
    - nuclear stratification is not as marked as in polypoidal dysplasia
    - nuclear atypia more pronounced than in polypoidal dysplasia
- Immuno: Bcl-2 and nuclear β-catenin +ve, p53 usu. −ve until late / severe dysplasia
- d/dg tangential cut of a hyperplastic polyp *vs.* low grade dysplasia (adenoma): distinction is important because adenoma / dysplasia indicates colonoscopic F/U (hyperplastic polyp does not)
- Other features that may affect Mx: ➢ severe dysplasia *or*
                                        ➢ dysplasia reaches the stalk (or <2mm from it)
                                        ➢ there is submucosal invasion ('polyp cancer') *vide infra*

Flat Dysplasia in Chronic idiopathic Inflammatory Bowel Disease (CIBD)
- options: 'indefinite for dysplasia', low grade, high grade
- features favouring dysplasia over regenerative / inflammatory atypia:
    - changes involve whole gland to surface
    - absence of active inflammation
    - irregular or giant villosity
    - elongated crypts (*cf.* atrophic in inflammatory atypia)
- High grade: ➢ severely distorted architecture (e.g. marked villosity)
                ➢ severe nuclear stratification
                ➢ 'basal cell dysplasia' of nuclei (flat adenoma-like nuclear abnormalities)
- Low grade: subjectively quantitatively less severe features *cf.* high grade
- Indefinite: if ① acute activity is present in the atypical glands or ② cannot see changes extending to surface or, some say, ③ ≤3 crypts only are involved
- Immuno: p53 often +ve in earliest stages / mild dysplasia (see table 11.2)

Dysplasia Associated with a Lesion or Mass (DALM) in CIBD
- Greatly increased risk of invasive carcinoma *cf.* flat dysplasia in CIBD

- Features favouring sporadic adenoma over DALM:
  - ➤ lesion is located in part of the bowel unaffected (and never affected) by CIBD
  - ➤ architecture fits one of the standard adenoma types (tubular/villous/tubulovillous)
  - ➤ no other foci of more typical flat dysplasia assoc[d] with the colitis[13]
  - ➤ Hx of CIBD for < 8 years
- Immuno: ➤ p53: >50% nuclei staining = definite +ve; <10% = −ve
  - ➤ Bcl-2 staining is more towards the crypt base (restricted to the base in normal mucosa)

TABLE 11.2 Immuno in lower GI dysplasia

	p53	*Bcl-2*	*β-catenin*
DALM	nuclear +ve	−ve	cell membrane +ve
Sporadic adenoma	−ve	cytoplasmic +ve	nuclear +ve

Colorectal Carcinoma

Diagnosing colorectal carcinoma

- Invasion beyond the muscularis mucosae is required to diagnose carcinoma in the UK because we do not recognise intramucosal CA in the colon (unlike in the stomach where intramucosal CA is a valid diagnosis). (See Appendix for a note on pseudoinvasion)
- 'Early colorectal cancer' = invasion not beyond the submucosa (± mets); if seen in a polyp = 'malignant polyp' or 'polyp cancer' and endoscopic resection may suffice unless high risk for LN mets ∴ look for: level of invasion (see Figure 11.4), lymph or blood vascular invasion, any poorly diff / undiff focus incl. signet ring – even if only at the advancing edge, small buds of cells at the invasive front ('budding'), tumour at the resection margin

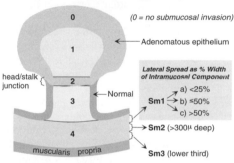

Haggitt Levels 0-4 and Kikuchi Submucosal Levels for Polyp Cancers Limited to the Submucosa
(sessile polyps start at Haggitt 4, Sm1)

(0 = no submucosal invasion)

← Adenomatous epithelium

head/stalk junction

← Normal

Lateral Spread as % Width of Intramucosal Component

Sm1 → a) <25%
      b) ≤50%
      c) >50%

Sm2 (>300μ deep)

muscularis propria

Sm3 (lower third)

FIGURE 11.4 Haggitt and Kikuchi levels

- d/dg *colitis cystica profunda* in which the glands are not dysplastic or angulated and a thin investment of lamina propria (± haemosiderin) may be present

Grading colorectal carcinoma

- For major resections grade according to the predominant pattern (by area – ignoring the advancing edge of the tumour) but for local excisions (wedge, endoscopic, etc.) grade by the worst focus
- Well diff: well-formed glands with tubular arch. and basal nuclei ('adenoma-like')
- Moderately diff: less regular but easily recognised glands, larger non-basal nuclei
- Poorly diff: glands difficult to discern (irregularly folded and distorted small tubules or solid) / SmCC
- Undiff. (medullary): NE-like but no glands, mucin or NE markers, pushing edge, lymphocytes may be numerous – has a good prog. unlike d/dg anaplastic CA (sarcomatoid / spindle and giant cell histology)

Neoadjuvant Rx (Pre-op RadioRx ± ChemoRx)

- Changes incl.: necrosis, fibrosis, mucin pools, radioRx vessel changes, lymphoid atrophy (incl. ↓LN yield and Jass score is meaningless) ± *colitis cystica profunda* (! d/dg well-diff mucinous carcinoma)
- Residual cancer should only be diagnosed if viable tumour epithelium is present (acellular mucin pools, etc. show where cancer most probably had been prior to neoadjuvant therapy)

Immuno

For additional immuno, see p. 17

- Cancers that stain +ve for EGFR (with a specific Dako® PharmDX™ kit) may be treated with cetuximab (a therapeutic EGFR-blocking Ab)
- CDX-2 nuclear +vity is seen in many GI adenocarcinomas (may help in identifying mets)
- Loss of nuclear +vity for MLH1, PMS2, MSH2, MSH6 is suggestive of HNPCC (requires genetics to confirm) – assoc[d] with: proximal site, high grade, mucinous type, lymphoid stroma, younger patients

---

[13] if the endoscopist suspects a DALM they should take biopsies from around the lesion as well as from the lesion

Appendix

- Normal structures incl. small groups of EC-cells and Schwann cells in the l.p; focal loss of the m.m. (and the author has also seen rare serosal Walthard rests – ! d/dg lymphangitis carcinomatosa)
- Diagnose 'acute appendicitis' only if there are transmural PMN – otherwise just give a description
- L-cell carcinoid: these are usu. CgA −ve (but CgB +ve) so do CD56 / synaptophysin / NSE etc.
- Balloon cell / clear cell carcinoid: usual arch., pale cytoplasm (−ve for AB and DPAS and PAS)
- Tubular carcinoid: ➤ infiltrative arch., squashed tubules ± some lumenal AB and DPAS +ve mucin
  - ➤ CEA and glucagon +ve but no sig. intracellular mucin, CgA weak / −ve
  - ➤ d/dg mucinous / goblet cell 'carcinoids' (worse prog.)
- 'Mucinous carcinoid' / 'goblet cell carcinoid' (crypt cell carcinoma):
  - ➤ more aggressive *cf.* other carcinoids but less so *cf.* mucinous adenocarcinoma
  - ➤ low grade nuclei and typical carcinoid arch.: islands, ribbons, anastomosing cords ± mucin pools; they typically form little clusters of goblet cells and these clusters infiltrate (*cf.* single cells)
  - ➤ lack an *in situ* component and have a mix of cell types incl. goblet cells, mucinous columnar cells in glandular acini (d/dg non-mucinous rosettes or 'pseudoglands' of NE cells in other carcinoids) ± Paneth cells and usu. some NE cells (! but some may have no NE cells)
  - ➤ poor prog. architectures = diffuse / single file / signet ring or gland fusion / cribriform / solid sheet
  - ➤ mitoses (>2/10 hpf) and extracellular mucin pools containing fused glands lacking lumena are also poor prognostics (mucin pools with separate acini with preserved lumena are OK)
  - ➤ CEA +ve, usu. glucagon −ve, cytoplasmic mucin +ve (AB & DPAS) – *cf.* d/dg tubular carcinoid, p53 is usu. not over-expressed (immuno is −ve) but p53 mutations occur in 25% of cases
  - ➤ ! proper signet ring carcinoma may be mixed with it (= '*mixed carcinoid-adenocarcinoma*')
  - ➤ d/dg: tubular carcinoid, balloon cell/clear cell carcinoid (*vide supra*) – also, mucinous carcinoids often lack the hyperplasia of the infiltrated muscularis propria seen in usual type carcinoids
  - ➤ d/dg metastatic adenoca: low grade nuclei, mixture of cell types, carcinoid growth patterns
- Hyperplastic polyp: only diagnose if it is localised and the epithelium is typical (not mucinous)
- Diffuse hyperplasia: must have typical (not mucinous) serrated bland epithelium (but, like dysplasia, the underlying lymphoid tissue may be absent and diffuse hyperplasia is assoc[d] with colorectal CA elsewhere). Most cases are probably examples of sessile serrated polyp (see p. 150).
- Non-neoplastic mucocoele: (take multiple sections to rule out cystadenoma / adenocarcinoma)
  - ➤ unilocular, completely flat and bland epithelium and usu. < 1cm ∅
  - ➤ may have mucin pools in wall but leakage → localised pseudomyxoma (resolves after excision)
  - ➤ d/dg cystadenoma: any multilocularity, epithelial crenation or papilloid / 'hyperplastic' projections (esp. if assoc[d] with loss of underlying lymphoid tissue) = cystadenoma (at least)
- Mucinous cystadenoma: (take multiple blocks to look for invasion)
  - ➤ assoc[d] with synchronous colorectal carcinoma (∴ the diagnosis indicates colonic Ix) and PMP
  - ➤ epithelium may be very bland and flattened or look like focal hyperplasia (but with mucinous cells) so use the low threshold criteria discussed above for non-neoplastic mucocoele
  - ➤ invasion should be definite (not just mucin displacement under an intact m.m.) otherwise call it '*mucinous tumour of undetermined malignant potential*')
  - ➤ pseudoinvasion is suspected if there is: herniation (e.g. near lymphoglandular complexes or appendicular diverticula), mucin displacement (usu. with a l.p. investment or inflam[n]), no desmoplasia or lack of a phenotypic change in the 'invading' glands

Anal Canal

- Normal: the dentate line (= pectinate line) is at the level of the anal valves (i.e. the lower ends of the vertical anal folds; may be marked by papillae). Histologically it is ≈ the junction of the transitional zone and squamous zone. Perianal skin is defined by the presence of hair and sweat gland adnexae
- AIN: histological criteria for AIN are similar to CIN but *NB*: the normal proliferative zone in the transitional mucosa (by Ki-67) is just *above* the basal layer ∴ ! do not overdiagnose low grade AIN (= AIN 1). Cytological atypia should be present (and squamous metaplasia is helpful)
- Carcinoma: SCC, basaloid carcinoma, adenoca and others (e.g. 1° small cell malignant melanoma)

Peritoneum

Simple Cysts
- Usu. young people
- Cysts are of lymphatic origin (lymphangioma)

Sclerosing Peritonitis
- Assoc[d] with practolol, Le Veen shunt, CAPD and a variant of luteinised thecoma (with focal microcystic change, small luteinised cells, cellular stroma and often bilateral involvement)
- Usu. small bowel ($\pm$ obstruction); no retroperitoneal fibrosis
- $\pm$ Focal surface fibrin
- Laminated sub-mesothelial dense fibrosis
- Focal lymphohistiocytic infiltrate deep to this

Multicystic Mesothelial Proliferation
- Benign reactive condition $\pm$ PMHx surgery / inflam[n]; the condition also occurs in the pleura
- Multicystic mass
- Cyst lining is monolayered $\pm$ papillaroid infoldings
- Immuno: as for reactive mesothelium (see pp. 89–90)

Papillary Mesothelioma (Well-Differentiated Papillary Mesothelioma)
- Benign papilloma, 0.5 to 5cm max. $\varnothing$, lined by single layer of bland mesothelium without mitoses (not asbestos-related)
- Basal vacuoles in between mesothelial cells
- Loose stroma (may be myxoid) containing a few lymphocytes but usu. no psammoma bodies
- Multiple (rarely and usu. in women) – must rule out cytol. atypia as these may be more aggressive
- d/dg mucinous carcinoma (due to the stroma), serous tumours, malig. mesothelioma (but these malig conditions may have atypia, invasion, desmoplasia, necrosis, mitoses $\pm$ psammoma bodies ++)

Epithelioid Mesothelioma vs. Serous Carcinoma of the Peritoneum / Ovary
- +vity for calretinin (nuclear $\pm$ cytoplasmic) and podoplanin / D2-40 and –vity for Ber-EP4 and MOC-31 favours mesothelioma [cytoplasmic (only) calretinin may be seen in other things incl. serous CA]
- EM can be very helpful, esp. if immuno is equivocal

For more information see p. 90, pp. 244–245 and p. 255.

Retroperitoneal Fibrosis
See p. 311.

Pseudomyxoma Peritonei and Müllerian Conditions
See pp. 254–255.

Myopathies

General considerations
- Myopathies may be 1° (early onset/congenital or late onset) or 2° to systemic disease or local insult
- Consider taking fresh samples for freezing (for molecular / histochemistry) and EM (glutaraldehyde)

See Martin *et al.* (1999 and 1990) and other specialist texts.

Gastroparesis
- Usu. younger adults (F>M) with diabetes (*gastroparesis diabeticorum*) / post-viral / other
- No gross hypertrophy
- Variable fibre size and NCR ($\pm$ occ. pyknoses) } in both muscularis propria
- Variable muscle fibre atrophy with interstitial fibrosis } and muscularis mucosae
- M-bodies in muscularis propria (5–25μ, eosinophil globules, PAS –ve)
- Normal vessels, neural plexi and nerves and no inflam[n]

Polyglucosan inclusion myopathy of the internal anal sphincter
- May have familial hypertrophy of the sphincter with obstructive effects
- Endomyseal fibrosis, muscle fibre vacuoles and whorling (*cf.* normal concentric fascicles)
- Inclusions are 2–30μ, intracellular, ovoid, eosinophilic, DPAS and retic +ve with typical EM

Autoimmune plexopathy

* ± Assoc^d with CTD
* Plasma cell infiltrate in myenteric plexus
* d/dg infection (e.g. Strongyloidiasis)

Bibliography

Attanoos, R.L., Webb, R., Dojcinov, S.D. and Gibbs, A.R. (2002) Value of mesothelial and epithelial antibodies in distinguishing diffuse peritoneal mesothelioma in females from serous papillary carcinoma of the ovary and peritoneum. *Histopathology*, **40** (3), 237 –244.

Bacon, C.M., Du, M-Q. and Dogan, A. (2007) Mucosa-associated lymphoid tissue (MALT) lymphoma: a practical guide for pathologists. *Journal of Clinical Pathology*, **60** (4), 361–372.

Bariol, C., Hawkins, N.J., Turner, J.J. *et al.* (2003) Histopathological and clinical evaluation of serrated adenomas of the colon and rectum. *Modern Pathology*, **16** (5), 417–23.

Barrett, A.W. and Speight, P.M. (2001) Diagnostic problems in oral mucosal pathology and how to approach them. *CPD Bulletin (Cellular Pathology)*, **3** (1), 17–21.

Biddlestone, L.R., Bailey, T.A., Whittles, C.E. and Shepherd, N.A. (2001) The clinical and molecular pathology of Barrett's oesophagus, in *Progress in Pathology*, vol. 5 (eds.N. Kirkham and N.R. Lemoine), Greenwich Medical Media Ltd, London, pp. 57–80.

Bouquot, J.E., Speight, P.M. and Farthing, P.M. (2006) Epithelial dysplasia of the oral mucosa – diagnostic problems and prognostic features. *Current Diagnostic Pathology*, **12** (1), 11–21.

Brien, T.P., Farraye, F.A. and Odze, R.D. (2001) Gastric dysplasia-like epithelial atypia associated with chemoradiotherapy for esophageal cancer: a clinicopathologic and immunohistochemical study of 15 cases. *Modern Pathology*, **14** (5), 389–396.

Caneiro, F. (1997) Classification of gastric carcinomas. *Current Diagnostic Pathology*, **4** (1), 51–59.

Cerio, R. (ed) (2001) *Dermatopathology*, Springer–verlag, Berlin.

Chu, P.G. and Weiss, L.M. (2002) Keratin expression in human tissues and neoplasms. *Histopathology*, **40** (5), 403–439.

Day, D.D., Jass, J.R., Price, A.B., Shepherd, N.A., Sloan, J.M., Talbot, I.C., Warren, B.F. and Williams, G.T. (2003) *Morson & Dawson's Gastrointestinal Pathology*. 4th edn, Blackwell Science Ltd, UK.

Dickson, B.C., Streutker, C.J. and Chetty, R. (2006) Coeliac disease: an update for pathologists. *Journal of Clinical Pathology*, **59** (10), 1008–1016.

Dixon, M.F. (1995) Progress in gastric cancer, in *Progress in Pathology*, vol. 1 (eds N. Kirkham and P. Hall), Churchill Livingstone, Edinburgh, pp.13–29.

Duerden, B.I., Reid, T.M.S., Jewsbury, J.M. and Turk, D.C. (1987) *A New Short Textbook of Medical Microbiology*. 1st edn, Edward Arnold (Hodder & Stoughton), London.

Dworak, O., Keilholz, L. and Hoffmann, A. (1997) Pathological features of rectal cancer after preoperative radiochemotherapy. *International Journal of Colorect Disease*, **12** (1), 19–23.

Eckstein, R. and Shepherd, N. (Chairs) (2004) SYMPOSIUM 24—GASTROINTESTINAL TRACT: Iatrogenic and drug induced pathology of the gastrointestinal tract. *Pathology International*, **54** (Suppl. 1), S177–S192.

Ejskjaer, N.T., Bradley, J.L, Buxton-Thomas, M.S. *et al.* (1999) Novel surgical treatment and gastric pathology in diabetic gastroparesis. *Diabetic Medicine*, **16** (6), 488–495.

Farthing, P.M., Bouquot, J.E. and Speight, P.M. (2006) Problems and pitfalls in oral mucosal pathology. *Current Diagnostic Pathology*, **12** (1), 66–74.

Fisher, C. (2005) Gastrointestinal stromal tumours, in *Recent Advances in Histopathology*, vol. 21 (eds M. Pignatelli and J.Underwood), The Royal Society of Medicine Press, London, pp. 71–88.

Fletcher, C.D., Berman, J.J., Corless, C. *et al.* (2002) Diagnosis of gastrointestinal stromal tumors: A consensus approach. *Human Pathology*, **33** (5), 459–465.

Goepel, J.R. (1981) Benign papillary mesothelioma of the peritoneum: a histological, histochemical and ultrastructural study of six cases. *Histopathology*, **5** (1), 21–30.

Haggitt, R.C., Glotzbach, R.E., Soffer, E.E. and Wruble, L.D. (1985) Prognostic factors in colorectal carcinomas arising in adenomas: implications for lesions removed by endoscopic polypectomy. *Gastroenterology*, **89** (2), 328–336.

Hallak, A., Baratz, M., Santo, M. *et al.* (1994) Ileitis after colectomy for ulcerative colitis or carcinoma. *Gut*, **35** (3), 373–376.

Hamilton, S.R. and Aaltonen, L.A. (eds) (2000) *WHO Classification of Tumours: Pathology & Genetics Tumours of the Digestive System*, 1st edn, IARC Press, Lyon.

Isaacson, P. (1982) Biopsy appearances easily mistaken for malignancy in gastrointestinal endoscopy. *Histopathology*, **6** (4), 377–389.

Jenkins, D., Balsitis, M., Gallivan, S. *et al.* (1997) Guidelines for the initial biopsy diagnosis of suspected chronic idiopathic inflammatory bowel disease. The British Society of Gastroenterology Initiative. *Journal of Clinical Pathology*, **50** (2), 93–105.

Joensuu, H., Fletcher, C., Dimitrijevic, S. *et al.* (2002) Management of malignant gastrointestinal stromal tumours. *Lancet Oncology*, **3** (11), 655–664.

Kaifi, J.T., Strelow, A., Schurr, P.G. *et al.* (2006) L1 (CD171) is highly expressed in gastrointestinal stromal tumors. *Modern Pathology*, **19** (3), 399–406.

Kirsch, R., Pentecost, M., Hall, P de M. *et al.* (2006) Role of colonoscopic biopsy in distinguishing between Crohn's disease and intestinal tuberculosis. *Journal of Clinical Pathology*, **59** (8), 840–844.

Lee, F.D. (1997) Drug-related intestinal disease. *Current Diagnostic Pathology*, **4** (3), 128–134.

Lucas, R.B. (1984) Pathology of Tumours of the Oral Tissues, 4th edn, Churchill Livingstone, Edinburgh.

MacDonald, D.G. and Browne, R.M. (1997) Tumours of odontogenic epithelium, in *Recent Advances in Histopathology*, vol. 17 (eds P.P. Anthony, R.N.M. MacSween and D.G Lowe), Churchill Livingstone, Edinburgh, pp. 139–166.

Mainprize, K.S., Mortensen, N.J. McC. and Warren, B.F. (1998) Early colorectal cancer: recognition, classification and treatment. *British Journal of Surgery*, **85** (4), 469–476.

Martin, J.E., Smith, V.V. and Domizio, P. (1999) Myopathies of the gastrointestinal tract, in *Recent Advances in Histopathology*, vol. 18 (eds D.G. Lowe and J.C.E. Underwood, Churchill Livingstone, Edinburgh, pp. 43–62.

Martin, J.E., Swash, M., Kamm, M.A. *et al.* (1990) Myopathy of internal anal sphincter with polyglucosan inclusions. *Journal of Pathology*, **161** (3), 221–226.

Misdraji, J. (2005) Neuroendocrine tumours of the appendix. *Current Diagnostic Pathology*, **11** (3), 180–193.

Montgomery, E.A. (2006) *Biopsy Interpretation of the Gastrointestinal Tract Mucosa.* Lippincott Williams & Wilkins, Philadelphia.

Morson, B.C (ed) (1987) Alimentary Tract in *Systemic Pathology*, Vol.3, 3rd edn, (ed W. St C. Symmers), Churchill Livingstone, Edinburgh.

Mudhar, H.S. and Balsitis, M. (2005) Colonic angiodysplasia and true diverticula: is there an association? *Histopathology*, **46** (1), 81–88.

Mueller, J., Mueller, E., Hoepner, I. *et al.* (1996) Expression of Bcl-2 and p53 in *de novo* and *ex–adenoma* colon carcinoma: a comparative immunohistochemical study. *Journal of Pathology*, **180** (3), 259–265.

Nagao, T., Serizawa, H., Iwaya, K. *et al.* (2001) Keratocystoma of the parotid gland: a report of two cases of an unusual pathologic entity. *Modern Pathology*, **15** (9), 1005–1010.

Ng, W-K. (2003) Radiation-associated changes in tissues and tumours. *Current Diagnostic Pathology*, **9** (2), 124–136.

Odze, R.D, (2006) Diagnosis and grading of dysplasia in Barrett's oesophagus. *Journal of Clinical Pathology*, **59** (10), 1029–1038.

Ordóñez, N.G. (2006) The diagnostic utility of immunohistochemistry and electron microscopy in distinguishing between peritoneal mesothelioma and serous carcinomas: a comparative study. *Modern Pathology*, **19** (1), 34–48.

Parfitt, J.R., Gregor, J.C., Suskin, N.G. *et al.* (2006) Eosinophilic esophagitis in adults: distinguishing features from gastroesophageal reflux disease: a study of 41 patients. *Modern Pathology*, **19** (1), 90–96.

Price, A.B. (1996) Indeterminate colitis – broadening the perspective. *Current Diagnostic Pathology*, **3** (1), 35–44.

Rindi, G., Azzoni, C., La Rosa, S. *et al.* (1999) ECL cell tumour and poorly differentiated endocrine carcinoma of the stomach: prognostic evaluation by pathological analysis. *Gastroenterology*, **116** (3), 532–542.

Rosai, J. (2004) Mandible and Maxilla, in *Rosai and Ackerman's Surgical Pathology*, 9th edn (ed J. Rosai), Mosby, Edinburgh, pp. 279–304.

Rossi, G., Valli, R., Bertolini, F. *et al.* (2005) PDGFR expression in differential diagnosis between KIT-negative gastrointestinal stromal tumours and other primary soft-tissue tumours of the gastrointestinal tract, *Histopathology*, **46** (5), 522–531.

Schlemper, R.J., Riddell, R.H., Kato, Y. *et al.* (2000) The Vienna classification of gastrointestinal epithelial neoplasia. *Gut*, **47** (2), 251–255.

Serra, S. and Jani, P.A. (2006) An approach to duodenal biopsies. *Journal of Clinical Pathology*, **59** (11), 1133–1150.

Shepherd, N.A. (1997) Polyps and polyposis syndromes of the intestines. *Current Diagnostic Pathology*, **4** (4), 222–238.

Shepherd, N.A., Jass, J.R., Duval, I., Moskowitz, R.L., Nicholls, R.J. and Morson, B.C. (1987) Restorative proctocolectomy with ileal reservoir: pathological and histochemical study of mucosal biopsy specimens. *Journal of Clinical Pathology*, **40** (6), 601–607.

Simpson, R.H.W. (1997) Salivary gland tumours, in *Recent Advances in Histopathology*, vol. 17 (eds P.P. Anthony, R.N.M MacSween and D.G Lowe), Churchill Livingstone, Edinburgh, pp.167–190.

Simpson, R.H.W. and Sarsfield, P.T.L. (1997) Benign and malignant lymphoid lesions of the salivary glands. *Current Diagnostic Pathology*, **4** (2), 91–99.

Sjölund, K., Sandén, G., Håkanson, R. and Sundler, F. (1983) Endocrine cells in human intestine: an immunocytochemical study. *Gastroenterology*, **85** (5), 1120–30.

Sternberg, S.S. (ed) (1997) *Histology for Pathologists*, 2nd edn, Lippincott Williams & Wilkins, Philadelphia.

Takubo, N., Nakagawa, H., Tsuchiya, S. *et al.* (1981) Seedling leiomyomas of the esophagus and esophago-gastric junction zone. *Human Pathology*, **12** (11), 1006–1010.

Talbot, I.C. (2001) Dysplasia in the lower gastrointestinal tract in *Recent Advances in Histopathology*, vol. 19 (eds D.G. Lowe and J.C.E. Underwood), Churchill Livingstone, Edinburgh, pp.211–225.

Tanaka, M. and Riddell, R.H. (1990) The pathological diagnosis and differential diagnosis of Crohn's disease. *Hepato-Gastroenterology*, **37** (1), 18–31.

Torlakovic, E. and Snover, D.C. (1996) Serrated adenomatous polyposis in humans. *Gastroenterology*, **110** (3), 748–755.

Warren, B.F and Shepherd, N.A. (1995) Iatrogenic pathology of the gastrointestinal tract, in *Progress in Pathology*, vol. 1 (eds N. Kirkham and P. Hall), Churchill Livingstone, Edinburgh, pp. 30–54.

Warren, B.F. and Shepherd, N.A. (1999) Surgical pathology of the intestines: the pelvic ileal reservoir and diversion proctocolitis, in *Recent Advances in Histopathology*, vol. 18 (eds D.G. Lowe and J.C.E. Underwood), Churchill Livingstone, Edinburgh, pp. 63–88.

Willis, R.A. (1952) *The Spread of Tumours in the Human Body*, Butterworth & Co. Ltd, London.

Wong, N.A.C.S., Yong, R., Malcomson, R.D.G., *et al.* (2003) Prognostic indicators for gastrointestinal stromal tumors: a clinicopathological and immunohistochemical study of 108 cases resected of the stomach. *Histopathology*, **43** (5): 118–126.

Wyatt, J. (2001) Routine reporting of non–neoplastic gastric biopsies, in *Progress in Pathology*, vol. 5 (eds N. Kirkham and N.R. Lemoine), Greenwich Medical Media Ltd, London, pp.121–134.

Web Sites

Park, L. (2004) Common variable immunodeficiency. http://www.emedicine.com/ped/topic444.htm (accessed March 2007).

Royal College of Pathologists (July 2006) Standards and Datasets for Reporting Cancers. www.rcpath.org.uk (accessed August 2007).

12. Liver, Biliary Tract and Pancreas

Normal Liver and Artefacts

Acinar Zones and Lobular Regions
- Zones 1+2 ≈ the periportal region (with clover-like extensions between central veins)
- Zone 3 ≈ the pericentral region (with spurs and connections to adjacent zones 3)

Parenchymal Changes
- From birth to 3 months old: Cu and Fe are normally 'increased'
- Upto 5 years old the hepatocyte plates are normally two cells thick
- Any age: fibrosis and necrosis are accentuated in subcapsular/ perihilar regions
- Glycogenated nuclei are common in adolescents and the elderly

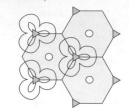

FIGURE 12.1   Zones and regions

Intrahepatic Interlobular Bile Ducts
- 10–30% (higher in pre-term babies) of PT arteries are devoid of an accompanying BD
- Most PTs have just under 1 to 2 BDs per artery of similar ∅ (! don't count periph. proliferated ductules)
- Biliary epithelium can be selectively stained (*cf.* hepatocytes) with CK (7, 19 or AE1/AE3), pCEA and CD10 stain intercellular canaliculi and CD56 stains ductules (e.g. at the edge of PTs)

Other
- PTs in the left lobe are usu. larger than the right
- Post-op changes: PMN, focal necrosis, bland zone 3 canalicular cholestasis
- Some fine needle (e.g. TJ) or aspiration Bx samples may fragment – ! does not imply cirrhosis

Iron, Copper, α_1-Antitrypsin (α_1AT) and Mallory Hyaline

Iron Predominantly in Hepatocytes (± Kupffer cells)
- Type 1 haemochromatosis (AR, 6p HFE c282y): predom. zone 1 ± in BD epithelium, no sig. inflam[n]
- Porphyria cutanea tarda (PCT) – usu. mild in periportal hepatocytes (assoc[d] with HCV)
- Iron overload of advanced liver disease e.g. cirrhosis
- Haematological disease with ↑ Fe absorption (HS/β-thalassaemia minor) – *not* transfusion related
- Chronic haemolysis (get hepatocyte as well as Kupffer cell Fe)
- Familial iron overload (not HFE-linked)
- Neonatal iron overload (the rare *neonatal haemochromatosis*) and similar condition in Down's
- Gilbert's syndrome shows mild hepatocyte iron and no cholestasis
- Grading: I   periportal hepatocytes only
             II   more than grade I but not in all hepatocytes
             III all but still have a gradient ⎤ grades 3 & 4 = significant
             IV   all with no P-C gradient   ⎦ iron overload

Iron Predominantly in Kupffer Cells (± Hepatocytes)
- ↑ Dietary Fe absorption (potentiated by alcohol)
- Post viral hepatitis you may see scattered Kupffer cells and endothelial cells laden with Fe
- Post haemolysis/blood transfusion/some haematological disorders
- Variants of haemochromatosis e.g. the ferroportin disease (= Type 4 haemochromatosis)

Wilson's Disease (Hepatolenticular Degeneration) and d/dg
- Chromosome 13, defective Cu ATPase in biliary epithelium → can't excrete Cu ∴ liver Tx = cure
- Pre-cirrhotic: steatosis, lipofuscin ++, glycogen nuclei, thin fibrous partial septa
- later: as above + chronic hepatitis, Mallory hyaline, PMN (! d/dg alcoholic or viral hepatitis)
- Cirrhotic: as above + broad vascular fibrous septa with interface activity, ballooning[1], cholestasis

---

[1] i.e. cell swelling with rounding but retaining a central nucleus and having reticular pale cytoplasm

- May present as fulminant disease with necrosis $++$ and liver failure (stain $+$ve for Cu/CuBP)
- Cu: ➢ ! failure to stain doesn't exclude it (except in the fulminant variant)
            ➢ ! exclude other causes of $\uparrow$ Cu (PBC, Indian childhood cirrhosis, normal neonatal liver, etc.)
            ➢ Cu / CuBP may be distributed throughhout the lobule (*cf.* zone 1 in biliary disease)

Alpha-1-Antitrypsin Deficiency ($\alpha_1 AT \downarrow$)
- AR, may present as cholestasis in infancy or as progressive hepatitis or incidentally in adulthood
- Neonate: canalicular cholestasis and neonatal GC hepatitis but no $\alpha_1 AT$ globules till $\approx$ 6 months old
- Later: mild PT inflam^n and fibrosis $+$ zone 1 irreg. globules ($+$ve for DPAS, PTAH & $\alpha_1 AT$ immuno)
- Other: BD prolif^n or loss, cirrhosis (esp. biliary type in children, viral-type in adults) $\pm$ HBV/HCV
- d/dg: any cause of neonatal hepatitis or chronic hepatitis/cirrhosis
- d/dg $\alpha_1 AT$ globules are also seen in hepatocellular neoplasia/hyperplasias, ischaemia/congestion: but in these the globules may not have such a predilection for periportal hepatocytes
- d/dg α_1-antichymotrypsin globules: $\therefore$ do $\alpha_1 AT$ immuno for confirmation

Mallory Hyaline (Mallory Bodies)
- Paranuclear eosinophilic hyaline material ($+$ve for p62, CK & ubiquitin)
- Wilson's disease, PBC, PSC, HCV, alcohol/ASH/NASH
- Some tumours and tumour-like lesions: HCC, MRN, FNH and dysplastic nodules
- Biliary causes give Mallory bodies mainly in zone 1; others have them scattered in the lobule

Steatosis and Steatohepatitis (incl. Alcoholic Hepatitis)

Macrovesicular Steatosis
- Large (some say $> \varnothing$ of a nucleus) pauci-droplet, displaced nucleus; causes incl. some IEM and:
    ➢ nutritional (starvation/cachexia/old age, obesity/NIDDM, TPN, CIBD)
    ➢ toxic (alcohol, methotrexate and other drugs)
- Simple steatosis (incl. OH & NAFL) lacks lobular inflam^n, fibrosis and evidence of liver cell damage but spilled lipid can cause lipogranulomas ($\pm$ assoc^d fibrous reaction) that persist if steatosis resolves
- Some grade steatosis as mild, mod., severe $\propto$ the amount of the lobule involved ($< \frac{1}{3}$, $< \frac{2}{3}$, $> \frac{2}{3}$)
- d/dg steatohepatitis – this must have some liver cell damage (Mallory hyaline, ballooning, etc.), fibrosis (often pericellular) or inflam^n

Microvesicular Steatosis
- $\approx 1\mu$ poly-droplet, nucleus not displaced, usu. with liver cell damage/necrosis $\pm$ giant mitochondria
- Not always detectable on routine H&E ($\therefore$ consider staining a FS for fat)
- Causes incl. metabolic e.g. Reye's syndrome (panacinar $\pm$ aspirin), drugs (*q.v.*), alcohol (perivenular, reversible), infective (e.g. Salmonella, HAV, HDV) and others (for acute fatty liver of pregnancy and HELLP syndrome, see p. 385)

Alcoholic Hepatitis/Steatohepatitis (ASH)
- Clinical biochcmistry: $\uparrow$ AST $>$ ALT, $\uparrow$ total de-sialated transferrin
- Liver cell damage (ballooning, Mallory, necrosis, apoptosis) with a PMN infiltrate is assoc^d with OH
- $\pm$ Mononuclear cells (but 'satellitosis' refers to *PMN* surrounding hepatocytes with Mallory hyaline)
- Steatosis is macrovesicular (but a microvesicular component may co-exist) $\pm$ giant mitochondria
- Pericellular fibrosis and perivenular fibrosis (may result in veno-occlusion ! d/dg VOD)/lymphocytic phlebitis
- All changes tend to be worse in the perivenular region
- d/dg other conditions with steatosis and giant mitochondria e.g. DM

Non-alcoholic Steatohepatitis (NASH)
- Clin.: $\uparrow$ALT $>$ AST, transferrin ratios may help in d/dg ASH; better prog. *cf.* ASH (fewer cirrhotics)
- 1° NASH (NASH 1): assoc^d with the metabolic syndrome (NIDDM, obesity, HT, $\downarrow$HDL, $\uparrow$LDL)
- 2° NASH (NASH 2): other causes e.g. drugs (e.g. amiodarone) and SI blind loops/diverticula
- Steatosis, fibrosis, liver cell damage (ballooning $+/$ Councilman), $\pm$ lobular PMN, etc. as for ASH
- Glycogen nuclei and lack of venocentricity is more typical of *some* NASH *cf.* ASH
- Biliary changes (biliary interface activity, bilirubinostasis) favour ASH (! but exclude other causes)
- Any of these are assoc^d with progression (to cirrhosis or a liver death): Mallory, fibrosis, ballooning

- d/dg *isolated portal fibrosis* of the morbidly obese (BMI $\geq 40 Kg/m^2$): portal/periportal fibrosis $\pm$ septa/P-P linking $\pm$ steatosis $\pm$ PT/panacinar 'inflam^n' (but no zone 3 fibrosis, ballooning, necrosis)

Neonatal (Giant Cell) Hepatitis

- PT: lymphocytic inflam^n and variable fibrosis (but not usu. marked and no ductular prolif^n)
- Lobules: widespread multinucleated hepatocytes (giant cells) and variable retic collapse due to necrosis
- Many causes: TORCH, HBV, α_1AT$\downarrow$, Wilson's, galactosaemia, Down's, etc.
- d/dg extrahepatic BD atresia (p. 164 – important because atresia requires early surgery)

Acute Viral Hepatitis

Classical Acute Hepatitis ('Acute Hepatitis with Spotty Necrosis')
- Perivenular: ➤ hepatocyte damage (apoptosis, swelling, regenerat^n incl. rosettes) → lobular disarray
  - ➤ canalicular cholestasis
  - ➤ mononuclear cell infiltrate and Kupffer cell hyperplastic groups (DPAS +ve, Fe $\pm$ve)
- Portal: ➤ chronic inflam^n incl. follicles (d/dg HCV) and interface activity
  - ➤ hepatitic damage to bile ducts (i.e. irregular staining, vacuolation, (pseudo)stratification assoc^d with lymphocytes, esp. near follicles, but no granulomas) – d/dg sepsis or 1° biliary disease
  - ➤ aggregates of DPAS/Fe +ve Mϕ
- Variants: ➤ giant cell (d/dg variants of active AIH and neonatal GC hepatitis of $\approx$ any cause)
  - ➤ cholestatic: liver cell damage *not* confined to cholestatic areas (*cf.* 2° cholestasis)

Acute Hepatitis with Bridging Necrosis
- Features as for classical acute hepatitis plus portal-central bridging necrosis
- $\pm$ C-C linking necrosis (but this is not included in the definition)
- d/dg necrosis *vs.* chronic fibrosis (p. 159)

Acute Hepatitis with Pan-Acinar/Pan-Lobular/Massive/Sub-massive Necrosis
- Extent (multilobular *vs.* massive hepatic necrosis) cannot be determined on needle Bx
- Neocholangioles proliferate around PTs
- Variable collapse (as judged by retic and extent of approximation of adjacent PTs)
- $\uparrow\uparrow$ Ceroid-laden Mϕ (! do not confuse for hepatocytes)
- $\pm$ Central venulitis

Acute Hepatitis with Periportal Necrosis
- Lymphocytes and plasma cells (esp. in HAV). Plasma cells may be numerous but entrapped hepatocytes scant (*cf.* CAH/AIH)
- Perivenular changes may be mild (esp. in hepatitis A) → ! misdiagnosed as CAH (∴ need CPC)
- Don't confuse P-P linkage with true bridging necrosis (i.e. P-C)

Hepatitis A (HAV) and Hepatitis E (HEV)
- Acute hepatitis with PT plasma cells and interface activity (d/dg AIH), zone 3 cholestasis, $\pm$ little hepatocyte damage $\pm$ microvesicular steatosis
- HAV $\approx$ never progresses to a clinically chronic hepatitis
- HEV can be esp. lethal in pregnancy and show prominent cholestasis and phlebitis $\pm$ BD proliferation

Differential Diagnosis of Acute Hepatitis
- EBV: no/mild liver damage; atypical lymphocytes in sinusoids and PTs
- HSV/CMV: confluent necrosis (*cf.* spotty); minimal lymphocytes in sinusoids; inclusions
- Drugs: ➤ poor/absent PT inflam^n
  - ➤ PMN, eos., granulomas

- ➢ paracetamol: *sharply defined perivenular necrosis* with little inflam[n]
    - ➢ mixed hepatitic/cholestatic picture *with duct damage* (e.g. flucloxacillin/paraquat)
- Alcohol: perivenular ballooning with PMN (*cf.* lymphocytes) ± Mallory hyaline/steatosis/fibrosis
- Biliary disease:
    - ➢ may show granulomas in PBC (but ! d/dg IVDA)
    - ➢ relative lack of lobular disease
    - ➢ CuBP (black dots with orcein or blue dots with a Victoria blue stain)
    - ➢ greater ductular proliferation ± ductopaenia with relative lack of cholestasis
    - ➢ CPC (autoAbs, etc.)
- 2° cholestasis: liver cell damage confined to cholestatic areas, lack of spotty necrosis
- AIH: hard to distinguish from acute hepatitis (esp. HAV) ∴ need CPC (auto/viral Abs, etc.)
- Chronic hepatitis/cirrhosis: distinguish bridging/confluent necrosis from fibrosis (*vide infra*)

Features Favouring Necrosis cf. Fibrosis
- Other assoc[d] features of acute hepatitis
- Elastic is absent (elastic takes time to develop so is a sign of chronicity)
- Residual hepatocyte plate structure is preserved (although collapsed) on reticulin stain
- Stroma is more haemorrhagic with more Mφ (! don't confuse ceroid Mφ for hepatocytes)
- Bile ductular proliferation and PMN

Chronic Viral Hepatitis

General Points
- Def[n] of chronic hepatitis: continuing clinicopathological disease for ≥6 months
    - ➢ excludes PBC, PSC, α_1AT deficiency and Wilson's disease.
    - ➢ usu. due to viruses, autoimmunity and drugs
- Traditional classification into CAH, CPH and CLH is no longer used because all may co-exist and the difference depends on interface activity whereas other factors (confluent necrosis, fibrosis, etc.) may be more significant – hence the current vogue for histological grading and staging schemes
- 'Activity' has two aspects: interface and lobular.

Portal Inflammation and Interface Activity
- Predominantly T4 cells and some plasma cells (T8 cells at the advancing front of interface hepatitis/activity)
- Interface activity = spill-over of inflam[n] beyond the PT limiting plate (± hepatocyte apoptosis) with lymphocytes closely adhered to (peripolesis) or apparently within (emperipolesis) hepatocytes. It is helpful to see lymphocytes at the hepatocyte-hepatocyte interface (otherwise it could just be sinusoidal infiltration)
- Hepatitic damage to bile ducts ± portal phlebitis (*cf.* the *central* phlebitis in acute hepatitis)
- It is no longer necessary to see dead/dying hepatocytes to diagnose interface activity

Lobular Activity
- Focal spotty necrosis: this term includes perivenular parenchymal inflam[n2] or acute-type necrosis – not just apoptoses (Councilman bodies), although these are also included
- Confluent necrosis: may be linking +/ bridging (C-C +/ P-C but only P-C is used in the Ishak grade) ± hepatitic rosettes (surrounded by inflam[y]/connective tissue and usu. lack a lumen *cf.* d/dg cholestatic rosettes that *may* also show a connection to bile ductules, contain bile and stain for biliary CK)

Viral Co-Infection
- HBV: if serology +ve for HBV with tissue immuno −ve for HBsAg, suspect co-HCV or co-HDV
- HIV and HBV: a higher % progress to chronicity but they show lower histological activity. May get 'reactivation' lobular hepatitis in severe AIDS, even if +ve for HBsAb (may even get FCH)
- HIV and HCV: synergistic – both the HIV and HCV pursue a worse course (incl. ↑ risk of HCC)

Hepatitis B (HBV)[3]
- Ground glass hepatocytes (eccentric nucleus ± clear rim around the ground glass cytoplasmic inclusion *cf.* d/dg oncocytic change) ± lymphocyte emperipolesis

---

[2] does *not* include inflam[y] cells only in the sinusoids; ! exclude cross-cuts of inflamed PT septa
[3] HBV is the only one out of A, B, C, D, E that is a DNA virus

- Sanded nuclei (core Ag or HDV), ↑ anisonucleosis ± large cell dysplasia (*q.v.*)
- ↑ Replication (and ↑ histological activity unless immunosuppressed) if immuno shows:
    - ① membranous staining for HBsAg (not just cytoplasmic)
    - ② HBcAg +vity (esp. if there is cytoplasmic staining)
- 90% of cases become e & s Ag −ve, Ab +ve: this indicates protective Ab virus elimination
- 10% of cases become e & s Ag +ve, Ab −ve: this indicates chronic hepatitis (active)
- 50% of chronic hepatitics *seroconvert* to eAg −ve, Ab +ve (assoc[d] with clinical and histological exacerbation) to become chronic carriers
- mutants: ① pre-core: eAg not expressed, eAb +ve despite ongoing replication and active disease
    - ② sAg: vaccine resistant

Hepatitis C (HCV)
- Bx changes do not correlate with clinical/biochemical severity ∴ Bx gives independent information
- Lymphoid follicles (1° or 2° – germinal centres are esp. characteristic) ± hepatitic BD damage
- Mild-moderate steatosis (macro and microvesicular)
- Sinusoidal lymphocytes (d/dg EBV)
- Synergistic with OH: suggest OH if *severe* fat or pericellular/venular fibrosis or ballooning and PMN
- Fe in Kupffer ∝ poor response to Rx; Fe in parenchyma: ① PCT ② cirrhosis ③ haemochromatosis
- Granulomas (PT or lobular) – but not assoc[d] with chronic ductopaenia and not causing BD destruct[n]
- Extrahepatic effects: cryoglobulinaemia, GN[4], Sjögren's; PAN, LP, PCT, lymphoma (low grade B-cell e.g. LPL, MZL and MALTomas incl. hepatic/salivary 1° – not TCL or HL), autoAb e.g. ALKM, anti-thyroid, ANA (a false +ve due to cross-reactivity with HCV Ags) and antiphospholipid (but usu. without the TMA of antiphospholipid Ab syndrome)

Hepatitis D (Delta Agent, HDV)
- Co-infection/super-infection with HBV is assoc[d] with active/fulminant disease (recurrent acute hepatitis is characteristic), cirrhosis and HCC; may see periportal morule cells (multivacuolated hepatocytes)
- Immuno (nuclear +vity for delta agent) is more reliable than serology
- Inhibits HBV replication → ① HBV immuno can become −ve, ② ↓ mortality in Tx patients
- Chronic HDV may have an ALKM-3 AIH component

The Modified Histological Activity Index (HAI) for Chronic Hepatitis – Table 12.1
- ! Sub-capsular/peri-hilar biopsies show unrepresentative accentuation of fibrosis +/ necrosis

The Royal College of Physicians/BSG categories for HCV hepatitis
- Mild: stage ≤ 2 AND *either* ➤ combined grade ≤3/18
    - *or* ➤ **A** grade ≤ 1 AND **C** grade ≤ 1 AND **B** grade = 0 (**D** grade = any)
- Moderate: stage 3–5 AND/OR combined grade >3/18
- Cirrhotic: stage = 6 (any grade)

Differential Diagnosis of Chronic Viral Hepatitis
- Acute hepatitis A: interface activity and plasma cells ++ can give impression of AIH or chronic viral hepatitis ∴ look for lobular changes and CPC
- AIH: ➤ serology, plasma cells ++, interface ++ with rosetting, parenchymal collapse
    - ➤ ! HCV can give false +ve ANA
    - ➤ ! an AIH component may accompany hepatitis B, C and D
    - ➤ ! d/dg drug-induced AIH-like disease
- Metabolic: ➤ α₁AT deficiency: DPAS +ve globules (! exclude concomitant viral infection)
    - ➤ Wilson's disease: Mallory hyaline, fat, Cu, broad vascular fibrous septa
- Drug-induced: viral-type chronic hepatitis is rare but can occur (e.g. with α-methyldopa – but AIH-like chronic hepatitis is commoner with this drug)
- PBC: early lesions difficult to distinguish from HCV which may show bile duct damage and loss. Later: ① granulomatous BD destruct[n]; ② ductular prolif[n], ③ chronic cholestasis periportal/septally
- PSC, PBC and other biliary diseases: deposition of Cu/CuBP at an early stage of liver disease favours a biliary disease (but any cause of *end-stage* liver disease can cause CuBP to accumulate)

---

[4] membranoproliferative or ADP (both may be due to cryoglobulins)

TABLE 12.1   Grade and stage in heptatitis

SCORE	INFLAMMATORY INFILTRATE WITHIN SEPTA & PORTALTRACTS (% of septa/PTs affected)	ACTIVITY Interface (% of septal PTs affected)	Lobular (foci per x10 objective)[*]	CONFLUENT NECROSIS (% of acini with confluent necrosis in a zonal pattern)	FIBROSIS (% of PTs expanded)
	D Grade	A Grade	C Grade	B Grade	Stage
0	none	none	none	none	none
1	mild (in ≤ 100%)	focal & <50%	≤1	focal (not zonal)[†]	<50% ± short septa[‡]
2	moderate (in ≤ 100%)	focal & >50%	2–4	<50% (zone 3 only)	>50% ± short septa
3	100%, some with a severe infiltrate	continuous around <50%	5–10	>50% (zone 3 only)	>50% & occ. P-P links
4	100%, all with a severe infiltrate	continuous around >50%	>10	occasional bridging to zone 1 (P-C)	marked linking/bridging (P-P +/ P-C)
5				multiple P-C bridges	as for score 4 plus occasional nodules[x]
6				≥ 1 acinus shows zonal necrosis in all 3 zones	cirrhosis (even if only probable)[**]

This grading & staging system is a modification of Knodell's HAI & is based on Ishak K, Baptista A, Bianchi L, *et al.*
J Hepatol (1995); 22:696-9
[*]i.e. focal inflam^n/apoptosis/'lytic' cell dropout. Focal inflam^n does *not* include diffuse sinusoidal infiltration by inflam^y cells. It is 'interface'-type inflam^n but in a pericentral location.
[†]i.e. contiguous groups of hepatocytes are necrotic (not apoptotic) but without a clear zonal pattern (d/dg HSV or TB).
[‡]septa due to interface activity tend to be curved, cellular & stain for retic but not type I collagen until mature.
[x]this is sometimes called 'incomplete cirrhosis' which, here, appears to mean 'not quite fully cirrhotic' rather than the more tightly defined entity of *incomplete septal cirrhosis* (q.v.).
[**]! Avoid overcalling cirrhosis due to artefactual Bx fragmentation.

- Leukaemia/lymphoma: no true piecemeal *necrosis*; lymphoid cells may look 'clonal'/'pure culture' (i.e. not mixed inflam^n); some claim scarring is absent while others describe possible fibrosis incl. P-P linking

Autoimmune Hepatitis (AIH)

- Type 1: classic lupoid CAH: ANA/ASGP-R/ANCA, assoc^d with other system autoimmunity
- Type 2: idiopathic in children (in adults it is usu. due to HCV = Type 2b), ALKM-1, ALC
- Type 3: assoc^d with SLP auto-Abs (also called SLA), no other system autoimmunity
- Type 4: assoc^d with anti F-actin smooth muscle Abs (ASMA)
- ↑ Globulinaemia and autoAbs (>1:80 adult or 1:20 child) though some may be −ve at presentation and many auto-Abs e.g. ANA or ASMA are not specific to AIH so other features must be present
- Plasma cells ++, interface hepatitis ++, ± cholestasis/bile duct damage; in acute AIH there is also severe lobular plasma cell-rich inflam^n ± giant cells and ballooning
- ± Central necrosis ± bridging, ± acute/fulminant hepatitis (d/dg HAV) esp. in childhood type 2 AIH
- Zone 3 variant: centrilobular necroinflam^n, usu. with plasma cell clusters ± congest^n ± PT inflam^n
- d/dg AMA −ve PBC: in AIH inflam^n is more uniform and intense, shows lobular activity and lacks typical PBC duct damage
- d/dg zone 3 variant *vs.* venous outflow obstruction
- 'Probable AIH'(→trial of steroids) if: ① mild changes *or*

    ② lack typical Abs *or*

    ③ other possible aetiological factors are present

Overlap Syndromes
- Steroid-responsive cholangiopathic autoimmune hepatitides (! long-term steroids may *worsen* PBC)
- Mixed AIH/PSC: uncommon, often in children
- Mixed AIH/PBC[5]: ① AMA −ve, ANA/ASMA +ve and the inflam^n has some PBC-like features *or*

    ② AMA +ve with AIH-type inflam^n *or*

    ③ clinically, any patient with ≥ 2 features of AIH and ≥ 2 features of PBC

---

[5] AMA -ve types are sometimes called '*autoimmune cholangiopathy*' or 'immunocholangitis'.

Intrahepatic Bile Ducts

Cholestasis
- Perivenular canalicular bilirubinostasis (seen in acute hepatitis, drugs, ischaemia, post-op, etc.)
- Cholestatic liver cell rosettes (usu. have a lumen and are surrounded by other hepatocytes)
- Biliary interface activity (biliary piecemeal necrosis):
  - ➤ is the main clue to diagnosing a 1° biliary disorder (obstructive, inflam[y], etc.)
  - ➤ is defined by three features: ① cholate stasis, ② ductular react[n], ③ fibroplasia
  - ① *Cholate Stasis:*
    - ☞ feathery degeneration of periportal hepatocytes which acquire Cu and CK7/19 +vity
    - ☞ later bilirubin and Mallory hyaline (in zone 1) also accumulate ± xanthomatous Mϕ
  - ② *Ductular Reaction:*
    - ☞ proliferation of ductules and neocholangioles at the limiting plate[6]
    - ☞ ± PMN due to irritant effect of bile (not seen in other causes of ductular proliferation e.g. infection, alcohol, venous outflow obstruction or *isolated ductular hyperplasia)*[7]
  - ③ *Fibroplasia:* accompanies the ductular reaction and is loose/oedematous and at the periphery of the PT/septum (→ clear 'halo' effect around septa/PTs)
- Biliary cirrhosis: monolobular arch. (i.e. retained central venule ± 'jig-saw' parenchyma), clear halo around septa, *lots* of zone 1 Cu/CuBP and loose lamellar fibrosis in the septa suggest a biliary origin

Vanishing Bile Duct Syndrome

Adequacy of sampling
- 10 PTs are needed (some say 20) to diagnose ductopaenia by the 50% rule (i.e. $\geq$50% of PT arteries are unaccompanied by a BD). Also, sig. BD loss is present if <80% of PTs have a BD
- However there is evidence that, for BD loss to be statistically significant, the minimal % BD loss required varies with the nõ. of PTs in the Bx e.g. for a Bx with 4 PTs you need 100% loss, for 8 PTs you need $\geq$75% loss, etc. (see Tadrous and Goldin, 1997)

(Sub)acute BD loss
- Acute cholestasis with little or no biliary interface activity
- Causes incl. GVHD, liver Tx rejection, some drugs, treated HL

Chronic BD loss
- Little cholestasis but prominent biliary interface activity → cirrhosis
- Causes incl. PBC, PSC/SSC, liver Tx rejection, sarcoid, ischaemia, some drugs and infections

Septal/large duct disease
- PSC and childhood extrahepatic biliary atresia may cause ductopaenia

Other causes
- Idiopathic adulthood ductopaenia (diagnosis of exclusion, some are progressive like PSC/PBC)
- Infantile/childhood:　➤ syndromic e.g. Alagille, Zellweger, α_1AT ↓, CF, Down's, etc.
　　　　　　　　　　　➤ non-syndromic e.g. PFIC (cholestasis, cholate stasis, inflam[n] and cirrhosis), d/dg BRIC (canalicular cholestasis only)

Staging of PBC and PSC
- In a Bx, report the highest stage present (not the predominant stage). Some recommend using the HAI
  - I　changes confined to the PT
  - II　interface activity (chronic inflam[y] and biliary) ± short radiating septa
  - III　scarring, incl. significant septa or P-P linkage ('biliary fibrosis')
  - IV　biliary cirrhosis

Primary Biliary Cirrhosis (PBC)
- Clin.: F≫M (9:1), anti-M2 AMA +ve in >95%, ± Sjögren's, PSS, coeliac, etc.
- Early:　➤ mixed chronic inflam[y] infiltrate in PT (predom. lymphoid) with granulomas ⎫ = *'florid bile*
　　　　　➤ small BD epithelial damage and regeneration, intraepithelial lymphocytes ⎬ *duct lesion'*
　　　　　➤ patchy changes (! sampling may result in non-specific PT inflam[n] only) ⎭

---

[6] ductular prolif[n] (often lumenless) is seen in many conditions with limiting plate hepatocyte damage
[7] isolated ductular hyperplasia (i.e. with no other lesion) is a cause of prolonged ↑ in ALT +/ γGT

- Medium term: ➢ vestigial CK7/19 or PAS +ve elements
                  ➢ condensation of fibrous tissue   } where BDs used to be
                  ➢ lymphoid aggregates ± foamy Mφ
- Late: ➢ progressive BD loss (the smaller the duct the more likely it is to be lost)
            ➢ biliary interface activity
            ➢ biliary cirrhosis and cholestasis
- Other: ➢ mild lobular inflam^n incl. sinusoid lymphocytosis ± small granulomas
            ➢ lymphocytic interface hepatitis ± occ. plasma cells and the odd germinal centre (d/dg viral/AIH)
            ➢ ± Councilman bodies (some say that hepatocyte damage or other sig. lobular activity is not typical of PBC and should suggest a superimposed process or an overlap syndrome)
- d/dg: sarcoid (*vs.* AMA −ve PBC) granulomas are not targeted at BDs, may cluster and are ≈ bare
- d/dg: drugs, PSC, viral or AIH, HL and any cause of vanishing BDs

Primary Sclerosing Cholangitis (PSC)

- Clin.: M>F, ± colonic CIBD, pancreatitis, multifocal fibrosclerosis, osteopaenia, cholangioCA
- Radiol: abnormal MRI cholangiogram or ERCP (otherwise = 'small duct PSC')
- Macro: normal → dilated irregular ducts → segmental/hemi cirrhosis (i.e. more uneven *cf.* PBC)
- Largest BDs: ➢ periduct fibrosis extending to fat, prolif^n of periductal glands
                  ➢ severe (mainly lymphoplasmacytic) inflam^u (! d/dg severe hepatitis)
                  ➢ ulceration (± acute inflam^n and bilirubin impregnation) ± dysplasia
- Large BDs: ➢ tortuosity ± mixed inflam^n ± follicles ± interface activity (biliary ± AIH-like)
                  ➢ d/dg PBC but PSC has: ☞ less inflam^n but more oedema
                                             ☞ sparse/no intraepithelial lymphocytes/granulomas
                                             ☞ concentric lamellar ('onion skin') and hyaline fibrosis
                                             ☞ nodular scarring ± adjacent parenchymal collapse
                                             ☞ larger ducts also involved
                                             ☞ ± cholangitis
                                             ☞ earlier cholestasis
- Small BDs: ➢ BDs vanish (replaced by a hyaline/fibrous scar)
                  ➢ PT arteries appear to proliferate (due to tortuosity 2° to PT fibrous shrinkage)
- Gallbladder: l.p. lymphocytic + plasma cell inflam^n (esp. if diffuse and acalculous) ± fibrosclerotic vasc. changes
- d/dg SSC (HIV, post-op ischaemia, mastocytosis, HX, etc.): can't distinguish from PSC by histol.
- d/dg: PBC and any other cause of vanishing bile duct syndrome (*q.v.*)
- d/dg extrahepatic or large duct obstruction (*q.v.*) from any cause incl. PSC (they may coexist) or recurrent suppurative cholangitis (healing → fibrous scar replaces duct) due to *Clonorchis*/ascarids

Dubin-Johnson Syndrome

- Variably-sized lipofuscin-like granules in (predom. zone 3) hepatocytes but no cholestasis

Caroli Disease and Syndrome

- Clin.: *disease* is sporadic, no portal HT; *syndrome* (= disease + congenital hepatic fibrosis) is usu. AR
- Dilated bile ducts (upto 2cm ⌀) with thickened walls and marked chronic inflam^n
- Lining: BD epithelium (bland or reactive atypia or dysplasia) or denuded with bile encrustation ± Mφ
- ± Surrounding small duct proliferation: d/dg atresia (*q.v.*)
- Assoc^d with autosomal recessive polycystic kidney disease, choledochal cyst(s) and cholangioCA
- d/dg biliary ectasias 2° to PSC

Congenital Hepatic Fibrosis

- Usu. AR (but AD occurs) ± Caroli disease ± portal HT, cholangitis, cholangioCA, polycystic kidney disease (AR and AD types), TS, Meckel-Gruber and many more syndromes
- Liver carved up into irregular islands ('jig-saw') by fibrous tissue
- Elongated irregular BD-like structures at the limiting plate and separate BDs centrally within the septa
- No cholestasis or sig. inflam^n unless complicated by ascending cholangitis (or Caroli)
- ± Mallory hyaline but no sig. lobular activity/necrosis
- Assoc^d with malformation of intrahepatic portal vein branches (may be small/absent)
- d/dg cirrhosis: this has regenerative nodules ± inflam^n/necrosis

Alagille's Syndrome (Arteriohepatic Dysplasia)
- Sporadic/AD, dysmorphic baby, CVS anomalies, ± portal HT
- Canalicular cholestasis ± hepatocellular giant cells, biliary interface activity and evidence of biliary epithelial damage (lymphocytes, PMN, ± lumenal fibro/epithelial obliteration)
- Chronic BD loss (for def[n.] see 'Vanishing Bile Duct Syndrome', p. 162)

von Meyenburg Complexes (vMC or Bile Duct Hamartoma)
- Para-PT, usu. <5mm, ± multiple; assoc[d] with cavernous haemangioma, cholangioCA, ADPCKD[8]
- Round with irregular (branched, angulated, ectatic) and inter-connected ducts in cellular fibrous stroma
- Cytology: bland, ± inflam[y] atypia if intralumenal PMN, ± bile plugs, ± intralumenal mucin (rare and not intracellular as in d/dg adenoCA or BD adenoma) or amorphous eosinophilic proteinaceous secretions
- Immuno: mCEA has a lumenal pattern (*cf.* cytoplasmic in adenocarcinoma)
- d/dg adenocarcinoma: good circumscription, bland cytology, bile plugs, vMC gland architecture and lack of intracellular mucin all favour vMC
- d/dg multiple vMC *vs.* congenital hepatic fibrosis: use CPC
- d/dg BD adenoma (*q.v.*) is bigger with less stroma, smaller (and more packed) ducts and no bile plugs

Extrahepatic and Large Bile Ducts

Large Duct Obstruction in Neonates (Extrahepatic Biliary Atresia)
- Early: PT oedema, BD (and ductular) prolif[n] ± PMN ± inspissated bile (d/dg sepsis *q.v.*)
- Lobules may show cholestasis (esp. zone 3) ± a few zone 1 multinucleated hepatocyte GC
- Later: BD loss progressing to 2° biliary cirrhosis (see section on Cholestasis, p. 162)
- Obliterated extrahepatic duct(s) show fibrosis ± chronic inflam[n] ± residual epithelial cells
- FS during Kasai procedure:[9] ➤ are there genuine BDs (*cf.* para-scar blind saccules)?
  ➤ BD lumen of $\geq$100–200 μ $\varnothing$ at the proximal resection margin suggests likely success (else the procedure may be abandoned)
- d/dg incl. many things (so definitive diagnosis should not be solely histological):
  ➤ neonatal hepatitis: atresia has ductular prolif[n], sig. PT fibrosis, less retic collapse/lobular disarray, fewer GC (and these tend to be in zone 1 *cf.* widespread) and more cholestasis
  ➤ prolonged TPN ($\geq$ 3 weeks) and obstructive choledochal cyst show similar histology $\therefore$ need CPC
  ➤ some cases of CMV or α_1AT↓ or other IEM

Large Duct Obstruction in Adults
- Early changes: zone 3 cholestasis with enlarged Kupffer cells, PT oedema
- Later in PT: mixed inflam[n] incl. PMN ± eos., ± concentric BD fibrosis (d/dg PSC, which may coexist)
- Later in lobules: feathery degeneration and *mild* changes reactive to bile: apoptosis, mitosis and inflam[n]
- $\approx$ Specific changes (helpful in the d/dg but not always present):
  ➤ para-PT lobular bile infarcts: a bile infarct is an area of pale/foamy/rounded/pyknotic or dead hepatocytes (! d/dg Mϕ) and fibrin ± bile-staining
  ➤ PT bile extravasates with Mϕ response ± giant cells
  ➤ marginal bile ductular prolif[n] with the ductules orientated $\approx$ parallel to the limiting plate
- If untreated → cholate stasis → 2° biliary cirrhosis
- d/dg drug reaction (if eos. prom.): obstruction rarely shows bland cholestasis without ductular prolif[n]
- d/dg alcohol (ASH) (if PMN prom.): OH has more *lobular* activity (incl. PMN, Mallory and steatosis)
- d/dg acute hepatitis: necrosis (without bile infarcts) with bridging favours hepatitis
- d/dg ductular prolif[n] of cholate stasis: biliary piecemeal necrosis has more irregular ductules, many without lumena and not arranged $\approx$ parallel to the limiting plate (as may occur in marginal prolif[n])
- d/dg space occupying lesions may show similar changes but with sinusoid dilatation
- d/dg TPN can also be a mimic in adults but more commonly it shows steatosis and less/no PT changes
- d/dg sepsis and 2° ascending cholangitis (*q.v.*)
- d/dg autoimmune pancreatitis: plasma cells in liver are +ve for IgG4 and patients have ↑ serum IgG4

---

[8] The lesions of ADPCKD are thought to arise by dilatation of vMCs and peribiliary glands.
[9] some say it makes no difference if ducts are found at FS or what their $\varnothing$ is - the procedure may still work. Others say that a total lumenal area (of all hilar ducts) $\geq$ 100000 μm^2 is a good prognostic.

HIV Cholangiopathy (= AIDS Cholangiopathy)
- Occurs in late HIV with low CD4 count
- Due to Cryptosporidium/microsporidium/CMV infection
- MRI, ERCP and histology are all similar to that seen in PSC (*q.v.*)

Liver Transplant Pathology

FS of Potential Donor Liver
- Exclude contraindications to Tx: severe macrovesicular steatosis, neoplasia or chronic hepatitis
- Mild portal triaditis is acceptable provided there is no clinical/serological evidence of viral disease

Reperfusion Injury (e.g. in the Baseline Bx at $\frac{1}{2}$ hour)
- Cholestasis (intrahepatocyte and canalicular) lasts a few weeks
- Ballooning without necrosis is also transitory
- Mild focal endothelialitis is acceptable without implying rejection
- ± Lipopeliosis (fatty expansion of sinusoids) may occur in steatotic transplants
- Tiny foci of hepatocyte necrosis ± local PMN (usu. resolve within days)
- Widespread PMN or zones 1&3 necrosis with subcapsular accentuation is a poor prognostic

Transplant Rejection

Hyperacute (humoural) rejection
- Occurs hours to 1 week after Tx
- Early: sinusoid engorgement, fibrin, PMN, Ig and C3
- Later: extensive zone 3 haemorrhagic coagulative necrosis

Acute rejection
- Occurs in the first 2 months (after Tx or after reduction in immunosuppression); requires ≥2 of:
    ① venular endothelialitis (predom. PT but, if severe, extends to zone 3 necrosis ± regenerat^n/ congest^n)
    ② mixed PT inflam^n (eos., lymphocytes [usu. T8], blasts, Mφ, plasma cells, PMN) ± interface if severe
    ③ BD epithelial vacuolation/regenerative atypia ± lymphocytes +/ PMN (! d/dg ascending cholangitis)
- ± Arterial endothelialitis/fibrinoid ⎫ indicate severe rejection and
- ± Zone 3 necroinflam^n not 2° to venular endothelialitis ⎬ ↑ risk of chronic rejection
- Atypical acute rejection has zone 3 necroinflam^n, congestion ± dropout but no sig. PT anomaly
- In early rejection PT inflam^n is predominantly lymphocytic, other cells (esp. eos.) ↑ with severity
- Immunosuppression Rx quickly removes endothelialitis and decreases eos. and mononuclear cells ∴ if Rx started prior to initial Bx look for BD epithelial damage and be wary of grading severity
- Grade (via the Banff Rejection Activity Index – see Bibliography and www.tpis.upmc.edu)
    ➤ ≥ moderate rejection (i.e. RAI ≥6 or infiltrate expanding most PTs) requires additional Rx
    ➤ only grade if rejection is the predominant cause of the abnormalities
    ➤ only grade if Bx is adequate: ≥5 PTs available, ≥2 H&E sections at each of ≥2 levels
- d/dg: recurrent viral hepatitis (esp. HCV): HCV chronic hepatitis occurs >4 months post Tx and is favoured by high serum HCV RNA, predominantly lymphocytic inflam^n, ↑ interface, ↑ fibrosis, sig. lobular activity (steatosis, sinusoidal dilatat^n, necroinflam^n, etc.) and lack of venular endothelialitis. If features are equivocal, consider simultaneous HCV and rejection.
- d/dg other causes of endothelialitis e.g. severe HCV (i.e. endothelialitis alone is not proof of reject^n)
- d/dg: other causes of zone 3 necroinflam^n: reperfusion injury, chronic reject^n, viral hepatitis, AIH, calcineurin inhibitors, vasc. occlusion (any vessel) and idiopathic chronic hepatitis

Chronic rejection
- Occurs ≥ 60 days (post Tx or reduction in immunosuppression)
- Medium and larger arteries: prolif and obliterative endarteritis with foam cells → ischaemia (*q.v.*)
- PT early changes:
    ➤ cytologically atypical BD atrophy (nuclei: irregular distribution, drop-out, ↑ size and hyperchromasia; cytoplasm: eosinophilia and syncytia) with ↓ inflam^y infiltrate as rejection progresses
    ➤ mild BD loss (≥50% of PTs have a BD) and mild PT artery loss (≥75% of PTs have an arteriole)

- PT late: marked BD loss (<50% of PTs have a BD), PT artery loss (<75% of PTs have one)
- Zone 3 early: necroinflam^n ($\pm$ pigment Mϕ, cell dropout and mild fibrosis)
- Zone 3 late: ballooning, cholestasis, severe fibrosis $\pm$ foam cells in sinusoids/smaller vessels
- d/dg recurrent chronic biliary disease (PBC/PSC): rejection has $\downarrow$inflam^n in PT, no florid BD granulomas, no ductular prolif^n or PT fibrous expansion. PSC/PBC usu. recur late ($\geq$ 1 year)
- d/dg: other causes of zone 3 necroinflammation or vanishing BD syndrome (*vide supra*)

Idiopathic chronic hepatitis
- Occurs >1 year post Tx, $\downarrow$ endothelialitis, $\downarrow$ BD damage, $\uparrow$ interface, $\uparrow$ zone 3 spotty necrosis
- Not obviously viral, AIH or drug-related. (? is a form of delayed acute reject^n)

Recurrent and De Novo Disease in the Graft
- Most look similar to the disease in the native liver but may be modified by immunosuppression
- PSC must be distinguished from chronic rejection (*vide supra*) and ischaemic SSC (which usu. presents <6 months post Tx unlike recurrent PSC)

Infection post Liver Tx:
- Opportunistic (e.g. CMV): look for mini-microabscesses (PMN aggregates) +/ granulomas
- Fibrosing Cholestatic Hepatitis (FCH) may occur in the 1st few months of recurrent HBV/HCV with widespread viral immunopositivity. It shows: ① PT ductular reaction with fine reticular fibrosis, ② florid hepatocyte ballooning but minimal inflam^n, ③ cholestasis.
- New/recurrent HBV: usual acute/chronic hepatitis ($\pm$ more aggressive) or steatosis +/ FCH
- New/recurrent HCV: usual histology ($\pm$ ductular reaction/confluent necrosis) or predominantly lobular apoptoses with mild PT changes or FCH

Other Post Tx Complications
- Vascular thromboses can lead to infarcts (usu. in the 1st 2 weeks post Tx) – ! exclude d/dg fungi
- SSC/biliary anastomotic obstruction (cholestasis + ductular reaction + PT oedema and PMN)
- Drug effects incl. cholestasis +/ zone 3 necrosis/fibrosis – d/dg acute rejection/ischaemia
- PTLD may present as a mass lesion or as PT infiltrates d/dg acute rejection infiltrate (which is EBV & HHV8 −ve)

Graft vs. Host Disease (GVHD)

- Due to foreign lymphocytes from BMTx, non-irradiated blood or solid organs (e.g. SI or liver Tx). Maternal lymphocytes can produce similar pathology in the immunocompromised fetus
- Clin.: changes occur in the liver (jaundice and cholestatic LFTs), skin & gut (and, if chronic, also in LN, muscle, lung, lacrimal & salivary glands)
- 1st month: lobular focal inflam^n, focal necrosis and Councilman bodies (d/dg viral hepatitis, CMV, etc. – but these usu. have less BD damage *cf.* GVHD)
- 2nd month: ➤ PT lymphocytes (T8 and CD56 +ve NK cells) – mild (*cf.* liver Tx reject^n)
  ➤ BD atypia (incl. stratificat^n, hyperchromasia, vacuolat^n and $\uparrow$ NCR), distort^n and loss
  ➤ parenchymal bilirubinostasis without biliary interface activity
- 3rd month: BD loss, PT fibrosis, endothelialitis ($\approx$ diagnostic if present, in the absence of other causes)
- Longer term: $\pm$ connective tissue plugs in veins, $\pm$ 2° biliary cirrhosis (clin./radiol. d/dg SSC)
- Other BMTx assoc^d disease: viral hepatitis, transfusion siderosis, VOD, NRH, infection, PTLD

Sepsis and Infections

Sepsis
- *Cholangiolitis lenta*: periportal cholangioles dilated with bile plugs with PMN in +/ around them
  ➤ without suppurative cholangitis = sepsis
  ➤ with suppurative cholangitis = ascending cholangitis (*q.v.*) or toxic shock syndrome
- Any bile plug may be a sign of sepsis, the larger the plug (from canaliculus to portal tract bile duct) the stronger the association
- Other features: steatosis, perivenular necrosis, microabscesses, clumps of cocci and PMN

Ascending Cholangitis (Suppurative Cholangitis)
- 2° to obstruct^n, bacteria, helminthes (*Clonorchis*, ascarid or schistosomal), opportunistic infect^n, etc.
- Affects the smaller (portal tract) bile ducts; large ducts may look normal

- More PMN (*cf.* biliary irritation alone) and PMN aggregates within BD walls and lumens
- ± Bacterial colonies ± PT abscesses ± portal pyelephlebitis/thrombosis ± cholangiolitis lenta
- ± Lobular changes: PMN in sinusoids; parenchymal necrosis

Some Specific Causative Organisms

Salmonella (Typhoid)
- Sinusoid lymphocytosis,[10] Kupffer cell hyperplasia, erythrophagocytosis
- Granulomas that may necrotise (but no Langhans giant cells)
- Microvesicular steatosis

Brucella
- Kupffer cell hyperplasia ± focal hepatocyte necrosis
- Granulomas (anything from microgranulomas to tuberculoid type)

Coxiella burnetii (Q-Fever)
- Fibrin-ring granuloma (small, PMN, Mϕ, ring of fibrin) are typical but non-specific (see 'Drugs')
- Non-specific granulomas, foci of necrosis, steatosis, inflam^n and fibrosis ± cirrhosis

Listeria
- Viral hepatitis-like
- Microabscesses with Gram +ve rods
- Granulomas

Francisella tularensis (Tularaemia)
- Granulomas may be indistinguishable from TB or sarcoid

Bartonella
- Cat scratch granuloma i.e. irregular shape with periph palisaded Mϕ and central PMN/necrosis
- *Bacillary peliosis hepatis* is the equivalent to bacillary angiomatosis (see p. 319) and not the bland blood filled cystic dilatations of ordinary *peliosis hepatis* (this may also occur with infections, be idiopathic or be assoc^d with drugs, cachexia, Tx (liver/renal), asphyxia and tumours)

HIV (and AIDS)
- May get a mild lobular hepatitis upon seroconversion ± sinusoidal lymphocytosis (d/dg EBV)
- Children may show a giant cell hepatitis or a GVHD-like picture with lobular and PT lymphocytes
- Hepatocyte and Kupffer cell Fe (± EMH) is usu. 2° to transfusions/haemolysis
- Reaction to opportunists may be suppressed and microbes may roam free within the sinusoids ∴ should always stain for opportunists (DPAS, ZN ± Grocott/CMV immuno)
- *Peliosis hepatis* (ordinary and bacillary types)
- Tumours: HCC (due to HCV), 1° DLBCL, 2° HL, KS (d/dg bacillary angiomatosis/peliosis), etc.
- *Vide supra* for association with HBV/HCV and cholangiopathy; *vide infra* for drug reactions

Other viruses (EBV, CMV, etc.)
See 'Acute Hepatitis' (p. 158) and 'Infection post Liver Tx', (p. 166).

Drugs/Iatrogenic

Generalities (with examples)
- Clin.: *usu.* subside on removing the drug (or persist if taken for >6 months) & relapse if restarted
- Eosinophils – but ! these may be present in small Nõs in other things e.g. AIH, HCV, etc.
- Zone 3 cholestasis alone ['bland cholestasis'] *(anabolic steroids, oral contraceptives,* [pregnancy])
- Cholestatic hepatitis [zone 3 bile, lobular inflam^n, ± eos] *(phenothiazines, Augmentin®, erythromycin)*
- Cholestatic acute hepatitis [≈ d/dg HAV-type with necrosis] *(halothane, isoniazid)*
- Ascending cholangitis *(phenothiazines, allopurinol)*
- Vanishing bile ducts ± PBC-like *(flucloxacillin, paraquat, ibuprofen, erythromycin, phenothiazines)*
- SSC (ischaemia, post-op/post liver Tx, intra-arterial *floxuridine*)
- Granulomas esp. if atypical, of NST (d/dg idiopathic or 2° to lymphoma) or accompanied by eos. Some specific types are linked to drugs (e.g. fibrin-ring granuloma with *allopurinol* d/dg Q-fever, HL, viruses, CTD, leishmaniasis, Toxoplasma, etc. and lipogranulomas *with oral mineral oils – usu. para central venules* cf. d/dg steatohepatitic ones)
- Chronic hepatitis *(α-methyldopa, zidovudine-like anti-retrovirals, isoniazid, nitrofurantoin, aspirin)*
- AIH-like, type 1 (ANA +ve, ASMA −ve) *(minocycline, α-methyldopa)*

---

[10] d/dg of lymphocytes in dilated sinusoids include: typhoid, EBV (infectious mononucleosis), HCV, HIV, malaria (tropical splenomegaly syndrome) and CLL.

- Macrovesicular steatosis *(OH, cortisone, oestrogens, methotrexate)*
- Microvesicular steatosis *(i.v. tetracyclines)*
- Mixed steatosis (microvesicular and macrovesicular) ± giant mitochondria (2° to mitochondrial damage due to *OH, valproate*, antivirals e.g. *zidovudine and* Reye's syndrome initiated by *salicylates)*
- NASH *(TPN, oestrogens & tamoxifen, nifedipine, didanozine, amiodarone, cortisone)*
- Fibrosis/cirrhosis *(OH, vitamin A, methotrexate)*
- Zone 1 necrosis [d/dg PET] *(cocaine, phosphorus, ferric sulphate, aflatoxin & other toxins)*
- Zone 2 necrosis [d/dg VHF] *(frusemide)*
- Zone 3 necrosis [coagulative necrosis ± ductular prolif^n] *(cocaine, paracetamol – aggravated by OH, CCl$_4$)*
- Veno-occlusive disease *(chemo/radioRx, bush teas, OH* may cause veno-occlusion)
- Hepatic vein thrombosis → Budd-Chiari (prolonged *progesterone* e.g. *OCP*, pregnancy)
- *Peliosis hepatis (azathioprine, tamoxifen)*
- Siderosis *(ribavirin* causes haemolysis hepatocyte and Kupffer cell Fe, *OH* may cause haemolysis)
- Lamellar inclusion phospholipidosis *(co-trimoxazole, amiodarone)*
- Neoplasia *(oestrogens, androgens, vinyl chloride monomer, aflatoxin, thorotrast, post-Tx/immuno-suppression)*

Methotrexate
- Damage ∝ dose, interval, cumulative dose, OH, obesity, diabetes, reason for Rx (psoriasis > RhA)
- Nuclear hyperchromasia, glycogenation and anisonucleosis
- Steatosis, ballooning, necrosis
- Fibrosis → micronodular cirrhosis (cirrhosis is rare with cumulative dose <1.5g)
- PT show a mixed infiltrate (lymphocytes, Mφ, PMN)
- Grading is via the classification of Roenigk *et al.*, 1982 – see table 12.2

TABLE 12.2   Grading methotrexate liver damage

Grade	Steatosis	Nuclear variability	Liver cell necrosis	Portal inflam^n	Fibrosis
I	none/mild	mild	none	mild	none
II	moderate/severe	moderate/severe	moderate/severe	moderate/severe	none or mild PT expansion without septa or limiting plate disruption
IIIa	any	any	any	any	mild with septa
IIIb	any	any	any	any	moderate to severe with septa
IV	any	any	any	any	cirrhosis

Vascular Disorders

General Features of Ischaemia
- Zone 3 accentuated changes ± patchy/sharp demarcation depending on cause
- Cholestasis, ballooning, hepatocyte atrophy or dropout of hepatocyte clusters
- If more chronic: perivenular and pericellular fibrosis ± cirrhosis (! d/dg alcohol)
- If severe and acute: infarction (coagulative ± haemorrhagic necrosis)

Portal Vein Thrombosis
- Large portal vein (Virchow's triad: alterat^n in endothelium/flow/coagulat^n) e.g. MPD, sepsis, tumour
- Small portal vein: local PT disease (e.g. cirrhosis, schistosomiasis, hepatitis, PBC, PSC, vasculitis, sarcoid)
- May be 2° to systemic venous HT (e.g. Budd-Chiari syndrome/VOD, CCF)
- May be idiopathic (small vein obliteration is particularly marked)
- Veins: large – thromboses/recanalisation; small – obliterat^n/dilatat^n (to give 'ectopic' PT veins)
- Acute thrombosis → (pseudo)infarct of Zahn (= a wedge of congest^n & atrophy) ± ↑ apoptoses
- Other: partial atrophy of lobe, partial nodular transformation, NRH or no histological abnormality
- If portal vein thrombosis extends to occlude splenic vein ostium → venous bowel infarction

Portal Hypertension
- Many causes or idiopathic, Bx may be normal or show variable anomalies:
- Perisinusoidal sclerosis, dilated ('ectopic') PT veins or fibrotic PT with small, inconspicuous veins
- Incomplete septal cirrhosis +/ NRH
- ↑ Visibility and dilatation of PT lymphatics

Veno-Occlusive Disease (VOD)
- Minor hepatic veins (i.e. <1mm $\varnothing$ and commonly $<\frac{1}{2}$mm $\varnothing$)
- Plant extracts/bush teas, chemo/radioRx, azathioprine, immune$\downarrow$/AIDS, heroin, arsenicals, etc.
- Youths, acute (pain, jaundice, ascites), chronic (insidious, cirrhosis-like)
- Subintimal oedema/haemorrhage → heal with concentric fibrosis and obliteration/multilumena
- Perisinusoidal fibrosis ± cholestasis (the latter esp. in chemo/radioRx-induced VOD)
- Perivenular congestion (± severe) → regenerative nodules → venocentric[11] cirrhosis (spared PTs)
- ± Bile ductular proliferation
- d/dg VOD-like change in Budd-Chiari, hepatic haemangioendothelioma and constrictive pericarditis

Budd-Chiari Syndrome
- Major hepatic vein thrombosis (due to Virchow's triad, CIBD, CTD, coeliac, etc.)/obstruct^n at the level of the IVC (! exclude d/dg constrictive pericarditis); ± 2° portal vein thrombosis (varices and cirrhosis)
- Dilatat^n of central veins and sinusoids, RBC extravasat^n and variable necrosis
- ± Regenerative nodules (may be FNH-like)
- ± Bile ductular proliferation
- ± Thrombosis of smaller veins (VOD-like) → fibrosis → venocentric cirrhosis with dilated PT veins
- 2° Portal vein thrombosis → venoportal cirrhosis and parenchymal extinct^n with obliterated PT veins
- Patchy distribution and caudate may be spared/hyperplastic (because its veins drain directly into the IVC)
- Bx (bilateral) to guide therapy (fibrosis → Tx; necrosis → shunt) and monitor its success

Tumours and Nodules

Incomplete Septal Cirrhosis
- Fibrous septa are very thin (not obvious on H&E) and often broken/incomplete/blind ended
- Nodules are vague and regenerative with PTs and central veins (but unevenly spaced w.r.t. each other)
- Inflammation/necrosis is sparse or absent; ± sinusoidal dilatation

Nodular Regenerative Hyperplasia (NRH)
- F = M, $\frac{1}{3}$ die a liver death, assoc^d with autoimmune/vascular disease, MPD, drugs, portal HT
- Nodules 1mm to few cm in $\varnothing$ (clin. d/dg cirrhosis/mets)
- Hyperplastic nodules (± periportal) } not obvious until retic is done, but the presence of two
- Internodular atrophy and congest^n } populations of cells (large and small) is suggestive
- ± Cholestatic rosettes
- d/dg cirrhosis or incomplete septal cirrhosis: NRH shows a paucity of fibrosis – but ! a cirrhotic nodule may contain several NRH-like nodules within it
- CPC is important as focal NRH-like change may occur in HCC, cirrhosis or in pre-cirrhotic PBC

Focal Nodular Hyperplasia (FNH, 'mixed hamartoma of childhood')
- F≫M, vascular malformations, age: 20^s/30^s; incidental finding/mass
- Macro: subcapsular, well-circ., <5cm $\varnothing$, fibrous septa from stellate scar(s) – *no bile stains*
- Multinodular ('focal cirrhosis'), hyperplastic hepatocyte cords <3 cells thick
- Septa contain: bile ductules (± surrounding cholate stasis ± Mallory hyaline), arteries, inflam^n
- Central scar contains thick-walled vessels (or multiple and dilated channels in telangiectatic FNH)
- Lobules: liver cells like HCA with Kupffer cells, ± cholestasis but no mitoses/pleomorphism
- Multiple FNH: assoc^d with vascular anomalies in other organs and brain tumours
- d/dg cirrhosis, BD obstruction: use CPC and the radiological information of a discrete mass
- d/dg haemangioma/peliosis *vs.* the telangiectatic variant of FNH
- d/dg MRN: surrounding liver is usu. normal in FNH
- d/dg HCA (*vide infra*) ! *NB*: bile ductular structures may be hard to find in some FNH

Hepatocellular Adenoma (HCA)
- F>M, age 20^s/30^s, acute abdomen (± haemorrhage/rupture)/mass/incidental; ≈ all cases have a source of hepatic stimulation: OCP, anabolic androgens, DM, childhood IEM (also have ↑ risk of HCC)

---

[11] i.e. 'reversed lobulation' – regeneration of periportal hepatocytes → parenchymatous nodule with a PT at the centre rather than a central vein

- Subcapsular ± pedunculated, right lobe, solitary (except androgenic/metabolic), well-circ., a few cm to >10cm ⌀, variegate cut surface (haemorrhage, infarct, bile) ± central fibrosis (! d/dg FNH)
- Cytology: ➢ normal sized hepatocytes (± pigments, fat, glycogen, α_1AT bodies)
  - ➢ ± fat (d/dg focal fatty change, but this mass lesion has normal architecture)
  - ➢ inconspicuous nucleoli
  - ➢ no nuclear vacuoles
  - ➢ ± multi-(bland)nucleate forms
  - ➢ Kupffer cells present but fewer than in normal liver
- Arch.: cords (<3 cells thick), rosettes with bile but *no BDs or PTs* (except for trapped normal PTs)
- Mitoses are rare and vascular/capsular invasion is *absent*
- Androgenic ones may show cytol. atypia and pseudogland formation (with ↓NCR) or HCC-like foci and are diagnosed as 'atypical adenoma' or 'hepatocellular neoplasia of uncertain malignant potential'
- Multiple HCA: >10 tumours, older, no steroid association, d/dg NRH (different clinical background)
- Degenerative changes: ➢ peliosis/haemorrhage (inside tumour or in adjacent liver)
  - ➢ epithelioid granulomas
  - ➢ extramedullary haemopoiesis
  - ➢ necrosis and infarction → fibrous scars: d/dg FNH (but FNH septa contain BDs); d/dg fibrolamellar HCC (different cytology)
- d/dg MRN: in HCA the surrounding liver is ≈ normal and there is no ductular proliferation
- d/dg FNH: even spacing of arteries and lack of BD favour HCA
- d/dg HCC – see Table 12.3:

TABLE 12.3 Adenoma or carcinoma?

Feature	HCC	HCA
Plate thickness	>3 cells	<3 cells
Invasion (vasc./capsular)	may be present	absent
Reticulin	weak or absent	good staining (except infarcts)
Kupffer cells	sparse or absent	present
Mallory hyaline	often present & may be clustered	rare
Mitoses	±	rare
Immuno (typical)	AFP +ve, CD34 shows diffuse & continuous +vity in sinusoids	AFP −ve, CD34 is focal

Tyrosinaemia
- Cholestasis, cholestatic rosettes, siderosis
- Fibrosis (pericellular, PT and cirrhosis), fatty nodules
- MRN, liver cell dysplasia (large cell and small cell), dysplastic nodules, HCC
- d/dg HCC *vs.* large MRN can be problematic

Liver Cell Dysplasia

General definitions
- Dysplasia = altered prolif^n/genetics that *may* manifest abnormal histology in a cluster/nodule of cells
- Single cells or small groups with these features are not considered diagnostic of dysplasia
- If the cluster is <1mm ⌀ = *dysplastic focus* (else = *dysplastic nodule* and this is usu. in a background of cirrhosis)
- Associations: cirrhosis, HBV, HCV, HCC, α_1AT↓ and tyrosinaemia
- Dysplastic nodules may be low grade (≈ MRN) or high grade (≈ AAN) or NOS if insufficient tissue/features are present on Bx to grade reliably (HCC cannot be excluded on Bx – even with low grade)

Large cell dysplasia (= large cell change)
- No ↑ prolif^n (some demonstrate aneuploidy *cf.* normal polyploidy) and occurs in 1% of normals
- Large cells (upto 4 × normal) with large nuclei (≈ normal NCR) and prom nucleoli ± multinucleation
- ± Hyperchromasia with patchy chromatin clearing, abnormal nuclear shapes and multiple nucleoli

Small cell dysplasia (= small cell change)
- ↑ Proliferative activity (? pre-cancerous)
- Smaller, amphophilic cells with ↑NCR form irregular crowded trabeculae ± multinucleation

Low grade dysplastic nodule
- ≈ Normal hepatocytes in plates ≤2 cells thick (discounting tangential sections)

- ± Mallory hyaline, small cell/large cell dysplastic foci, displacement of nuclei towards sinusoids
- d/dg NRH: no central PT and no peripheral compressed rim

High grade dysplastic nodule
- As for low grade plus any focus showing any of: Fe resistance, rare mitoses, pseudoglands, nuclear anomalies ($\uparrow$ NCR, irregular membrane, hyperchromasia), basophilic cytoplasm, plates >2 cells thick
- d/dg HCC: no invasion or other, more subjective, features favouring HCC (i.e. $\uparrow$ mitoses, $\downarrow$ retic, marked atypia, clustering of Mallory bodies, floating trabeculae, lack of PTs, $\uparrow$ non-PT arteries)

Macro-Regenerative Nodule, Atypical Adenomatous Nodule (MRN/AAN)
- Def[n]: a nodule of $\geq$ 0.5 cm $\varnothing$ (some say $\geq$ 0.8 cm) in a background of cirrhosis/chronic liver disease
- Contains PTs ($\pm$ ductular reaction) but no stellate scar with septa and not AFP +ve
- $\pm$ Infarction with regenerative mitoses (mitoses should not be present in other circumstances)
- Large hepatocytes with mostly low NCR and plates $\leq$2 cells thick; no tumour necrosis
- AAN: this is an MRN with dysplastic areas ('nodule within nodule') or wholly dysplastic showing:
  - cells are usu. smaller and show liver cell dysplasia (*q.v.*)
  - trabeculae may be 2 or 3 cells thick $\pm$ pseudoglandular acini but PTs are still present
  - different H&E/Perls characteristics *cf.* rest of liver $\pm$ AFP +vity
- Clustering of Mallory bodies and clearing of haemosiderin suggests 'early HCC' (to these some add a 'nodule within nodule' pattern, cytoplasmic basophilia and the features mentioned for well diff HCC *q.v.*) – the term 'early HCC' is no longer recommended, consider 'small HCC' defined as <2cm $\varnothing$
- d/dg HCA/FNH (see those entities above)

Mesenchymal Hamartoma
- Myxoid stroma with PMN and blood vessels
- Irregular/branching BD-like structures that may be lined by bland cuboidal epithelium or be unlined
- Admixed areas of normal hepatocytes (not seen within d/dg bile duct adenoma – *q.v.*)

Hepatocellular Carcinoma (HCC)
- Clin: cirrhosis/hepatitis/IEM, pain/mass, $\pm$ $\uparrow$ AFP (for details and d/dg, see p. 19)
- Macro:
  - cut surface: haemorrhage, necrosis, bile staining, [and background liver disease]
  - border: expanding, infiltrating, multifocal
  - invasion: capsule, BD, veins (portal, hepatic, IVC)
  - record: size, nõ. of nodules, capsule ($\pm$), capsular invas[n] ($\pm$), venous invas[n] ($\pm$)
- Background liver usu. shows cirrhosis/chronic hepatitis,
- Cytology: polygonal cells, well-defined membrane, $\uparrow$NCR, round/irregular/hyperchromatic nuclei $\pm$ nuclear pseudoinclusions $\pm$ eosinophilic cytoplasmic inclusions
- Cytological variants: giant/clear/spindle/oncocytoid fibrolamellar
- Patterns: **p**elioid, **c**lear cell, **s**olid/sclerosing(scirrhous)[12], **t**rabecular (trabeculae >3 cells thick, lined by endothelium $\pm$ widely separated or isolated – 'floating'), **a**cinar[13] (may contain cell debris or be thyroidal with fibrin instead of colloid), **g**iant cell, **s**pindle cell (mets are more common), fibrolamellar, HCC with lymphoid stroma (T8-rich, plasma cells, follicles and 'piecemeal necrosis'-like reaction – good prognosis) and regressing HCC
- Sinusoids: CD34 is uniformly +ve $\pm$ perisinusoidal fibrosis (capillarisation), Kupffer cells $\downarrow$/lost
- Grading:
  - very well diff: PT or vasc. invasion by near normal hepatocytes
  - well diff: mitoses <5/10 hpf, plates $\leq$3 cells thick, $\pm$ good retic staining
  - mod. diff: mitoses >5/10 hpf, plates >3 cells thick, poor retic staining
- For small, well diff HCC, good diagnostic criteria are lacking; features suggesting HCC include:
  - $\uparrow$cellularity (nuclei per mm^2) of $\geq$2x the surrounding non-neoplastic cirrhotic liver
  - clear cell change (due to glycogen, water or lipid)
  - diffuse and uniform CD34 staining of sinusoidal endothelium
  - portal tract or vascular invasion
- Fibrolamellar:
  - younger, no cirrhotic background ($\therefore$ better prog. *cf.* conventional HCC with cirrhosis)

---

[12] sclerosing HCC are considered to be due to compression or chemo/radioRx artefact and not a specific subtype – more typical HCC should be present elsewhere otherwise the diagnosis should be reconsidered

[13] the preferred term is pseudoglandular in the liver (so as not to confuse with the liver acinus)

> calcification and pale bodies (ground glass fibrinogen *cf.* d/dg IIBsAg)
> lamellar fibrosis
> large oncocytic cells, vesicular nucleus and prominent nucleolus
> immuno: CK7 and CK19 +ve (*cf.* usual type HCC which are mostly −ve)

Features of hepatocellular differentiation

- pCEA (and CD10) +ve canaliculi are pathognomonic of hepatocellular differentiation in a tumour
- Intracellular bile is pathognomonic of hepatocellular differentiation in a tumour
- Mallory hyaline (+ve for ubiquitin, CK & p62) is nearly pathognomonic of hepatocellular differentiation
- Cu/CuBP (rhodanine/Shikata orcein +ve) are nearly pathognomonic of hepatocellular differentiation
- DPAS +ve globules (usu. α_1AT, albumin or fibrinogen) and AFP are suggestive but not specific
- Hep Par 1 is useful but not specific (many gastric and some cholangioCA are +ve)
- ISH for albumin: +vity occurs in cells with hepatic/hepatoid differentiation – highly specific

d/dg cholangiocarcinoma

- Mucin is −ve in pure HCC (but can be +ve in mixed HCC-cholangioCA)
- Features of hepatocellular differentiation are usu. −ve in cholangioCA (esp. if 'pathognomonic' – *vide supra*)
- MOC-31, mCEA, amylase, CK7 and CK19 are +ve in cholangiocarcinoma but −ve in HCC (! some pseudoglands in HCC may show CK7 +vity but not usu. CK19 unless fibrolamellar variant)
- Trabeculae are separated by desmoplastic stroma in cholangiocarcinoma (*cf.* sinusoids in HCC)
- EM: glandular features in cholangiocarcinoma

Other differentials

- d/dg NE tumour: NE tumour has smaller cells, inconspicuous nucleoli and prominent vascularity
- d/dg clear cell HCC *vs.* RCC: cytoplasmic +vity for TTF-1 favours HCC (see table 19.1 p. 276)
- d/dg HCA, MRN & AAN: (see respective sections above)
- d/dg metastasis from 1° hepatoid carcinoma of stomach, lung or ovary

Combined Hepatocellular and Cholangiocarcinoma
- There must be both proper glands with mucin and features of hepatocellular differentiation (*vide supra*) not based on immuno alone (if just ambiguous immuno = adenocarcinoma NOS)
- May be collision-type (most common), admixed or cells of dual differentiation (intermediate cells ± c-kit +ve)
- Prog. is worse than with either HCC or cholangiocarcinoma

Bile Duct Adenoma (Peribiliary Gland Hamartoma) and Bile Duct Adenofibroma
- Well-circ., para-PT, subcapsular, many small ducts/ductules in mature fibrous stroma, no bile plugs
- Glands have rounded edges, bland cytology and no mitoses or vascular invasion *cf.* d/dg adenoCA
- Admixed inflam^y cells (lymphocytes, PMN) ± follicles at periphery, ± PTs incorporated at periphery
- ± Focal mucinous or NE differentiation (d/dg NET), α_1AT globules or, rarely, clear cells (d/dg CCC)
- Adenofibroma has tubular, branching and cystic spaces ± bile ± apocrine metaplasia ($\approx$ FA of breast)
- d/dg metastatic adenoCA: as above; CA may also show the surrounding mass effect triad of ① PT oedema with polymorphs, ② atypical bile ductular prolif^n, ③ focal sinusoidal dilatation

Mucinous Cystic Lesions (Biliary Cystic Lesions)
- Simple cysts are usu. unilocular and perihilar with simple bland epithelium
- Benign cystadenoma is usu. multilocular [may be large] with simple bland epithelium ± small papillae
- Borderline cystadenoma/CIS has polyps or solid areas with cytol. atypia, mitoses, stratification
- Cystadenocarcinoma: must show stromal invasion by definition (∴ need extensive sampling to exclude it) – d/dg cholangiocarcinoma *ex* cystic BD malformation (more aggressive)
- Generally: stroma may be fibrous or (in women) ovarian-like ± focal cyst ulceration/Mϕ response

Dysplasia in the Gallbladder and Large Extrahepatic Bile Ducts
- Nuclear changes: enlargement (↑with NCR), broadening and hyperchromasia
- Loss of polarity ± some cells rising to the surface ± intestinal metaplasia
- d/dg reactive: > pseudostratification and nuclear elongat^n without the above are considered reactive in biliary epithelium (*cf.* pancreatic ducts where such changes are considered mild dysplasia)

> ➤ admixed pencil cells favour reactive over dysplasia
> ➤ adjacent nuclear inflam^{n}/ulcerat^{n} favour reactive esp. if not much hyperchromasia
> ➤ p53 +vity (–vity means nothing), abrupt transition and mitoses favour dysplasia

Cholangiocarcinoma
- Macro: intrahepatic (peripheral or hilar) and extrahepatic (periampullary CA being the most distal)[14]
- Growth patterns: ① mass forming (radial mass with well-defined border), ② periductal infiltration and ③ intraductal (= CIS – often multifocal, papillary ± stalk invasion or mucinous; dysplasia may extend into peribiliary glands ! d/dg periductal infiltration); types① and ② may occur together
- Usu. scirrhous adenoCA (mucin +ve) or other (e.g. mucinous, signet ring, ASC, SCC, sarcomatoid)
- Arch. is usu. tubulopapillary or cords or small narrow ductules (i.e. 'cholangiocellular' type)
- Adjacent major bile duct hyperplasia/dysplasia/CIS (! d/dg Pagetoid spread of metastatic carcinoma)
- Peribiliary glands may show adenomatoid hyperplasia ± CIS (! d/dg invasive carcinoma)
- Immuno: +ve for cytoplasmic mCEA, CA-19.9, CK7, CK19, amylase
- d/dg HCC: *vide supra*, ! hepatocyte bile may be incorporated into the periphery of cholangioCA
- d/dg metastatic adenocarcinoma – this may be impossible to differentiate:
    > ➤ clin. associat^{n}s of cholangioCA (PSC, CIBD, liver fluke, BD malformat^{n}s, Hx of thorotrast, etc.)
    > ➤ multifocality in the liver, peritoneal carcinomatosis and ↑ serum CEA occur in both cholangioCA and some mets – so these features are not helpful
    > ➤ presence of a likely 1° elsewhere – esp. if it is of a type that has characteristic immuno
    > ➤ Hep Par 1 +vity is strong evidence against cholangiocarcinoma
    > ➤ +vity for both CK7 and CK19 favour cholangioCA but are not absolute (see pp. 14–15)
    > ➤ perineural invasion or CIS (! not d/dg Pagetoid spread) favour cholangiocarcinoma
- d/dg benign malformation/fibrous stricture e.g. on FS – features that favour malignancy incl.:
    > ➤ ↑ nuclear size, marcronucleoli and pleom. (may not help if very well diff), intracytoplasmic lumena
    > ➤ cribriform glands, sharp/jagged gland profiles (! some glands of vMC may be angulated)
    > ➤ cellular debris in the lumen of glands
    > ➤ perineural or vascular invasion (or LN mets – esp. useful for lower BD tumours with much desmoplastic stroma and sparse malignant cells ∴ consider requesting a local LN sample if FS)
    > ➤ cytoplasmic mCEA in cholangiocarcinoma (*cf.* lumenal surface staining in benign epithelium)
    > ➤ nuclear p53 +vity (using heat-based antigen retrieval)
- d/dg benign intraductal papilloma *vs.* intraductal cholangioCA: papilloma has low grade cytology and lacks mitoses/stalk invasion (cholangiocarcinoma may also lack stalk invasion)
- d/dg biliary papillomatosis: a synonym for papillary intraductal cholangioCA of the extrahepatic BDs
- d/dg adenoma of the extrahepatic BDs *vs.* intraductal cholangioCA: adenomas have similar histology to those found elsewhere in the GIT but the lining may be of biliary, pyloric or intestinal epithelium

Other Tumours/Tumour-like Lesions of the Biliary Tree
- Serous cystadenoma: as for pancreatic (not ovarian) counterpart – see p. 177
- Granular cell tumour, traumatic neuroma, adenomyoma (! d/dg invasive adenoCA), botryoid RMS
- Almost anything else (e.g. melanoma, epithelioid haemangioendothelioma, etc.) can occur but is rare
- Lymphomas may be assoc^{d} with a degree of fibrosis incl. P-P linking

Gallbladder

Acute Cholecystitis
- An ischaemic dilatation that may be calculous or acalculous (e.g. *Salmonella*) ± CTD vasculitis
- Haemorrhage, oedema, fibrosis, myofibroblasts ± necrosis (gangrene) of the wall ± mucosal ulcerat^{n}

---

[14] some authors do not use 'cholangioCA' for extrahepatic BD tumours (which include gall bladder CA). Carcinoma of the ampulla of Vater are of biliary or intestinal histol. (some call only the former 'periampullary')

- ± Prior chronic cholecystitis may be superimposed
- Any PMN are usu. 2° to necrosis/ulcerat^n/infection and are not essential for the diagnosis

Effects of Salmonella on the Gallbladder
- None (normal histology)
- Carcinoma
- Mucosal lymphoid polyps +/ follicular cholecystitis
- Acute acalculous cholecystitis (*vide supra*)

Polyps
- Adenomyoma usu. occurs at the fundus and glands may surround nerves (! pseudo neural invasion)
- Adenomatous: may be tubular, papillary (usu. villous) or tubulopapillary with a range of dysplasia and be of pyloric, intestinal (≈ colonic adenomas) or biliary cytological type
- Low grade pyloric tubular adenomas are distinguished from metaplastic polyp by size >5mm
- Biliary types are rare and have ≈ normal biliary epithelium with ↑ apical mucin – d/dg pap. hyperplasia in chronic cholecystitis or cholesterol polyp (stroma filled with foamy Mφ)
- Others: metaplastic (e.g. pseudopyloric), heterotopic, lymphoid, cholesterol and inflam^y pseudotumour

Flat Dysplasia
- See pp. 172–173 for features: if high grade/CIS this may indicate further Rx post cholecystectomy
- More likely to be assoc^d with invasive CA (*cf.* adenomas) ∴ take more blocks if dysplasia is found
- d/dg colonisation of Luschka ducts or Rokitansky-Aschoff sinuses *vs.* invasive carcinoma

Carcinoma
- Associations: old age and gallstones; most occur in the fundus, then body
- Spread: direct (e.g. to liver), LN (cystic duct ± beyond), transcoelomic, blood vasc. → distant mets
- Usu. adenocarcinoma (pancreatic ductal-like but with less cellular mucin, even if well diff)
- Other types of adenoCA: intestinal, colonic, cribriform, mucinous, papillary
- Other types of carcinoma: ASC, carcinosarcoma, SCC, CCC, spindle cell, giant cell, SmCC
- Well-diff variant: papillary carcinoma (has a predom. intralumenal exophytic growth + invasion)
- Poorly diff variants: ➤ signet ring
                          ➤ spindle cell
                          ➤ giant cell (pleomorphic giant cells constitute the bulk of the tumour)
                          ➤ small cell undiff: focal mucin production, no NE markers
                          ➤ SmCC: as for pulm. SmCC, may be combined with adenoCA/carcinoid

Neuroendocrine Neoplasia
- Paraganglioma, carcinoid and SmCC
- Features are as for these tumours elsewhere (see pp. 93–94, pp. 139–140 and p. 279)

Exocrine Pancreas

Normal Histology
- The sphincter of Oddi is comprised of longitudinal and circular muscle coats of the main (Wirsung) pancreatic duct and common bile duct that thicken as they enter the duodenum. The bile duct component (= *sphincter choledochus*) is usu. more prominent than the Wirsung duct component
- Features near the ampulla of Vater:
  - ➤ all main ducts have valves of Santorini (long bland papillary folds)
  - ➤ accessory ducts insinuate through the duodenal musculature – d/dg adenocarcinoma (esp. on FS): these ducts form lobules encased in definitely formed fibrous tissue and lack cytological atypia
- Pancreatic ducts have a smooth (non-papillary) lining and an adventitial sheath of bland fibrous tissue which is esp. prominent in extralobular and larger ducts (the latter having periductal glands)
- Pancreatic acini differ from salivary acini in that they have eosinophilic apical cytoplasm, basophilic basal cytoplasm and lack myoepithelial cells. They contain central pale centroacinar cells
- *Pancreas divisum*: the Wirsung and Santorini duct systems do not fuse. They may drain separately into the major and minor duodenal papillae.

Acute (Haemorrhagic) Pancreatitis
- Ductal damage   ➢ alcohol, gallstones/other obstruction
                   ➢ periductal necrosis, acute inflam^n ± haemorrhage
- Vascular insufficiency   ➢ shock/dehydration/hypothermia
                            ➢ perilobular necrosis

Secondary changes occurring in either type
- Autodigestion → thromboses → infarction and pan-lobular necrosis, haemorrhage
- Surrounding fat necrosis ± chemical (± bacterial) peritonitis
- Abscess/pseudocyst formation

Autoimmune Pancreatitis (= Lymphoplasmacytic Sclerosing Pancreatitis)
- Clin: ↑ serum IgG4 (≫70 mg/dl), low CBD stricture + pancreatic mass (d/dg carcinoma); Rx − steroids
- Periductal inflam^n (lymphocytes, plasma cells ± eos., peripheral lymphoid follicles) with epithelial preservation, fibrosis, obliterative phlebitis with arteriolar preservation, loss of exocrine parenchyma, no fat necrosis
- Multi-organ involvement (salivary glands, GIT, liver, gallbladder, etc.) – ? related to multifocal fibrosclerosis
- Immuno: plasma cells +ve for IgG4 (>10 per hpf counting 10 hpf) in all affected organs

Chronic Pancreatitis
- Histology ∝ cause, stage of evolution and degree of atrophy and may get these changes adjacent to CA
- Early changes of perilobular fibrosis ± chronic inflam^n may cause enhanced lobulation
- Later there is fibrosis within (and atrophy of) acini with residual ducts in lobular configuration (i.e. centrally there are larger, possibly branched, ducts with peripheral smaller ones) – albeit distorted.
- Duct lumena may contain Ca^{2+}/protein plugs with some aetiologies (! not d/dg necrotic cell debris)
- Irregular duct ectasia ('retention cysts') ± mucinous metaplasia/hyperplasia/dysplasia (*vide infra*)
- Mucinous (pyloric) metaplasia can occur which may not retain lobular arch. but has benign cytology (with flattened basal nuclei); if there are mild anomalies of pseudostratification, uniform nuclear enlargement and distinct (but not macro) nucleoli = *mucinous hyperplasia*; if it also shows focal loss of polarity, anisonucleosis ± micropapillae = atypical hyperplasia; if extensive loss of polarity/arch./cytol. atypia (chromatin ± macronucleoli) ± ↑ mitoses = *dysplasia* (= CIS if severe)
- Other metaplasias include multilayered ('squamous'), goblet cell, acinar and oncocytic
- Advanced atrophy affects ducts as well as acini and results in changes that can mimic carcinoma incl.:
  - ➢ simulation of partial lumena in atrophic ducts
  - ➢ islet cell aggregation (d/dg NET *vide infra*)
  - ➢ islets extending into fat (d/dg extrapancreatic invasion) ⎫ d/dg adenoCA but these cells
  - ➢ ductuloinsular complexes (endocrine cells apposed to ducts) ⎬ are NE, not glandular, and do
  - ➢ diffuse islets (cords/trabeculae) infiltrating around nerves ⎭ not have malignant cytology
- d/dg adenoCA (*vide infra*): cytology is important, lack of desmoplasia is no help as some CA are not desmoplastic, presence of a two-duct-type (one benign, one atypical) helps, CEA is −ve in benign ducts, perineural invasion/sharply angulated ducts (esp. if infiltrating muscle/fat) favour malignancy

Other Non-Neoplastic Lesions
- Mucinous cyst (developmental/retention)
- Inflammatory pseudotumour (see p. 310)
- Pancreatic pseudocyst: non-epithelial fibroinflammatory and granulation tissue lining ± haemorrhagic/necrotic contents. d/dg cystic epithelial tumour or GIST (∴ may get a FS)
- Lymphoepithelial cyst/lymphoid hyperplasia

Ductal Mucinous Metaplasia, Hyperplasia, PanIN, Dysplasia and CIS
- *Mucinous metaplasia* (pyloric type) has tall apical mucin and bland flat basal nuclei (= PanIN 1A)
- *Hyperplasia* has mild anomalies of pseudostratification, uniform nuclear enlargement and distinct (but not macro) nucleoli; it may also have a papillary arch. (= PanIN 1B)
- *Atypical hyperplasia* also shows focal/partial loss of polarity, up to mod anisonucleosis ± micropapillae (= PanIN 2)
- *Dysplasia* (= PanIN 3) shows ↑ mitoses and extensive loss of polarity/papillae ± cribriformity and more severe cytol. abnormalities (incl. chromatin ± macronucleoli); = *CIS* if the changes are severe

Ductal Adenocarcinoma
- ↑Nõ of irregular tubular and ductal structures irregularly distributed in a desmoplastic stroma
- Infiltration does not respect lobular boundaries and non-neoplastic structures may be entrapped (d/dg close apposition of islet cells to benign ducts in chronic pancreatitis = ductuloinsular complex)
- Carcinomatous infiltration of duodenal muscle shows single/sparse atypical glands in between muscle fibres *without* well-formed stroma around them
- Lumenal anomalies: partial lumens, irregular branching, cribriformity, dirty necrotic contents
- Higher grade: poorly-formed glands, less mucus, ↑mitoses, ↑pleomorphism, perineural invasion
- Adjacent ducts may show papillary or flat *in situ* changes (= dysplasia) ± CIS (*vide supra*)
- Immuno: +ve for CK (liver *and* biliary – i.e. CK8,18,7,19), CEA (benign ducts may be CEA −ve), EMA, CA-19.9; usu. −ve for pancreatic enzymes (trypsin, amylase) and NE markers; α_1AT ±ve
- WHO (Klöppel) grading is based on the worst grade present (*not* the predominant grade):
  - ➢ the original series (of pancreatic head tumours) used Bouin's fixation and a very small hpf[15]
  - ➢ an even more marked correlation was found between nuclear circumference and survival (<24 μ did best, >31 μ did worst) but this measure is not part of the grading system.
  - **Grade 1** (Well diff): well-formed ducts, relatively large (*cf.* benign ducts) with some microcystic foci and smaller tubular glands; regular cells with minimal pleomorphism, basal nuclei; marked mucin production; mitoses <5/10 hpf. Cytoplasm is often clearer *cf.* normal or mod diff carcinoma
  - **Grade 2** (Mod diff): predominantly smaller tubular glands with some larger well-formed ducts; loss of polarity; some prominent nucleoli; variable mucin; mitoses 5–10/10hpf.
  - **Grade 3** (Poorly diff): irregular/poorly formed/compact aggregates of tubules or microglandular formations ± solid areas/mucoepidermoid foci (larger ducts are rare); marked pleomorphism and chromatin clumping; minimal mucin; mitoses >10/10hpf
- d/dg intraductal papillary hyperplasias/neoplasia/intraductal (Pagetoid) spread of invasive adenoCA
- d/dg gangliocytic paraganglioma/hamartoma (p. 179)
- d/dg accessory pancreatic ducts that penetrate duodenal muscle: these usu. occur in packets/lobules within a definitely formed stroma
- d/dg mimics of perineural invasion: closely apposed/perineural islet NE cells in chronic pancreatitis or true benign glandular perineural and intraneural inclusions
- d/dg ductal atrophy in chronic pancreatitis *vs.* incomplete lumen formation in carcinoma

FS diagnosis of pancreatic ductal adenocarcinoma
- Adenocarcinoma is rare under 40 years of age, it should have (at least):
  - ① many glands haphazardly distributed *and*
  - ② abnormal duct shapes and cytology (partial lumena, nuclear size variation of ≥ 4:1 and large irreg. nucleoli)
- The surrounding fat should be checked for free, lymphatic or perineural invasion (also look for this in CBD resection margin FS)
- d/dg chronic pancreatitis which:
  - ➢ shows residua of normal lobules within fibrosis (i.e. respect for lobular architecture that may manifest as central larger [possibly branched] ducts with smaller ducts around them)
  - ➢ shows Ca^{2+} and protein plugs in ducts (unlike CA which may have dirty necrotic cellular debris)
  - ➢ is not mitotically active and does not have dirty necrosis in duct lumena
  - ➢ may have islet cell remnants apposed to nerves/benign ducts (! not d/dg perineural/ periductal invasion by grade 3 adenoCA because of the lack glandular structure or high grade cytology)
  - ➢ may be impossible on FS due to distortion of entrapped ducts in a small sample (do levels)
- d/dg gangliocytic paraganglioma (p. 179)

Intraductal Papillary Mucinous Neoplasms (IPMN)
- Predominantly intraductal growth of complex villopapillary fronds in dilated main duct ± tributaries
- Benign (intraductal papillary adenoma): mild or no dysplasia
- Borderline: moderate dysplasia ± invasion of stalks but not into the surrounding pancreatic stroma
- CIS: severe dysplasia ± extraductal invasion (ductal adenocarcinoma NST or mucinous CA)

---

[15] the stated area of an hpf was 1356 μ^2 (= a diameter of 41.6 μ = 0.0416 mm). Most modern microscopes' hpf have a diameter ≈ 0.5 mm. Furthermore, it seems that the mitotic count was 2° to the architectural and cytological grade (e.g. grade 1 tumours had, on average, a mitotic count of <5 per 10 hpf) and a later study showed that cytological and architectural grading was more predictive than the Ki-67 LI.

Mucinous Cystic Tumours
- F≫M (rare in men and rare in head of pancreas); curable by resection unless invasive CA is present
- Usu. has ovarian-like stroma (unless in men) – not a feature of d/dg ectatic IPMN
- Benign: no/mild dysplasia, often flat lining; if not excised may progress to malignant type
- Borderline: moderate dysplasia ± papillaroid lining
- Malignant: severe dysplasia ± invasion ± mural nodules[16] (focal changes, needs extensive sampling)
- Immuno as for ductal carcinoma but may also have some NE marker + vity ± goblet & Paneth cells
- d/dg ectatic IPMN, but cystic tumours are not connected to the main duct system

Serous Cystic Tumours (Microcystic Adenoma and Serous Microcystic Carcinoma)
- Microcystic (d/dg acinar cell CA variant) or macro/oligocystic (assoc^d with VHL) ± stellate scar
- Cysts lined by glycogenated clear cells (unlike serous tumours of the ovary or acinar cell carcinoma)
- Bland compact nuclei with small or absent nucleoli (more irregular/larger nuclei in some VHL)
- Stroma is composed of vascular dense fibrous bands ± Ca^{2+}
- Usu. benign and amitotic ± focal tufting (malignancy is defined by invasion ± metastases)
- Immuno: +ve for CK, EMA, CA-19.9; −ve for CEA
- VHL: AD; other assoc^{n}s include: supratentorial haemangioblastoma, granular renal cysts, RCC, phaeochromocytoma, pancreatic NET, endolymphatic sac tumours, etc.

Atypical Acinar Cell Nodules (Acinar Cell Dysplasia)
- Compact aggregates (d/dg islets of Langerhans) of atypical acinar cells
- Basophilic type: loss of apical granules with nuclear (⊥ nucleolar) enlargement (↑NCR)
- Eosinophilic type: larger cells with loss of basal basophilia and with normal/dark nuclei ± cytoplasmic vacuoles

Acinar Cell Carcinoma
- Usu. late adulthood, poor prog. esp. if >10cm ∅ regardless of histology (except childhood ones)
- Macro: solid/cystic, haemorrhagic, fleshy; nodular with nodules separated by thick fibrous septa
- Arch.: acinar, microglandular (dilated acini), trabecular, solid; rich vasculature but sparse stroma
- Cytology: DPAS +ve granular apical cytoplasm, uniform basal round nucleolated nuclei, clumpy chromatin
- Variable mitoses, usu. >1/10 hpf (more in solid, less in pure acinar variants)
- Variant: solid – has less cytoplasm, more mitoses and is more likely to show nucleoli
- Variant: acinar cystadenoCA – has many large (mm to cm) cysts (d/dg serous microcystic tumours)
- Immuno/stains: +ve for lipase, amylase, trypsin, chymotrypsin, α_1AT and CAM5.2; CEA ± ve
- d/dg NET vs. solid variant: see p. 178 – also, NE markers are diffusely +ve in NET
- d/dg pancreatoblastoma: usu. children, has squamoid nests ± mesenchymal prolif^{n}s
- d/dg solid pseudopapillary CA has myxoid fibrovascular stroma and different immuno (*vide infra*)

Solid Pseudopapillary (= Solid / Cystic, Solid and Papillary Epithelial) Tumour
- Young, F≫M, large partly solid and cystic haemorrhagic/necrotic mass; rarely metastasise
- Uniform cells with eosinophilic or vacuolated cytoplasm and rare mitoses/nucleoli (d/dg NET)
- Necrosis with blood/myxoid cysts, cholesterol clefts in GC and papillae with loose fibrovascular cores; there are also solid areas and admixed collections of foam cells ± eosinophilic globules
- Immuno: α_1AT, vimentin +ve; CK, CEA, CA-19.9 usu. −ve; NSE, CgA and lipase only focal +vity
- d/dg NET but lack diffuse CgA +vity and have foamy Mφ, vimentin and α_1AT +vity (unlike NET)

Other Tumours
- A special type must comprise >50% of the tumour to qualify as that type
- Carcinomas with mixed differentiation (e.g. mixed ductal-endocrine or mixed acinar-endocrine): the minor type should comprise ≥30% of the tumour and both types intimately admixed to qualify
- ASC must have ≥30% of the tumour as squamous to qualify, else = NST: *NB*: the tumour may be predominantly squamous ! do not misdiagnose as d/dg SCC – take more blocks
- Mucinous non-cystic carcinoma (i.e. colloid carcinoma = the usual type mucinous CA [e.g. colonic])
- Signet ring carcinoma
- Carcinoma with osteoclast-like giant cells: mononuclear elements are pleomorphic ± spindled
- Undiff CA (= anaplastic CA): may have pleomorphic giant cells (*cf.* bland osteoclast-like giant cells)
- Clear cell carcinoma (d/dg metastatic RCC/ACC)

---

[16] similar to the mural nodules seen in ovarian mucinous cystadenocarcinoma (see p. 246)

- Oncocytic carcinoma
- Hepatoid carcinoma
- Microglandular adenocarcinoma

Endocrine Pancreas

Normal Histology
- Islets of Langerhans are CD99 +ve, usu. lack mitoses, may show dilated blood-filled spaces (*peliosis insulis*) and come in two main forms:

    (a) diffuse islets: found in the head, predom. PP cell, have an 'infiltrative' boundary (! d/dg CA on FS), form loose trabeculae and gland-like structures and have cells with distinct nucleoli ± columnar cells

    (b) compact islets: found in the dorsal pancreas are well-circ. with compact trabeculae of cells with typical NE nuclei and a mixture of alpha (glucagon, peripheral), beta (insulin, central), delta (somatostatin) and PP (very few) cells. Other peptides are usu. found only in tumours (e.g. gastrin)

Diabetes Mellitus
Type I (juvenile onset)
- Early: lymphohistiocytic insulitis of the islets of Langerhans
- Late: no inflam^n but loss of β-cells
Type II (adult onset)
- No inflam^n, β-cells preserved
- Amylin amyloid in islets

Well-Differentiated Endocrine Tumours
- Risk of malignancy (defined by gross invasion of adjacent organs or mets e.g. to LN, liver or distant) is related to:
    ① hormone produced (by immuno/EM) – *vide infra*
    ② tumour size[17] ≥ 2cm ∅
    ③ vascular/perineural invasion (large vessel invasion can be seen as a form of gross invasion)
    ④ coagulative tumour cell necrosis
    ⑤ high proliferation (mitoses ≥2/10 hpf or Ki-67 LI ≥2%)
- WHO (2004) distinguishes 'neoplasm' from 'carcinoma' by the presence of extrapancreatic spread and splits 'neoplasms' into 'benign behaviour' or 'uncertain behaviour' by the presence of any one of ②, ③ or ⑤ above.
- Carcinoid-like cells and arch. (± small nucleoli) ± gland-like formations of columnar NE cells
- Admixed fibrous stroma with delicate vessels ± amyloid (e.g. amylin in insulinomas)
- Variants: clear cell (esp. in VHL) and oncocytic
- Insulinoma (→ hypoglycaemic attacks); >95% are benign
- ACTH or PTHrP producing tumour are ≈ always malignant
- Glucagonoma (→ diabetes and necrolytic migratory erythema)   ⎫ these are
- Somatostatinoma (psammoma bodies and glandular structures)   ⎬ mostly
- Non-functioning[18] (∴ they may present at a later stage)   ⎭ malignant
- gastrinoma (→ ZE syndrome, ± MEN 1)   ⎫ 50 % of
- VIPoma (→ Verner-Morrison WDHA syndrome)   ⎬ these types
- GHRH producing tumours   ⎭ are malignant
- Other peptides or multihormonal tumours (e.g. PP + other peptides in MEN-1)
- EM may be characteristic in some (esp. for granule contents, if immuno is −ve)
- Immuno: for characteristic peptide(s) + NE markers (CD56, CD57, chromogranins, synaptophysin, NSE, PGP 9.5); many pancreatic NET may also be CD99 +ve; CAM5.2 +ve; CK7 is usu. −ve
- d/dg solid acinar cell carcinoma: has acinar foci and lacks NE nuclei or fibrous stroma within lobules
- d/dg solid pseudopapillary carcinoma (p. 177)

---

[17] called microadenoma if < 5 mm ∅ (if ≤ 0.3 mm = 'large islet' provided the distribution of peptide-producing cells is normal; a partial fibrous capsule favours microadenoma)
[18] non-functioning is meant clinically, the cells may be immuno +ve e.g. calcitonin, PP and neurotensin

- d/dg islet aggregations in atrophic chronic pancreatitis may reach upto a few mm in ⌀ but have multiple cell types by hormone immuno and it is rare for these islets to *completely* merge
- d/dg metastatic midgut carcinoids may be +ve for serotonin and substance P (unlike pancreatic 1°)
- d/dg metastatic RCC (esp. with clear cell/oncocytic variants): CK, EMA and vimentin +ve
- d/dg pancreatoblastoma: has acinar cell differentiation, squamous corpuscles ± mesenchymal stroma
- d/dg gangliocytic paraganglioma (*vide infra*)

Gangliocytic Paraganglioma/Hamartoma

① epithelioid NE cells   may have a strikingly infiltrative pattern
② spindle cell component   (! d/dg carcinoma on FS) but this does not
③ ganglion cells   equate to aggressive/malignant behaviour
- d/dg adenocarcinoma/carcinoid

Poorly-Differentiated Endocrine Carcinoma
- Like pulmonary SmCC (see pp. 93–94) or with larger cells
- d/dg PNET, lymphoma, metastasis, etc.

Pancreatic Transplant Pathology

Acute Rejection
- Mixed septal inflammation: lymphocytes, plasma cells, eos.
- Lymphocytic infiltration of the ducts (ductitis) and endothelialitis
- Acinar cell loss
- Islets spared or have 'spillover' infiltrates (recurrent 'auto'immune insulitis is rare)

Chronic Rejection
- Chronic graft vasculopathy (similar feature as for renal Tx see p. 208)
- Almost complete loss of parenchyma

Bibliography

Abrams, G.A., Kunde, S.S., Lazenby, A.J. and Clements, R.H. (2004) Portal fibrosis and hepatic steatosis in morbidly obese subjects: A spectrum of non-alcoholic fatty liver disease. *Hepatology*, **40** (2), 475–483.

Arora, D.S., Ramsdale, J., Lodge, J.P.A. and Wyatt, J.I. (1999) p53 but not bcl-2 is expressed by most cholangiocarcinomas: a study of 28 cases. *Histopathology*, **34** (6), 497–501.

Burt, A. (2001) Steatosis and steatohepatitis. *Current Diagnostic Pathology*, **7** (2), 141–147.

Burt, A.D., Portmann, B.C., Ferrell, L.D. (eds) (2006) *MacSween's Pathology of the Liver* (5th edn), Churchill Livingstone, London.

Chetty, R. and Vajpeyi, R. (2005) Lymphoplasmacytic Sclerosing Pancreatitis. *Current Diagnostic Pathology*, **11** (2), 95–101.

Davies, S.E. (1997) An update on chronic hepatitis, in *Progress in Pathology*, vol. 3 (eds N. Kirkham and N.R. Lemoine), Churchill Livingstone, NY, pp. 59–85.

Davies, S.E. (1997) Drugs and the liver. *Current Diagnostic Pathology*, **4** (3), 135–144.

DeLellis, R.A., Lloyd, R.V., Heitz, P.U. and Eng, C. (eds) (2004) *WHO Classification of Tumours: Pathology and Genetics Tumours of Endocrine Organs*, 1st edn, IARC Press, Lyon.

Demetris, A.J., Adams, D., Bellamy, C. *et al.* (2000) Update of the international Banff schema for liver allograft rejection: working recommendations for the histopathologic staging and reporting of chronic rejection. *Hepatology*, **31** (3), 792–799.

Demetris, A.J., Batts, K.P., Dhillon, A.P. *et al.* (1997) Banff schema for grading liver allograft rejection: an international consensus document. *Hepatology*, **25** (3), 658–663.

Fleming, M.D. (1998) Hepatic iron overload in the age of hereditary haemochromatosis mutation analysis. *American Journal of Clinical Pathology*, **109** (5), 505–507.

Gerber, M.A., Thung, S.N., Bodenheimer, H.C. Jr, *et al.* (1986) Characteristic histologic triad in liver adjacent to metastatic neoplasm. *Liver,* **6** (2), 85–88.

Goldin, R.D. (1997) Diagnosis of biliary ductopaenia. *Histopathology*, **31** (5), 397–399.

Goldin, R.D. (1998) Non-alcoholic steatohepatitis. *Current Diagnostic Pathology*, **5** (1), 44–49.

Goldin, R.D. and Lloyd, J. (2002) HIV and hepatobiliary disease. *Current Diagnostic Pathology*, **8** (3), 144–151.

Haugk, B. and Burt, A. (2005) Non-alcoholic fatty liver disease, in *Recent Advances in Histopathology*, vol. 21 (eds M. Pignatelli and J. Underwood), The Royal Society of Medicine Press, London, pp. 1–17.

Henson, D.E., Albores–Saavedra, J. and Corle, D. (1992) Carcinoma of the gallbladder. *Cancer*, **70** (6), 1493–1497.

Hübscher, S.G. (1994) Transplant pathology of the liver. *Current Diagnostic Pathology*, **1** (2), 59–69.

Hübscher, S.G. and Demetris, A.J. (2000) Pathology of liver transplantation: an update. *Current Diagnostic Pathology*, **6** (4), 229–241.

International Working Party (1995) Terminology of nodular hepatocellular lesions. *Hepatology*, **22** (3), 983–993.

Ishak, K., Baptista, A., Bianchi, L. et al (1995) Histological grading and staging of chronic hepatitis. Journal of Hepatology, 22 (6), 696–699.

Kakar, S. and Burgart, L.J. (2005) Tumours of the biliary system. Current Diagnostic Pathology, 11 (1), 34–43.

Kakar, S., Muir, T., Murphy, L.M. et al. (2003) Immunoreactivity for Hep Par 1 in hepatic and extrahepatic tumours and its correlation with albumin in situ hybridization in hepatocellular carcinoma. American Journal of Clinical Pathology, 119 (3), 361–366.

Klöppel, G., Lingenthal, G., von Bülow, M. and Kern, H.F. (1985) Histological and fine structural features of pancreatic ductal adenocarcinoma in relation to growth and prognosis: studies in xenografted tumours and clinico-histopathological correlation in a series of 75 cases. Histopathology, 9 (8), 841–856.

Knisely, A.S. (2002) Paediatric biliary tract disease. Current Diagnostic Pathology, 8 (3), 152–159.

Knodell, R.G., Ishak, K. and Black, T.S. et al. (1981) Formulation and application of a numerical scoring system for assessing histological activity in asymptomatic chronic active hepatitis. Hepatology, 1 (5), 431–435.

Krishna, M. and Nakhleh, R.E. (2005) Primary non-neoplastic diseases of the extrahepatic bile ducts. Current Diagnostic Pathology, 11 (1), 1–6.

Lack, E.E. (2003) Pathology of the pancreas, gallbladder, extrahepatic biliary tract and ampullary region. Oxford University Press, Oxford.

Lai, R. and Weiss, L.M. (1998) Hepatitis C virus and non-Hodgkin's lymphoma. American Journal of Clinical Pathology, 109 (5), 508–510.

Lau, S.K., Prakash, S., Geller, S.A. and Alsabeh, R. (2002) Comparative immunohistochemical profile of hepatocellular carcinoma, cholangiocarcinoma, and metastatic adenocarcinoma. Human Pathology, 33 (12), 1175–1181.

Lefkowitch, J.H. (2005) Hepatobiliary pathology. Current Opinion in Gastroenterology, 21 (3), 260–269.

Loquvam, G.S. and Russel, W.O. (1950) Accessory pancreatic ducts of the major duodenal papilla: structures to be differentiated from cancer. American Journal of Clinical Pathology, 20 (4), 305–313.

Lucas, S. (2000) Update on the pathology of AIDS. Current Diagnostic Pathology, 6 (2), 103–112.

Lüttges, J., Schemm, S., Vogel, I., Hedderich, J., Kremer, B. and Klöppel, G. (2000) The grade of pancreatic ductal carcinoma is an independent prognostic factor and is superior to the immunohistochemical assessment of proliferation. Journal of Pathology, 191 (2), 154–161.

Matteoni, C.M., Younossi, Z.M., Gramlich, T. et al. (1999) Nonalcoholic fatty liver disease: a spectrum of clinical and pathological severity. Gastroenterology, 116 (6), 1413–1419.

Nagato, Y., Kondu, F., Kondu, Y. et al. (1991) Histological and morphometrical indicators for a biopsy diagnosis of well differentiated hepatocellular carcinoma. Hepatology, 14 (3), 473–478.

Nakanuma, V. and Ohta, G. (1979) Histometric and serial section observations of the intrahepatic bile ducts in primary biliary cirrhosis. Gastroenterology, 76 (6), 1326–1332.

Ojanguren, I., Castella, E., Ariza, A. et al. (1997) Liver cell atypias: a comparative study in cirrhosis with and without hepatocellular carcinoma. Histopathology, 30 (2), 106–112.

Owen, D.A. and Kelly, J.K. (2001) Pathology of the gallbladder, biliary tract and pancreas. W.B. Saunders Co., Philadelphia.

Paterson, A.C. and Cooper, K. (2005) Tumours and tumour-like lesions of the hepatic parenchyma. Current Diagnostic Pathology, 11 (1), 19–33.

Portmann, B.C. (2002) Primary biliary cirrhosis and sclerosing cholangitis. Current Diagnostic Pathology, 8 (3), 133–143.

Quagla, A., Bhattacharjya, S. and Dhillon, A.P. (2001) Limitations of the histopathological diagnosis and prognostic assessment of hepatocellular carcinoma. Histopathology, 38 (2), 167–174.

Roenigk, H.H., Auerbach, R., Maibach, H.I. and Weinstein, G.D. (1982) Methotrexate guidelines – revised. Journal of the American Academy of Dermatology, 6 (2), 145–155.

Scheuer, P.J. and Lefkowitch, J.H. (2006) Liver Biopsy Interpretation. 7th edn, W.B. Saunders Co., London.

Solcia, E., Capella, C. and Klöppel, G. (1995) Tumors of the Pancreas, fascicle 20 in Atlas of Tumor Pathology, 3rd series, AFIP, Washington D.C.

Standish, R.A. and Davies, S.E. (2002) Bile duct tumours. Current Diagnostic Pathology, 8 (3), 160–171.

Stephenson, T.J. (1997) Criteria for malignancy in endocrine tumours, in Recent Advances in Histopathology, vol. 17 (eds P.P. Anthony, R.N.M. MacSween and D.G. Lowe), Churchill Livingstone, Edinburgh, pp. 93–111.

Tadrous, P.J. and Goldin, R.D. (1997) How many portal tracts are necessary to make a diagnosis of significant bile duct loss (SBDL)? Journal of Pathology, 181 (Suppl.), 11A.

Tsui, W.M.S. (2003) Drug-associated changes in the liver. Current Diagnostic Pathology, 9 (2), 96–104.

Waters, B.L. and Blaszyk, H. (2005) Disorders involving intrahepatic bile ducts. Current Diagnostic Pathology, 11 (1), 7–18.

Web sites

Booth, J.C.L., O'Grady, J. and Neuberger, J. (2001) Clinical guidelines on the management of hepatitis C, Royal College of Physicians and British Society of Gastroenterology, www.bsg.org.uk (accessed April 2007).

13. Central Nervous System and Skeletal Muscle

CNS (Non-Neoplastic)

Dementia

General
- Def[n]: chronic persistent global reduction in previously attained higher cognitive functions but with normal consciousness, and of sufficient severity to increase dependency for normal daily activities
- Normal ageing: ➤ normal weight (see p. 391) decreases after 65 years
  - ➤ ↓cortex, ↓white matter, ↑ventricles, cerebellum is usu. spared
  - ➤ neuron loss, plaques, tangles
  - ➤ hippocampus: *rare* cells with granulovacuolar degeneration and Hirano bodies

For anatomy, see figure 4.1 (p. 36); for block-taking, see pp. 381–382.

Histological features seen in the most common dementias
- Neuritic plaques (+ve for tau protein with A4 (β) amyloid core and more speckled A4 (β))
- Intraneuronal tangles (tau protein) – the term 'tauopathy' is applied to conditions with abnormal tau protein inclusions including Alzheimer's, Pick's disease and corticobasal degeneration
- Granulovacuolar degeneration of Simchowicz (multiple intraneuronal 3–5μ clear vacuoles each with a basophilic argyrophil central granule)
- Hirano bodies: eosinophilic oval/rod-like pyramidal cell intracytoplasmic inclusions (= crystalline actin)
- Pick bodies: argyrophil and tau +ve neurofilament inclusions in superficial cortex neurons
- Lewy bodies: two-tone concentric eosinophil cytoplasmic inclusions with dense core and pale rim (+ve for α-synuclein and ubiquitin). H&E morphology is less well defined in cerebral ones
- Congophilic amyloid angiopathy (CAA): +ve for A4 (β) ± evidence of previous haemorrhage
- MND inclusions: ubiquitin +ve inclusions in cortical neurons and hippocampal dentate granule cells
- Spongiform degeneration i.e. grey matter microvacuolation and reactive gliosis (= '*status spongiosus*' if advanced)

Mixed dementias
- Alzheimer's + vascular dementia or Alzheimer's + DLB
- Vascular dementia + other neurodegenerative disease (DLB, basal ganglia, Pick, etc.)

Primary dementias
- Alzheimer's (± Familial Alzheimer's)
  - ➤ exaggerated ageing changes (esp. in hippocampus, amygdala, thalamus, neocortex, olfactory bulb & basal ganglia); more than 1 or 2 hippocampal cells containing Hirano bodies or granulovacuolar degeneration are suspicious (and lots of them are ≈ only seen in dementia)
  - ➤ CAA (see p. 72)
  - ➤ plaques containing tau protein (*cf.* A4 (β) amyloid only plaques) occurring together with neocortical tangles favour Alzheimer's over ageing changes
  - ➤ in the USA, the National Institute on Aging, and the Reagan Institute Working group issued diagnostic guidelines based on the CERAD protocol which gives an age-related probability of Alzheimer's ('definite', 'probable' or 'possible') based on semiquantitative impressions of plaque nõs (none, mild, moderate, severe), and likewise tangle nõs. The disease may be 'staged' according to the nõ of brain sites involved using the 'Braak stage' criteria. For these articles, see Bibliography; for UK autopsy and sampling guidelines, see pp. 381–382
- Diffuse Lewy body disease (= dementia with Lewy bodies (DLB))
  - ➤ psychiatric Sx +/ 1° dysphagia; neuroleptics are contra-indicated (they can be fatal)
  - ➤ Lewy bodies esp. in cingulate gyrus, hippocampus, amygdala and substantia nigra
  - ➤ paucity of plaques and tangles (unless combined Alzheimer's + DLB)
- Frontotemporal dementias
  - ➤ affective / disinhibitive Sx prior to memory problems
  - ➤ atrophy of superficial layers of frontotemporal cortex
  - ➤ Pick's disease: ± superficial cortex neuronal Pick bodies ± ballooned eosinophilic 'Pick cells' (neurons containing tau and αβ crystallin by immuno)

Diagnostic Criteria Handbook in Histopathology: A Surgical Pathology Vade Mecum by Paul J. Tadrous
Copyright © 2007 by John Wiley & Sons, Ltd.

> MND inclusion dementia: MND inclusions in cortical neurons and hippocampal dentate gran-
ule cells ± clinical MND/AMLS
> others: e.g. 'corticobasal degeneration' and 'non-specific frontotemporal dementia'
- Basal ganglia degenerations e.g. Huntingdon's (selective caudate atrophy) / Parkinson's (depigmentation of substantia nigra and Lewy bodies in substantia nigra, locus ceruleus and cortex)

Secondary dementias
- Vascular (multi-infarct dementia and Binswanger's disease)
  > suspect if younger patient (*cf.* pure Alzheimer's) with step-wise clinical progression and PMHx of IHD, HT, smoking, vasculopathy, SLE, etc.
  > features incl.: softening of white matter, lacunar spaces around small vessels in basal ganglia, microinfarcts of the cortex and arteriosclerotic vessels
  > multi-infarct dementia shows cortex and white matter predominant damage – usu. with a total ≥50–100ml brain volume lost
  > Binswanger's disease shows basal ganglia and white matter predominant damage ± Parkin-sonian Sx.
- Post-traumatic (e.g. chronic subdural haematoma / *dementia pugilistica*)
- Post-infective:
  > AIDS (cognitive and motor complex, see 'HIV encephalopathy', below)
  > post-encephalitic
  > GPI (syphilis)
  > prion: (→ grey matter spongiform degeneration) suspect if rapid onset and progression (<2 years), motor Sx e.g. myoclonus/cerebellar, ± characteristic EEG (absent in vCJD), prior psychiatric +/ sensory disturbance (esp. in vCJD), FHx (in GSS/FFI/familial CJD)
- Others: e.g. toxic, metabolic, 'normal' pressure (i.e. intermittent) hydrocephalus

Ischaemic Hypoxic Injury
- Seen in sensitive brain areas after global circulatory collapse (shock, MI, etc.) or CO poisoning
- Sensitive areas: sulci, CA1, deep white matter, striatum, boundary zones (see figure 4.1 on p. 36)
- Macro: laminar dark/discoloured areas (esp. in CA1 and cerebral neocortex layers 3 & 5[1])
- Neurons: shrink, ↑ cytoplasmic eosinophilia, nuclear pyknosis and angulation
- Glia: gliosis (GFAP immuno: ↑cells in cerebral cortex layers 3 & 5, vertical processes in cerebellar cortex)
- Later: neuron loss, demyelination (due to oligodendroglial damage)

HIV Encephalopathy
- Degree of synaptic damage and global ↓ in neuronal numbers correlates with 'AIDS dementia'
- Macro: ± ventricular dilatation and widened sulci
- *Multinucleated Giant Cell Encephalitis* (in deep white/grey matter and corticomedullary junction):
  > microglial nodules (cellular foci)
  > multinucleated giant cells (most probably derived from glia)
  > prominent endothelial cells
  > demyelination and perivascular foamy Mφ (lipid)
  > HIV is detectable (e.g. by p24 immuno) in microglia (which are CD4 +ve), GC and endothe-lium
- Lymphocytic meningitis: leptomeningeal and perivasc. heavy lymphoid infiltrate (but no bugs)
- Leucoencephalopathy: multifocal/diffuse demyelination, Mφ, gliosis, GC, sparse lymphocytes
- Cerebral granulomatous angiitis: mixed chronic inflam[n] and GC in vessel walls ± necrosis
- Diffuse poliodystrophy: astrocytosis of the grey matter (of bainstem nuclei, basal ganglia and cerebral cortex)
- IRDS encephalopathy: intense perivasc. Mφ (lipid, Fe and p24) and T-cells with severe demyelination
- 2° pathology: severe immuno↓ → CMV, PML, NHL; milder→ toxoplasmosis, VZV, HSV

Multiple Sclerosis
- Onset in youth (optic neuritis), chronic relapse/remit or continuous → *ataxic paraplegia*
- CSF: ↑lymphocytes, ↑ γ-globulin:albumin ratio, oligoclonal bands
- Acute: > yellow and soft, peri-axial (e.g. angles of lateral ventricles), around small veins
           > lymphoplasmacytic cuffing (of vessels) ± vesicular oedema and fibrin if acute/active
           > lipid foamy MΦ, esp. perivascular (may contain stainable myelin)

---

[1] layers 3 & 5 (of total 6) are the two layers that contain pyramidal neurons. They are in the mid cortex separated by a narrow band (= layer 4, composed of stellate cells)

- Chronic:
  - ➤ grey and sclerotic, demarcated irregular areas (confluence) shadow plaques
  - ➤ paucicellular, gliosis, survival of neurons
  - ➤ axons survive initially then undergo Wallerian degeneration
- Variants:
  - ➤ *Neuromyelitis Optica (= Devic's disease 2° to MS)*: adults, rapid blindness and paraplegia (brain, optic nerve, spinal cord). d/dg Devic's disease 2° to a necrotic TB lesion in the spinal cord
  - ➤ *Sudanophilic Diffuse Sclerosis*: children, acute and progressive, esp. occipital (MΦ aggregates and neuron loss)

Acute Disseminated (Perivenous) Encephalomyelitis
- Post viral (measles, mumps, rubella, chickenpox, resp. infection)/vaccination (rabies/smallpox)
- Acute onset
- Diffuse perivenular demyelination and PMN → mononuclear cells later
- It is considered an EAE-type reaction / reaction to a virus. Similar lesions may be seen in Behçet's

Acute Haemorrhagic Leucoencephalopathy/Leucoencephalitis/Leucoencephalomyelitis
- Post viral (incl. influenza)/resp. infection/shock/drugs/cerebral malaria. Rapidly fatal
- Swollen brain, perivenular demyelination, venular necrosis, ball and ring haemorrhage
- Initially PMN → mononuclear cells later
- It is considered to be a hyper-acute EAE-type reaction

Other Forms of Paraxial Demyelination
- *Central pontine myelinolysis*: due to too rapid correction of plasma $[Na^+]$ in alcoholics/malnourished/generally ill patients
- *Toxic demyelination*: due to tin/carbon monoxide poisoning (subcortical white matter may be spared)
- Viral infection:
  - ➤ *PML*: polyoma (JC), immunosuppression, abnormal oligodendrocytes (viral inclusions)
  - ➤ *SSPE*: measles (years before)/rubella, age <20, death within six months, meningoencephalitis, neuronophagia, inclusions

Miscellaneous Demyelinations
- Subacute combined degeneration of the cord (vitamin B12↓): lateral and posterior columns affected
- Alcoholic, diabetic and Guillain-Barré peripheral neuropathy: segmental myelin loss in periph. nerves
- RadioRx (via toxic effects on oligodendrocytes)

CNS (Neoplasms)

Differential Diagnosis by Site and Age

TABLE 13.1 Tumours by site and age

Tumour \ Site	level of the foramen magnum	brain stem	cerebellopontine angle	cerebellum	cerebrum	corpus callosum	pineal	pituitary	optic nerve & chiasm	lateral ventricle	4th ventricle	3rd ventricle (within)	3rd ventricle (around)
astrocytoma (G1, G2)		C, A		C, A	C, A	C, A			C, A				C (pilocytic & fibrillary), A
astrocytoma G3		C, A			C, A	C, A							A
astrocytoma G4		C, A			A	A							A
adenoma								C, A					
AVM					A								
choroid plexus papilloma			C, A							C, A	C, A	C	
craniopharyngioma								C, A					
cysts			A (epidermoid)	C (dermoid)								A (colloid)	
ependymoma			C		A					C, A	C, A	C, A	A
germ cell							C, A	C, A					
glomus jugulare			A										
haemangioblastoma				A									
lipoma						C, A							
medulloblastoma				C, A									
meningioma	A		A		A		A	A	A	A			
metastatic				A	A								
neurofibroma	A												
oligodendroglioma					C, A	C, A							C, A
sarcoma					A								
Schwannoma	A		A (acoustic)										
subependymoma											A		

Not all tumours are represented C = occurs in children, A = occurs in adults, G1-4 = tumour grade.

Neuroblastoma, Ganglioneuroblastoma, Ganglioneuroma
See p. 59.

Schwannoma, Neurofibroma, MPNST
See pp. 315–316.

Pineal Tumours
- Neuronal (well-diff to poorly diff, mitotic count is prognostic – worse if >6/10hpf.):
  - ➤ pineocytoma: usu. adults; sheets of uniform cells with small nuclei are punctuated by pockets of eosinophilic fibrillar material (pineocytomatous rosettes) – these may interconnect
  - ➤ pineal parenchymal tumour: intermediate differentiation and features between pineocytoma & pineoblastoma, ± lobulation
  - ➤ pineoblastoma: usu. children; sheets of pleomorphic SBRCT ± rare retinoblastomatous rosettes
- Germ cell: germinoma (≈ seminoma, OCT4 +ve), teratoma (mature ones more common than immature)

Craniopharyngioma
- Adamantinomatoid (see ameloblastoma on p. 128) – have an ill-defined 'pseudo-invasive' boundary with the brain
- Squamoid (papillary arch., not calcific or cystic – see d/dg) – are well circumscribed
- ± Ghost epithelium, Ca^{2+}, cystic change (± cholesterol crystals) +/ xanthogranulomatous inflam^n
- Immuno: +vity for CK5/6, CK17, CK19, CK7, 34βE12 and hCG (may help in d/dg), −ve for CK20
- d/dg pilocytic astrocytoma (because craniopharyngioma may have adjacent chronic astrocytosis with Rosenthal fibres, etc.)
- d/dg Rathke's cleft cyst: lined by cuboidal/columnar epithelium with goblet cells, cilia and focal squamous metaplasia (hence the possibility for confusion)
- d/dg: epidermoid cyst: these tend to be unilocular, non-papillary squamous lesions with keratin
- d/dg squamous metaplasia of the pars intermedia of the pituitary: ∴ do not diagnose craniopharyngioma just because you see some squamous tissue !

Chordoma
- Axial notochordal sites – esp. extremes (sacrum or clivus)
- Lobulated architecture on low power with fibrous septa and myxoid background (± chondroid)
- Cords of eosinophilic cells with interspersed physaliphorous (bubble-bearing) cells
- Variants: dedifferentiated (has spindle sarcomatoid areas) and chondroid: both show brachyury +vity
- Immuno: brachyury nuclear +vity (very specific for notochord differentiation); for d/dg see Table 13.2:

TABLE 13.2 Immuno in the d/dg of chordoma

	S100	CK	Brachyury	Other Features
chordoma	+	+	+	GFAP (30%), galectin-3 (75%), CAM5.2, EMA & MNF116 +ve; CK7, CK20, CEA & D2-40 −ve
chondrosarcoma	+	−	−	site is helpful, +ve for D2-40, −ve for EMA & galectin-3
liposarcoma	+	−	−	fibrous septa unusual (refers to myxoid/round cell type)
RCC	−	+	−	fibrous septa/lobulation unusual in 2° CA; vascularity
myxopapillary ependymoma	±	−	−	GFAP & vimentin +ve; AE1/AE3 ±ve; CgA, CEA, EMA & CAM5.2 −ve; d/dg also includes paraganglioma
meningioma	±	±	?	refers to the chordoid variant of meningioma

Olfactory Neuroblastoma
- Lobulated blue cell tumour in the sinonasal region presenting usu. in teens or middle-aged adults
- Grade 1: obvious neurofibrillary material, no mitoses/necrosis, small uniform round cells, ± Ca^{2+}
- Grade 2: few mitoses, no necrosis, little pleom., less neurofibrillar material, ± Ca^{2+}
- Grade 3–4: ↑mitoses, necrosis, pleom.; ↓neurofibrillar material (≈ absent in G4), no Ca^{2+}
- Immuno: NSE +ve, CK ±ve, −ve for CD99, desmin, HMB45, EMA, CEA; NE granules on EM
- d/dg G3-4 *vs.* sinonasal undiff carcinoma (see Chapter 8: Respiratory and Mediastinum)

Astrocytomas

Immuno
- GFAP: +ve in low grades, weak or variable +vity in higher grades; D2-40 +ve in glioblastoma
- Prognostic markers: p53, pRb (p105), p16

Pilocytic astrocytoma (grade I)
- Child, posterior fossa, curable by resection ∴ best prognosis
- Relatively well-circumscribed *cf.* other types
- Bipolar cells: have long ('matted hair') fibrillar processes ± elongated nuclei
- Biphasic pattern: compact (bipolar cells) and loose/spongy/microcystic (multipolar/stellate cells)
- Eosinophilic carrot-shaped Rosenthal fibres and rounded granular/cytoid bodies (intra/extra-cellular) differentiate them from *most* higher grade gliomas (but not gliosis); calcispherules may be present
- If cystic, a vascular *mural nodule* may be present – d/dg haemangioblastoma (lipid +ve, GFAP and calcispherule –ve)
- Nuclear atypia, infarct-like necrosis, microvascular proliferation[2] and subarachnoid space infiltration are *not* poor prognostics
- Malignant degeneration is rare and usu. post radioRx (hypercellularity, multiple mitoses per hpf, palisaded necrosis ± microvascular proliferation)
- d/dg chronic astrogliosis adjacent to some other lesion ∴ check representativeness of Bx and CPC

Sub-ependymal giant cell astrocytoma (grade I)
- Grade I by definition; usu. occur in TS; well-circumscribed and periventricular; ± cysts / Ca^{2+}
- The GC are astrocytic, usu. mononuclear and show variable neuronal differentiation; HMB45 is –ve
- Smaller cells are admixed resulting in a hetrerogenous picture
- Good prognosis even if: mitoses, microvascular proliferation and necrosis

Astrocytoma (grade II)
- Not pilocytic and not anaplastic. This is also called '*Diffuse Astrocytoma*'
- Mitoses should be ≈ absent: if >1 mitosis is seen over many hpf = anaplastic astrocytoma (*q.v.*)
- Ki-67 LI is usu. <2%
- Includes: ① *Fibrillary* (most common)

     ② *Gemistocytic* (must have >20% gemistocytes [abundant eosinophilic cytoplasm without Nissl substance and eccentric nucleus ± pleom.], also has perivascular lymphoid infiltrate; d/dg *Sub-ependymal Giant Cell Astrocytoma*)

     ③ *Protoplasmic* (rare)

Anaplastic astrocytoma (grade III)
- Mitoses and ↑cellularity (*cf.* grade II). (The exact boundary between grade II & III is blurred)
- No coagulative necrosis/microvascular proliferation (unless part of a focus of oligodendroglioma differentiation)

Glioblastoma multiforme – GBM – (grade IV)
- Clin./radiol.: supratentorial ring-enhancing lesion (grade III astrocytomas are not ring-enhancing)
- Generally, as for Grade III plus coagulative necrosis +/ microvascular proliferation (this manifests as ↑cellularity of vessel walls or glomeruloid multilumena on H&E and broadening of capillary outlines on retic)
- Cytological pleomorphism and mitoses may not be prominent on small Bx
- Variants: ① *Gliosarcoma* (GFAP –ve spindle sarcomatoid component ± collagen production)

     ② *Giant cell glioblastoma* (multinucleate giant cells ++)

     ③ *Small cell glioblastoma*
- d/dg anaplastic oligodendroglioma/oligoastrocytoma (esp. since oligo may have necrosis and ↑vessels, small cell GBM may look like oligo and any GBM may have minor foci of true oligo differentiation). Glioblastoma cytology varies more within any given tumour *cf.* oligo (hence 'multiforme')
- d/dg other lesions with necrosis/microvascular proliferation (e.g. sub-ependymal giant cell astrocytoma (*vide supra*), ependymoma (*vide infra*), metastatic carcinoma, lymphoma and abscess)
- d/dg meningioma *vs.* gliosarcoma (look for more typical GBM components)
- d/dg radioRx effect: the necrosis is not palisaded, the atypical glial cells are not mitotic and the vascular changes are those of radiation (see p. 72) not microvascular proliferation

---

[2] 'microvascular proliferation' is the newer term for 'vascular endothelial proliferation' used in the older literature. See the section on Glioblastoma Multiforme for a description of its morphology.

Oligodendroglioma/Oligoastrocytoma (Grade II) and Anaplastic Oligo/Oligoastro (Grade III)
- An important diagnosis to get right because these are sensitive to chemoRx (esp. if there is del. 1p or 19q) and may mimic high grade astrocytomas
- Evenly-spaced cells with central round nuclei (with chromocentres ± small nucleoli) and clear cytoplasm
- ± Microgemistocytes (GFAP +ve, vimentin −ve) and reactive astrocytes (GFAP +ve, vimentin +ve)
- Prominent chicken-wire capillaries (! do not confuse with true microvascular – endothelial – prolif^n, although this may also occur focally in grade II lesions)
- ± Mucin microcysts (proteinaceous microcysts also occur in astrocytomas) ± focal calcifications
- Mixed tumours (oligoastrocytoma) must have a 'prominent component' of each type (oligo and astrocytoma) that may be well-defined or diffusely admixed. Some suggest >30% astrocytoma and >50% oligo but this is not universally agreed. (d/dg astro component *vs.* microgemistocytes and reactive astrocytosis [*vide supra*])
- Mitoses are sparse (Ki-67 LI is usu. <5%)
- High grade (anaplastic) features: { ① ↑ cellularity, ② ↑mitoses and ③ nuclear pleom.} – may be focal or diffuse (= grade III if diffuse). Microvascular prolif^n +/ necrosis in the oligo component don't change anything but if in the astrocytoma component = 'GBM with an oligo component' (grade IV)
- Immuno: GFAP +ve in microgemistocytes but ±ve in oligo component, CD57 +ve, vimentin −ve, EMA −ve, MAP-2 +ve.
- d/dg other clear-cell/epithelioid neoplasms: meningiomas (have well-defined boundaries and opposite immuno for CD57, EMA, vimentin and GFAP), pituitary adenoma (site and peptides), RCC/other carcinoma (sharp demarcation + immuno), haemangioblastoma (lacks Ca^{2+}), clear cell ependymoma
- d/dg high grade astrocytomas esp. small cell GBM (*vide supra*)
- d/dg reactive lipid Mϕ have foamy cytoplasm and bland, vesicular, eccentric, bean-shaped nuclei

Meningiomas

Typical meningiomas (WHO grade I)
- Sites: spinal/cranial/ectopic; also in intra-osseous (petrous), intraorbital and intraventricular sites
- Meningothelial meningioma:
  - ➢ epithelioid cells with poorly defined cell borders ('syncytial')
  - ➢ whorls of cells, sometimes around vessels
  - ➢ ovoid nuclei with bland chromatin ± intranuclear cytoplasmic inclusions
  - ➢ ± psammoma bodies (may be numerous in *psammomatous meningioma = psammoma*)
- Local invasion: into dura and bone → ↑risk of local recurrence; into brain → see Grade II, below
- Variants (mesenchymal): fibroblastic, angiomatous, metaplastic (contains bone/cartilage/adipose/ myxoid/xanthomatous components)
- Variants (epithelioid): microcystic, secretory (PAS +ve)
- Immuno: vimentin +ve, GFAP −ve, S100 variably +ve (usu. mesenchymal types), CK variably +ve (esp. epithelioid types), EMA usu. +ve but may be patchy, CD57 −ve. CEA +ve in secretory type. Some are D2-40 +ve; Ki-67 LI may be prognostic

Atypical meningioma (WHO grade II)
- Aggressive epithelioid variants: clear cell (PAS +ve), chordoid, oncocytic
- Any type with the following are features of atypicality (even if only focal):
  - ➢ mitoses ≥4 per 10 hpf (with an hpf area defined as $0.16mm^2 \approx 0.45mm$ Ø)
  - ➢ foci of geographic necrosis (not surgically induced)
  - ➢ hypercellularity
  - ➢ sheet-like growth
  - ➢ nuclear pleomorphism (incl. prominent nucleoli)
  - ➢ small cells with ↑NCR
- Atypical meningioma may be diagnosed on the mitotic criterion alone or on the presence of 3 of the non-mitotic criteria if mitotic count is low. Brain invasion is not considered a defining criterion for Grade II tumours but if present in a grade I tumour it connotes grade II-like behaviour so it should be sought (do GFAP immuno).

Malignant (anaplastic) meningioma (WHO grade III)
- Aggressive epithelioid variants:
  - ➢ papillary (elongated cells, pattern may be focal, d/dg adenocarcinoma)
  - ➢ rhabdoid (may not be aggressive if only a minor focal component, d/dg oncocytic)
- Any type with ≥20/10hpf mitoses or marked cytological atypia ± exaggerated atypical features listed above

Other 1° Meningeal Tumours
- Soft tissue tumours: benign (e.g. lipoma), HPC, SFT, sarcomas (osteosarcoma, chondrosarcoma esp. mesenchymal chondrosarcoma, RMS, etc.)
- Haemangioblastoma
  - usu. infratentorial/spinal cord (unless assoc^d with VHL), often cystic
  - epithelioid foamy lipidised and glycogenated 'stromal' cells + fine branching vessels
  - ± haemosiderin, mast cells
  - retic: pericellular and perivascular staining
  - immuno: NSE, vimentin and D2-40 +ve, EMA and CK −ve
  - d/dg meningioma / metastatic RCC / astrocytic lesion (because there may gliosis and Rosenthal fibres adjacent to a haemangioblastoma)
- Melanoma

Lymphomas
- Most are high grade large cell lymphomas e.g. DLBCL, ALCL
- Any other type can occur but 1° HL is almost unheard of

Per-operative Diagnosis (Brain Smear/Frozen Section)
Differentiating glioma from gliosis
- Usu. only a problem at the *margin* of a glioma ∴ if unsure at frozen section ask for a deeper Bx
- Mitoses and Ca^{2+} suggest glioma but these are rare at the margins
- Nuclear hyperchromasia and pleomorphism suggest glioma
- Density:
  - gliosis = uniform or gradient (in white matter) or banded with neurons (in grey matter)
  - glioma = uneven distribution, palisades, 2° structures of Scherer[3]
- Nuclei touch / indent each other in glioma (but nuclei don't touch in gliosis)
- Characteristic features of specific glioma types e.g. proteinaceous microcysts in astrocytoma
- Immuno: *widespread* p53 +vity favours neoplasia over gliosis
Features suggesting 1° neoplasia
- Coagulative tumour cell necrosis (esp. if geographic and palisaded[4]) is the hallmark of a high grade neoplastic lesion (! exclude d/dg e.g. abscess or infarct with pseudopalisading necrosis)
- Birefringent fibrils may be seen in astrocytomas (Rosenthal fibres are not birefringent)
- Nuclear features:
  - hyperchromasia
  - pleomorphism
  - bare nuclei
  - nucleoli (!but can get regular nucleoli in reactive astrocytes and oligodendrocytes)
  - nuclear crowding (hypercellularity)
- Microvascular proliferation (! not capillary proliferation) – this is rarely seen in metastases and is a hallmark of 1° brain tumours (although not necessarily malignant – see 'Astrocytomas', above)
- ! Vascularity and variable numbers of Mφ may be seen in space occupying infarcts
- ! Mitoses can be seen in reactive conditions
Some typical lesions
- Meningioma – *vide supra*, helpful features in per-operative diagnosis are:
  - intranuclear cytoplasmic inclusions
  - psammoma bodies
  - epithelioid cells / whorls
  - ± bundles of spindle cells (d/dg Schwannoma)
- Gliomas – *vide supra* – *NB*: the cytoplasmic clearing of oligos may not be seen in FS/smear but oligos tend to have a uniform distribution of cells (*cf.* perivascular accentuation in astrocytomas)
- Central Neurocytoma:
  - usu. young (20s), intraventricular, low grade and surgically curable
  - salt and pepper nucleus and perinuclear halos
  - embryonal neuropil-like areas
  - immuno: GFAP +ve, synaptophysin +ve in ≈ all cells (only focal in oligos)
  - d/dg oligodendroglioma/ependymoma

---

[3] these are (almost organoid) aggregates of neoplastic glial cells in perivascular, perineuronal or sub-pial locations
[4] i.e. aggregation of tumour cell nuclei at the periphery of the infarct *appear* palisaded at low power. Because these nuclei are not actually lined up this appearance is also called 'pseudopalisading necrosis'

- Ependymoma:
  - ➤ papillary formations and rosettes: true (ependymal) and pseudo (perivascular)
  - ➤ nuclei have coarse, clumped chromatin and are more uniform (*cf.* astrocyte nuclei)
  - ➤ degenerative changes: hyaline vessels, myxoid, cartilage/bone/Ca^{2+}, haemorrhage, non-palisaded tumour necrosis (does not upgrade the tumour unless palisaded)
  - ➤ all are grade II except myxopapillary and sub-ependymoma (grade I) and anaplastic (III)
  - ➤ anaplastic features: ↑cellularity, mitoses ++, microvasc. prolif^n, palisading necrosis, D2-40 +ve
  - ➤ immuno: Ki-67 may be prognostic; +ve for GFAP, vimentin, EMA, S100; CK ±ve (focal)
  - ➤ variants: many, but ! distinguish tanycytic (Grade II, occurs within brain/cord parenchyma) from sub-ependymal (Grade 1, mural nodule in ventricle) because these both have similar histology of hyper and hypo cellular areas in a fibrillary background.
- Choroid plexus tumours:
  - ➤ papilloma (grade I): monolayer of amitotic bland cuboidal/columnar cells + brush border
  - ➤ carcinoma (grade III): ≥1 of the following: pleom., mitoses ++, necrosis, ↑NCR, ↑cellularity (incl. solid or spindle foci) – ! d/dg metastatic carcinoma (−ve for D2-40)
  - ➤ immuno: +ve for transthyretin, CK, vimentin, D2-40, S100; ±ve for GFAP and EMA
- Medulloblastoma (grade IV):
  - ➤ infratentorial (cerebellar) location – otherwise it's called a PNET
  - ➤ SBRCT of hyperchromatic cells (nuclei may be carrot-shaped) with ↑NCR
  - ➤ arch.: sheets and focal rhythmic palisaded architecture ± rosettes (*vide infra*)
  - ➤ neuropil fibrillary material emanating from the tumour cells (unlike d/dg lymphoma where the background fibrils belong to the invaded neuropil). In this context Homer-Wright rosettes (have fibrillary centres but no lumen) are useful if present (they are rarely seen in smears).
  - ➤ mitoses and apoptoses
  - ➤ immuno: ±ve for GFAP, synaptophysin, neurofilament protein, S100, NSE, D2-40
  - ➤ retic: intercellular fibres +ve (except in the hypocellular areas of the biphasic *Desmoplastic Medulloblastoma* variant)
  - ➤ d/dg (esp. on smears): granule cells of cerebellum and lymphoma

Pituitary

See pp. 277–279.

Skeletal Muscle

Normal Skeletal Muscle

Staining properties

TABLE 13.3 Muscle fibre staining properties

FIBRE TYPE	I	IIA	IIB
Morphology/Physiology	red, slow, fatigue resistant	white, fast, fatigue resistant	white, fast, fatigue sensitive
Myoglobin (eosinophilia)	+++	+	+
Glycogen (PAS)	+	+++	++
Gomori's trichrome	+++	+	+
Lipid (Sudan)	++	+	±
Mitochondrial enzymes (NADH & cytochrome oxidase)	+++	++	+
ATPase pH 9.4 - pH 9.9	±	++/+++	+++
ATPase pH 4.4 - pH 4.6	+++	±	++
ATPase pH 4.2 (or 4.3)	+++	±	±
Phosphorylase	±	+++	+++

'+ + +' means an intense reaction/'dark' staining whereas '±' means weak/'light' staining.

- Developing (undifferentiated) muscle fibres (= Type IIC) show similar staining properties to Type IIB but have no lipid and show greater ATPase activity at pH 4.2 and greater cytochrome oxidase and succinate dehydrogenase activity
- NADH is often stained for by the tetrazolium reductase method that gives a blue reaction product

Morphology

- Type I fibres are normally of similar size to type II fibres
- A *motor unit* = a single motor neuron (usu. an anterior horn neuron of the spinal cord) plus all the muscle fibres it supplies
- All fibres in a motor unit are of the same type
- Fibres from different motor units are intermingled as a mosaic in any given muscle
- Endomysial connective tissue is very sparse
- <3% of fibres should have central nuclei
- Fibre type proportions in *biceps brachii* and *quadriceps femoris*[5]:
  - ➤ adults = 33:33:33:1 (I:IIA:IIB:IIC)
  - ➤ children = 50:50 (I:II)
- Muscle fibre diameter is defined as the *minor axis diameter* (you first find the maximum diameter then use the longest diameter which is at right angles to this) of the fibre cut in transverse section. The mean measurement of ≥200 fibres is recommended (see Song *et al.*, 1963)
- Fibre diameter varies with age, gender, exercise and site: e.g. (all sizes are given in μ) for adult *quadriceps femoris* the mean diameter ranges from 62–65 (for Type 1 fibres) and 63–66 (Type 2) depending on the component e.g. superficial *vastus lateralis* has means of 63.1 (Type 1) and 63.2 (Type 2) while for deep *vastus lateralis* these become 64.6 and 63.7; for *sternocleidomastoideus* the means are 50.2 (Type 1) and 53.3 (Type 2); for *psoas* 54.5 and 51.7; for deep *biceps brachii* 49.8 and 52.1; for deep *triceps brachii* 57.2 and 62.8; for the 1st *dorsal interosseus* 50 and 67; for medial head of *gastrocnemius* 65 and 66 and for lateral head of *gastrocnemius* 48.4 and 50.5 (data from Polgar *et al.*, 1973)
- In a Bx with a mixed population of small and large fibres, perform the measurement on each population separately (to see if the smallest fibres are atrophic and the largest fibres hypertrophic)
- ! Beware artefacts of sampling (e.g. Bx from near a tendinous insertion may normally show fibrosis and fibre size variation)

Vacuolated Fibres

- Slow freezing artefact: widespread vacuoles of irregular polygonal form that vary in size and may show a gradation in size from one part of the section to another which was less affected
- May be insignificant if only a few and contain glycogen (esp. if not convex and central)
- If full of lipid (Sudan) they usu. connote a metabolic myopathy
- Small vacuoles are also part of inclusion body myositis (*q.v.*)
- Central multiloculated vacuoles (± Ca^{2+}) may be seen in the acute phase of periodic paralysis

Ragged Red Fibres

- Fibres with scattered red blotches by Gomori stain (mitochondria)
- Occur in some mitochondrial myopathies (± lipid vacuoles) and many other myopathies

Type I Fibre-selective Atrophy

- Myotonic dystrophy and other dystrophies
- In congenital myopathies Type I fibres may be small/atrophic but they may predominate numerically

Type II Fibre-Selective Atrophy

- Steroid (glucocorticoid) / thyroid hormone-assoc[d] myopathy
- Disuse atrophy, paraneoplastic atrophy
- MG: also focal lymphoid infiltrates, elongated endplates and (by EM) wide and shallow synaptic clefts
- CTD, polymyalgia rheumatica, polymyositis / dermatomyositis
- Some dystrophies (e.g. Type IIB fibre atrophy in limb girdle dystrophy)

Regeneration

- Central nuclei in small rounded fibres (becoming angulated with time)
- Cytoplasmic basophilia due to RNA (∴ will be pyroninophilic)
- Large vesicular nuclei with prominent nucleoli

---

[5] in the deltoid the proportions vary with depth of Bx

Metabolic Myopathies

Diabetes mellitus
- Thickening of vascular BM in a gastocnemius Bx is said to be diagnostic of diabetes

Others
- Hypothyroidism, mitochondrial myopathies, glycogenoses (types 2, 5 and 7), lipid storage diseases, malignant hyperpyrexia, periodic paralyses and other IEM.
- Histology may be 'suggestive of' or 'consistent with' (e.g. ragged red fibres +/ lipid vacuoles in mitochondrial myopathies) but is usu. not diagnostic – the diagnosis being based on CPC (e.g. oph-thalmoplegia, myoclonus, dementia, etc. in mitochondrial myopathies), biochemistry and genetics.

Neurogenic Myopathies (Denervation and Reinnervation)
- Causes: trauma, peripheral neuropathy (usu. with assoc[d] sensory Sx), CNS motor neuron damage (usu. no sensory Sx – e.g. SMA, MND, etc.)
- Early: +++ (dark) NSEst reaction
- Intermediate: disseminated atrophy: small angulated[6] fibres (that stain +++ with NADH, this is useful since non-neurogenic atrophic fibres do not usu. show this intense NADH reaction) are mixed in amongst normal fibres
- Late:
  - fibre type grouping (due to re-innervation) – some define a 'group' as $\geq$15 fibres of the same type being adjacent to each other – ! distinguish from fibre predominance (*vide infra*)
  - groups of pyknotic nuclei
  - target fibres (central pale zone *with accentuated dark rim* in fibres with NADH and succi-nate dehydrogenase – without the rim they are 'core fibres' that may also occur but are less characteristic of neurogenic atrophy and may be seen in other things incl. central core disease)
- d/dg non-neurogenic myopathies:
  - re-innervation produces groups of type I *and* groups of type II fibres whereas non-neurogenic myopathies show selective atrophy or predominance of one fibre-type that can give an impres-sion of grouping. Some define 'predominance' as >50% of fibres being type I or >80% Type II
  - similarly, neurogenic atrophy produces atrophic fibres of both types

Necroinflammatory and Destructive Myopathies
- Necrotic fibres are pale (on H&E), lack nuclei and striations and are +ve for NADH
- Phagocytosis
- 'Moth-eaten' fibres (i.e. show irregular partial staining for NADH)
- Variation in fibre size and features of regeneration (*q.v.*)
- Endomysial fibrosis
- Some examples:
  - dermatomyositis:
    - ☞ perifascicular necrosis or atrophy
    - ☞ B-cell-rich infiltrate with admixed T4 cells – predom. perivascular
  - polymyositis:
    - ☞ endomysial patchy necrosis
    - ☞ T8 predominant infiltrate – predom. within and around muscle fibres
    - ☞ d/dg facioscapulohumeral dystrophy – but this has hypertrophic fibres
    - ☞ d/dg HIV myopathy – may also show nemaline rods and giant cells
  - in both dermatomyositis and polymyositis the only changes may be Type II fibre atrophy or late changes (fibrosis and variable fibre atrophy). If a CTD vasculitic process is also present there may be superimposed changes of vascular damage (*vide infra*)
  - vascular damage:
    - ☞ features of the vascular lesion (atheroma, arteritis, etc.)
    - ☞ focal necrosis / infarction
    - ☞ neurogenic damage (*vide supra*) due to vasc. compromise of supplying nerves
  - trauma:
    - ☞ if extensive may get scarring
    - ☞ if repeated → continuous myoblast and myofibroblast prolif[n] and granulation tissue (= *proliferative myositis*) + ossification (= *myositis ossificans*). For details, see p. 309.

---

[6] atrophic fibres are rounded in Werdnig-Hoffman disease = infantile SMA (SMA type 1)

> inclusion body myositis:
>> ☞ proximal muscle wasting in middle-aged (clin. d/dg polymyositis unresponsive to steroids)
>> ☞ mixed abnormalities: ± lymphoid infiltrates, ± fibre grouping, fibre hypertrophy (± splitting), ragged red fibres
>> ☞ nuclear inclusions and cytoplasmic vacuoles: best seen on FS and contain smudged pale pink (H&E) material that may contain sparse β-amyloid filaments (Congo red is faint/−ve). Basophilic rimming of the vacuoles by Gomori is characteristic but not specific
> some dystrophies (e.g. Duchenne) – but these usu. have fibre hypertrophy and lack inflam^n
> viruses / drugs / toxins (e.g. influenza, Coxsakie B, HIV, alcohol, penicillamine, snake venom [snake and scorpion venom can also cause an acute ischaemic colitis])
> parasitic infections (e.g. *Trichinella spiralis*, *Echinococcus granulosus*, etc.) – look for eosinophils and parasite morphology (see Chapter 23: Infection and Immunity)
> sarcoidosis: granulomas may have prominent lymphoid infiltrate in early stages (d/dg TB)

Congenital Myopathies

General
- Although muscular dystrophies may be inherited they are not usu. manifest at birth but they are progressive with a poor prognosis. Congenital myopathies are usu. manifest as 'floppy baby' shortly after birth but tend to plateaux or resolve with good prognosis – hence the importance of making the distinction
- They have characteristic histological features but don't show dystrophy-like destructive changes

Centronuclear myopathy (= myotubular myopathy)
- Central nuclei in variably sized fibres. Prognosis may be poor in some infants

Congenital fibre type disproportion
- Atrophy and size variability of Type I fibres (usu. ≥12–15% smaller than Type II)
- Hypertrophy (or normal) Type II fibres

Nemaline rod myopathy
- Should have many rods in most fibres and an appropriate clin. Hx (because these rods are not specific)
- Nemaline rods are clusters of thread-like structures that stain red with Gomori (not obvious on H&E)

Other congenital myopathies
- These include central core disease, multicore disease (= minicore disease) and desmin myopathy

Muscular Dystrophies

General
- Prominent regeneration myocytophagia
- Fibre hypertrophy (± fibre splitting)[7]
- > 3% fibres with central nuclei
- No inflam^n (except in facioscapulohumeral dystrophy or in reaction to necrosis)

Duchenne muscular dystrophy
- Endomysial fibrosis ± adiposity
- Greater variability in fibre size (atrophic and rounded hypertrophic fibres)
- Scattered 'pre-necrotic' fibres (rounded, hypereosinophilic, hyaline)
- Loss of membranous +vity for dystrophin (may be focal)

Becker's muscular dystrophy
- Like Duchenne but less regeneration and necrosis

Myotonic dystrophy
- Type I fibre-selective atrophy
- Features of regeneration
- Ring fibres (a peripheral ring of radial striations seen in a transversely cut fibre) – these are also seen (in smaller numbers) in limb girdle dystrophy and other conditions

Other muscular dystrophies
- These include facioscapulohumeral, distal, scapuloperoneal and oculopharyngeal dystrophies and the ≈ 10 subtypes of limb girdle dystrophy

Tumours
See Chapter 21: Soft Tissues.

---

[7] hypertrophy is useful because non-dystrophy necroinflammatory myositides do not usu. show this (except inclusion body myositis)

Bibliography

Adams, C.W.M. (1989) *A Colour Atlas of Multiple Sclerosis and other Myelin Disorders*, 1st edn, Wolfe Medical Publishers Ltd, UK.

Ang, L.C. (2004) Skeletal Muscle, in *Rosai and Ackerman's Surgical Pathology*, 9th edn (ed J. Rosai), Mosby, Edinburgh, pp. 2663–2681.

Brett, F.M. (1998) Non-Alzheimer degenerative dementias. *Current Diagnostic Pathology*, **5** (3), 118–125.

Braak, H. and Braak, E. (1991) Review: Neuropathological stageing of Alzheimer-related changes. *Acta Neuropathologica*, **82** (4), 239–259.

Cotran, R.S., Kumar, V, and Collins, T. (eds) (1999) *Robbins Pathologic Basis of Disease*, 6th edn, W.B. Saunders Co., Philadelphia.

Farrell, M.A. (1998) The human transmissible encephalopathies. *Current Diagnostic Pathology*, **5** (3), 126–137.

Gearing, M., Mirra, S.S., Hedreen, J.C. *et al.* (1995) The CERAD. Part X. Neuropathology confirmation of the clinical diagnosis of Alzheimer's disease. *Neurology*, **45** (3 Pt 1), 461–466.

Gray, F., Chrétien, F., Vallat-DeCouvelaere, A.V. and Scaravelli, F. (2003) The changing pattern of HIV neuropathology in the HAART era. *Journal of Neuropathology and Experminental Neurology*, **62** (5), 429–440.

Gray, W. and McKee, T. (eds) (2002) *Diagnostic Cytopathology*, 2nd edn, Churchill Livingstone, Edinburgh.

Holloway, P., Kay, E. and Leader, M. (2005) Myxoid tumours: A guide to the morphological and immunohistochemical assessment of soft tissue myxoid lesions encountered in general surgical pathology. *Current Diagnostic Pathology*, **11** (6), 411– 425.

Ince, P.G. (2000) Autopsy in dementing disorders of the elderly. *Current Diagnostic Pathology*, **6** (3), 181–191.

Ironside, J.W. (1999) New variant Creutzfeldt-Jakob disease, in *Recent Advances in Histopathology*, vol. 18 (eds D.G. Lowe and J.C.E. Underwood), Churchill Livingstone, Edinburgh, pp. 1–22.

Kleihaus, P. and Cavenee, W.K. (eds) (2000) *WHO Classification of Tumours: Pathology & Genetics Tumours of the Nervous System*, 1st edn, IARC Press, Lyon.

Love, S. (2006) Demyelinating diseases. *Journal of Clinical Pathology*, **59** (11), 1151–1159.

Lowe, D. (2001) A practical approach to the autopsy in dementia, in *Recent Advances in Histopathology*, vol. 19 (eds D. Lowe and J.C.E. Underwood), Churchill Livingstone, Edinburgh, pp. 163–179.

Lucas, S. (2000) Update on the pathology of AIDS. *Current Diagnostic Pathology*, **6** (2), 103–112.

Mastaglia, F.L. and Walton, J. (eds) (1982) *Skeletal Muscle Pathology*. 1st edn, Churchill Livingstone, Edinburgh.

Nakamura, Y., Kanemura, Y., Yamada, T. *et al.* (2006) D2-40 antibody immunoreactivity in developing human brain, brain tumors and cultures neural cells. *Modern Pathology*, **19** (7), 974–985.

The National Institute on Aging, and Reagan Institute Working Group on Diagnostic Criteria for the Neuropathological Assessment of Alzheimer's Disease (1997) Consensus recommendations for the postmortem diagnosis of Alzheimer's disease. *Neurobiology of Aging*, **18** (4 Suppl.1), S1–S2.

Ng, T.H.K. and Leung, S.Y. (1991) Muscle biopsy: an overview. *Journal of the Hong Kong Medical Association*, **43** (1), 21–25.

Ng, W-K. (2003) Radiation-associated changes in tissues and tumours. *Current Diagnostic Pathology*, **9** (2), 124–136.

Parchi, P., Gambetti, P., Piccardo, P. and Ghetti, B. (1998) Human prion diseases, in *Progress in Pathology*, vol. 4 (eds N. Kirkham and N.R. Lemoine), Churchill Livingstone, Edinburgh, pp. 39–77.

Polgar, J., Johnson, M.A., Weightman, D. and Appleton, D. (1973) Data on fibre size in thirty-six human muscles. An autopsy study. *Journal of the Neurological Sciences*, **19** (3), 307–318.

Romeo, S. and Hogendoom, P.C.W. (2006) Brachyury and chordoma: the chondroid-chordoid dilemma resolved? *Journal Pathology*, **209** (2), 143–146.

Ruprecht, K.W. and Naumann, G.O.H. (1986) The Eye in Systemic Disease, in *Pathology of the Eye*, 1st edn (G.O.H. Naumann and D.J. Apple), Springer-Verlag, NY, pp. 873–956.

Song, S.K., Shimada, N. and Anderson, P.J. (1963) Orthogonal diameters in the analysis of muscle fibre size and form. *Nature*, **200** (Dec 21), 1220–1221.

Sternberg, S.S. (ed) (1997) *Histology for Pathologists*, 2nd edn, Lippincott Williams & Wilkins, Philadelphia.

Symmers, W. St. C. (ed) (1979) *Systemic Pathology*. vol. 5, 2nd edn, Churchill Livingstone, Edinburgh.

Vinters, H.V. (1998) Alzheimer's disease: a neuropathologic perspective. *Current Diagnostic Pathology*, **5** (3), 109–117.

Vujovic, S., Henderson, S., Presneau, N. *et al.* (2006) Brachyury, a crucial regulator of notochordal development, is a novel biomarer for chordomas. *Journal.of Pathology*, **209** (2), 157–165.

Weller, R.O. (1984) Muscle biopsy and the diagnosis of muscle disease, in *Recent Advances in Histopathology*, vol. 12 (eds P.P Anthony and R.N.M. MacSween), Churchill Livingstone, Edinburgh, pp. 259–288.

Wharton, S.B., Fernando, M.S and Ince, P.G. (2003) Neuropathology of hypoxia, in *Recent Advances in Histopathology*, vol. 20 (eds D. Lowe and J.C.E.Underwood), Royal Society of Medicine Press Ltd, London, pp. 129–143.

Young, J.A. (1993) *Fine Needle Aspiration Cytopathology*, 1st edn, Blackwell Scientific Publications, Oxford.

Web sites

Royal College of Pathologists (2004) *Standards and minimum datasets for reporting common cancers: Minimum dataset for the histopathological reporting of tumours of the central nervous system*. www.rcpath.org.uk (accessed May 2005).

14. Eye and Ear

Normal Eye

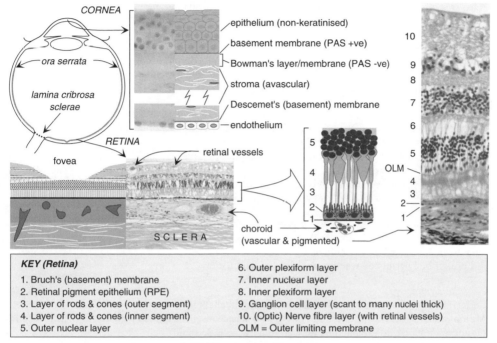

KEY (Retina)

1. Bruch's (basement) membrane
2. Retinal pigment epithelium (RPE)
3. Layer of rods & cones (outer segment)
4. Layer of rods & cones (inner segment)
5. Outer nuclear layer

6. Outer plexiform layer
7. Inner nuclear layer
8. Inner plexiform layer
9. Ganglion cell layer (scant to many nuclei thick)
10. (Optic) Nerve fibre layer (with retinal vessels)
OLM = Outer limiting membrane

FIGURE 14.1   Eye histology

Cysts and Developmental/Inflammatory Conditions

Pterygium
- A 'wing' of vascular granulation tissue encroaching (usu. from the nasal side) on the cornea
- Epithelial actinic changes (incl. upto marked dysplasia)
- Stromal elastosis, basophilic degeneration and hyalinisation
- Destroys Bowman's layer

Hamartia and Hamartoma
- A *hamartia* is a developmental lesion resulting in abnormal arrangements/proportions of tissues that would otherwise have been normally formed at that site. [From the Greek $\alpha\mu\alpha\rho\tau\iota\alpha$ = sin]
- When a hamartia takes the form of a mass it is called a *hamartoma*
- Haemangioma and neuroma/neurofibroma are common examples
- Assoc[d] with the phakomatoses and various syndromes

Chorista, Choristoma, Dermoid and Teratoma
- A *chorista* is a developmental lesion comprising tissue(s) not normally present at a site (i.e. ectopic)
- When a chorista takes the form of a mass it is called a *choristoma*
- Assoc[d] with the phakomatoses and various syndromes e.g. Goldenhar's = limbal dermoids + auricular appendages + vertebral anomalies (= oculoauriculovertebral dysplasia)
- A *dermoid cyst* is lined by epidermis-like epithelium and contains (pilo)sebaceous units ± sweat glands in its wall (unlike an epidermal cyst or an inclusion [= implantation] dermoid cyst) ± a foreign body reaction to spilled contents/keratin

Diagnostic Criteria Handbook in Histopathology: A Surgical Pathology Vade Mecum by Paul J. Tadrous
Copyright © 2007 by John Wiley & Sons, Ltd.

- Dermoids are usu. situated in the orbit (e.g. external angular dermoid) but can be epibulbar (scleral)
- Zimmerman's tumour is a phakomatous choristoma of the lid (made up of lens epithelium) – rare
- A simple choristoma contains a single tissue type (e.g. osteoma or the fibroadipose dermolipoma)
- A complex choristoma contains >1 tissue type (epidermal/dermal, smooth muscle, cartilage, neural, lacrimal, bone, etc.)
- A true *teratoma* is a choristoma containing representatives of all three germ layers (ectoderm, endoderm and mesoderm) and are usu. benign in the eye

Hordeolum (= Stye)
- Acute localised purulent inflammation ($\approx$ 'boil' of the eyelid)
- Centred on pilosebaceous glands of Zeiss (= external hordeolum)
- Centred on a Meibomian gland of the tarsal plate (= internal hordeolum)

Chalazion
- A lipogranuloma of the lid arising from a Meibomian or Zeiss gland or their ducts
- Focal granulomas and abscess around fat
- Giant cells ($\pm$ Schaumann or asteroid bodies), lymphocytes, plasma cells
- d/dg ! do not call it sarcoid or TB
- d/dg juvenile xanthogranuloma – this may occur on the eyelid, conjunctiva, orbit, iris

Amyloid
- Eyelid, conjunctiva, cornea, vitreous, perivascular (retina/choroid)
- Usual features of amyloid (see p. 11)
- May form an isolated *amyloid tumour*
- $\pm$ Foreign-body giant cell reaction & chronic inflammation

Cysts of the Eyelid
- Sudoriferous (apocrine gland of Moll): columnar epithelial lining
- Meibomium (sebaceous): epidermoid lining with sebaceous glands, filled with keratin. The sebaceous glands are not seen all around the cyst wall (otherwise = dermoid)
- Dermoid: epidermoid lining with sebaceous glands all around the cyst wall

Behçet's Disease
- Def^n: ① recurrent uveitis, ② oral aphthae, ③ genital ulceration. [Also get arthritis $\pm$ Crohn's-like ileocaecal disease or colitis]
- Retinal necroses 2° to retinal vasculitis with thromboses
- Vitreous haemorrhage
- Acute and chronic non-granulomatous inflammation of the uveal tract

Reiter's Disease
- Non-specific anterior uveitis
- Conjunctivitis (mixed PMN and lymphocytic with perivascular cuffing)

Juvenile Rheumatoid Arthritis (Still's Disease / Juvenile Chronic Arthritis)
- Granulomatous anterior uveitis (may be sarcoidal)
- d/dg other causes of granulomatous uveitis (*vide infra*)

Rheumatoid Arthritis (Adult)
- Granulomatous scleritis (rheumatoid nodules) $\pm$ perforation and PMN (*scleromalacia perforans*)
- Corneal stromal thinning $\pm$ perforation
- $\pm$ Uveitis

Ankylosing Spondylitis
- Acute iridocyclitis
- Non-granulomatous uveitis

Sjögren's Syndrome (Sjøgren's Syndrome)
- MESA of the lacrimal glands, parotid (see pp. 132–133), other glands and RhA/CTD
- d/dg Mikulicz syndrome = multigland enlargement due to any cause e.g. MESA, sarcoid ('uveo-parotid fever'), TB, lymphoma, lead poisoning, iodide excess, etc., and no CTD association

Granulomatous Uveitis
- Infection: *Brucella*, syphilis, TB, leprosy, Toxocariasis (incl. retinal involvement)
- Immunological: cutaneous tattoo ophthalmitis (cobalt blue pigments), sympathetic ophthalmitis
- Idiopathic: rheumatoid arthritis (adult/juvenile), sarcoidosis

HSV Keratitis
- Corneal epithelial ulceration
- Swelling and inclusions in corneal epithelium
- Disciform keratopathy: oedema and thickening of the stroma with thickening and corrugation of Descemet's membrane

Chlamydial Keratoconjunctivitis (TRachoma and Inclusion Conjunctivitis – TRIC)
- Follicular conjunctivitis
- Papillary hyperplasia of the conjunctiva
- Inclusions are ≈ nucleus-sized collections of Chlamydial elementary bodies in a glycogen matrix (Giemsa and PAS +ve)
- Trachoma: ➢ predominantly affects the upper tarsal
  - ➢ chronic inflam^n goes deep (includes tarsal glands) → scarring, atrophy and distortion
  - ➢ chronic follicular inflam^n at the limbus → trachomatous pannus (pterygium)
- Inclusion Conjunctivitis: ➢ predominantly affects the lower tarsal
  - ➢ superficial inflam^n and no scarring, limbic follicles or pannus
- d/dg other causes of follicular conjunctivitis e.g. adenovirus (this has no papillary hyperplasia, etc.)

Hypertensive Retinopathy

- Histological changes are recognisable in stage III & IV (IV = III + papilloedema)
- Haemorrhage in the nerve fibre layer ('flame') or deeper e.g. inner nuclear layer ('dot/blot')
- Microinfarcts of the nerve fibre layer with vacuolated dilatation of axons ('cytoid bodies')
- Hyaline protein and lipid (± foamy Mϕ) exudates in the outer plexiform layer

Diabetes Mellitus

Anterior Chamber and Ciliary Body

Diabetic iridopathy
- Lacy vacuolation (glycogen accumulation, PAS +ve) of the iris pigment epithelium
Rubeosis iridis
- Not confined to diabetics and seen in association with severe microvasc. disease elsewhere
- Leaky neovascularisation over the anterior iris
- Contractures, synechiae and haemorrhage are accompanying features
Ciliary body
- BM thickening (> expected for age) of the plicated part of the pigment epithelium
- Stromal fibrosis
- Neovascularisation

Diabetic Retinopathy

Non-proliferative retinopathy
- BM thickening ± hyaline arteriolosclerosis-like changes
- Loss of capillary pericytes
- Microaneurysms
- Prominent collateral networks 2° to local ischaemia (intraretinal microvascular anomalies – IRMA)
- Tortuosity and dilatation of veins
- Haemorrhage in the nerve fibre layer ('flame') or deeper e.g. inner nuclear layer ('dot/blot')
- Microinfarcts of the nerve fibre layer with vacuolated dilatation of axons ('cytoid bodies')
- Macular changes: florid oedema or cystoid degeneration (p. 197)
Proliferative retinopathy
- Also seen in oxygen toxicity (retrolental fibroplasia) and ischaemic states (e.g. sickle cell anaemia)
- Thin capillary glomeruloid loops and sheets start in the retina

- Progression involves extension into the vitreous together with fibroblasts & glial cells
- Haemorrhage, contraction and scarring → retinal detachment

Degenerative/Age-Related Changes

Xanthelasma
- Lipid foamy Mφ (as elsewhere)

Pinguecula
- Grey-white conjunctival thickening in the horizontal plane of the palpebral fissure
- Epithelial atrophy with loss of goblet cells ± actinic dysplasia or even hyperplasia
- Stromal elastosis ± granulomatous reaction
- Accumulation of amorphous hyaline material ± Ca^{2+}
- d/dg incl. Gaucher's disease (if the patient is young)

Keratoconus
- Conical bulging of the cornea, begins in teens, F≫M, Down's syndrome > sporadic, bilateral > unilateral
- Apex of cone shows stromal thinning, irregularity and scarring (hypercellularity) ± amyloid
- Bowman's (normally acellular hyaline) layer gets interrupted by cellular foci containing nuclei
- ± Breaks in Descemet's membrane: occur later but may be associated with oedematous thickening of the stroma (clinically presenting as *acute keratoconus*)
- The base/rim of the cone shows Fe deposition in the epithelium (i.e. a Fleischer ring – ! do not confuse with a Kayser-Fleischer ring which shows copper in Descemet's membrane)

Cornea Guttata
- F>M, bilateral, elderly; affects the central cornea; changes of Fuch's occur later (*q.v.*)
- Thickening of Descemet's membrane (with typical EM) in a linear, corrugated and knobbly pattern
- d/dg Hassall-Henle warts (a normal finding after age 20) are identical but are only found at the extreme periphery of the cornea so should not be present on surgically excised corneal specimens
- d/dg ageing results in a non-specific purely linear thickening of Descemet's membrane

Fuch's Combined Corneal Dystrophy
- Refers to the epithelial and subepithelial changes that occur in combination with cornea guttata (*q.v.*)
- Superficial stromal cells insinuate through Bowman's layer to lie horizontally in between that layer and the epithelial basement membrane – this can form a multicellular thick stromal pannus with time
- The overlying epithelial cells show variability in staining intensity
- Late changes: oedema of stroma and epithelium ± bullae (that may rupture)
- d/dg non-specific reactions to injury, oedema or inflam^n can cause a pannus +/ bullae

Corneal Stromal Deposits
- Ca^{2+} (called *bland keratopathy* it esp. affects the superficial stroma incl. Bowman's layer)
- Amyloid: may be familial (incl. TGFβ or gelsolin amyloid in *lattice corneal dystrophy*) or sporadic in many chronic eye diseases e.g. uveitis, sympathetic ophthalmitis, keratoconus, retrolental fibroplasia, glaucoma, trachoma and trauma
- Others: MPS (*macular corneal dystrophy*), actinic eosinophilic change (*climatic droplet keratopathy*)

Cataract
- Similar changes are seen in senile, diabetic and congenital forms but specific subtypes also exist
- Clefts (spaces) filled with the following:
- Eosinophilic globules of Morgagni
- ± Epithelial cells proliferate posteriorly (beyond the equator of the lens)
- ± Ca^{2+} deposition (= hypermature cataract)

Age-related Macular Degeneration (AMD)
- Similar changes are seen in rare genetic conditions
- Atrophy of the macular retina

- ± Fibrous plaque (organised previous haemorrhage from choroidal vessels that perforated up through Bruch's membrane) in the *disciform degeneration* variant
- Disruption of the retinal pigment epithelium ± some epithelial cell clusters remaining
- Accumulations of BM material on Bruch's membrane

Cystoid Degeneration of the Retina
- Similar changes are seen in ageing, diabetes, myopia, neoplasia and inflammatory conditions
- Is considered 'normal' in adults if restricted to foci at the ora serrata without complications
- Most prominent at the periphery/macula regions
- Mucopolysaccharide-filed cysts in the outer plexiform layer of the retina
- Cysts coalesce ± → clefting/retinal detachment/retinal perforation

Melanocytic Lesions

Melanocytic Naevi
- Rarely involve the corneal or tarsal conjunctiva (common at the limbus)
- Pigmentation and size may ↑ after puberty (does not imply malignancy)
- 50% have cyst-like spaces lined by conjunctival epithelium – rare in melanoma or acquired melanosis
- *cf.* skin, they have more chronic inflam[n] and epithelial hyperplasias (! do not misdiagnose as SCC)
- Junctional: ➢ the cords and nests may reach the surface (unlike most skin naevi)
                        ➢ naevocytes may be large
                        ➢ d/dg melanoma: occurrence in childhood and Hx of pre-existing naevus help
- Compound: ➢ junctional activity and apparent atypia may lead to misdiagnosis of melanoma
                        ➢ Spitz/Reed naevi equivalent:
                              ☞ spindle and epithelioid cells (which can be multinucleated)
                              ☞ mitoses more common than in skin
                              ☞ occur in children – !d/dg melanoma
                        ➢ d/dg melanoma: youth and downward maturation help (i.e. favour benignity)
- Subepithelial: ➢ occur in elderly patients
                        ➢ in the substantia propria (≈ lamina propria) – usu. with a Grenz zone
                        ➢ may be heavily pigmented
- Balloon cell: ➢ very large pale naevocytes with central small hyperchromatic nuclei
                        ➢ balloon cells may also be seen in blue naevi and malignant melanoma
- Blue: ➢ well-circumscribed area in conjunctival stroma
           ➢ spindle/dendritic melanocytes in the episclera (i.e. the loose connective tissue external to the sclera)
           ➢ = naevus of Ota if the surrounding skin is also involved (oculodermal melanocytosis)

Melanosis Oculi
- Without atypia: ↑ basal layer pigmentation or basal layer hyperplasia of non-atypical melanocytes
- With mild atypia: polygonal melanocytes with round nuclei and scant cytoplasm
- With moderate/severe atypia: epithelioid, dendritic or spindle melanocytes ± suprabasal extension
Congenital
- Unilateral, darker races, part of Ota's naevus
- Diffuse increase in melanocytes in uvea (incl. *heterochromia iridis*), sclera and episclera
- The conjunctiva is not involved (∴ clin. the pigmentation does not move with it when pulled)
Acquired (epithelial)
- Bilateral: age-related ↑ in conjunctival basal layer pigmentation (≈ ephelis in skin)
- Unilateral: ➢ age >40, pre-malignant[1], poorly-circumscribed irreg. pigmentation in conjunctiva
                   ➢ the melanosis fluctuates (due to variable inflam[n] and pigmentary incontinence)
                   ➢ ↑ pigmentation of conjunctival epithelium (most basally)
                   ➢ variable chronic inflammatory response in the stroma
                   ➢ lesion progression involves progressive lentiginous proliferation of junctional melanocytes with increasing pigmentation, nesting and invasion into the underlying stroma and may be classified by the Zimmerman stage

---

[1] ocular counterpart of *lentigo maligna*

- Zimmerman Stage: I (benign)
    - A. minimal lentiginous/junctional activity
    - B. excessive lentiginous/junctional activity

    II (cancerous – i.e. invasive melanoma, often shows junctional nesting)
    - A. with minimal invasion e.g. <1.5 mm deep (or pT2 i.e. ≤0.8mm deep)
    - B. with extensive invasive growth

Differential Diagnosis (Naevi vs. Melanoma vs. Melanosis)
- Naevi: intra/subepithelial, clinically stationary, cystoids[2] +ve, inflammation ±ve
- Melanoma: intra/subepithelial, clinically progressive, no cystoids, inflammation ++
- Melanosis:
    - ➤ acquired: intraepithelial, 'waxes and wanes', no cystoids, inflammation +
    - ➤ congenital: scleral/episcleral, stationary, heterochromia iridis, no cystoids, no inflammation
- Also, naevi can show any degree of pigmentation but acquired melanosis is heavily pigmented

Conjunctival Melanoma
- 50% arise *de novo*, and 50% from naevi/acquired melanosis
- Suspect melanoma developing in a naevus if there is a size increase not assoc[d] with:
    1. ↑ pigmentation at puberty/pregnancy ± UV/sun exposure
    2. enlargement of cyst-like spaces lined by conjunctival epithelium
    3. inflammation
- Similar histology to skin melanoma – usu. pleomorphic epithelioid cell type
- Depth is measured from the top of the conjunctival epithelium (Jakobiec-Breslow thickness)
- d/dg extension of a uveal melanoma through the sclera[3]

Uveal Melanoma
- Origin in choroid, ciliary body, iris
- There are four main histological types (the modified Callender classification):
    1. Spindle A: thin spindle cells, small elongated nuclei + longitudinal groove, no/inconspicuous nucleoli, ill-defined cell borders, few mitoses
    2. Spindle B: plump spindle cells, ovoid nuclei with coarser chromatin and prominent nucleoli, well-defined borders, mitoses ++
    3. Epithelioid: polygonal cells with pleomorphic nuclei, prominent nucleoli, multinucleate cells, mitoses ++
    4. Mixed (spindle and epithelioid): state % proportions of each type
- Prognostics: spindle types have a better prognosis than epithelioid; melanoma confined to the iris has a very good prognosis regardless of histological type; growth pattern (focal mass, diffuse or ring), trabecular meshwork involvement (for iris lesions), extracellular matrix pattern on PAS (heterogenous, rings or loop networks)

Conjunctival Tumours

- Squamous papilloma
- Squamous carcinoma: usu. exophytic, can be pigmented
- MEC
- Lymphomas: usu. MALTomas, d/dg follicular conjunctivitis, chronic dacroadenitis, chloroma, CLL
- Melanocytic tumours (*vide supra*)
- Sarcomas incl. RMS, leiomyosarcoma and KS
- Myxoma: stellate ± multinucleate myxoma cells (+ve for αSMA and vimentin, −ve for S100 & desmin) ± pale nuclear inclusions, mast cells & AB +ve hypovascular background

---

[2] i.e. cyst-like spaces lined by conjunctival epithelium
[3] conjunctival melanoma is rare *cf.* uveal which is the commonest adult intraocular malignancy

Tumours of the Orbital Tissues and Muscles

- Any soft tissue tumour incl. granular cell tumour, RMS, liposarcoma, endothelial tumours, etc.
- Mesenchymal chondrosarcoma
- Lymphoma: usu. extranodal MZL, other types occur (e.g. FCL, DLBCL) but are less common

Retinoblastoma

- Composed of neuroblasts from cellular layers of the retina
- Growth may be in towards the centre of the vitreous (endophytic) or out through the wall of the globe (exophytic) or both
- Mitotically active small blue oval cell tumour
- Solid sheets, necrosis with perivascular sparing, multifocality, Ca^{2+}
- $\pm$ Fibrillary rosettes with (Flexner-Wintersteiner) or without (Homer-Wright) central lumena
- Immuno: GFAP shows perivascular stromal astrocytes
- d/dg retinoma (retinocytoma) is usu. small, less cellular and is composed of better differentiated photoreceptor cells (more cytoplasm, smaller basal nuclei)

For details important for the report, see p. 44.

The Ear

Accessory Auricles (incl. Tragi)
- Clin: like a FEP near the ear but present at birth $\pm$ other anomalies
- Adnexa-containing skin and adipose $\pm$ central cartilage (d/dg FEP lacks adnexa/cartilage)

Chondrodermatitis Nodularis Helicis
- Clin: painful ulcer on the helix, rarely >1cm, d/dg BCC/SCC
- Ulcer with adjacent dermal vasc. ectasia $\pm$ actinic change $\pm$ PEH (! see clin. d/dg above)
- Underlying granulation tissue and inflam^n involves perichondrium with fibrinoid and eosinophilic degeneration of the cartilage

Malignant Otitis Externa (Necrotising External Otitis)
- *Pseudomonas aeruginosa* cellulitis with poor circulation and $\downarrow$ PMN function (e.g. DM/elderly)
- Acute and chronic inflam^n, necrotic tissue (incl. bone and cartilage when there is osteomyelitis / chondritis), granulation tissue, scarring, Gram $-$ve rods $++$
- Ulceration of the EAM $\pm$ PEH (! d/dg SCC which may also show necrotic tissue)

Aural Polyp (Inflammatory)
- Youths, arise in middle ear ($\pm$ non-ciliated columnar lining) but may protrude through the EAM
- Variably mature granulation tissue, mixed chronic inflam^n, plasma cells $\pm$ big Russell bodies, $\pm Ca^{2+}$
- Cholesterol granulomas may be present (! do not confuse with cholesteatoma, *vide infra*)
- Seek an infective aetiology (e.g. do a Gram and DPAS) and rule out the d/dg below
- d/dg: bacillary angiomatosis, HX, RMS, paraganglioma, other neoplasm

Cholesteatoma (of the Middle Ear)
- This is an acquired (epidermal) or congenital (epidermoid) inclusion cyst of the EAM or external tympanic membrane that erodes into the bone around the middle ear
- Bx usu. shows loose irregular flakes of keratin but stratified squamous epithelium (non-dysplastic) is required for diagnosis
- d/dg SCC is dysplastic and may show desmoplasia or an infiltrative margin
- d/dg *keratosis obturans* shows tightly-packed lamellar keratin flakes

Otosclerosis (of the Endochondral Part of the Temporal Bone)
- Early: resorption of the normal compact lamellar bone ($\pm$ cartilage islands) by vascular fibrous tissue $\rightarrow$ woven bone
- Later: hypercellular, dense, sclerotic, darker-staining woven bone fuses the stapes to its footplate

Neoplasms
- Salivary gland and Schneiderian-type, SCAP, SCC, adenoCA, paraganglioma and soft tissue lesions

External ear: ceruminal gland adenoma/carcinoma
- Apocrine-like cells containing intracytoplasmic brown pigment (ZN +ve and autofluorescent)
- Arch.: papillary, solid cords, cystic ± cribriform
- Adenoma: well-circ. (no capsule), 2-cell type seen focally, ± minor atypia and few mitoses
- Carcinoma: infiltrative, no myoepithelial layer, ± marked atypia/mitoses/ulcerat^n
- d/dg rare ∴ exclude metastatic (e.g. salivary) or middle ear 1°

Middle ear: middle ear adenoma
- Plasmacytoid cells, ± pleom. but rare mitoses, ± NE nucleus, ± AB & DPAS +ve secretions
- Arch.: single cell-lined acini, trabeculae, 'back-to-back', solid sheet; well-circ. (no capsule); sparse stroma
- Immuno: +ve for CK ± NE markers, −ve for vimentin (and −ve for S100 in 85% of cases)
- d/dg carcinoid if NE +ve: most think you should call this 'adenoma with NE differentiation'

Inner ear: endolymphatic sac papillary tumour (= 'low grade adenocarcinoma of probable endolymphatic sac origin')
- Clin: locally aggressive ∴ → radical surgery. May be assoc^d with VHL
- Simple papillae with simple lining (flat to columnar, may be clear ± intracytoplasmic DPAS +ve material; only mild pleom. and rare mitoses)
- Stroma: granulation tissue, haemosiderin ± Ca^{2+} (not psammomatous)
- Thyroid follicle-like areas with DPAS +ve 'colloid' (not thyroglobulin)
- Immuno: +ve for CK ± vimentin, EMA, S100, GFAP and NE markers; −ve for thyroglobulin
- d/dg: mets (RCC, thyroid), 1° middle ear adenoCA (more pleom., mitoses and infiltration; also use CPC − esp. radiol.)

Bibliography

Albert, D. and Syed, N., Cancer Committee, College of American Pathologists (2001) Protocol for the examination of specimens from patients with uveal melanoma. A basis for checklists. *Archives of Pathology and Laboratory Medicine*, **125** (9), 1177–1182.

Arnold, W.J., Laissue, J.A., Friedmann, I. *et al.* (1987) *Diseases of the Head and Neck*, 1st edn, Thieme Medical Publishers Inc., NY.

Berns, S. and Pearl, G. (2006) Middle ear adenoma. *Archives of Pathology and Laboratory Medicine*, **130** (7), 1067–1069.

Demirci, H., Shields, C.L., Eagle Jr, R.C. *et al.* (2006) Report of a conjunctival myxoma case and review of the literature. *Archives of Ophthalmology*, **124** (5), 735–738.

Domizio, P., Lowe, D. and McCartney, A. (1997) Eye, in *Reporting Histopathology Sections*, 1st edn (eds P. Domizio and D. Lowe), Chapman & Hall Medical, London, pp. 356–365.

Firkin, B.G. and Whitworth, J.A. (1987) *Dictionary of Medical Eponyms*, 1st edn, The Parthenon Publishing Group, Lancs., UK.

Hughes, G.R.V. (1977) *Connective Tissue Diseases*, 1st edn, Blackwell Scientific Publications, Oxford.

Norton, A.J. (2006) Monoclonal antibodies in the diagnosis of lymphoproliferative diseases of the orbit and orbital adnexae. *Eye*, **20** (10), 1186–1188.

Ruprecht, K.W. and Naumann, G.O.H. (1986) The Eye in Systemic Disease, in *Pathology of the Eye*, 1st edn, (eds G.O.H. Naumann and D.J. Apple), Springer-Verlag, NY, pp. 873–956.

Sternberg, S.S. (ed) (1997) *Histology for Pathologists*, 2nd edn, Lippincott Williams & Wilkins, Philadelphia.

Symmers, W. St. C. (ed) (1980) *Systemic Pathology*, Vol. 6, 2nd edn, Churchill Livingstone, Edinburgh.

Völcker, H.E. and Naumann, G.O.H. (1986) Conjunctiva, in *Pathology of the Eye*, 1st edn (eds G.O.H. Naumann and D.J. Apple), Springer-Verlag, NY, pp. 249–316.

Wheater, P.R., Burkitt, H.G. and Daniels, V.G. (1987) *Functional Histology: A text and colour atlas*, 2nd edn, Churchill Livingstone, Edinburgh.

Yanoff, M. and Fine, B.S. (1982) *Ocular Pathology: A text and atlas*, 2nd edn, Harper & Row Publishers, Ltd, Philadelphia.

15. Renal Medicine

Normal and Age-Related Changes

- The blood supply of the tubules is mainly from the efferent arteriole (∴ any scarring glomerular disease → ischaemic tubules → interstitial fibrosis and tubular atrophy)
- Cellularity (in a 3μ H&E section): capillary loops – 0 nuclei; mesangium – 2–4 nuclei
- Adequacy of a renal Bx: need ≥20 glomeruli not to miss focal disease
- Sclerosed glomeruli (= global acellular sclerosis): ≪5% till 30 years then [age/2]-10 gives the 90th centile (from Smith *et al.*, 1989). *Segmental* sclerosis is not normally seen
- Ageing: arterioles: hyaline change; arteries: fibrous intimal thickening and reduplication of the IEL

Clinical Presentation and Syndromes

Nephrotic Syndrome
- **P**roteinuria (3–10g/d), **O**edema, **H**ypoalbuminaemia: [HT, ↓renal function, hyperlipidaemia, infections]
- Macro: kidneys are large and pale (due to oedema) with yellow streaks in the cortex
- Micro: ➤ foamy Mφ ± cholesterol granulomas
              ➤ hyaline and fatty droplets in PCT
              ➤ hyaline casts in DCT
              ➤ EM: effaced foot processes (pedicel 'fusion') due to cytoplasmic swelling
- Causes: ➤ 1° glomerular (minimal change disease, FSGS and all GN but crescentic)
              ➤ 2° to systemic disease (D.A.S.H.I.N.)[1] and drugs

Nephritic Syndrome
- **O**edema (± effusions), **H**T (± encephalopathy), **O**liguria: [microhaematuria, protein, granular casts]
- Causes: usu. glomerulonephritis of ADP / RPC / focal and segmental types

Asymptomatic Proteinuria
- Causes: many, but if proteinuria is asymptomatic renal damage is usu. slight, early or not obvious

Painless Haematuria
- With dysmorphic erythrocytes on urine cytology
- Causes: IgA nephropathy and some hereditary nephritides (Alport's and thin membrane disease)

Hypertension
- Causes are many: renal, vascular and systemic

Renal Failure or Impaired Renal Function
- Causes of ARF: ATN, various GN, acute interstitial nephritis, vasculitides/CTD, Goodpasture's disease and myeloma
- Causes of CRF: advanced chronic renal disease may be difficult to diagnose but try to distinguish between glomerulonephritic (e.g. IgA nephropathy) or non-glomerulonephritic (e.g. DM)

General Points on Histological Interpretation and Reporting

- *Stage*: always give an estimate of the degree of irreversible chronic damage i.e. % scarring and tubule atrophy (see the Banff system on p. 209 for a method) – in any disease, not just Tx rejection
- *Grade*: give the nõ and % of glomeruli showing 'active lesions' (for an example, see SLE, p. 204)
- Report: a) what is present (cortex +/ medulla), b) the maximum nõ of glomeruli on any single section, the % sclerosed and a description of any glomerular lesions, c) any tubular lesion and % tubular loss, d) state of the interstitium, e) the nõ and type of blood vessels and any changes, f) immuno and EM, e) conclusions

---

[1] Diabetes, Amyloid, SLE, HSP, Infection, Neoplasia

Diagnostic Criteria Handbook in Histopathology: A Surgical Pathology Vade Mecum by Paul J. Tadrous
Copyright © 2007 by John Wiley & Sons, Ltd.

- Describe the location and *pattern* of immunostaining: linear / granular, mesangial / loops
- Some IgM often deposits in the mesangial matrix and doesn't mean much unless intense ($\rightarrow$FSGS)
  [*NB*: some regard FSGS as the severe end of a spectrum: minimal change disease $\rightarrow$ steroid dependent / resistant minimal change disease with mesangial IgM $\rightarrow$ mesangial expansion with IgM ($\pm$ C3 and minor amounts of IgA / IgD) + glomerular capillary hypercellularity (the so-called 'mesangioproliferative glomerulopathy'[2] or 'IgM nephropathy') $\rightarrow$ FSGS]
- IgG/M deposition is usu. not significant (= serum background-staining) unless the pattern is continuous and linear +/ complement is also deposited *but...*
- C3 can be unreliable with immunoperoxidase $\therefore$ use a panel that includes others e.g. C9 or C1q
- The odd glomerular PMN may be seen in any proliferative lesion – it does not imply ADP GN

Glomerulonephritis

Clinical Perspective on GN
- The nasty ones are RPC GN, membranoproliferative GN and FSGS. The others are usu. more indolent and prognosis depends on the underlying cause
- Look for cholesterol emboli (foam cells, fat stain +ve, birefringent fat on FS) if a 'vasculitic' FSGN is proposed or in the d/dg of TMA. Cholesterol emboli usu. occur in vasculopaths (e.g. IHD), following repair of an aortic aneurysm or following removal of a graft kidney from an atheromatous donor
- The commonest 1° glomerular causes of the nephrotic syndrome are:
  - ➢ (child) minimal change / FSGS
  - ➢ (adult) membranous / FSGS
- The commonest cause of an RPC GN is P-ANCA +ve microscopic polyarteritis
- HSP may present with an ADP GN picture (not just FSGN / RPC GN)
- For an urgent Bx you must decide if the kidney is viable, whether the disease is acute / chronic, and where the main seat of disease is (glomeruli, tubulointerstitium, vessels, etc.)

Chronic Glomerulonephritis
- Macro: granular contracted kidney (for d/dg reflux nephropathy, see p. 213)
- Hyalinised glomeruli
- Interstitial fibrosis, chronic inflammation and tubular atrophy
- The type of preceding GN is usu. not recognisable but most are thought to be IgA nephropathy

Acute Diffuse Proliferative GN (Post-infective ADP GN)
- Youths (but all ages), nephritic / subclinical, low C3, post infective (*Strep.*/EBV/HCV/malaria)
- Most youths recover but 50% of older patients develop RPC GN and die
- Rx: *not* steroids
- *Macro:* large and pale kidney with grey dot glomeruli in an expanded cortex.
- *Micro:* large hypercellular glomeruli (incl. PMN, esp. if $\geq$5), $\pm$ a few crescents, $\uparrow$ mesangial cells
- *Immuno:* granular IgG and C3
- *EM:* subepithelial 'humps' (nõ. $\propto$ severity)
- *Elsewhere:* protein and RBC casts $\pm$ ischaemic tubules

Rapidly Progressive Crescentic GN
- Older (but all ages), insidious malaise, oedema, dyspnoea
- 1° Pauci-immune GN (= idiopathic) / post *Strep.* $\frac{2}{3}$ have p-ANCA, $\frac{1}{3}$ c-ANCA
- 2°: Goodpasture's (young M) / vasculitides (WG, S.H.I.P.[3])
- Rx: immunosuppression $\rightarrow$ temporary remission else RF in days–months (ANCA +ve cases may be curable)
- *Macro:* $\pm$ large and pale kidney with grey dot glomeruli and petechiae
- Micro: ➢ diffuse segmental proliferation & cellular crescents (in >70% of glomeruli)
  - ➢ $\pm$ haemorrhagic necrosis of capillaries $\rightarrow$ scarring (d/dg TMA / HUS – see p. 207)
- *Immuno:* crescents contain fibrin but not Ig
- *EM:* crescents do not contain immune complexes

---

[2] !do not confuse with mesangioproliferative glomerulo*nephritis* (p. 203)
[3] SLE, HSP, Infective endocarditis, microscopic Polyarteritis (malaise, purpura, arthralgia)

- *Elsewhere:* as for ADP but more severe. Reporting of the vasculitides should incl. % active tubular inflam^n/necrosis and % glomeruli that are/have: ① normal, ② segmental scars, ③ crescents, ④ necrosis

Membranous GN
- Older men, insidious nephrotic syndrome, ± microhaematuria (never gross)
- 1° idiopathic (majority)
- 2° to **S**arcoid, **I**nfection (malaria, HBV, syphilis), **N**eoplasia, **D**rugs (gold, penicillamine, ACEI)
- Rx: diuretics *not* steroids; over 10 years 50% → CRF
- *Macro:* nephrotic changes (see p. 201)
- Micro: ➢ no proliferation
            ➢ hyaline BM thickening → narrow loop lumens → ↓ GFR
            ➢ silver 'spikes' in vertical section / bubbly 'chain-mail' in tangential section
- *Immuno:* peripheral granular IgG (± C3) *in situ* complex formation
- *EM:* multiple, almost confluent, subepithelial deposits
- *Elsewhere:* tubular atrophy and scarring, nephrotic changes (see p. 201), changes of any 1° disease

Membranoproliferative GN Types I – III (MPGN or 'Mesangiocapillary GN')
- nephrotic / nephritic (esp. type II) / asymptomatic proteinuria, low C3
- 1° (most are now known to be post HCV cryoglobulinaemia) / 2° (infective endocarditis, malaria, HCV)
- Type II may be familial (assoc^d with partial lipodystrophy and Factor-H deficient TMA)
- Rx: symptomatic, *not* steroids; most → CRF. Type II may recur in a transplanted kidney.
- Micro: ➢ (diffuse prolif^n, accentuated lobulation, narrowed loops) → ↓ cells, ↑ hyaline → GS
            ➢ double contour BM (also seen in PET and many causes of glomerular TMA)
            ➢ crescents are more common with type II
- *Immuno:* C3 and IgG +/ IgM, granular and peripheral (i.e. involving capillary loops)
- *EM:* I – discrete subendothelial immune complex deposits, mesangial interposition and subendothe-lial new BM formation
         II – 'dense deposit disease' – due to underlying defect of the BM. BM splits around *dense deposits* (= BM material damaged by circulating anti-C3bBb Ab i.e. 'nephritic factor'). *NB:* Only 25% show MPGN by LM – most show mesangial prolif^n, ADP or cresentic GN
         III – very rare, subendothelial and subepithelial deposits

Mesangial Proliferative GN (Mesangioproliferative GN)
- ↑ Cellularity ± ↑ matrix in the mesangium without capillary loop involvement
- Common with IgA nephropathy (more common than FSGN) and SLE
- Many other causes e.g. the healing phase of ADP GN

Focal Segmental GN (FSGN)
- 1° (= IgA nephropathy = Berger's disease),[4] common adult GN, recurrent haematuria ± nephritic syndrome, assoc^d with IgA mucositis / liver disease (some only diagnose Berger's in the absence of this)
- 2° to WG, S.H.I.P. and Goodpasture's; (**H**. is a variant of Berger's disease, **I**. is assoc^d with low C3)
- Rx: immunosuppression in some cases (!but see d/dg below); upto 50% → CRF
- *Micro:*   ➢ focal and segmental prolif^n ± fibrinoid necrosis / thrombosis (d/dg TMA/HUS *q.v.*)
              ➢ ± RBC in Bowman's space / tubules
              ➢ ± small cellular crescents
- *Immuno:* 1°: IgA and C3 (mesangial)[5] 2°: **H**. as for 1°, **I**. shows IgG, **P**. pauci-immune, **S**. full house
- *EM:* subendothelial and mesangial deposits
- *Elsewhere:* infarcts and vasculitis (in the case of microscopic polyarteritis)
- d/dg: cholesterol emboli: these can mimic vasculitic rash and give FSGN – !do NOT immunosuppress

---

[4] *IgA nephropathy* is also known as mesangial IgA disease as deposits are usu. mesangial and often large, appearing as eosinophilic PAS +ve tiny drops on LM. IgA/M in the capillary loops or mesangial IgG are poor prognostics. Grade should include % gloms with: ① cellular crescents, and ② segmental necrosis. Percent of cortical myofibroblasts by αSMA immuno correlates with advancing stage
[5] often with IgM, full house occurs in 25% of Berger's – then go by predominant staining: predominantly IgA favours Berger's, predominantly IgG favours lupus (a 'mixed' GN morphology also favours SLE)

Focal Segmental Glomerulosclerosis (FSGS)
- Nephrotic, HT and microhaematuria common (2° to parenchymal loss); FSGS circulating factor
- 1° (idiopathic) / 2° (HIV, IVDA 'heroin nephropathy'); most → CRF after years; recurs in Tx
- *Macro:* changes of the nephrotic kidney (see p. 201)
- *Micro:*   ➤ juxtamedullary large glomeruli with focal and segmental hyaline obliteration
  - ➤ becomes global and diffuse with time
  - ➤ silver stain highlights segmental scars
- *Immuno:* IgM and C3 granular/nodular. Lack of IgG helps exclude the resolving phase of ADP GN
- *Elsewhere:* nephrotic changes, tubule atrophy (and large thyroidal tubular casts and inflammation in the 'collapsing FSGS' variant often assoc^d with HIV)

Minimal Change Disease (Lipoid Nephrosis)
- Nephrotic syndrome, usu. in children, selective albuminuria, no HT / haematuria
- 1° (most) / 2° (atopy/allergy/lymphomas/other malignancy)
- Rx: spontaneous resolution or steroids; may relapse (and some may progress to FSGS)
- *Macro:* changes of the nephrotic kidney (see p. 201)
- *Micro:* fixed dilated capillaries and nephrotic changes (see p. 201)
- *Immuno:* −ve
- *EM:* pedicel 'fusion' or 'effacement' (= cytoplasmic swelling) assoc^d with loss of polyanion

The Kidney in Systemic Disease

Diabetic Nephropathy
- Clin. progression is: asymptomatic proteinuria → HT and nephrotic → CRF (granular contracted kidney)
- Hyaline arteriolosclerosis: worse in afferent *cf.* efferent (and both are worse *cf.* HT / old age)
- Nodular glomerulosclerosis (Kimmelstiel-Wilson lesion) is more characteristic of DM, but diffuse glomerulosclerosis is more ∝ to renal function. Sclerosis is assoc^d with microangiopathy elsewhere (e.g. retina)
- *Immuno:* glomerular and tubular BM: linear IgG (but not C3); sclerotic lesions: IgM, C3, κ and λ all ±ve
- *EM:* pedicel 'fusion', ↓ podocytes per glomerulus, ± mesangial bundled diabetic fibrillosis
- Other lesions: fibrin cap, capsular drop, mesangial expansion, glomerular capillary microaneurysm, renal artery atheroma, renal papillary necrosis, UTI / acute pyelonephritis, interstitial scarring
- d/dg nodular glomerulosclerosis: other hyaline deposits (e.g. amyloid, fibrillary glomerulopathy, MIDD, macro/cryoglobulins), advanced MPGN, idiopathic nodular glomerulosclerosis

HIV Nephropathy
- FSGS (*q.v.* – esp. the collapsing FSGS variant)
- EM: tubuloreticular structures and cylindrical confronting cisternae (esp. the latter)
- Rx-related effects and opportunistic infections e.g. CMV

Systemic Lupus Erythematosus and the 2003 ISN/RPS Lupus Nephritis Classes
Class 1: glomeruli normal by LM but immuno shows mesangial deposits
Class 2: mesangial disease only (hypercellularity) by LM with mainly mesangial deposits by immuno/EM
Class 3: focal GN: global/segmental, active (proliferative) +/ chronic (sclerosing)
Class 4: diffuse GN: global (≥1/2 the tuft is involved in ≥50% of the affected glomeruli)/segmental, active +/ chronic
Class 5: membranous GN ± advanced sclerosis
Class 6: chronic GN ('advanced sclerosis'): ≥90% of the glomeruli are totally sclerosed and inactive
- Rx: aims to transform 3/4 (proliferatives) to 1, 2 or 5
- There may be more than one class in a given biopsy (e.g. class 2 and 5)
- Any 'active lesions' make the class 2 (if focal) or 3 (if diffuse): i.e. PMN/leukocytoclasia, crescents with some cellularity, hyaline 'wire loop' lesions (due to massive subendothelial deposits), lilac haematoxyphile bodies, hyaline/fibrin thrombi or segmental fibrin
- 'Diffuse' disease is defined as ≥50% of glomeruli are involved (in the past, >80% was used)
- Give the nõ and % of glomeruli with: ① any active lesion, ② crescents and ③ fibrinoid necrosis
- Interstitial nephritis may be the more predominant disease

- ± Lupus vasculopathy: hyaline deposits and myocyte dropout in media and intima of terminal inter-lobular arteries and afferent arterioles, immuno +ve for Ig, complement and fibrin (d/dg TMA which may also occur due to antiphospholipid Abs but has a better prog.)
- Immuno: ➤ full house i.e. IgG/A/M, C3, C4, C1q complex (mesangial/subendothelial/epithelial)
            ➤ mixture of GN patterns favours LE (e.g. membranous with hypercellular mesangium)
            ➤ mesangial immune deposits favour LE (but IgA may be Berger's disease)
            ➤ presence of IgA/M without IgG is unlike lupus and the aetiology should be questioned

Renal Amyloidosis
- 1°/2°; pericapillary deposition and obliteration (nephrotic → CRF)
- Can get spiking of BM in amyloid (d/dg membranous GN)
- Nodular deposits (d/dg DM, light chain, advanced mesangiocapillary GN)
- Negative Congo Red does not rule out amyloid – even if properly done – ∴ need EM
- d/dg fibrillary and immunotactoid glomerulopathies, cryoglobulinaemia

Myeloma Kidney
- May lead to ARF/CRF

Myeloma cast nephropathy
- BJP is toxic to tubule epithelial cells and casts[6] erode tubules → giant cell[7] and PMN inflam^n
- d/dg innocuous hyaline casts: in myeloma at least some of the casted tubules will not have a flat, atrophic lining; these are the innocuous ones. Pure Tamm-Horsfall casts are intensely DPAS +ve (but weakly +ve if diluted by paraproteins)
- d/dg TORi toxicity post-Tx (see p. 210)

Paraprotein deposition
- Amyloid / κ light chains are deposited in vessels, glomeruli, tubules (light chain nephropathy)

Nephrocalcinosis
- Ca^{2+} in tubule epithelial cells and BM → interstitial fibrosis and chronic inflam^n → ± CRF

Associated features
- Plasma cell infiltrates, urate crystals (gout), nephrotoxic effects of drugs

Light Chain Nephropathy
- Due to *nonfibrillary* light chains (unlike amyloid)
- Nephrotic / proteinuria, HT, CRF; myeloma may or may not be present
- *LM:* lobular accentuation and PAS +ve[8] mesangial nodules (κ) [also in glomerular and tubule BM]
- *Immuno:* κ ≫ λ (may be −ve as Fc may be missing ∴ urine may also be −ve for light chains)
- d/dg membranous GN / DM nodular GS (if ?DM but no hyaline arterioles, consider light chain disease), amyloid, advanced mesangiocapillary GN
- d/dg other forms of MIDD i.e. heavy chain or mixed light chain and heavy chain deposition disease

Hereditary Nephritis

Alport's Disease
- AD/XL; both sexes: haematuria; males: proteinuria, ↓renal function, spherophakia, nerve deafness
- *LM:* normal / FSGN
- *Immuno:* −ve
- *EM:* multilamination / splitting / trabeculation / fragmentation of glomerular capillary, tubular and Bowman's capsular BM (! may be focal and also reported in d/dg post *Strep.* ADP GN, Berger's disease and thin membrane disease)

Thin Membrane Disease (Benign Familial Haematuria)
- Usu. AD but non-familial cases occur; variable haematuria, ↑ incidence of HT, ± other renal disease.
- *LM:* minimal change or ↑ sclerotic glomeruli / mesangial thickening
- *EM:* thin glomerular BM must be measured carefully (! tangential artefacts), *lamina densa* is preserved

---

[6] These acellular casts (BJP & Tamm-Horsfall protein) may stain for amyloid. The κ and λ immuno is hard to interpret. Glomerular capillaries may be involved ('hyaline thrombi') in Waldenström's

[7] giant cells can appear intratubular as well as interstitial

[8] silver stain negative (unlike d/dg ↑ mesangial matrix)

Fabry's Disease
- Treatable XL recessive lysosomal storage disease (glycosphingolipid accumulates in many organs – esp. epithelial, endothelial and smooth muscle cells incl. cornea, synovium and solid organs)
- *LM:* foam cells (podocytes) in the glomeruli, endothelial and epithelial (incl. tubular) cells show PAS +ve vacuoles; immuno is −ve
- *EM:* myeloid bodies (= irregular lamellated lipid inclusions) in the podocytes or tubular epithelium
- Is assoc^d with multiple angiokeratomas of the skin (*angiokeratoma corporis diffusum*)

MPGN II: (see p. 203)

Tubulointerstitial and Vascular Disease

Potassium Deficiency (Hypokalaemia)
- Macrovesicular vacuolation of PCT cells (unlike d/dg cyclosporin toxicity – p. 209)

Acute Pyelonephritis
- PMN in tubules

Acute Tubular Necrosis
- Clin.: ARF ± oliguria → normal in days/weeks (but 50% mortality)
- Aetiology: ischaemic (medical/surgical/obstetric), nephrotoxic (drugs/chemicals/pigments)
- Macro: pale oedematous cortex and dark congested medulla (enhanced corticomedullary differentiation)
- Micro:
  - interstitial oedema and focal Ca^{2+} (oxalate)
  - focally dilated tubules with sloughing of PCT brush border (PCTs look like DCTs)
  - ± necrosis of tubule epithelial cells ± tubulorrhectic inflam^n
  - after 1 week: mitoses and regenerative atypia
  - 'tubular cell unrest' (anisocytosis of tubular cells)
  - ± mild tubulitis (i.e. < 4 mononuclear cells, see p. 208)
  - casts in DCT (protein or granular)
  - in renal Tx kidneys, ATN may show:
    - more interstitial inflam^n and calcifications
    - less 'unrest', casts and brush border damage
    - foci of full-cross sectional tubule necrosis

Renal Papillary Necrosis (Causes)
① diabetes mellitus
② analgesic nephropathy
③ vascular occlusion e.g. sickle cell disease, leukaemia, etc.
④ urinary tract obstruction
⑤ haemorrhagic necrosis of papillae in the newborn

Interstitial Nephritis
- Interstitial scarring (fibrosis) as seen in any GN with a chronic component contains a chronic inflammatory infiltrate which does *not* imply interstitial nephritis
- Granulomas in the kidney are *not* usu. related to drugs (*cf.* in the liver)
- The three main aetiological categories are:
① Drugs
'Acute' interstitial nephritis
- For example, due to penicillin or quinine; mediated by anti-tubule Abs
- Mixed chronic inflam^y cell infiltrate (incl. eosinophils) with tubule destruction
- Glomeruli are spared (or involved by a drug-induced TMA)
Analgesic nephropathy
- Papillary necrosis with overlying chronic inflam^y infiltrate
- ± Metaplastic bone / Ca^{2+}
- Glomeruli are spared
② Radiation

Radiation nephropathy
- Vascular changes incl. fibrinoid necrosis (without severe HT) – see also p. 72
- Stromal fibrosis and tubular atrophy
- Glomerular capillary loop thickening and fusion
③ Metabolic:
Urate nephropathy (gout)
- Fibrosis, tubule atrophy and medullary stromal urate crystals ± renal urate calculi
- Medullary collecting tubule uric acid crystals and giant cell reaction
- Atrophy of corresponding nephrons ($\rightarrow$ granular contracted kidney)
- Superimposed HT changes
Nephrocalcinosis
- Intra- and extratubular Ca^{2+}
Cystinosis
- Multinucleated podocytes

Thrombotic Microangiopathy (TMA)
- TMAs are non-inflammatory thrombotic vasculopathies (d/dg vasculitis – ! although some TMA lesions may be seen downstream of classical vasculitides). The thrombi are +ve for FVIIIRA
- Clinically thrombocytopenia, red cell fragmentation and ↑LDH (due to tissue hypoxia) may be seen (= TTP if there is deficiency of FVIIIRA proteases or = HUS if there is ARF)
- May predominantly affect glomeruli, afferent arterioles and other small arteries/arterioles $\propto$ cause
- Arteriole-capillary TMA: platelet-rich thrombi ± lumenal microaneurysmal dilatation. May heal by re-endothelialisation ($\rightarrow$ subendothelial hyaline humps) ± recanalisation ($\rightarrow$ glomeruloid structures)
- Glomerular TMA:
  - ➤ normal cellularity or ↑ PMN but not otherwise inflam^y and no immune deposits. May lead to glomerular sclerosis or cortical necrosis if severe
  - ➤ bloodless glomeruli with fibrin thrombi and an eosinophilic 'double contour' on H&E (thickening of capillary wall and subendothelial space expansion – ! do not confuse with BM double contouring on silver stains [which, if present, usu. indicates a more chronic and less destructive course])
  - ➤ engorged and partly necrotic glomeruli ('glomerular paralysis') due to distal thrombosis
- Small artery-arteriole severe TMA ('malignant vascular injury') is essentially the same lesion as found in malignant HT with myxoid and proliferative endarteritis, fibrinoid necrosis and variable thrombosis and occurs in malignant HT, HUS and PSS renal crises (= PSS + HT + ARF). Assoc^d focal tissue ischaemia/necrosis is more common with this form
- Causes include: drugs (incl. quinine, OKT3, cyclosporin and tacrolimus), post Tx humoural rejection, Type II MPGN (and other causes of factor-H deficiency), bacterial toxins (*Shigella*, *E.coli* phage), radioRx, chemoRx (esp. mitomycin C), antiphospholipid Ab syndromes (± SLE) and anti-endothelial Ab states (e.g. post *Strep. pneumoniae*), viruses (HIV, CMV, parvovirus B19), pregnancy / puerperium, paraneoplastic, any cause of TTP / HUS and idiopathic
- In glomerular TMA, accompanying mesangiolysis and BM reduplication is not usu. seen with infective toxin-assoc^d cases but may be seen with the other causes (and also in PET)
- Effects ($\propto$ cause and severity): resolution, glomerular sclerosis, tubular damage ± RF
- d/dg: vasculitis (inflam^n, immune markers, CPC), chronic allograft glomerulopathy (also has other changes of chronic rejection), DIC (platelet poor, FVIIIRA −ve thrombi and moribund patient)
- d/dg PET (large and bloodless glomeruli due to endothelial swelling occluding the lumens, double contour BM due to mesangial interposition, glomerular capillary partial prolapse into the PCT – but no arterial/arteriolar changes of TMA, also PET changes resolve 3–6 months post partum)
- d/dg venous thrombosis (go by CPC if a thrombosed vein is not sampled)
- d/dg hyaline glomerular thrombi of light chain or Waldenström's type (glomerular hypercellularity and immuno for IgM/κ/λ and CPC)
- d/dg cholesterol emboli (*vide supra* under 'Clinical Perspectives on GN' on p. 202)

Renal Transplant and Rejection Pathology

General Considerations
- Rejection changes are widespread but can be focal ∴ consider sampling effect
- Some of the changes may have been present in the donor (! overrating rejection severity)

- Effect of opportunistic infections (e.g. CMV or polyoma)
- Effects of drugs (e.g. see CNI and TORi on pp. 209–210) $\Big\}$ incl. TMA ± HUS
- Recurrence of 1° renal disease in the graft
- Obstructive effects: lymphatics distended with protein, dilated ducts in the outer cortex ± a foreign body-type granulomatous response to disrupted tubules
- For details and illustrations see: http://tpis.upmc.edu/ and specialist texts

Tubulitis
- Defined according to the Nō. of mononuclear cells per 10 tubular epithelial cells (or per tubule cross section) in the worst affected tubules as:
  - ➢ mild tubulitis: 1–4 mononuclear cells
  - ➢ moderate tubulitis: 5–10 mononuclear cells
  - ➢ severe tubulitis: >10 mononuclear cells

  > do not include areas with interstitial fibrosis and tubular atrophy because these may have non-specific lymphocytic infiltration

- ! If patient is on CAMPATH1 anti-lymphocyte Rx, the above definitions may be meaningless
- d/dg: mild tubulitis (<4 cells) may occur in non-Tx kidneys and non-rejection states e.g. mild ATN or cyclosporin toxicity; other d/dg incl. viral infection (esp. CMV or polyoma)

Preservation Injury
- ATN-like changes in the tubules (see p. 206)

Hyperacute Rejection (hours–days)
- Ab-mediated (humoural) damage to endothelia → arterial thromboses
- Glomerular congestion and glomerular capillary thromboses, PMN ± necrosis
- Interstitial tissue infarcts and haemorrhage, PMN margination in peritubular vessels
- Immuno: −ve or linear deposits of IgG ± IgM; +ve for C3 and fibrin in small vessel walls (not limited to glomeruli)
- 'Accelerated acute rejection' is a variant of this humoural rejection manifesting as episodes of ↓ renal function over the first few days. 'Delayed accelerated acute rejection' is the same as accelerated rejection but starts after a few weeks (this happens when the prior exposure to the offending Ags occurred a long time before transplantation)
- d/dg other causes of thromboses: cold-ischaemia-induced graft vascular endothelial damage (shows less active inflam^n *cf.* rejection), systemic vasculitis, DIC, calcineurin-inhibitor toxicity (use CPC)
- ! Do not confuse with the acute and chronic forms of 'Humoural / Ab-Mediated Rejection' that occurs later and is defined by C4d deposition and circulating anti-donor HLA / ABO Abs described below

Acute Cellular Rejection (weeks–years)
- Glomeruli spared (unless co-existent vascular rejection – *vide infra*)
- Mixed mononuclear interstitial infiltrate (predom. T8) ± granulocytes
- Tubulitis (*vide supra*)
- Interstitial fibrosis and oedema

$\Big\}$ d/dg PTLPD which is destructive and B-cell predominant

Acute Vascular Rejection (weeks–years)
- Endothelialitis (MPS intimal thickening, lymphocytes, endothelial cell swelling and shedding)
- Transmural vasculitis (± fibrinoid necrosis)
- ± Glomerulopathy (endothelial swelling, fibrin thrombi, platelet aggregates)
- ± Acute cellular rejection changes (*vide supra*)

Chronic Rejection (months–years)
- Vascular changes: fibrous concentric intimal thickening hyperplasia not attributable to other causes (e.g. donor HT), variable lumenal narrowing ± IEL breach ± foam cells ± mononuclear cells (*NB*: acute vascular rejection changes may be superimposed). The changes may be segmental. d/dg HT: reduplicative multilayering of the IEL and lack of intimal foam / mononuclear cells all favour HT
- Tubular atrophy (i.e. thickened BM or ∅< 50% of normal) and interstitial fibrosis with lymphocytic infiltration
- Chronic allograft glomerulopathy (glomerular sclerosis, ± lymphocytic infiltration ± glomerular TMA-like changes; for Banff scoring look for ↑ mesangial matrix and thickened BM ± double contours in capillary loops [the latter increase with severity]) – d/dg mesangiocapillary GN (but the Tx lesions are usu. *focal*) or other lesions if your examination is by LM alone
- Banff criteria: EITHER new (non-pre-existent) vasc. lesions OR the glomerulopathy are sufficient to diagnose chronic rejection, but if LM alone is used then ONLY new vascular lesions are acceptable

Humoural Rejection ('Antibody-Mediated Rejection')
- A term used to indicate Ab-mediated vascular damage occurring in acute and chronic rejection
- Early ('Acute Humoural Rejection'): interstitial oedema, PMN margination and accumulation in capillaries (peritubular and glomerular), glomerular fibrin thrombi and endothelial swelling (= 'glomerular solidification'), peritubular capillary congestion. Fibrinoid necrosis and ischaemic tubular damage may also be seen
- Later ('Chronic Humoural Rejection'): continued peritubular and glomerular capillary damage (lumenal dilatation and BM thickening and reduplication) → tubular atrophy and interstitial fibrosis with ↑ intravascular mononuclear cells ± loss of peritubular capillaries
- Immuno: ➤ *linear* deposition of C4d lining the peritubular and glomerular capillaries (! may also be seen in, e.g., LE [usu. granular] ∴ not 100% specific, but it is usu. −ve in acute cellular rejection)
  ➤ alternatively, C3 +/ Ig may be +ve in arterial walls (but C4d in arteries is non-specific)
  ➤ glomerular C4d is normal in FS but is pathological in paraffin sections (although the pathology may be any immune complex deposition disease such as membranous GN)
- d/dg acute cellular rejection or other causes of TMA (e.g. HUS): these are C4d −ve
- Grading: ➤ Type 1: +ve serology for donor specific HLA Abs (indicates performing a renal Bx)
  ➤ Type 2: C4d deposition on Bx but no other changes
  ➤ Type 3: C4d deposition on Bx plus other histological changes
  ➤ Type 4: clinical evidence of allograft dysfunction ± Types 1–3 (indicates Rx)

Banff (1996–1997) Grading of Renal Allograft Rejection

Acute rejection
- Minor grades show acute cellular rejection (Borderline and Grades 1–2A)
- More severe types show acute vascular rejection (Grades 2B and 3)
Borderline: subtle changes not definitive for rejection → Rx based on clinical criteria alone
Grade 1A: >25% of interstitium inflamed + moderate tubulitis
Grade 1B: >25% of interstitium inflamed + severe tubulitis
Grade 2A: >25% of interstitium inflamed + arterial endothelialitis upto moderate degree
Grade 2B: severe arterial endothelialitis (defined as >25% lumenal area)
Grade 3: transmural or necrotising arteritis or interstitial haemorrhagic infarction without other cause
Chronic Allograft Nephropathy (chronic rejection)
- Grade each component separately on a 4 point scale (0–3) as follows:
Glomerulopathy: % non-sclerosed glomeruli affected (cg0 = 0%, cg1 ≤25%, cg2 26–50%, cg3 >50%)
Interstitial Fibrosis: % of cortical area (ci0 ≤5%, ci1 6–25%, ci2 26–50%, ci3 >50%)
Tubular Atrophy: % area of cortical tubules (ct0 = 0%, ct1 ≤25%, ct2 26–50%, ct3 >50%)
Vasculopathy: % narrowing of the lumen (cv0 = 0%, cv1 ≤25%, cv2 26–50%, cv3 >50%)
(= % lumenal narrowing by fibrous intimal thickening in the worst affected vessel taking the area enclosed by the IEL as the original lumen size)
Other changes
- For example: pre-existent / recurrent disease, venulitis, ATN, drug toxicity (*vide infra*)
- Infection e.g. polyoma tubulointerstitial nephritis: look for inclusions in tubule cell nuclei – confirmation is by immuno nuclear +vity for SV40 large T Ag in tubular cells but this may be lost later on (so stain a previous Bx if suspected)

Banff (2005) Changes Since 1997
- Chronic Allograft Nephropathy has been dropped
- Humoural Rejection (antibody-mediated rejection) has been included
- For details see: Solez *et al.*, 2007

Anti-Rejection Drug Toxicity

Calcineurin Inhibitors (= CNI, e.g. Cyclosporin and Tacrolimus [FK506])
- Nodular hyaline deposits in afferent arterioles (usu. more focal and peripherally sited in the media *cf.* arteriolosclerotic or DM changes which begin sub-intimally). Diffuse hyalinosis is non-specific
- Microvesicular vacuolation of the PCTs (unlike d/dg hypokalaemia *q.v.*) ± eosinophilic inclusions
- Myxoid and granular intimal thickening of arterioles

- Medial myocyte cytoplasmic vacuolation ± apoptosis
- HT-like arteriolosclerotic changes
- Alternating dense and rarefied ('stripy') stromal fibrosis or patchy fibrosis
- Stromal +/ tubular calcifications
- ± TMA (due to endothelial damage)
- ± Mild tubulitis (<4 cells)
- ± Renal changes of drug-induced DM
- Juxtaglomerular apparatus hyperplasia

Target of Rapamycin Inhibitors (= TORi, e.g. Rapamycin)

- Functional proteinuria
- Myeloma-cast-like nephropathy (but the casts stain for CK, not light chains)
- ± TMA

Bibliography

Alsaad, K.O. and Herzenberg, A.M. (2007) Distinguishing diabetic nephropathy from other causes of glomerulosclerosis: an update. *Journal of Clinical Pathology*, **60** (1), 18–26.

Bellamy, C.O.C. (2004) Microangiopathies & malignant vascular injury in the kidney. *Current Diagnostic Pathology*, **10** (1), 36–51.

Churg, J., Cotran, R.S., Sinniah, R. *et al.* (eds) (1985) *Renal Disease Classification and Atlas of Tubulo-Interstitial Diseases*, 1st edn, Igaku-Shoin, Tokyo.

Colvin, R.B. and Cornell, L.D. (2007) Renal transplant pathology: an update. *Current Diagnostic Pathology*, **13** (1), 15–24.

Corwin, H.L., Schwartz, M.M. and Lewis, E.J. (1988) The importance of sample size in the interpretation of renal biopsy. *American Journal of Nephrology*, **8** (2), 85–89.

Cotran, R.S., Kumar, V. and Collins, T. (eds) (1999) *Robbins Pathologic Basis of Disease*, 6th edn, W.B. Saunders Co., Philadelphia.

Furness, P.N. (2000) Renal biopsy specimens. *Journal of Clinical Pathology*, **53** (6), 433–438.

Ghadially, F.N. (1998) *Diagnostic ultrastructural pathology: A self-evaluation and self-teaching manual*, 2nd edn, Butterworth-Heinemann, Boston.

Howat, A.J., Thomas, C.M. and Coward, R.A. (2000) Immunoperoxidase for the demonstration of immune deposits in renal biopsies. *Current Diagnostic Pathology*, **6** (2), 125–129.

Howie, A.J. (2005) Approach to diagnosis and pitfalls: the renal biopsy, in *ACP Yearbook*, Association of Clinical Pathologists, Hove, pp. 37–38.

Howie, A.J. (2001) *Handbook of Renal Biopsy Pathology*, 1st edn, Kluwer Academic Press, Dordrecht.

Howie, A.J. (1997) Interstitial nephritis, in *Recent Advances in Histopathology*, Vol. 17 (eds P.P. Anthony, R.N.M. MacSween and D.G. Lowe), Churchill Livingstone, Edinburgh, pp. 219–231.

Lucas, S. (2000) Update on the pathology of AIDS. *Current Diagnostic Pathology*, **6** (2), 103–112.

Luu, J., Bockus, D., Remington, F. *et al.* (1989) Tuboloreticular structures and cylindrical confronting cisternae: a review. *Human Pathology*, **20** (7), 617–627.

Roberts, I.S.D., Furness, P.N. and Cook, H.T. (2004) Beyond diagnosis: stage and grade in inflammatory renal disease. *Current Diagnostic Pathology*, **10** (1), 22–35.

Roberts, I.S.D. and Solez, K. (2000) New developments in renal transplant pathology. *Current Diagnostic Pathology*, **6** (4), 219–228.

Smith, S.M., Hoy, W.E. and Cobb, L. (1989) Low incidence of glomerulosclerosis in normal kidneys. *Archives of Pathology & Laboratory Medicine*, **113** (11), 1253–1255.

Solez, K., Benediktsson, H. and Cavallo, T. (1996) Report of the third Banff conference on allograft pathology on classification of lesion scoring in renal allograft pathology, July 20–24, 1995, Banff, Canada. *Transplantation Proceedings*, **28** (1), 441–444.

Solez, K., Colvin, R.B., Racusen, L. *et al.* (2007) Banff '05 Meeting Report: Differential diagnosis of chronic allograft injury and elimination of chronic allograft nephropathy ('CAN'). *American Journal of Transplantation*, **7** (3), 518–526.

Walker, P.D., Ferrario, F., Joh, K. *et al.* (2007) Dense deposit disease is not a membranoproliferative glomerulonephritis. *Modern Pathology*, **20**(6), 605–616.

Weening, J.J., D'Agati, V.D., Schwartz, M.M. *et al.* (2004) The classification of glomerulonephritis in systemic lupus erythematosus revisited. *Kidney International*, **65** (2), 521–530.

Whittaker, M.A., Bass, P.S. and Rogerson, M.E. (2003) Systemic lupus erythematosus and the kidney-lupus nephritis, in *Progress in Pathology*, vol. 6 (eds N. Kirkham and N. Shepherd), Greenwich Medical Media, Ltd, London, pp. 29–50.

Web sites

University of Pittsburgh, Transplant Pathology Internet Service, http://tpis.upmc.edu/ (accessed April 2007).

Schrier, R. (ed) Atlas of Diseases of the Kidney, http://www.kidneyatlas.org/toc.htm (accessed March 2007).

16. Urological

Normal Testis

Normal Morphology of Spermatogenesis

Sertoli Cells
- Oval/triangular pale vesicular nuclei, may be folded
- Prominent central round to oval nucleolus
- Nucleolus flanked at poles by heterochromatin which accentuates the oval/fusiform shape
- Indistinct cytoplasm (± Charcot-Böttcher needle crystalloids basally in mature cells)

Spermatogonia
- Basally located, undergo mitosis
- Round-ovoid nucleus ($\approx 2\times$ the diameter of a lymphocyte)
- Type A: ➤ moderately condensed chromatin with small peripheral nucleoli +/ nuclear vacuole
   ➤ pale and dark subtypes
- Type B: more open chromatin with a central nucleolus, no nuclear vacuole

Primary Spermatocytes
- Larger than spermatogonia, span the thickness of the tubule and increase in size with meiotic stage
- Rounded nuclei show filamentous chromosomes with increasing degrees beadedness and thickness with meiotic stage (preleptotene, leptotene, zygotene, pachytene and diplotene)
- Abundant cytoplasm

Secondary Spermatocytes
- Too short-lived for reliable identification, look similar to early spermatids

Spermatids
- Central location, smaller than 1° spermatocyte ($\approx$ diameter of a lymphocyte)
- Condensed chromatin, round to oval nucleus

Spermatozoa
- Small pointy nuclei, very condensed chromatin

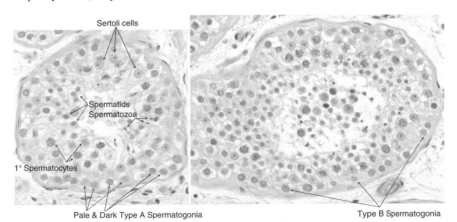

FIGURE 16.1   Spermatogenesis

Sertoli and Leydig Cells
- Leydig cells may normally be found within tubules, within the *tunica albuginea testis* and in the paratesticular soft tissues around nerve twigs
- Immuno: (see Table 16.1)
- See also sections on Sertoli Cell Nodule/'Adenoma', p. 227

TABLE 16.1   Immuno of Sertoli and Leydig cells

Antibody	Leydig	Sertoli
inhibin A, S100, calretinin	+	+
PGP 9.5, NSE	+ (& spermatogonia)	−
3βOHSD	+	−
WT1	−	+ (mature & immature)
p27kip	−	+ (mature only)

Diagnostic Criteria Handbook in Histopathology: A Surgical Pathology Vade Mecum by Paul J. Tadrous
Copyright © 2007 by John Wiley & Sons, Ltd.

Epididymis and Vas Deferens
* Post-pubertal epithelium may show eosinophilic DPAS +ve nuclear inclus[n]s (! these are not viral)

Johnsen's Score for Seminiferous Tubules (Assessment for Infertility/Subfertility)
* Adequacy: a Bx with <50 tubules is considered inadequate for scoring by some authorities
* The score correlates with sperm count and certain sub-fertility conditions
* The average score over all tubules in the section should be calculated (excluding tangential cuts and damaged tubules at the edge of the Bx)
* The original study used a ×10 objective in general (×25 to confirm spermatozoa or if poor fixation)
* The term 'many' is not defined numerically but >10 per tubule cross section is a reasonable guide

TABLE 16.2   Johnsen scoring

Score	Spermatozoa	Spermatids	Spermato-scytes	Spermato-gonia	Sertoli Cells	Other Features
10	many	many	present	present	present	open lumen & uniform germinal layer
9	many	many	present	present	present	disorganised germinal layer (sloughing / lumen obliteration*)
8	<5–10/tubule	many	present	present	present	
7	none	many	present	present	present	
6	none	<5–10/tubule	present	present	present	
5	none	none	≥5/tubule	present	present	
4	none	none	<5/tubule	present	present	
3	none	none	none	present	present	
2	none	none	none	none	present	
1	none	none	none	none	none	= acellular tubule

Based on: Johnsen SD. Testicular biopsy score count - a method for registration of spermatogenesis in human testes: normal values and results in 335 hypogonadal males. *Hormones* (1970); **1**:2–25.
* said to be indicative of distal obstruction

Developmental Anomalies

Renal Dysplasia (Multicystic Dysplasia, Cystic Dysplastic Kidney)
* Neonate/infant, usu. unilateral; most are obstructive (assoc[d] with valves/atresia/reflux), a minority are syndromic/inherited
* Macro: irregular nodularity
* Lobular disarray (jumbled mix of cortical and medullary structures)
* Stromal cartilage (helpful but not always seen)
* Primitive tubules
* Ducts/ductules lined by simple cuboidal/columnar epithelium and surrounded by fibromuscular or mesenchymatous stroma. Some may be cystic hence the alternative names for this condition
* ± Nodules of blastema (may be preneoplastic → Wilms' tumour)
* Some residual normal parenchyma may be present

Renal Hypoplasia
* Small kidney
* ≤5 calyces
* Normal histology

Autosomal Dominant Polycystic Kidney Disease (ADPCKD, Adult-type)
* Children/middle-aged, ± infection, HT (± complications), nephrolithiasis, renal failure
* Bilateral huge kidneys with surface bosselations
* Spherical cysts enlarge throughout the cortex and medulla
* Lined by flattened or PCT-like epithelium ± papilloid hyperplasia
* Filled with serous/haemorrhagic/gelatinous material ± superposed infective changes/stones
* Occ. glomeruloid tufts project into the lumen from the cyst wall (this feature may predominate in childhood cases = one form of 'glomerulocystic disease')
* Normal parenchyma in between

- $\pm$ Cysts in other organs (liver, pancreas, spleen, lung)
- $\pm$ Berry aneurysms
- d/dg renal dysplasia: can be a problem if young and asynchronous development (i.e. unilateral)

Autosomal Recessive Polycystic Kidney Disease (Infantile-type)
- Less severe form: infant/children, $\pm$ HT ($\pm$ complications), $\pm$ portal HT due to liver changes
- Severe (fatal) form: $\pm$ Potter's triad (oligohydramnios, pulmonary hypoplasia, uro/renal dysgenesis)[1]
- Bilateral huge kidneys without surface bosselations and without lobular disarray
- Elongated, slit-like cysts radiate from medulla to cortex ($\pm$ medullary dilatation)
- Lined by flattened or cuboidal (collecting-duct) epithelium
- Normal (but fibrotic/atrophic) parenchyma in between
- $\pm$ Cysts in liver (but usu. not other organs – else consider a different diagnosis)
- $\pm$ Berry aneurysms
- Liver shows dilated biliary structures and fibrosis (periportal and perivenular) and may amount to congenital hepatic fibrosis or Caroli disease $\pm$ 2° ascending cholangitis/sepsis changes

Medullary Sponge Kidney
- Adults, bilateral, urinary Sx $\pm$ nephrolithiasis/pyelonephritis
- Cysts in renal papillae (may contain calcific concretions)
- Simple cuboidal/columnar lining

Epididymal Cysts and Testicular Appendage Anomalies
- The *appendix epididymis* is cystic with a low columnar internal lining and fibrovascular wall lined externally by serosa
- The *appendix testis* (Morgagni) is a solid polyp with a fibrovascular core and columnar (non-ciliated) external lining
- They are located close to each other on the superior pole of the testicle and may tort/enlarge

Maldescended Testis (Cryptorchid Testis)
- $\approx$ Normal histology until after puberty but may show:
  - fibrous thickening of the *tunica albuginea testis*
  - reduced numbers of germ cells
  - small $\pm$ annular tubules
- Small size (and small seminiferous tubules)
- Fibrous thickening of the *tunica albuginea testis*
- Atrophy and loss of spermatogenic cells with persistence of Sertoli cells
- $\pm$ Tubules lined by immature (long and thin with small nucleus) Sertoli cells – may form aggregates (Pick's tubular 'adenomata' – *vide infra* under 'Sertoli Cell Nodule', p. 227)
- Stromal fibrosis with 'apparent' Leydig cell hyperplasia
- Peritubular fibrosis
- $\pm$ Germ cell neoplasia (intratubular germ cells may be sparse but can be seen at any age)

Inflammatory Conditions

Chronic Pyelonephritis and Reflux Nephropathy
- Interstitial fibrosis and chronic inflam^n $\pm$ intratubular PMN
- Loss of some tubules and dilatation of others with hyaline casts ('thyroidisation')
- Glomeruli show periglomerular fibrosis and clusters of obsolete glomeruli
- d/dg reflux nephropathy *cf.* chronic GN:
  - changes worst at the poles in reflux nephropathy
  - reflux show dilated, distorted and thickened calyces apposed to scarred parenchyma
  - in reflux the scarring is asymmetrical and irregular

---

[1] inability to contribute to the amniotic fluid volume by urination $\rightarrow$ oligohydramniotic restrictive environment $\rightarrow$ squashed face (Potter's facies with beaked nose, etc.) and squashed thorax $\rightarrow$ pulmonary hypoplasia (respiratory distress of immature lungs prevents these neonates surviving)

Xanthogranulomatous Pyelonephritis
- ! Can be misdiagnosed (clin. and pathologically) as RCC (clear cell and sarcomatoid types)
- ! Can co-exist with RCC or metastatic cancer
- Assoc^d with obstruction (e.g. calculus) and infection (*Proteus* spp. & *E.coli*)
- Macro: mass lesion, yellow, destroying renal parenchyma
- Micro: a mass of foamy Mϕ plus lymphocytes, plasma cells and occ. giant cells
- d/dg RCC: ➢ lack of reticular capillary vascular pattern of clear cell RCC
  - ➢ presence of a mixed inflam^y infiltrate
  - ➢ foamy rather than clear cytoplasm
  - ➢ Mϕ immuno rather than RCC immuno

Granulomatous Pyelitis
- A rare complicat^n of chronic renal outflow obstruction with some degree of pelvicalyceal dilatation
- Pelvis may contain calcific/necrotic material (−ve for TB/fungi by culture)
- Granulomatous inflammation in the pelvis (but not granulomatous interstitial nephritis)
- d/dg TB, fungi, other infective agents

Malakoplakia
- Lamina propria of bladder/ureter, substance of kidney, GIT/other organs ± assoc^d malignancy
- Mϕ with abundant granular eosinophilic cytoplasm (Hansemann cells) containing:
  - ① Michaelis-Gutmann bodies: ➢ lamellar, haematoxyphile and refractile
    - ➢ mineralised (von-Kossa) and iron
  - ② non-mineralised, PAS +ve globules
  - ③ iron granules
- Other chronic inflam^y cells are also present
- d/dg: signet ring carcinoma on FS (but mucin vacuoles are not refractile)

Interstitial Cystitis (± Hunner's Ulcer)
- Diagnosis of exclusion with characteristic clin. and cystoscopic features
- Urothelial denudation ± ulceration
- Lamina propria oedema, congestion, fibrosis ± focal RBC extravasation
- Chronic inflam^n: lymphocytes ± Mϕ, eos., plasma cells
- ↑ Mast cells in muscle and lamina propria: some say the ratio count (detrusor muscle *vs.* lamina propria) is helpful, others report that it is useless in distinguishing interstitial cystitis from controls

Painful Bladder Syndrome
- Def^n: >3 months of urinary Sx with suprapubic pain and sterile urine
- Apparent discontinuity of the BM
- ↑ T-cells in the lamina propria
- ↑ Blood vessels in the lamina propria
- ↑ Perimuscular collagen (EVG)

Eosinophilic Cystitis
- Assoc^d with allergy or prior trauma
- Transmural eosinophils + fibrosis

Granulomatous Cystitis
- TB
- BGC (non-caseating, lymphoid follicles, ± crystals in the giant cells)
- Schistosomiasis

Chemotherapy-Induced Change in the Bladder

Haemorrhagic cystitis
- Haemorrhage ++, oedema and congestion of the lamina propria
- Ulceration/sloughing of the urothelium
- Urothelial atypia (*vide infra*)
- Regenerative changes: fibroblastic/histiocytic reaction in the stroma, mitoses in the epithelium (!)

Urothelial atypia
- Cytomegaly
- Nuclear pleomorphism and hyperchromasia
- d/dg CIS: ➢ upper layers worst affected (*cf.* full-thickness in CIS)
  ➢ good cohesion (! but not in haemorrhagic cystitis)
  ➢ lack of mitoses (! but get mitoses in regenerative phase of haemorrhagic cystitis)

Radiation Cystitis

Acute (months)
- Epithelial sloughing and cytological atypia:
  ➢ cytomegaly with ill-defined hyperchromatic chromatin
  ➢ nuclear and cytoplasmic (mucin −ve) vacuolation
  ➢ d/dg carcinoma (*vide infra* under urothelial CIS, pp. 219–220)
- Lamina propria oedema (→ cystoscopic cobbles = 'bullous cystitis')
- Microvascular engorgement and dilatation

Chronic (years)
- Fibrinoid ulcers ± focal cytol. atypia (a rare PEH-like proliferation may be seen. This is limited to the superficial lamina propria, has variable squamous metaplasia, normal NCR and no ↑ in mitoses)
- Stromal fibrosis (incl. muscularis propria)
- Bizarre stromal cells (multinucleated radiation fibroblasts)
- Proliferative endarteritis

Granulomatous Prostatitis
- Idiopathic (most common type, 70%)
- Iatrogenic (TURP/Teflon/silicone)
  ➢ xanthoma/xanthogranuloma – d/dg hypernephroid Gleason 4/5 adenocarcinoma
  ➢ others: reactive atypia and ↑ cellularity d/dg high grade carcinoma
- Infective (TB, Brucella, Histoplasma, Schistosoma, VZV)
- Systemic disease (Wegener's, Churg-Strauss, Sarcoid, RhA)
- Malakoplakia (see p. 214)
- Wegener's, RhA and post-TURP can look similar to each other with palisaded granulomas

Granulomatous Orchitis
- Adult, pain, ± PMHx UTI/trauma. Clinical d/dg neoplasia
- Macro: homogeneous (d/dg lymphoma)
- Tubulocentric mixed chronic inflam^y infiltrate with epithelioid Mφ ± giant cells
- ± Focal necrosis
- Granulomatous nature of the inflam^n may not be obvious
- d/dg: lymphoma (but lymphoma has relative sparing of the tubules and is more monotonous)
- d/dg: granulomas associated with seminoma or a specific infection
- d/dg: idiopathic (spermatogenic) – exclude other causes first

Penile Lesions

Zoon's balanitis (Balanitis circumscripta plasmacellularis)
- Red patch(es) in old uncircumcised men (clin. d/dg erythroplasia of Queyrat)
- Plasma cell-rich band-like dermal inflam^n ± siderophages

Lichen sclerosus (Balanitis xerotica obliterans, BXO)
- White plaques on glans +/prepuce; assoc^d with phimosis, CIS and some forms of invasive SCC
- Early: lichenoid (± vacuolar) interface change, orthohyperkeratosis, atrophy of stratum spinosum
- Later: band-like or patchy lymphoid-rich inflam^n descends to the mid-dermis leaving the intervening dermis hyalinised, oedematous (± dilated microvasculature) and epidermis atrophic or hypertrophic
- Other sites incl. the vulva and breast in women and back where follicular plugging is also a feature
- d/dg: other lichenoid inflammatory dermatoses (pp. 297–298), morphoea (p. 301)

Syphilis
See p. 296.

Renal Tumours (Benign)

Renal Oncocytoma
- Solid, tubular, tubulocystic or trabecular nests of oncocytes (mitochondia $+++$ on EM)
- Stroma: abundant oedematous, hyaline/myxoid
- Acceptable: ➤ focal nuclear pleomorphism and large nucleoli (grading is inappropriate)
                  ➤ a few cases invade the perinephric fat
                  ➤ microvascular invasion
- Unacceptable: ➤ mitoses are *very* rare and *never* atypical or present in an area of nuclear atypia
                  ➤ clear cell *areas*, papillary growth pattern, sarcomatoid change
- Immuno/stain: $-$ve for CK7, 'RCC MA', MOC31 and mucin (by Hale's); $\pm$ve (weak/patchy) for CD10 and vimentin; $+$ve for EMA, AE1/AE3 and c-kit; Ber-EP4 is usu. weak/$-$ve
- d/dg chromophobe carcinoma or oncocytic conventional Renal Cell Carcinoma (RCC)

Cystic Nephroma (Multicystic Nephroma)
See 'Renal Cell Carcinoma (Conventional)', below

Renal Adenoma
- <5 mm $\varnothing$ and is of papillary non-clear cell type (by definition)
- No clear cell/chromophobe/collecting duct areas and no sig. atypia/mitoses
- Cytogenetics same as papillary renal cell carcinoma
- Most common tumour at PM, often in scarred areas ($\therefore$ most do not progress to pap. RCC)

Angiomyolipoma
- HMB45 $+$ve PEComa (for a more complete description, see p. 326)
- ① abnormal vessels ② myoid spindle cells ③ fat (but can lack fat spaces and can be very cellular)
- Can mimic RCC and some foci can be pigmented (d/dg pigmented RCC, melanoma)
- Epithelioid variant may show malignant behaviour
- 50% have tuberose sclerosis (TS), 75% of TS have angiomyolipoma

Metanephric Adenoma
- F $\gg$ M, middle age, incidental
- Macro: upto 8 cm $\varnothing$
- Packed round tubules in the renal cortex
- Empty lumens
- May have papillary areas (and spindle fibrous component $=$ *metanephric adenofibroma*)

Renal Tumours (Malignant)

Renal Cell Carcinoma (Conventional)
- Cells (clear/granular/oncocytic/spindle): contain glycogen, fat, $\pm$ abnormal mitochondria, *no mucin*
- Arch.: solid, alveolar, glandular ($=$ tubular), papillary (in $<75\%$ of the tumour)
- Sarcomatoid change is 'RCC MA' $-$ve and may incl. osteosarcoma, chondrosarcoma and RMS areas
- May have extensive rhabdoid features (! do not confuse with RMS-like sarcomatoid change)
- Pushing margin (else consider sarcomatoid change)
- Stroma: inconspicuous with a rich delicate microvascular network
- Focal cystic change has no prognostic significance
- Multilocular cystic variant (good prog.):
    ➤ no expansile solid clear cell nodules present
    ➤ little groups of clear cells in the septa
    ➤ d/dg multicystic nephroma (benign): no little groups clear cells in the septa
- d/dg simple cysts lined by a single layer of clear cells $=$ simple cysts *not* RCC
- d/dg melanoma: ! some RCC are pigmented (have Fe $-$ve lysosomal pigment, not melanin)
- d/dg mucinous tubular spindle cell CA (*vs.* sarcomatoid change): this has bland spindle cells in fascicles $\pm$ myxoid with a minor component of epithelium (tubules are rare). It is low grade malig. and its d/dg incl. mixed epithelial stromal tumour and xanthogranulomatous inflam^n

Papillary Renal Cell Carcinoma (= Chromophil Carcinoma)
- Def[n]: the tumour must be >70–75% papillary (*cf.* clear cell) and ≥5 mm ∅. (*NB:* the 'solid variant' has alveolar/glomeruloid areas which are taken as 'papillary' for the purposes of this percentage as are other papillary variant architectures such as elongated trabeculoid papillae)
- Cells: low grade nuclei with cuboidal cytoplasm (Type 1) or columnar ± higher grade, focal necrosis and more mitoses (Type 2, worse prog.). The cytoplasm is usu. eosinophil, amphophil or basophil
- Stroma: foamy Mφ in papilla cores ± psammoma bodies; not desmoplastic (*cf.* collecting duct CA)
- Extensive haemorrhage/cyst formation
- Complicates end stage kidneys (dialysis/post Tx) – these also predispose to ureteric carcinoma
- d/dg conventional RCC (most are CK 7 −ve *cf.* papillary which are usu. CK 7 +ve incl. solid type)
- d/dg collecting duct CA, chromophobe CA, papillary TCC, papillary mets

Differential Diagnosis of Conventional Renal Cell Carcinoma
- Immuno for clear cell/papillary RCC: ➢ +ve for CK, EMA, vimentin, CD10 and 'RCC MA'
                                          ➢ c-kit, MOC31, S100 and CEA are *usu.* −ve
- 'RCC MA' is also +ve in breast and parathyroid epithelial tumours, cystic nephroma, mesothelioma
- Adrenocortical carcinoma: EMA +ve favours renal cell and excludes adrenal, CK +vity too but less so. For an immuno panel and more information, see table 19.1 on p. 276.
- Melanoma: EMA +ve and CK +ve favour renal cell and excludes melanoma
- Other carcinomas: CK and vimentin +vity is unusual in other carcinomas (except endometrial)
- Translocation carcinoma: esp. in children, pale/clear cells but with nests/papillae ± psammoma bodies; has der(17)t(X;17)(p11.2:q25) and has nuclear immuno +vity for *TFE3* (related to ASPS)

Collecting Duct Carcinoma
- Macro: the tumour is centred on the medulla
- Cells: high grade (unlike papillary carcinoma), eosinophilic cytoplasmic globules, hobnailing
- The rare low grade type has cuboidal cells with prom. nucleoli, tubulocystic arch. ± lumenal mucin
- Mixed solid and tubulopapillary pattern
- Dysplastic changes in adjacent collecting ducts
- Stroma: desmoplastic (± PMN) associated with an infiltrating ductal carcinoma component
- Its metastases may be microcystic
- Stains: +ve for mucin, some HMW CK and *Ulex europaeus* lectin; −ve for vimentin and 'RCC MA'
- d/dg: ➢ any papillary lesion (*vide supra*) esp. pelvic TCC spreading up ducts
           ➢ metastatic carcinoma
           ➢ overlap with renal medullary carcinoma

Renal Medullary Carcinoma
- Variant of collecting duct carcinoma seen in association with sickle *trait* (not sickle cell disease)
- Inflammatory stroma
- Infarcts/ischaemic areas

Chromophobe Carcinoma
- Macro: oncocytoma-like (i.e. brown with central stellate scar[2]), cystic change is rare
- Two cell types: ➢ oncocytic (may have high grade nuclei but often low grade)
                     ➢ cells with pale staining granular cytoplasm (unless eosinophilic subtype), perinuclear halo (koilocytoid) and peripheral condensation to highlight cell borders (= plant-like in the paler ones)
- Nuclei: wrinkled ± grooved, always find at least some binucleate/multinucleate forms
- Cells are of variable size ('mosaic' pattern)
- Microvessels are of variable thickness (with some thick vessels)
- May have a papillary pattern and sarcomatoid change is relatively common
- Stains: Hale's colloidal iron (mucin) diffuse strong reticular cytoplasmic staining (*cf.* focal, weak, dust-like for all others), also AB +ve; lipid and glycogen −ve
- Immuno: vimentin −ve; Ber-EP4 and MOC31 usu. +ve. CK and EMA *patchy* +ve (incl. 'membranous' +vity for CK7). *Diffuse cytoplasmic* MUC1 +ve (*cf.* membranous in papillary/conventional)[3]. CD10

---
[2] a central scar just means its a slow growing tumour and can be seen in any type
[3] see Llinares *et al.*, 2004

−ve except in an aggressive subset (*cf.* +ve for papillary/clear cell or ±ve in others incl. oncocytoma). 'RCC MA' is *usu.* −ve (95% of cases). c-kit and Kidney-specific cadherin +ve (−ve in most other renal tumours except oncocytoma)
- EM: perinuclear microvesicles (? mitochondrial membrane derived). These don't survive wax processing so take fresh tissue directly into glutaraldehyde at time of cut-up

Prognostic Factors
- Stage (esp. LN/mets), grade (Fuhrman), margins, histotype:
- ?14q- in clear cell (a bad prognostic); ?proliferation status

good   chromophobe
papillary
clear cell
bad   collecting duct

Cytogenetics
- Oncocytoma : Y-, 1-
- Papillary adenoma/carcinoma : Y-, trisomy 7, trisomy 17
- Clear cell : 3p- (VHL oncosuppressor – not seen in other histotypes)
- Collecting duct : 1-, 6-, LOH on 8p/13q
- Chromophobe : 1-, 2-, hypodiploid

Fuhrman Grading of Nuclei
- The original study was based on 103 patients with a minimum of 4 years F/U
- Nuclear grade predicted mets better than (each of): size, stage, cell type, cytoarchitecture
- Grade according to the worst focus (not the predominant grade)

TABLE 16.3 Fuhrman grading

Grade	Nuclear size	Nuclear shape	Nucleoli
I	≈ 10 μ	round & uniform	small/absent
II	≈ 15 μ	irregularity visible with ×40 objective	frequently seen with ×40 objective
III	≈ 20 μ	obvious irregularity	large (seen with ×10 objective)
IV	≥ 20 μ	as for III + bizarre/multilobed forms and heavy chromatin clumps	large (seen with ×10 objective)

Based on: Fuhrman SA, Lasky LC, Limas C. Prognostic significance of morphologic parameters in renal cell carcinoma. *Am J Surg Pathol.* (1982); **6**:655-663.

Metastatic Tumours
- Common sources are lung/stomach; also pancreas, adrenal (by direct spread), contralateral kidney (via renal veins), breast and melanoma (± glomerular emboli)
- There may be interstitial infiltration with glomerular sparing
- Extensive vascular invasion favours a 2° origin
- Coexistence of usual-type 1° tumour or preneoplastic metaplasia favours 1°

Frozen Sections
- Usu. done for margins on partial nephrectomies or to diagnose a mass in a potential donor kidney
- Problems include crushed tubules/detached groups of cells ?benign/malignant: go by architecture and cytology (esp. nuclear features of atypia)
- Cysts: if clear cell lining more likely RCC (! but see 'd/dg simple cyst' on p. 216) but if granular eosinophilic cells consider 'atypical cyst' (the patient need not have VHL)
- Fatty masses: d/dg angiomyolipoma (look for eosinophilic granular cells), fat necrosis, angiosarcoma
- If not confident request additional tissue

Urothelial Tumours

Nephrogenic Adenoma / Metaplasia (NA)
- Affects any urothelial-lined structure, esp. bladder and urethra and may extend into prostate
- Immuno: +ve (PAX2, AMACAR, CK7, EMA, CA-19.9, CA-125); ±ve (CK20, 'RCC MA', CD10); −ve for basal cells and p53, p63, Ki-67, PSA / PSAP
- d/dg prostatic CA: NA has oedematous/inflam^y stroma, *intracellular* mucin +ve, PSA/PSAP −ve
- d/dg clear cell carcinoma: +vity for Ki-67 and p53 favours CCC. See also table 16.4

Inverted Papilloma
- Clin.: male, 50's, BOO/haematuria; macro: polypoid/nodule
- Normal overlying urothelium, minimal exophytic component
- Anastomosing trabeculae with palisading, eddies, cysts and glandular areas

TABLE 16.4   Nephrogenic adenoma or clear cell carcinoma?

Clear cell carcinoma	Nephrogenic adenoma
>40 years, large size → clinical presentation	younger, small, incidental (unless urethral)
No PMHx of GU surgery/trauma/calculi	often PMHx of GU surgery/trauma/calculi
tubules, cysts, papillae and diffuse sheets	*ditto* - but no big diffuse sheets
clear (glycogen) cells + flat + hobnail cells	*ditto* - but glycogen not as abundant
prom. nucleoli, nuc. pleomorphism + mitoses	bland cytology - but some may have nuc. atypia

- d/dg TCC has a prominent exophytic component, sig. atypia and mitoses, ± keratinisation, infiltration (but beware TCC extending into von Brunn's nests)

Small Cell Carcinoma of the Bladder
- Polyp/nodule ± ulcerated, mitoses ++, NE nuclei, nests, necrosis, Azzopardi/crush effect ± rosettes
- Usu. mixed with a conventional CA (usu. TCC) – this is good evidence of 1° *cf.* metastatic SmCC
- Synaptophysin and CD56 (NCAM) +ve, CgA ±ve, CAM5.2 +ve in $\frac{2}{3}$ of cases (paranuclear dot-like)
- Poor prognosis ∴ must mention a SmCC component no matter how little is present

Transitional Cell Carcinoma (TCC)
- Immuno: hCG +vity is a bad prognostic, p63 +vity suggests urothelium (see also p.18)
- Features suggestive of stromal invasion: cytoplasmic eosinophilia, lack of basal palisading, ± desmoplasia, ± retraction clefts (! not d/dg vasc.) [*NB*: adipose may occur in normal lamina propria]
- d/dg papillary nephrogenic adenoma (which, in turn, must be differentiated from nested carcinoma of the bladder with tubular differentiation). NA is p63 −ve.
- d/dg paragangliomas of the bladder are often misdiagnosed as invasive TCC on biopsy/curettings
- d/dg poorly diff TCC *vs.* high grade prostatic adenocarcinoma
- d/dg 'transitional cell papilloma': this has fibrovascular cores but no cytol. atypia or urothelial disorganisation/frond fusion (*cf.* TCC) and no increase in cell layers (although some say thickness is not important); it is a small and isolated lesion and is rare; younger patients may be affected
- d/dg transitional cell hyperplasia: this has marked ↑ cell layers (e.g. >7) but not disorganisation/atypia and is either flat or tufted/undulating (= 'papillary' but lacks well-developed fibrovascular cores)

Grading TCC by the 1973 WHO Scheme (currently recommended in the UK)

G1 ↑ cell layers (often > 7), mild atypia, mitoses rare	solid areas are rare, ± papillary fusion
G2 focal moderate atypia, more than an occasional mitosis	fusion of papillae may be seen
G3 focal high-grade nuclei (at least), mitoses easy to find	solid areas more common, ± necrosis

G4 undiff CA (if total, can only call it 'TCC' by assumption, e.g. previous Bx showed G1–3 TCC)
- Grade by worst area (not predominant grade) and avoid tangential cuts through basal urothelium
- The 2004 WHO papillary TCC grades ('PUNLMP', 'low grade', 'high grade') are not quite the same ('low grade' includes some G2 and those G1 cases that are not 'PUNLMP'; 'high grade' includes G3 and some G2 cases)

Micropapillary TCC
- High grade and usu. high stage with vascular invasion
- Mets look similar to the primary
- Prognosis is similar to poorly diff TCC

SCC Bladder
- Exclude 2° from cervix – esp. when it is in the trigone
- Concurrent squamous metaplasia favours 1°

Adenocarcinoma
- 2° tumours are just as common as 1° (and either may be intestinal, clear cell or signet ring type)
- 1° usu. arise in urachus or an exstrophic bladder
- d/dg: endocervicosis, nephrogenic adenoma (*vs.* CCC)
- Urachal carcinomas arise within the muscle hence there is controversy over significance of depth of invasion and the importance of establishing a urachal origin (dome location, intestinal histotype, lack of mucosal involvement and exclusion of a colonic 1° [CEA is nearly always +ve in colonic adenocarcinoma but may be −ve in urachal so a −ve result helps but a +ve result means nothing])

Flat Carcinoma in situ of the Urothelium (CIS)
- Types: small cell, large cell (with moderate cytoplasm), Pagetoid variant of large cell type
- Dilapidated brick wall (dyscohesion) and disorganised orientation of cells (± extension into von Brunn nests)

- Proliferated microvasculature in the superficial lamina propria
- Full-thickness dysplasia and ↑ cell layers are NOT required for diagnosis
- Nuclei: pleomorphism, hyperchromasia, coarse chromatin, prominent angulated nucleoli
- Mitoses common and abnormal
- Immuno:
  - ➢ CK20 (umbrella cells only in normal, full thickness staining in CIS)
  - ➢ CEA +ve (−ve in normal)
  - ➢ Ki-67 +ve (not limited to basal layers in CIS; weak, patchy and basal in normal)
  - ➢ p53 strong +ve in >30% of cells in CIS *cf.* weak and <20% (usu. 10%) in normal
- d/dg chemo/radioRx atypia – these show:
  - ➢ worse atypia than expected for CIS
  - ➢ cytomegaly more than ↑ NCR
  - ➢ smudged chromatin detail rather than crisp coarseness
  - ➢ lack of mitoses (esp. given the degree of atypia)
  - ➢ associated stromal changes (and appropriate Hx)
- d/dg inflammatory atypia (apply criteria ± immuno above)
- d/dg urothelial atypia/dysplasia not amounting to CIS – this is diagnosed by the following:
  - ➢ urothelium still cohesive
  - ➢ architectural distortion – clustering of nuclei
  - ➢ some but not all cells are dysplastic
  - ➢ chromatin is fine, nucleoli small and mitoses rare

Secondary Tumours of the Bladder
- Usu. by direct spread from cervix/colon, else blood-borne from melanoma/breast
- Extensive vascular invasion favours a 2° origin
- Coexistence of usual-type 1° tumour or preneoplastic metaplasia/dysplasia favours 1°

Prostatic Carcinoma and its Mimics

Prostatic Adenocarcinoma (of Conventional Acinar Type)
- Infiltrative arch. (if > Gleason 2) between benign glands and esp. perineural/intravascular
- Single layered glands (in lower grades) with absent basal cells ± glomeruloid tuftings ± mitoses
- Nuclear enlargement, nucleolomegaly ± hyperchromasia
- Intralumenal: collagenous micronodules (specific but rare), crystalloids, wispy blue mucin
- Immuno: for AMACAR, PSA, PSAP and basal cell markers, see p. 18

Adenomatous Polyp of the Prostatic Urethra (Prostatic-Type Polyp)
- Usu. young, at verumontanum, haematuria/haemospermia
- Two architectures:
  - ➢ prostatic glands covered by smooth urothelium
  - ➢ slender villoglandular (or stubbier rounded) fronds lined by typical prostatic epithelium
- A basal cell layer is present and the cytology is bland
- d/dg prostatic duct carcinoma (*q.v.*)

Normal Seminal Vesicle/Ejaculatory Duct (vs. d/dg Prostate Carcinoma)
- Closely packed glands (resembling low grade prostatic adenocarcinoma)
- Lipofuscin and scattered 'monster' cells; nuclei may be apical; muscle may have hyaline globules
- Monster cells have hyperchromatic degenerative-like pleomorphic nuclei adjacent to benign appearing nuclei in well formed glands
- Immuno: PSA and PSAP −ve; 34βE12 +ve (i.e. the opposite to prostatic adenocarcinoma)

Atypical Adenomatous Hyperplasia (Adenosis)
- Mostly occurs in the transitional zone   } so AAH should be a rare diagnosis
- Well-circumscribed ± minimal peripheral infiltration } on core Bx (need to see whole lesion)
- Closely packed small acini lacking epithelial infoldings
- Acini may appear to bud from the adjacent benign glands/merge with a usual hyperplastic nodule
- Cells: clear cytoplasm, lack malignant nuclear features (but prominent nucleoli occur in 20–30% of cases)

- A disrupted basal cell layer is present (by immuno)
- d/dg adenocarcinoma: ➤ basal layer present in AAH
  - ➤ architectural features
  - ➤ nucleoli usu. $<1\mu$ ($>3\mu$ is incompatible with AAH)
- Cases that don't fulfil AAH criteria and have some features suspicious for adenoCA = ASAP (*q.v.*)
- AAH has uncertain malignant potential

Sclerosing Adenosis
- Well formed glands and cellular spindled stroma
- Limited foci on TURP chips (*cf.* d/dg high grade adenocarcinoma)
- Infiltrative but still relatively circumscribed (*cf.* d/dg high grade adenocarcinoma)
- Benign nuclei (although some may be moderately enlarged with prominent nucleoli)
- Hyaline sheath-like structure around some of the glands
- Basal cell layer present (discontinuous): αSMA and S100 +ve (i.e. myoepithelial phenotype) unlike prostate basal cells (for immuno profiles of basal *vs.* myoepithelial cells, see p. 18)
- Spindle cells of the stroma show focal CK and αSMA +vity (myoepithelial differentiation)
- No association with carcinoma

Sclerotic Atrophy and Postatrophic Hyperplasia
- Low power shows basophilia due to shrunken cytoplasm (gland-forming prostate carcinomas are not so basophilic due to their more abundant cytoplasm); $\pm$ residual periglandular chronic inflam^n
- Postatrophic hyperplasia shows arbitrarily more acini; they have variable shape and size (mostly small)
- Hyperchromatic nuclei, occasional small nucleoli, $\uparrow$ nuclear size and minimal pleomorphism
- Fibrosis imparts an infiltrative appearance but the glands appear infiltrative as a patch – not individual glands infiltrating between larger benign glands (like carcinoma)
- Immuno: partial atrophy can be AMACAR +ve with focal loss of basal cells (! d/dg adenoCA)
- d/dg atrophic carcinoma (rare):   ➤ truly infiltrative
  - ➤ presence of ordinary (less atrophic) carcinoma
  - ➤ greater cytological atypia

Prostatic Intraepithelial Neoplasia (PIN)
- Mostly occurs in the peripheral zone, high grade is usu. seen in association with peripheral cancers
- The level of serum PSA does not correlate with the volume of PIN
- $\uparrow$ PSA and high grade PIN on Bx $\rightarrow$ re-Bx (or process rest of chips); close F/U with PSA and rectal exam
- Low power: basophilia; 4 main arch.: flat (single layer), tufting, micropapillary, cribriform
- Cytol. features are often abrupt (stratificat^n, $\uparrow$ nuclear and nucleolar size, anisonucleosis, coarse chromatin)
- Grade 1: $\uparrow$ nuclear size and anisonucleosis are the main features   } = Low grade
- Grade 2: hyperchromasia, chromatin margination, $\uparrow$ nucleolar size   } = High grade
- Grade 3: many large nucleoli, nuclear crowding, less anisonucleosis   } = High grade
- Some diagnose high grade PIN without prominent nucleoli provided there is: marked pleomorphism, hyperchromasia, mitotic activity and a cribriform or micropapillary architecture
- A basal cell layer (even discontinuous) must be identified to exclude invasive carcinoma (! but small cribriform foci of PIN on Bx may lack a basal layer due to unrepresentative sampling)
- d/dg   ➤ invasive cribriform carcinoma (Gleason 3–4): but in PIN the lobular architecture is retained
  - ➤ primary duct (endometrioid) CA may mimic micropapillary PIN: but PIN is usu. peripheral, shows a central maturation effect and lacks endometrioid columnar cells or true papillae
  - ➤ TCC is usu. PSA −ve
  - ➤ post radiotherapy changes: main d/dg with this is invasive CA but a basal layer will remain
  - ➤ cribriform hyperplasia will lack the nuclear atypia of PIN
  - ➤ basal cell hyperplasia (*q.v.*) has oval regular nuclei with (usu.) small nucleoli and is LP34 +ve
  - ➤ reactive epithelium (post trauma/inflam^n) is hyperchromatic but lacks other nuclear features
  - ➤ 'intraduct carcinoma': basal layer +ve but has necrosis and pleom. $\gg$ that of high grade PIN. This may actually be cancerisation associated with an aggressive invasive CA nearby rather than CIS

Other Mimics of Prostatic Adenocarcinoma
- Normal structures (esp. if adjacent to nerves) e.g. small prostatic glands, Cowper's glands (mucinous acini) and paraganglia (have their own internal capillary network – unlike cancer)
- Hyperplasias: basal cell (*q.v.*), clear cell cribriform, transitional cell, verumontanum mucosal gland
- Stromal hyperplasia with atypical giant cells
- Inflammatory: malakoplakia, granulomatous prostatitis
- Other tumours: TCC (e.g. micropapillary pattern), nephrogenic adenoma (rare, but can be AMACAR +ve and is basal cell –ve; PSA/PSAP is either –ve or only focal and weakly +ve)

Gleason Grading and Scoring of Prostatic Adenocarcinoma
- Gleason Score = predominant grade + next most abundant grade (provided the latter constitutes >5% of the tumour – otherwise just double the predominant grade)
- WHO (1999): also record the % of tumour that is high grade (= Gleason 4 or 5)
1) Closely packed uniform glands without intervening normal glands. Well-circumscribed. Glands tend to have even lumenal surface and more crystalloids. These tumours are small and occur in transition zone (periurethral area) ∴ rare on needle Bx. A few small malig. glands on needle biopsy with intervening normal glands may be mistaken for low grade (1–2) cancer but this is obviously wrong as low grade does not have intervening normal glands.
2) More separation, more variation and irregular outline to the group of pale glands but still no intervening normal glands. Same comments re needle biopsy as above.
3) The malignant glands, while single and separate, are smaller than the glands in 1 and 2. They infiltrate between normal glands. A few small (i.e. size of a normal gland) *well-circumscribed* cribriform glands may be present which are difficult to distinguish from cribriform PIN. Ragged cribriform areas indicate grade 4 as does fusion of cribriform acini (= acinus elongated to ≥4:1 length:width).
4) The glands are no longer single and separate. In cribriform carcinoma the cribriform areas are larger than the size of a normal gland, have a more ragged edge and less well developed composite gland spaces (*cf.* the punched out holes of the small cribriform foci seen in some grade 3 cases). The lack of stroma within the cribriform unit means that they tend to fragment on Bx. Another pattern is that of loss of individual gland formation with only focal lumenal differentiation. ± Clear cell change.
5) Individual cells lacking glandular lumenal differentiation. Solid sheets of cells ± focal rosetting (poor attempts at gland formation). Cords of cells. Comedo necrosis in solid nests of cells. ± Clear cell change (= hypernephroid variant).
- d/dg for grades 2 and 3 with dilated gland architecture: benign prostatic hyperplasia
- d/dg for grades 4 and 5 includes: NEC, TCC, (xantho)granulomatous prostatitis and malakoplakia

Criteria for Extraprostatic Extension of Prostatic Carcinoma
- Extraprostatic spread up-stages the tumour; intra-capsular infiltration is not sufficient
- Tumour must infiltrate periprostatic fat OR seminal vesicle muscle or glands
- ! Some *intraprostatic* skeletal muscle (of the urogenital diaphragm) may be seen at the apex

Atypical Small Acinar Proliferations (ASAP and ASAPUS)
- A small (i.e. <24 acini and usu. <12) atypical lesion which, after levels, immuno, etc., cannot be diagnosed as adenoCA with sufficient confidence to form the basis of definitive cancer Rx
- Report level of suspicion for CA ('suspicious' or 'highly suspicious') and advise re-Bx
- The term ASAPUS suggests a lower suspicion of CA *cf.* ASAP (it is of 'uncertain significance')
- d/dg 'minimal cancer' = definite CA involving <5% of the tissue

Prostatic Duct Carcinoma (includes Endometrioid/'Endometrial' Carcinoma of the Utricle)
- Usu. >60 years, haematuria/BOO, PSA may be normal, poor prognosis
- Columnar cells ± glycogen clearing (not mucin)
- Endometrioid subtype has dark cytoplasm ± subnuclear vacuoles +/cilia
- High grade nuclei with prominent nucleoli (except some type A cases), mitoses ++, loss of nuclear polarity (nuclei may be elongated/stratified)
- Two architectures (may be a mixture):
    - ➤ A (1° duct type – less common): tall, complex papillae
    - ➤ B (2° duct/endometrioid type): cribriform, comedo, low papillae
- Immuno: PSA and AMACAR +ve, CEA ±ve, 34βE12 basal cells *mostly* absent

- d/dg:
  - ➤ adenomatous polyp (low grade simple epithelium, basal layer ++, architecture, age)
  - ➤ verumontanum hyperplasia (as for adenomatous polyp, above, also AMACAR is −ve)
  - ➤ TCC (does not usu. have glands, has different immuno)
  - ➤ high grade PIN (basal layer ++ but ! ductal adenoCA can spread intraductally – see Pickup and Van der Kwast, 2007)

Basal Cell Hyperplasia (BCH), Basal Cell Adenoma and Basal Cell Adenomatosis
- Associations: BPH of the transitional zone, anti-androgen Rx, edge of infarcts
- Basaloid cells (little cytoplasm, bland oval non-grooved nuclei, small nucleoli), sparse mitoses
- Well-circumscribed at low power with lobular architecture ± some intermingling with normal glands at the periphery in florid forms ('pseudoinfiltrative'), may merge into normal glands
- Con/eccentric prolif^n around lumenal cells or solid nests ± cribriform areas ± peripheral palisading
- ± Central Ca^{2+} +/ intracytoplasmic (α_1AT/AFP +ve) globules (useful if present)
- Stroma: cellular but otherwise normal prostatic type
- Variants:
  - ➤ 'sclerosing BCH' has sclerotic stroma (d/dg sclerosing adenosis – αSMA/S100 may help)
  - ➤ 'BCH with prominent nucleoli' = 'atypical BCH': larger nucleoli and focal chronic inflam^n
  - ➤ 'florid BCH': ① mostly solid nests with little intervening stroma, pseudoinfiltration, nuclear and nucleolar enlargement and ↑ mitoses *or*
    ② BCH forming a nodule of >100 acini in one slide
  - ➤ 'basal cell adenoma' = BCH forming an expansile nodule (= 'adenoid basal tumour' if cribriform areas ++ or 'adenomatosis' if multifocal)
- Immuno: +ve for LP34, 34βE12, CK7; −ve for CK20, AMACAR; ±ve for PSA, αSMA, S100
- d/dg: PIN, adenocarcinoma, sclerosing adenosis (*q.v.*)
- d/dg urothelium (more cytoplasm, grooved nuclei, CK20 +ve), TCC (as for urothelium plus more pleomorphic and ↑ mitoses *cf.* BCH)
- d/dg BCC: invasion (incl. perineural and extraprostatic), necrosis and higher Ki-67 LI

Basal Cell (Basaloid/Adenoid Cystic) Carcinoma
- Infiltration (outside prostate/around nerves/around retained glands)
- Foci of necrosis ± desmoplastic reaction
- No metastases reported to date
- d/dg basal cell hyperplasia/basal cell adenoma (*vide supra*), TCC

Other Types of Prostatic Carcinoma
- Neuroendocrine tumours (carcinoid and SmCC subtypes): have eosinophilic granules:
  - ➤ NE differentiation in any tumour may be mis-interpreted as poorly diff adenocarcinoma
  - ➤ Gleason 5 adenocarcinoma may be misinterpreted as an NET (∴ do immuno)
- SmCC may be 1° or 2° (usu. from lung):
  - ➤ co-existing usual-type adenocarcinoma favours 1°, extensive vascular invasion favours 2°
  - ➤ immuno for TTF-1 is not helpful as 1° prostatic SmCC may be +ve
- Mucinous carcinoma/signet ring carcinoma
- SCC/ASC
- Lymphoepithelioma-like carcinoma ('like' because EBV cannot be demonstrated)
- Sarcomatoid carcinoma
- Carcinoma with oncocytic features

Secondary Tumours of the Prostate
- Usu. by direct spread from bladder/rectum
- Extensive vascular invasion favours a 2° origin
- Coexistence of usual-type 1° tumour or preneoplastic metaplasia favours 1°

Effects of Radiotherapy

Benign prostatic tissue
- Cytological atypia: nucleolar enlargement, nuclear enlargement and vacuolated/hazy chromatin, nuclear pyknosis, cytoplasmic eosinophilia ± vacuolisation
- Lumenal haematoxyphil mucin
- Glandular atrophy

- Metaplasias: mucinous, squamous and Paneth-like
- Atypical basal cell hyperplasia (nuclear vacuoles, powder-like chromatin and cytoplasmic vacuolation help identify radioRx as the likely cause)
- Xanthogranulomatous foamy Mφ
- Immuno: basal layer strongly +ve for 34βE12, lumenal cells weak/−ve for PSA

Prostatic adenocarcinoma

- Poorly-formed glands with single cells and haphazard arrangement (!Gleason grade inflation – but post-radioRx Bx grade still correlates with subsequent prostatectomy findings)
- Hyperchromatic nuclei with less visible nucleoli (! d/dg benign/atrophy)
- Cytoplasmic vacuoles (d/dg signet ring)/reticulated texture
- Immuno: PSA +ve, 34βE12 −ve
- ∴ Rely on architecture, invasion (e.g. perineural) and immuno rather than cytology to identify CA

Effects of Androgen Blockade Therapy

- Benign glands: simplification of gland architecture (loss of hyperplastic papillations), basal cell hyper-plasia, squamous metaplasia
- Malignant: ↓ extent of PIN and CA, loss of gland lumens and ↓ crystalloids, ↓ intensity of PSA staining
- Both: cytoplasmic vacuolation; nuclear shrinkage, hyperchromasia, pyknosis and apoptosis with ↓ mitoses and loss of nucleolar prominence
- Stroma: focal hypercellularity and chronic inflam^n ± foamy Mφ

Testicular Tumours

Histological Classification in Practice

- Germ cell tumour: 1. Seminoma (must be 100% pure[4] ± syncytiotrophoblastic cells)
  2. NSGCT (list the histological components present)
  3. Combined (give % of seminoma and NSGCT)
  4. Spermatocytic seminoma
- Non-germ cell tumours: sex cord/stromal, lymphoma, sarcomas, etc.

Germ Cell Tumours

Immunocytochemistry and tumour markers

- Serum AFP and hCG must both be measured because they are produced by different cell types, fluctuate independently of each other and frequently only one is elevated
- A patient with an apparently pure seminoma but a raised AFP must be treated as though he had an undiagnosed teratoma in addition (because tumours in these circumstances behave aggressively)
- AFP: YST (see also p. 19)
- hCG: trophoblastic elements (may also be +ve in MTU)
- NSE (serum and immuno), PLAP (membranous +vity), c-kit: seminomas (not spermatocytic), ITGCNU, (PLAP may also be +ve in borderline seminoma/teratoma)
- CD30: MTU (esp. if membranous +vity; may become −ve after chemoRx ∴ Hx is important) and non-neoplastic cells (e.g. activated lymphocytes/Mφ) in any tumour/lesion
- CK: MTU (CAM5.2), YST but not seminoma unless aggressive (anaplastic/borderline) types
- OCT4 (an octamer-binding transcription factor showing nuclear +vity by immuno in germ cells and stem cells): +ve in ITGCNU, non-spermatocytic seminoma, germinomas and MTU but −ve in better differentiated tumours such as YST, ChC and MTD. Positivity occurs at all 1° sites (pineal, ovary, retroperitoneum, mediastinum, etc.)
- Podoplanin: +ve (membrane) in germinomas but −ve in NSGCT (incl. YST, MTU and ChC) in the CNS

Intratubular germ cell neoplasia unclassified (ITGCNU)

- Is the precursor of all germ cell tumours except spermatocytic seminoma
- A single Bx is usu. sufficient since ITGCNU is usu. diffuse ∴ a −ve Bx is a sign of very low risk
- Tumour patients should have a contralateral Bx if the testis is of poor quality (soft/small)

---

[4] some accept rare foci of MTU (with just a few cells per focus, max.) in a seminoma but report that finding

- Cells: large, vacuolated cytoplasm with irregular nuclei and nucleoli (some say you must see these contiguously around at least 1 whole tubule cross-section to make the diagnosis)
- Partially involved tubules may show residual spermatogenesis
- Immuno/stains: glycogen, PLAP, c-kit, OCT4, NSE +ve (rarely: CAM5.2 +ve, also in Sertoli cells)
- 'Unclassified' distinguishes ITGCNU from intratubular embryonal CA/spermatocytic seminoma

Classical seminoma

- Macro: homogeneous, grey-white, no haemorrhage/necrosis
- Poorly-defined solid lobules of seminoma cells (± focal tubular arch./Pagetoid spread in *rete testis*)
- Delicate septa/dense scarring, T-cell infiltrates, granulomas
- Cells: uniform, large, polygonal-round, clear cytoplasm, well-defined cell borders, central large round nucleus with delicate hyperchromatic chromatin strands and multiple (usu. 1–2) prom. nucleoli
- Immuno/stains: contain glycogen ± lipid. PLAP, c-kit, OCT4 and NSE +ve; AFP −ve; CK (AE1/AE3) −ve in $\frac{2}{3}$ cases; some tumours have hCG +ve syncytiotrophoblastic cells; CD68 −ve; [i(12p)] +ve
- d/dg: spermatocytic seminoma, MTU (which may be focally PLAP +ve), Sertoli cell tumour (esp. if the seminoma has tubular areas), lymphoma, granulomatous orchitis – *q.v.*
- d/dg vascular invasion *vs.* tumour smearing artefacts or intravascular histiocytes
- d/dg ChC may have sheets of cytotrophoblast that mimic seminoma – look for more typical areas

Anaplastic seminoma

- Variant of classical seminoma defined as seminoma with ≥3/hpf mitoses
- More pleomorphic and less lymphoid *cf.* classical seminoma
- Stage for stage it has the same prognosis as classical *but* presents at a later stage more often

Spermatocytic seminoma

- Older patients (but rare, so classical seminoma is still more common), mets are rare, excision is curative
- Macro: large, grey, gelatinous and cystic
- Sheets of mitotic, cells with moderate-abundant cytoplasm (plasmacytoid if Bouin's fixed) with ≈ round nuclei showing 'nemaline'/'spireme' chromatin (i.e. evenly-dispersed large elongated clumps)
- These cells vary in size (more than shape) from large (± multinucleated) to small (lymphocyte-like) and textbooks describe this as an admixture of '3-cell types: large, intermediate and small'
- 'Anaplastic spermatocytic seminoma' has areas where the large cells predominate (but is otherwise typical)
- Stromal oedema/myxoid change (there is a lack of true lymphocytes, sclerosis and granulomas)
- May spread along tubules (= intratubular spermatocytic seminoma) thereby mimicking ITGCNU
- No trophoblastic elements but may develop spindle sarcomatous transformation ± RMS
- d/dg anaplastic seminoma: spermatocytic has sparse lymphocytes and is −ve for PLAP, c-kit, ITGCNU and [i(12p)]
- *Only* occurs in the testis (*cf.* seminoma/germinoma arising in mediastinum, pineal, etc.)

Borderline seminoma/teratoma (anaplastic germ cell tumour)

- Features favouring undiff teratoma: overlapping nuclei, multiple nucleoli
- Features favouring seminoma: lack of the above and lymphocytes in the stroma
- Highly aggressive
- Immuno: CD30 +ve (EMA −ve); CK (AE1/AE3 or CAM5.2), PLAP and NSE +ve (> 80%); c-kit +ve in 40% of cases; AFP +ve cells and hCG +ve syncytial cells may be present

Differentiated teratoma (MTD)

- Teratomas are germ cell tumours with differentiation towards all 3 somatic germ layers (ectoderm, mesoderm, endoderm) or predominantly 1 (= 'monodermal teratoma') or 2 of them
- MTD is a BTTP term that encompasses both mature and immature teratomas and any admixture of the two because prog. ∝ age, not the presence of immature elements (*cf.* ovarian teratomas):
  - ➤ pre puberty: these are benign (do not metastasise) even if there are immature elements. They are usu. pure teratomas *without* associated ITGCNU. [∴ best omit the 'malignant' bit of 'MTD' in a report]
  - ➤ post puberty: these are malignant (may metastasise), often have accompanying ITGCNU and are rarely pure teratomas (they tend to occur with MTU +/other germ cell tumour elements)
- Some elements may show cytological atypia or glandular complexity (∴ do not diagnose somatic carcinoma arising in a MTD without good evidence of invasion)
- A 'dermoid cyst' is a subset of MTD containing skin and adnexa only (some authors allow cartilage/bone and ciliated/GI epithelium in the wall provided that there is no cytological atypia, abnormal spermatogenesis or ITGCNU elsewhere) – it is benign (in all age groups). d/dg epidermoid cyst (does not show adnexa or surrounding ITGCNU – see 'Frozen Section' p. 228 for details)

- $2°$ malignancy arising in MTD = overgrowth of a single component to fill >50% of a low power field ($\times 4$ objective) or forming an expansile mass (of ≥ 1 cm $\varnothing$ for neuroectodermal tumours). Unlike in the ovary, sarcomas (esp. RMS) and PNET are more common than carcinomas
- d/dg monodermal (or predominantly monodermal) MTU *vs.* metastatic tumour of that type (e.g. carcinoid): presence of ITCGNU or other differentiated tissues favour MTU; multiple/bilateral lesions, vascular invasion ++ and clin. evidence of possible $1°$ lesion(s) elsewhere favour a metastasis

Undifferentiated teratoma (MTU = embryonal carcinoma)

- Rare alone but occurs in 45% of composite tumours. Macro: haemorrhage and necrosis
- Sheets, alveolar, glandular patterns $\pm$ papillary projections
- Cells are pleomorphic and epithelial-like (basophil to amphophil non-clear cytoplasm) with ill-defined cell borders $\pm$ overlapping nuclei; (d/dg seminomas can be pleomorphic, so use all these features)
- Separate tumour nodules in the tunica or hilum suggest vascular invasion (which should be sought)

Malignant teratoma intermediate (MTI)

- A mixture (any proportions) of MTU and MTD. It is the commonest subtype of teratoma in adults

Trophoblastic differentiation and Malignant teratoma trophoblastic (MTT)

- For morphology of trophoblasts and ChC, see pp. 65–66
- Isolated syncytiotrophoblastic elements are assoc^d with hCG +vity in tissue and serum but does NOT influence tumour behaviour. This may line degenerate cysts post chemoRx in retroperitoneal LN
- Syncytio and cytotrophoblast = 'choriocarcinomatous elements'
- Syncytio and cytotrophoblast *forming a villous or papillary pattern* is required to diagnose MTT (thus, MTT is just a villo/papillary architectural subtype of ChC [there are no stromal cores])
- ChC/MTT/high serum hCG are assoc^d with haematogenous mets, aggressive behaviour and good response to chemoRx

Yolk sac tumour (YST) / yolk sac elements

- Children: usu. pure YST; adults: usu. YST with other germ cell elements
- Variable patterns: reticular (= microcystic), **solid**, **glandular** (alveolar, intestinal and endometrioid-like), macrocystic, **polyvesicular vitelline** (= irregular vesicles [with constrictions] partly lined by flattened and partly by columnar epithelium in a cellular or loose mesenchyme), **hepatoid**, papillary, myxoid, adenofibromatous, **parietal** (= abundant extracellular eosinophilic confluent BM material), **mesenchyme-like**, YST with $2°$ neoplasia (e.g. RMS or NET)
- Those in **bold** constitute special variants if they occupy >50% of the tumour (have Mx implications)
- $\pm$ Schiller-Duval bodies (= cuboidal/columnar epithelial papilla with a single vessel in the core and projecting into a space lined by flattened cells). If numerous or predominant the term endodermal sinus pattern/tumour is used. It also has labyrinthine spaces amid branching loose fibrous cores festooned with epithelium
- Variable cytology ($\propto$ arch.): flat to columnar, clear to hepatoid, blastematous, $\pm$ basal vacuoles, $\pm$ intestinal differentiation, $\pm$ mucin glands, $\pm$ EMH foci (!d/dg syncytiotrophoblast which is rare in YST)
- Variable stroma ($\propto$ arch.): primitive spindle, mesenchymal, heterologous elements, luteinisation
- Intra and extracellular DPAS +ve hyaline globules are common but non-specific (AFP/α_1AT +ve)
- Nuclei: bland or large, hyperchromatic and irreg. with prominent nucleoli; $\pm$ vacuoles, $\pm$ mitoses ++
- Immuno: $-$ve for EMA and OCT4; +ve for CK (AE1/3 or MNF116), AFP, α_1AT, PLAP [and canalicular CD10/pCEA in hepatoid]
- AFP is +ve in: YST, teratoma (liver/skin/nerve/tubular epithelial structures), hepatoblastoma/HCC
- d/dg ChC may have sheets of cytotrophoblast that mimic YST – look for more typical areas
- d/dg hyperplasia of the rete testis with hyaline globules and MTU [for other d/dg, see p. 252]

Prognostic indicators and response to therapy

- Pure seminoma: radioRx/carboplatin
- Non-seminomatous and mixed germ cell tumours: vascular invasion +ve: $\rightarrow$ chemoRx / vascular invasion $-$ve: $\rightarrow$ F/U
- ChC elements/high serum hCG: risk of haematogenous spread
- YST elements: more likely to present at stage I (confined to testis)
- MRC Prognostic Score for Stage I Teratoma (see box on the right – add to give score out of 4):

1: presence of MTU
1: absence of YST elements
1: presence of blood vasc. invasion
1: presence of lymphatic invasion

Gonadoblastoma, polyembryoma, diffuse embryoma, malignant mixed germ cell tumour
See p. 252.

Sex Cord/Stromal Tumours

Immunocytochemistry
(Also see 'Normal Testis' section and table 16.1 on p. 211)
- Melan A (A103) may be +ve in Sertoli/Leydig tumours (and, to a lesser extent, stromal tumours)
Leydig cell tumour
- No familial tendency; liberate testosterone, oestrogens or other hormones
- Intracellular lipofuscin and Reinke's crystalloids are typically present
- May be calcifying
- Immuno: S100 +ve in some cases
- Features of malignancy (never occurs in children):
  - >5cm $\emptyset$
  - infiltrating margins
  - prominent foci of necrosis
  - 3/10 lpf mitoses (not sufficient on its own)
  - vascular invasion
  - metastases
  - do not respond to chemo/radioRx
- d/dg: large cell calcifying variant of Sertoli cell tumour
- d/dg Leydig cell hyperplasia (microscopic, multifocal and preserves underlying architecture)
Sertoli cell nodule (= Pick's adenoma/tubular adenoma/Sertoli cell adenoma)
- Usu. microscopic in maldescended testis but may be upto a few mm $\emptyset$ and in a descended testis
- Not neoplastic and no malignant potential ∴ terms using 'adenoma' are inappropriate
- Unencapsulated nodule of well-formed tubules of Sertoli cells with an immature phenotype (i.e. focal CK18 +vity with vimentin, cells usu. tall and thin with indistinct cytoplasm and bland dark round/oval nuclei)
- Simple tubules or 'cribriform'-like aggregates
- May have hyaline eosinophil blob in lumens (= 'Call-Exner-like bodies') may anastomose ± lamellar Ca^{2+}
- Usu. have interstitial Leydig cell aggregates (if not, some call it *Sertoli cell adenoma*)
- ± Intratubular spermatogonia or ITGCNU (! d/dg gonadoblastoma)
- d/dg Sertoli cell tumour: features that favour nodule over tumour are:
  - small and may be multifocal (! but a rare 'giant' variant, 1cm $\emptyset$, has been described)
  - tubules well-formed throughout (even if some do not show a lumenal space)
  - immature Sertoli cells with occ. spermatogonia *throughout* the lesion (*cf.* focal/peripheral)
  - not encapsulated / pseudoencapsulated or expansile in nature
  - presence of Call-Exner-like hyaline blobs and interposed Leydig cells (if present)
  - lack of typical Sertoli cell tumour stroma/stromal changes
Sertoli cell tumour and Sertoli-Leydig cell tumour
- Adult, present with mass (endocrine effects only if there is a Leydig component)
- Well-circumscribed and usu. 3–4cm $\emptyset$
- Tubular differentiation (at least focally):
  - a lumen is not always present (i.e. solid tubules, cords and strands)
  - simple lining or pseudostratified (endometrioid)
  - architecture: simple, irregular or complex (reteform)
- ± Solid areas (may look like Leydig cell islands or, if poorly diff., like a spindle sarcoma)
- ± Heterologous elements: mucinous cysts (may dominate the tumour), muscle, fat, bone, cartilage. These may be the source of sarcomatous overgrowth in some tumours
- The cells have moderate eosinophil cytoplasm (± lipid foam/globules)
- Mild nuclear pleomorphism and few mitoses unless poorly differentiated
- Poorly diff. tumours have (at least focal) solid spindle-sarcoma-like areas with mitoses ++
- Stroma: fibrous/hyaline with dilated vessels (and Leydig cells in Sertoli-Leydig cell tumours)
- Sclerosing variant: sclerotic stroma without the vessels, small atrophic tubules or solid areas
- Large cell calcifying variant: younger, smaller (1–2cm), ± multifocal, larger eosinophil cells with nucleoli, stromal Ca^{2+}, myxoid ± PMN, assoc^d with Carney syndrome, (d/dg Leydig cell tumour)
- Prognostics: size (esp. $\geq$5cm), mitoses (esp. $>$5/10hpf), necrosis, vascular invasion
- d/dg: Leydig cell tumour, adenomatoid tumour (but this is usu. paratesticular not intratesticular), Sertoli cell nodule (*vide supra*), tubular seminoma (look for lymphocytic stroma, granulomas ITGCNU and more classical seminoma morphology elsewhere), carcinoid (morphology and immuno)
- For more d/dg, see p. 249.

Testicular Lymphoma
- Usu. painless and in older patients with other organ involvement (e.g. CNS, MALT)
- Macro: homogeneous/nodular (d/dg seminoma)
- Interstitial infiltrate with relative tubular sparing
- DLBCL is the most common but others occur (e.g. HL, Burkitt's and T-cell in younger people)
- ± Vascular invasion
- d/dg: granulomatous orchitis (p. 215), leukaemia (late stage, usu. bilateral, PB findings)

Metastases from Testicular Tumours
- 1° tumours with YST elements have a worse prognosis if metastatic disease is present (stages II–IV)
- NSGCT: prior to cisplatin the mets looked like the 1°, but now they mature (mature elements are resistant) – MTD may be seen in the metastasis even if this was not seen in the 1°
- In a retroperitoneal LN dissection state:
    1) whether identifiable LN or surrounding tissues are present
    2) the presence and type of any residual tumour incl. if any somatic malignancies have developed (carcinoma [must be invasive, dysplasia only = teratoma or d/dg chemoradioRx atypia]/sarcoma/leukaemia/lymphoma/Wilms'/PNET/NB) – these may need different Rx.
       d/dg sarcoma *vs.* immature teratoma mesenchyme (look for destructive invasion, lack of organoid structure and the presence of abnormal mitoses)
       d/dg carcinoma (very rare) *vs.* YST glandular elements.
    3) completeness of excision
- d/dg met from a somatic malignancy (non-testicular): use CPC (incl. serum markers and testicular USS), EMA and mucin +vity is unlikely to be seen in an MTU, [i(12p)] favours seminoma and NSGCT

Metastases to the Testis
- Sources: prostatic adenoCA, relapse of ALL after (testicle-sparing) radioRx, RCC, melanoma
- There may be interstitial infiltration with tubular sparing
- Extensive vascular invasion favours a 2° origin
- Coexistence of usual-type 1° tumour or preneoplastic metaplasia favours 1°

Frozen Section of the Testis
- The usu. problem is d/dg epidermoid cyst *cf.* well diff. teratoma (→ radical orchidectomy and LN dissection)
- Also, distinguish Sertoli cell nodule (→ no action) from Sertoli cell tumour (→ radical orchidectomy)

Epidermoid cyst of the testis
- Benign but uncommon; usu. unilocular; should have all of the following *Price criteria* for diagnosis:
    ➢ intraparenchymal and without surrounding ITGCNU
    ➢ keratin contents and squamous lining (may be incomplete)
    ➢ fibrous (dermis-like) wall/capsule but no testicular parenchymal scarring
    ➢ no other elements (adnexa, endodermal tissues, mesodermal tissues, etc.)
- d/dg dermoid cyst: has adnexa (pilosebaceous) structures in the wall in normal skin-like orientation
- d/dg teratoma: macro is irregular ± multiloculated; micro has other tissues and not so well organised, ± cytological atypia/ITGCNU/testicular atrophy/scar; serum tumour markers may be elevated

Paratesticular Tumours

- Malignant: ➢ mesothelioma (! d/dg florid mesothelial hyperplasia of tunica vaginalis)
              ➢ RMS: usu. spindle/embryonal subtypes
              ➢ leiomyosarcoma: usu. well-diff; look for necrosis and mitoses
              ➢ liposarcoma: usu. well-diff (lipoma-like) – may need many blocks
              ➢ fibrosarcoma: usu. well-diff (! d/dg fibromatosis)
              ➢ others: extra-abdominal Wilms', ovarian/Müllerian-type carcinoma, KS, etc.
- Benign: ➢ adenomatoid tumour and (benign) papillary mesothelioma
              ➢ Brenner tumour
              ➢ *most* myxoid lesions are benign (myxoid variants of sarcomas are very rare here)
              ➢ developmental (adrenal rests, splenic-testicular fusion)
              ➢ inflammatory (fibrous pseudotumour, sperm granuloma, sclerosing lipogranuloma)
              ➢ any benign soft tissue tumour (lipoma, proliferative fasciitis, etc.)

- d/dg mets or testicular tumours extending to the paratesticular region: e.g. carcinoma of the rete testis or epididymis

Penile Neoplasia

Squamous Dysplasia
- Any grade can occur (low grade: $\leq$ basal $\frac{1}{3}$ of epithelium affected, high grade: $> \frac{1}{3}$). Full-thickness lesions (CIS) are termed Erythroplasia of Queyrat, Bowen's disease or Bowenoid papulosis (*vide infra*)
- Morphological subtypes: squamous, warty, basaloid
- Definitive diagnosis should be by CPC since prognosis differs (upto 20% of Bowen's disease and Erythroplasia progress to SCC $\pm$ mets whereas Bowenoid papulosis rarely progresses, usu. responds to local Rx and may spontaneously regress)

Erythroplasia of Queyrat
- Typical age 50 years; well-defined red velvety plaque on the glans; usu. single
- Irregular acanthosis; high grade dysplasia $\pm$ dyskeratoses; ($\pm$ parakeratotic hyperkeratosis)
- Chronic inflam^n and prominent capillarity in the underlying fibrous tissue

Bowen's disease
- Typical age 40 years; usu. paler (*cf.* Queyrat's erythroplasia) scaly lesion on the shaft; usu. single
- CIS also extends down pilosebaceous epithelium, hyperkeratosis is common (*cf.* erythroplasia)

Bowenoid papulosis
- Typical age 30 years; multiple papules on the shaft ($\pm$ glans/prepuce)
- Irregular acanthosis, $\pm$ warty features, $\pm$ more pigmented (melanin)
- The dysplastic cells, although full-thickness, may be more spaced out *cf.* Bowen's disease with some surface maturation and pilosebaceous units are usu. spared.

Squamous Cell Carcinoma
- Differentiate verrucous carcinoma from other types (see p. 285)
- Grading is as for skin (Broders' classification – see p. 284)
- Note local satellite nodules (discontinuous spread) – a poor prognostic feature
- d/dg PEH (as elsewhere)
- See also p. 42 and p. 51

Bibliography

Abrahams, N.A., Moran, C., Reyes, A.O. *et al.* (2005) Small cell carcinoma of the bladder: a contemporary clinicopathological study of 51 cases. *Histopathology*, **46**, 57–63.

Amin, M.B., Ro, J.Y., El-Sharkawy, T. *et al.* (1994) Micropapillary variant of transitional cell carcinoma of the urinary bladder. Histologic pattern resembling ovarian papillary serous carcinoma. *American Journal of Surgical Pathology*, **18**, 1224–1232.

Amin, M.B., Tamboli, P., Varma, M. *et al.* (1999) Postatrophic hyperplasia of the prostate gland: A detailed analysis of its morphology in needle biopsy specimens. *American Journal of Surgical Pathology*, **23** (8), 925–931.

Baithun, S.I. (1998) Prostatic neoplasia: the importance of PIN, biological markers and screening tests for diagnosis. *Current Diagnostic Pathology*, **5** (4), 180–187.

Barghorn, A., Alioth, H-R., Hailemariam, S. *et al.* (2006) Giant Sertoli cell nodule of the testis: distinction from other Sertoli cell lesions. *Journal of Clinical Pathology*, **59** (11), 1223–1225.

Bates, A.W. and Baithun, S.I. (2003) Secondary neoplasms of the urinary tract and male genital tract: a differential diagnostic consideration, in *Progress in Pathology*, Vol. 6 (eds N. Kirkham and N.A. Shepherd), Greenwich Medical Media, Ltd, London, pp.145–162.

Bates, A.W. and Baithun, S.I. (1998) The differential diagnosis of secondary and unusual primary tumours of the bladder. *Current Diagnostic Pathology*, **5** (4), 188–197.

Berney, D.M. (2005) A practical approach to the reporting of germ cell tumours of the testis. *Current Diagnostic Pathology*, **11** (3), 151–161.

Bostwick, D.G. (2006) Atypical small acinar proliferation in the prostate: clinical significance in 2006. *Archives of Pathology & Laboratory Medicine*, **130** (7), 952–957.

Bostwick, D.G. and Dundore, P.A. (1997) *Biopsy Pathology of the Prostate*, 1st edn, Chapman & Hall Medical, London.

Bostwick, D.G. and Eble, J.N. (eds) (1997) *Urologic Surgical Pathology*, 1st edn, Mosby, St Louis.

Cheng, L., Sung, M-T., Cossu-Roca, P. *et al.* (2007) OCT4: Biological functions and clinical applications as a marker of germ cell neoplasia. *Journal of Pathology*, **211** (1), 1–9.

Cheung, L., Cheville, J.C. and Bostwick, D.G. (1999) Diagnosis of prostate cancer on needle biopsies after radiation therapy. *American Journal of Surgical Pathology*, **23** (10), 1173–1183.

Cotran, R.S., Kumar, V. and Collins, T. (eds) (1999) *Robbins Pathologic Basis of Disease*, 6th edn, W.B. Saunders Co., Philadelphia.

Cormack, D.H. (1987) *Ham's Histology*, 9th edn, J.B. Lippincott & Co., Philadelphia.

Denholm, S.W., Webb, J.N., Howard, G.C. *et al.* (1992) Basaloid carcinoma of the prostate gland: histogenesis and review of the literature. *Histopathology*, **20**, 151–155.

Dundore, P.A., Schwartz, A.M. and Semerjian, H. (1996) Mast cell counts are not useful in the diagnosis of nonulcerative interstitial cystitis. *Journal of Urology*, **155** (3), 885–887.

Jones, E.C., Pins, M., Dickersin, G.R. and Young, R.H. (1995) Metanephric adenoma of the kidney. *American Journal of Surgical Pathology*, **19** (6), 615–625.

Epstein, J.I., Amin, M.B., Reuter, V.R. *et al*. (1998) The World Health Organization/International Society of Urological Pathology consensus classification of urothelial (transitional cell) neoplasms of the urinary bladder. *American Journal of Surgical Pathology*, **22** (12), 1435–1448.

Epstein, J.I. (1995) *Prostate Biopsy Interpretation*, 2nd edn, Lippincott-Raven, Philadelphia.

Ferry, J.A. and Young, R.H. (1997) Malignant lymphoma of the genitourinary tract. *Current Diagnostic Pathology*, **4** (3), 145–169.

Fisher, C. (2000) Paratesticular tumours and tumour-like lesions. *CPD Bulletin Cellular Pathology*, **2** (1), 13–16.

Fleming, S. (2005) Recently recognized epithelial tumours of the kidney. *Current Diagnostic Pathology*, **11** (3), 162–169.

Fleming, S. (2001) New classification of renal neoplasms, in *Recent Advances in Histopathology*, Vol. 19 (eds D. Lowe and J.C.E. Underwood), Churchill Livingstone, Edinburgh, pp. 99–114.

Fleming, S. (1995) Molecular genetics of renal neoplasia, in *Progress in Pathology*, Vol. 2 (eds N. Kirkham and N.R. Lemoine), Churchill Livingstone, Edinburgh, pp. 142–159.

Foster, C.S. and Ke, Y. (1998) Prostate cancer – current developments, in *Progress in Pathology*, vol. 4 (eds N. Kirkham and N.R. Lemoine), Churchill Livingstone, Edinburgh, pp. 137–164.

Fuhrman, S.A., Lasky, L.C. and Limas, C. (1982) Prognostic significance of morphologic parameters in renal cell carcinoma. *American Journal of Surgical Pathology*, **6** (7), 655–663.

Gaudin, P.B., Zelefsky, M.J., Leibel, S.A. *et al*. (1999) Histopathologic effects of three-dimensional conformal external beam radiation therapy on benign and malignant prostate tissues. *American Journal of Surgical Pathology*, **23** (9), 1021–1031.

Gleason, D.F. (1992) Histologic grading of prostate cancer: a perspective. *Human Pathology*, **23** (3), 273–279.

Gleason, D.F. and the veterans administration cooperative urological research group (1977) Histologic Grading and Clinical Staging of Prostatic Carcinoma, in *Urologic Pathology: the prostate*, 1st edn (ed M. Trannenbaum), Lea & Febiger, Philadelphia, pp. 191–218.

Gleason, D.F., Mellinger, G.T. and the veterans administration cooperative urological research group (1974) Prediction of prognosis for prostatic adenocarcinoma by combined histological grading and clinical staging. *Journal of Urology*, **111** (1), 58–64.

Gonlusen, G., Truong, A., Shen, S.S. *et al*. (2006) Granulomatous pyelitis associated with urinary obstruction: a comprehensive clinicopathologic study. *Modern Pathology*, **19** (8), 1130–1138.

Grigor, K.M. (1992) Germ cell tumours of the testis, in *Recent Advances in Histopathology*, Vol. 15 (eds P.P. Anthony, R.N.M. MacSween and D.G. Lowe), Churchill Livingstone, Edinburgh, pp. 177–194.

Humphrey, P.A. (2007) Diagnosis of adenocarcinoma in prostate needle biopsy tissue. *Journal of Clinical Pathology*, **60** (1), 35–42.

Iczkowski, K.A. and Bostwick, D.G. (1998) The pathologist as optimist: cancer grade deflation in prostatic needle biopsies. *American Journal of Surgical Pathology*, **22** (10), 1169–1170.

Johnsen, S.D. (1970) Testicular biopsy score count – a method for registration of spermatogenesis in human testes: normal values and results in 335 hypogonadal males. *Hormones*, **1** (1), 2–25.

Jones, T.D., Ulbright, T.M., Eble, J.N. *et al*. (2004) OCT4 staining in testicular tumors: a sensitive and specific marker for seminoma and embryonal carcinoma. *American Journal of Surgical Pathology*, **28** (7), 935–940.

Junqueira, L.C., Carneiro, J. and Long, J.A. (1986) *Basic Histology*, 5th edn, Appleton-Century-Crofts (Prentice-Hall), Norwalk, CT.

Llinares, K., Escande, F., Aubert, S. *et al*. (2004) Diagnostic value of MUC4 immunostaining in distinguishing epithelial mesothelioma and lung adenocarcinoma. *Modern Pathology*, **17** (2), 150–157.

Mallofre, C., Castillo, M., Morente, V. *et al*. (2003) Immunohistochemical expression of CK20, p53, and Ki-67 as objective markers of urothelial dysplasia. *Modern Pathology*, **16** (3), 187–191.

Martignoni, G., Pea, M., Brunelli, M. *et al*. (2004) CD10 is expressed in a subset of chromophobe renal cell carcinomas. *Modern Pathology*, **17** (12), 1455–1463.

McHale, T., Malkowicz, S.B., Tomaszewski, J.E. *et al*. (2002) Potential pitfalls in the frozen section evaluation of parenchymal margins in nephron-sparing surgery. *American Journal of Clinical Pathology*, **118** (6), 903–910.

Mishima, M., Kato, Y., Kaneko, M.K. *et al*. (2006) Podoplanin expression in primary central nervous system germ cell tumors: a useful histological marker for the diagnosis of germinoma. *Acta Neuropathologica*, **111** (6), 563–568.

Montironi, R. and Schulman, C.C. (1998) Pathological changes in prostate lesions after androgen manipulation. *Journal of Clinical Pathology*, **51** (1), 5–12.

Montironi, R., Mazzucchelli, R., Stramazzotti, D. *et al*. (2005) Basal cell hyperplasia and basal cell carcinoma of the prostate: a comprehensive review and discussion of a case with c-erbB-2 expression. *Journal of Clinical Pathology*, **58** (3), 290–296.

Montironi, R., Thompson, D. and Bartels, P.H. (1999) Premalignant lesions of the prostate, in *Recent Advances in Histopathology*, Vol. 18 (eds D.G. Lowe and J.C.E Underwood), Churchill Livingstone, Edinburgh, pp. 147–172.

Ng, W-K. (2003) Radiation-associated changes in tissues and tumours. *Current diagnostic Pathology*, **9** (2), 124–136.

Oxley, J.D., Sullivan, J., Mitchelmore, A. *et al*. (2007) Metastatic renal oncocytoma. *Journal of Clinical Pathology*, **60** (6), 720–722.

Pan, C-C., Chen, P. C-H., and Ho, D. M-T. (2004) The diagnostic utility of MOC31, BerEP4, RCC marker and CD10 in the classification of renal cell carcinoma and renal oncocytoma: an immunohistochemical analysis of 328 cases. *Histopathology*, **45** (5), 452–459.

Parkinson, M.C. (1995) Pre-neoplastic lesions of the prostate. *Histopathology*, **27** (4), 301–311.

Petersen, R.O. (ed) (1986) *Urologic Pathology*, 1st edn, J.B. Lippincott Co., Philadelphia.

Pickup, M. and Van der Kwast, T.H. (2007) My approach to intraductal lesions of the prostrate gland. *Journal of Clinical Pathology*, **60** (8), 856–865.

Poulos, C.K. and Cheng, L. (2005) Epidermoid Cyst of the Testis. *Pathology Case Reviews*, **10** (4), 212–216.

Rahemtullah, A. and Oliva, E. (2006) Nephrogenic adenoma: an update on an innocuous but troublesome entity. *Advances in Anatomic Pathology*, **13** (5), 247—255.

Rosai, J. (ed) (2004) *Rosai and Ackerman's Surgical Pathology*, 9th edn, Mosby, Edinburgh.

Roth, L.M. (2005) Variants of Yolk Sac Tumor. *Pathology Case Reviews*, **10** (4), 186–192.

Sheaff, M. and Baithun, S.I. (1997) Pathological effects of ionising radiation. *Current Diagnostic Pathology*, **4** (2), 106–115.

Sun, W., Zhang, P.L. and Herrera, G.A. (2002) p53 Protein and Ki-67 Overexpression in Urothelial Dysplasia of Bladder. *Applied Immunohisto-chemistry & Molecular Morphology*, **10** (4), 327–331.

Symmers, W. St. C. (ed) (1978) *Systemic Pathology*, Vol. 4, 2nd edn, Churchill Livingstone, London.

Theaker, J.M. and Mead, G.M. (2004) Diagnostic pitfalls in the histopathological diagnosis of testicular germ cell tumours. *Current Diagnostic Pathology*, **10** (3), 220–228.

Thilagarajah, R., Witherow, R.O. and Walker, M.M. (1998) Quantitative histopathology can aid diagnosis in painful bladder syndrome. *Journal of Clinical Pathology*, **51** (3), 211–214.

Trainer, T.D. (1997) Testis and Excretory Duct System, in *Histology for Pathologists*, 2nd edn (ed S.S. Sternberg), Lippincott Williams & Wilkins, Philadelphia, pp. 1019–1037.

Ulbright, T.M., Amin, M.B. and Young, R.H. (1999) Tumors of the Testis, Adnexa, Spermatic Cord and Scrotum, in *Atlas of Tumor Pathology Fascicle Nō 25*, 3rd series, Armed Forces Institute of Pathology, Washington DC.

Wheater, P.R., Burkitt, H.G. and Daniels, V.G. (1987) *Functional Histology: A text and colour atlas*, 2nd edn, Churchill Livingstone, Edinburgh.

Willis, R.A. (1952) *The Spread of Tumours in the Human Body*, Butterworth & Co Ltd., London.

Young, R.H., Srigley, J.R. and Amin, M.B. *et al.* (2000) Tumors of the Prostate Gland, Seminal Vesicles, Male Urethra and Penis, in *Atlas of Tumor Pathology Fascicle Nō 28*, 3rd series, Armed Forces Institute of Pathology, Washington DC.

17. Gynaecological

Vulva

Kraurosis Vulvae (Lichen Sclerosus)
See p. 215 under 'penile lesions'

Bartholin Gland Cyst
- Lining may be squamous, mucinous or transitional (similar to other vestibular gland cysts)
- d/dg the small (<2mm) apocrine gland retention cysts + hair follicle keratin plug of Fox-Fordyce disease

Squamous Cell Carcinoma (the Two Clinicopathological Types)
① older women, well-diff, keratinising, arising on a background of dystrophies
② young, basaloid, arising on a background of VIN with HPV; risk of synchronous/metachronous CA
- FIGO Stage 1A (≤2cm ∅, ≤1mm stromal invasion – from adj. dermal papilla) → conservative Mx

Extramammary Paget's Disease
- Sites (rich in apocrine glands): male or female perineum, external auditory meatus, eyelid, axilla
- ! An accompanying atypical squamous proliferation may mask the underlying Paget's
- Stromal invasion limited to <1mm = 'minimally invasive' (local excision may be curative)
- Immuno/stains: +ve for mucin (AB, DPAS), LMW CK (CAM5.2), CK7 (CK20 favours colonic/bladder 1°); ±ve for EMA, CEA, GCDFP15, AR, HER2, CD5; −ve for ER, PgR, PSA, Melan-A, HMB45
- d/dg Bowen's (+ve for HMW CK, −ve for mucin, CK7, GCDFP15) *vs.* anaplastic Paget's: Paget's spares the basal layer, may form small ducts and is +ve for mucin with a different immuno profile
- d/dg melanoma or metastasis from a visceral malignancy: use CPC, morphology and immuno

Vagina

Vaginal Intraepithelial Neoplasia (VAIN)
- Grading criteria for VAIN are the same as for CIN
- d/dg transitional cell metaplasia/epithelium

Effects of Diethylstilboesterol Exposure in utero
- Fibrotic anomalies: bands, septae, fornix obliteration, etc.
- ↑risk of squamous VAIN
- Vaginal adenosis (usu. affects the upper vagina):
  - ➢ Müllerian glands (endocervical, tubal/endometrial) in submucosa (may extend to the surface)
  - ➢ variable architectures including cystic (d/dg Nabothian follicles) and papillary (d/dg CCC, but CCC contains glycogen rather than mucin)
  - ➢ squamous metaplasia may occur (and may be the only feature if a superficial section is cut ∴ get levels if you see squamous epithelium dipping down deeper than usual into the stroma of a vaginal Bx)
  - ➢ may undergo Arias-Stella reaction (!d/dg atypical adenosis or CCC)
  - ➢ d/dg endometriosis (endometrial stroma and siderophages are absent in adenosis)
  - ➢ d/dg Wolffian remnants: occur deeper, no mucin (see Gartner's duct remnants p. 236)
- Atypical adenosis: adenosis with cytological atypia (prominent nucleoli, etc.) and no evidence of invasive architecture. Seen adjacent to (and thought to be the precursor of) CCC
- Carcinoma: CCC type, occurring in adolescent to young adult age group (always <40 years)

Other Mass Lesions
- Fibroepithelial polyp ± atypical ('bizarre') stromal cells
- 'Mesonephric' papilloma (young girls) – slender papillae lined by bland cuboidal-to-columnar non-mucous cells ± squamous metaplasia. Thought to be Müllerian rather than mesonephric

Diagnostic Criteria Handbook in Histopathology: A Surgical Pathology Vade Mecum by Paul J. Tadrous
Copyright © 2007 by John Wiley & Sons, Ltd.

- Rhabdomyoma (middle-aged): fibromyxoid stroma, elongated (strap-like) cells with vesicular nuclei & focal cross-striations by LM/EM. No cytol. atypia. Poorly circumscribed but usu. small (<3cm ∅)
- RMS botryoides (see p. 58)
- Many other very rare things incl. lymphoma, melanoma, leiomyosarcoma, ectopic rests, etc.

Cervix Uteri

FIGO Staging of Cervical Carcinoma (Old = 1988; New = 1995)

I confined to the uterus (corpus extension does not change the stage but worsens the prognosis)

II extracervical but not to the pelvic walls/lower third vagina (IIB = parametrial involvement)

III confined to pelvis but extends to walls/lower vagina or causes hydronephrosis/non-functioning kidney

IV *mucosa* of bladder/rectum involved or extrapelvic spread (IVB = distant mets)

- Stage IA = detectable by microscopy only ('microinvasive')[1] AND ≤7mm ∅ (i.e. ≤3 blocks)
  - ➤ IA1 = ≤3mm deep[2]
  - ➤ IA2 = 3–5mm deep
  - ➤ old IA1 = depth unmeasurable = <1mm ('early stromal invasion'), no ∅ limit
  - ➤ old IA2 = depth measurable = 1–5mm deep, ≤7mm ∅
- Stage IB: >1A or if clinically apparent (even if old IA1); Old IB: > old IA2
- Retain and distinguish the 'early stromal invasion' group as a subgroup of the new IA1 because treatment may be conservative provided the diameter is ≤7mm (if >7mm ∅, Rx is individualised)
- It is misleading to diagnose IA carcinoma if a lesion is incompletely excised. In such cases measurements should be qualified 'measuring *at least* . . .'
- Ulcerated lesions should not be staged as IA – their management should be individualised
- Small cell carcinoma should not be called 'microinvasive' – even if they are stage IA
- Vascular invasion does not affect the staging but should be mentioned

Cervical Squamous Intra-epithelial Neoplasia (CIN) and Early Invasive Squamous Carcinoma

- BAUS = basal layer nuclear abnormalities without full-thickness changes
- For CIN there must be nuclear abnormalities all the way to the surface epithelium for all grades 1–3
- Grading CIN: grades 1–3 show nuclear atypia (= enlargement, pleom., ↑NCR, variable hyperchromasia, irregular nuclear membranes, coarse chromatin and usu. *lack of* prominent nucleoli) & evidence of maturation lack occupying no more than the 1st, 2nd or 3rd thirds of the epithelial thickness respectively. Full thickness atypia (± slight surface flattening) is CIS (a subtype of CIN3)
- Mitoses: high mitoses and abnormal figures are helpful (2-group and 3-group forms – i.e. straggling/isolated chromosomes at the spindle poles – are more common than multipolar mitoses). For CIN1 the presence of mitoses (unless abnormal) is not helpful but some degree of nuclear enlargement and pleom. are essential. CIN in immature squamous metaplasia may not be gradable (= 'CIN ungradeable')
- In high grade lesions the basal layers are often vertically orientated (lateral crowding) and the epithelium, in general, has a tendency to strip off. Nuclear and cytoplasmic p16 +vity is typical
- Iodine artefact can result in under-grading CIN3 because it causes a pallor of staining in the superficial half of the epithelium with a sharp demarcation from the deeper half (nuclear morphology, apart from staining intensity, is not affected)
- Immuno: Ki67 +ve in the superficial levels, strong cytopl. and nuclear p16[INK4a] +vity (but may be −ve in low grade lesions)
- *ISH* for high risk[3] HPV: nuclear dot +vity ① indicates integrated virus, ② is seen in ≈ all cases of high grade CIN (i.e. CIN 2/3), and ③ may identify those cases of CIN 1 at risk of progression
- Features of impending invasion: extensive crypt involvement with distension, comedonecrosis and focal eosinophilic squamoid maturation (→ do levels); ! d/dg CIN3-like invasive SCC (p. 234)
- Features of early/microinvasion: irregular buds of cells (usu. arise from crypts *cf.* surface) with squamoid maturation (± pearls), nucleoli, stromal reaction (incl. chronic inflam[n] ± neovascularisation), bizarre giant basal cells (upto 5× normal size) and lack of basal palisading

---

[1] Both IA1 and IA2 are included in this category by the Working Party drawing up the UK National Dataset but some other authorities exclude the new IA2 from the 'microinvasive' category

[2] measured from the nearest stromal-epithelial junction – surface or crypt – from which the tumour arises

[3] = subtypes **16, 18, 31, 33, 35, 39, 45, 51, 52, 58, 59, 66, 68** (according to Kalof *et al.* 2005, all but 59 and 68 were used in their study)

- d/dg ! transitional cell metaplasia of the cervix can be misdiagnosed as CIN 3 but metaplasia:
  - ➢ has vertically (perpendicular to the BM) orientated nuclei in the deeper layers becoming transverse superficially (! but this may also be seen in high grade CIN)
  - ➢ smooth, oval nuclei with neat nuclear grooves *cf.* the nuclear atypia of CIN3 (*vide supra*)
  - ➢ lacks mitoses
- d/dg: ! do not mis-diagnose CIN3-like invasive SCC (irreg. islands of solid/comedo tumour) as CIN3
- d/dg postmenopausal atrophy: some advocate 'CIN ungradeable' if there are <4 cell layers with all horizontally orientated atypical cells; (mitoses or ↑Ki-67 LI help to confirm CIN)
- d/dg reactive/inflam^y/immature metaplasia (look for nucleoli and mucus cells but ! see SMILE, below)

Grading and Variants of SCC
- Large cell keratinising (well diff/G1): bridges and keratinising squamous pearls
- Large cell non-keratinising (moderately diff/G2): no pearls but may have single cell keratinisation
- Small cell non-keratinising (poorly diff/G3) and CIN3-like SCC: high grade cytology ± necrosis ± large pleomorphic cells with giant bizarre nuclei ± surrounding invasive squamoid tongues
- Squamotransitional cell CA (papillary SCC): the superficial part looks like urothelial G1/G2 pTa TCC but deeper it can be widely invasive (d/dg squamous papilloma which is rare esp. postmenopause)
- d/dg CIN3-like SCC *vs.* SmCC:
  - ➢ SCC has a solid pattern of infiltrative growth: 'back-to-back' islands showing comedonecrosis
  - ➢ SmCC: ☞ irregular loose/dyscohesive aggregates
    - ☞ organoid +/rosettes/acini
    - ☞ lack of a lymphoid response
    - ☞ vascular invasion more common than with SCC
  - ➢ immuno: 34βE12, p63, CK14 +ve in SCC; CD56 +ve in SmCC; CgA ±ve in SmCC and SCC

Adenoid Basal Carcinoma/Epithelioma
- Elderly, not mass-forming, assoc^d with surface CIN2-3 but on its own it has a good prognosis
- Basaloid islands (BCC-like cells with palisading) ± columnar cell rosettes within them ± mucin
- Few mitoses and no desmoplastic stromal reaction
- Islands with abrupt keratinisation
- Immuno: basaloid cells +ve for reserve cell CK (14, 17 and 19); columnar cells +ve for CEA, EMA
- d/dg CIN3-like SCC, adenoid cystic carcinoma, ASC with adenoid basal-like areas
- d/dg postmenopausal basaloid reserve cell change: buds, nests and interconnecting cords of basaloid reserve cells around endocervical glands without a stromal reaction (! do not call it cancer)

Cervical Glandular Intra-epithelial Neoplasia (CGIN) and Invasive Adenocarcinoma
- Classified into: low grade (CGIN I) and high grade (CGIN II and III = ACIS)
- CGIN often co-exists with CIN (but a cervical smear is *not* sensitive for detecting CGIN)
- High grade CGIN (but not low grade) is assoc^d with HPV 18

Histology of dysplasia
- *Abrupt* change from normal to abnormal areas in a gland is a feature of dysplasia (! or metaplasia)
- Hyperchromasia, pleomorphism, (abnormal) mitoses, aberrant (gastric neutral) mucin, apoptoses
- Goblet cells (not seen in non-neoplastic conditions)
- Low grade: nuclear abnormalities limited to the lower $\frac{2}{3}$ of the epithelium; apical mucin persists
- High grade: abnormal mitoses and apoptoses are common, arch. anomalies more usual *cf.* low grade (gland clustering, outpouchings, papillary formations, cellular bridging, etc.)
- d/dg: if ?dysplasia but can't tell whether squamous/glandular consider 'atypical reserve cell hyperplasia'
- d/dg: stratification is normal (cyclical) in endocervical cells so is insufficient for diagnosis in the absence of nuclear abnormalities; likewise cribriform change *per se* is not specific to neoplasia

Features of stromal invasion
- Oedema, fibrosis, inflammation and squamoid change are indicative of invasion
- Extension beyond the normal glandular field (presence of medium-sized arteries or >7.8mm deep)
- Large irregular 'crab-like' glands/dysplastic glands with 'stretched' areas and stromal oedema/inflam^n
- Solid growth patterns (see Figure 17.1 on p. 245) and adenosquamoid areas

Variants
- Endocervical, endometrioid, enteric, clear cell, adenosquamous, ciliated, microcystic adenoCA

Immuno

- CEA +ve (−ve in non-dysplastic structures in d/dg)
- EMA and CA-125 cytoplasmic staining (lumenal staining in non-dysplastic glands)
- CA-19.9 +ve in 50% of CGIN/adenocarcinoma (negative in non-dysplastic glands)
- p16 is diffusely +ve (nuclear and cytoplasmic) in high grade CGIN and some adenocarcinomas but usu. negative in non-neoplastic glands
- Bcl-2 −ve
- Ki-67 LI > 67% (some use a MIB1 of <10% and >50% as cut-off points for reactive *vs.* dysplasia)

Minimal Deviation Adenocarcinoma (Endocervical Type MDA = Adenoma Malignum)
- Clin: worse prognosis *cf.* other adenocarcinomas and is assoc[d] with Peutz-Jeghers and mucinous ovarian tumours (even in the absence of Peutz-Jeghers multifocal SCTAT)
- Deep infiltration (beyond the middle third/>7.8mm/presence of medium-sized arteries)
- 'Finger-in-glove'/'crab-like' complex outlines with pointy angles to glands
- Columnar mucinous cells with minimal/focal atypia
- Desmoplastic response focally (± vascular invasion): periglandular stromal cells become αSMA +ve, ER −ve (the opposite of periglandular stromal cells in benign glandular conditions)
- Immuno: −ve for ER, PgR and diffuse CA-125 and +ve for CEA (focal) and EMA (cytoplasmic)
- Contains pyloric-type mucin (neutral sialomucin) *cf.* normal glands (sulphomucins – mixed purple/violet on ABDPAS) – but ! exclude d/dg simple pyloric metaplasia using morphology
- d/dg: endometrioid variant MDA (good prognosis, pseudostratified glands) ! d/dg CGIN/TEM
- d/dg Fluhman Type A tunnel clusters (undilated, branched/budded hyperplastic glands). Type B tunnel clusters are like deep Nabothian polyfollicles (can also get deep Nabothian follicles proper)
- d/dg lobular glandular hyperplasia/deep crypts (rounded glands, lobular, no desmoplasia, immuno)
- d/dg mesonephric remnant hyperplasia (p. 236)
- d/dg endocervicosis (in the cervix there must be a gland-free zone between superficial and deep glands)
- d/dg florid cystic endosalpingiosis lacks atypia or stromal response

Other Tumours
- AdCC: S100 −ve (unlike other sites), may co-exist with adenocarcinoma or SCC, poor prognosis
- Glassy cell carcinoma: ASC variant with vesicular nuclei and prominent nucleoli, poor prognosis
- Clear cell ASC: like glassy cell but no prominent nucleoli, poor prognosis
- SmCC: occurs with adenocarcinoma or SCC – ! DO NOT misdiagnose as ASC. Aggressive
- Benign: Müllerian papilloma of childhood, adenomas (tubular, villous, TV, villoglandular)

Metaplasias and Other Lesions in the Differential Diagnosis of CGIN

Tuboendometrioid metaplasia (TEM)
- Assoc[d] with trauma (cone, birth, prolapse)
- Mixture of cell types: intraepithelial lymphocytes and tubal epithelium (alternating ciliated/secretory)
- Cilia (favour a metaplastic rather than neoplastic process, esp. if well-formed)
- Apoptoses are rare (likewise mitoses – and there should be no abnormal mitoses)
- Immuno: p16 −ve/focal +vity; Bcl-2 +ve (diffuse cytoplasmic) } opposite to high grade CGIN
- Pseudostratification (*cf.* true stratification in CGIN – requires EM to distinguish)
- Atypical: variation in nuclear size (after accounting for the 3 cell types)
- d/dg ciliated CGIN: CGIN lacks multiple cell types, has more complex arch., ↑Ki-67 LI, etc.

Microglandular endocervical hyperplasia (MGH)
- Usu. (but not necessarily) assoc[d] with pregnancy or pill – can occur postmenopausally
- PMN
- Vacuolated cells, not stratified
- Lacy columnar reserve cells present (MGH may coexist with reserve cell hyperplasia)
- Normal mitoses and lack of apoptoses (*cf.* CGIN)
- Immuno: p16 −ve (and Bcl-2 −ve)
- Hyalinised stroma (pseudoinfiltrative), solid sheets, hobnail/signet cells → d/dg clear cell CA (but CCC has nuclear atypia, ↑ mitoses and intracellular glycogen predominantly [± a little mucin])
- d/dg microglandular endometrial adenoCA – this lacks lacy reserve cells and has endometrial stroma

Stratified mucinous intraepithelial lesion (SMILE)
- This is considered a form of unstable reserve cell hyperplasia

- Mucous vacuoles in stratified epithelium showing nuclear atypia and a high proliferation index
- Assoc^d with CIN, CGIN, adenoca or SCC ∴ do levels/embed more tissue if only SMILE is seen

Oxyphil metaplasia (OMEE)
- Large nuclei with nucleoli but normochromatic, normal mitoses and inflammation in lumena

Florid cystic endosalpingiosis
- Lacks atypia or stromal response

Papillary endocervicitis
- Blunt-tipped papillae, not dysplastic or proliferative (*cf.* d/dg: villoglandular/papillary carcinoma)

Gartner's duct remnants
(Gartner's duct is the intra-cervical part of the Mesonephric [Wolffian] system)
- Acinar/lobular architecture
- Eosinophil secretions (DPAS and AB +ve) but no intracellular mucin
- Large vesicular nuclei (not hyperchromatic)
- Immuno: CD10 +ve
- d/dg SCC (CIN may extend into mesonephric remnants, esp. after conisation d/dg invasive SCC), MDA (but this has columnar mucous cells and complex glands), metastatic breast carcinoma (but this is usu. diffusely infiltrative – ! may be overlooked as 'stromal hypercellularity')

Lobular glandular hyperplasia/deep crypts
- Bland glands ± foreign body granulomatous reaction to spilled mucin

Arias-Stella reaction
- May affect endometriotic or native cervical glands (see section on Arias-Stella, p. 237, for details)
- ! do not confuse the stromal decidualisation for d/dg SCC

Radiation atypia
- Nuclear hyperchromasia is rare
- Stromal radiation changes are also present
- Lack of mitoses – esp. in relation to the degree of atypia
- ! cytoplasmic CEA may be +ve

Corpus Uteri

Normal Endometrium
- Simple glands i.e. no branching or budding (complexity)
- The deep *stratum basalis* does not cycle: ➢ weakly prolif. & minimally tortuous glands
  ➢ dense stroma intermingled with myometrium
- The *stratum functionalis* (= mid *stratum spongiosum* and superficial *stratum compactum*) undergo morphological changes with the hormonal status/menstrual cycle
- There is synchronous proliferation of blood vessels, glands and stroma – except that:
  ➢ glands predominate in late secretory/early menstrual
  ➢ stroma predominates in decidua/atrophy
- The changes are uniformly developed across the uterine cavity (except the isthmus)
- The lower uterine segment/isthmus has: ① spindled stromal cells with collagen fibres in between, ② hybrid endometrial/endocervical glands, ③ less marked hormonal effects
- Typical immunoprofile: epithelial cells are +ve for CK, EMA, vimentin; CEA −ve; S100 −ve unless in early pregnancy (i.e. <12 weeks); stromal cells are CD10 +ve

Dating Secretory Endometrium – see table 17.1

Diagnosing Pregnancy
- Only a placental site reaction is diagnostic of intrauterine gestation:
  ➢ layer of (Nitabuch's) fibrinoid and intermediate (esp. multinucleate) trophoblasts in the endometrium
  ➢ ± trophoblastic invasion of vessels (replace endothelium) and fibrinoid vascular change
  ➢ ± villi or any of the other features described below
- Coincidence of gestational endometrium with ↑hCG suggests a gestation (at any site)

Gestational endometrium (= 'gestational hyperplasia')
- Hypersecretory glands: vacuolated cytoplasm, prominent pap. infolds ('ferning'), secretions ++
- Arias-Stella reaction (*vide infra*) ± nuclear clearing (! not d/dg HSV inclusions)
- Prominent oedema (mid-secretory-like)

TABLE 17.1 Dating Secretory Endometrium

	Early features		Mid. features		Late features	
POD	Vacuoles	Mitoses	Secret"s	Oedema	Pre-decidual change	Other
1	uniform & subnuclear <50% of glands	++	–	–	–	
2	uniform & subnuclear >50% of glands (ovulation confirmed)	++	–	–	–	
3	well-aligned (↓ pseudostratification)	±	–	–	–	
4	move to lumenal aspect	rare	±	–	–	
5	sparse	–	+	–	–	
6		–	+++	–	–	
7	–	–	+++	++	–	
8	–	–	+++	+++	–	
9	–	stromal +	+++	++	first appears	spiral arteries become prominent
10	–	stromal ++	+++	+	thick cuffs around arteries	
11	–	stromal +	+++	+	superficial islands	
12	–		++	+	islands start to merge	
13	–		++	+	maximal confluence	granulocytes become prominent
14	–		+	±	+	RBC extravasation
mens.	–	+	exhaust^n	±	halos	crumbling

- Decidual reaction of pregnancy (*decidua vera*)
  - ➢ thick-walled spiral arteries (± atherosis/necrosis/inflam^n – all *suggest* intra-uterine gestation)
  - ➢ abundant, *well defined* eosinophilic to clear cytoplasm (glycogen and lipid)
  - ➢ large ovoid vesicular pale bland nuclei and well-defined nucleoli
  - ➢ ↑stromal granulocytes (K-cells) in early gestation (but these are ≈ absent by term)
  - ➢ d/dg mononuclear intermediate trophoblasts (these are hPL, CD146 and CK +ve)
- Decidual glands and Fallopian tube epithelium become S100 +ve in early pregnancy (i.e. <12/40)

Arias-Stella Reaction (= focal polyploid change)
- Affects endometrium, cervix, Fallopian tube or endometriosis and may be 2° to any cause of ↑hCG (gestation, mole, tumours, etc) or hormone therapy or a *corpus luteum* (cyst or persistent)
- Cytoplasm: clear, eosinophil or vacuolated ++ (*NB*: there is cytomegaly such that NCR is preserved)
- Nuclei (active phase): ↑size, irregular outline, granular chromatin ± prominent nucleoli
- Nuclei (degenerate phase): smudged nuclear hyperchromasia and pleomorphism ± hobnailing
- d/dg CCC: focality, background of gestational changes, normal NCR and lack of mitoses all favour benignity

Menstrual Endometrium
- Stromal fibrin and fibrin thrombi
- Stromal crumbling forming balls with surrounding halos of pre-decidual cells
- Glands showing 'secretory exhaustion' (dilated, flattened cells with frayed borders)
- Glandular apoptotic bodies and PMN infiltrates in glands
- The *stratum basalis* is normal

Variants of Secretory

Under-developed secretory (Luteal phase defect = LPD)
- Clin.: infertility/recurrent miscarriage (= habitual abortion i.e. ≥3 consecutive pregnancy losses)
- Morphologically abnormal: ➢ inadequate gland coiling (proliferative phase deficiency)
  - ➢ inadequate secretions/decidualisation (luteal phase deficiency)

- Normal but delayed development (i.e. Out Of Phase = OOP)
  - ≥3 days OOP occurring more than sporadically
  - asynchronous development of glands *vs.* stroma (e.g. due to some drugs)
- Normal morphology but luteal phase lasts ≤ 11 days
- Causes of LPD: ➢ hyperprolactinaemia, weight-loss and exercise-induced endocrinopathies
  - ovarian (age extremes)
  - endometrial (steroid receptor deficiency overlying leiomyoma)
  - ovulation-inducing drugs

Mixed secretory pattern
- Def^n: >2 days discrepancy between fragments

Secretory changes in other conditions
- For example, in hyperplasia/carcinoma

Variants of Proliferative

Atrophic/inactive/weakly proliferative
- Clin: occurs pre-puberty/postmenopause/due to drugs
- Epithelial mitoses: absent (atrophy/inactive) or scant (weakly proliferative)
- Cuboidal/flattened nuclei (atrophy) or elongated/pseudostratified (weakly proliferative)
- ±Cystic glands (± budding)
- Variably collagenised stroma: d/dg normal lower uterine segment endometrium (p. 236)

Persistent proliferative
- Def^n: proliferative endometrium in postmenopausal women

Disordered proliferative
- Clinical: anovulatory cycles/exogenous oestrogens; Mx is as for simple non-atypical hyperplasia
- Poorly developed thin-walled vessels
- Fibrin thrombi and stromal haemorrhage if shedding
- Asynchronous growth: normal/cystic glands with shallow buds
- Metaplasias (esp. ciliated) but no cytological atypia
- Volume occupied by glands *cf.* stroma is < 3:1 (this glands:stroma ratio is a subjective evaluation)
- d/dg simple hyperplasia: this is a continuum, diagnose hyperplasia if there are lots of dilated glands

Endometrial Hyperplasia
- Glands:stroma ratio usu. ≥ 3:1 (may be very high in complex hyperplasia or ≈ normal is simple)
- Gland architecture: simple (dilated glands ± occ. buds/infolds); complex (more crowding and irregular shapes with branches, 'hand-in-glove', etc. but still with stroma between glands)
- Nuclear cytology: non-atypical/atypical (↑size, rounding, vesicular, irregular membrane, prominent nucleoli, coarse chromatin, normal mitoses, ± marked $stratificat^n$) – compared to uninvolved glands
- d/dg adenoCA is favoured by: non-squamous solid/cribriform arch., central necrosis/PMN, desmoplasia

Endometrial Polyps
- Glands orientated parallel to the surface endometrium are a useful sign of polyp (any type)

Functional polyps
- Composed of cycling endometrioid glands (but often OOP *cf.* the background endometrium)
- Fibrotic spindled stroma
- Large thick-walled vessels
- ±Irregularly distributed and mis-shapen glands ± metaplasias ± $prolif^n$ (even postmenopausally)
- Some consider features of simple non-atypical hyperplasia to be 'normal' in functional polyps so should not be reported as hyperplasia unless they involve the background endometrium as well

Tamoxifen polyps
- Usu. long fibrous talk
- Complex and cystic glands
- Glandular metaplasias (squamous, mucinous, papillary, clear cell, apocrine, tubal, etc.)
- Fibrous/fibromyxoid stroma with focal stromal condensation around glands
- ±Infarction/ulceration/polyp-cancers
- d/dg adenosarcoma: polyp has only focal periglandular stromal condensates and stromal mitoses are sparse and not atypical
- See also p. 254 for other effects.

Neoplastic polyps (incl. polyp-cancers)
- Submucosal leiomyoma
- *Adenomyoma:* smooth muscle predominant stroma with normal glands
- *Atypical polypoid adenomyoma:* adenomyoma with atypical glands and squamoid morules
- Adenofibroma
- Polyp-cancers (e.g. MMMT, CCC, serous CA/CIS [= serous surface carcinoma], endometrioid CA)

Endometriosis
- Diagnosis *usu.* requires at least two out of three criteria: 1) glands 2) stroma 3) siderophages
- Variants (have different natural history, origin and behaviour):
Pelvic peritoneal endometriosis
- Due to retrograde menstruation (+/metaplasia), often regress, a minor amount is considered normal
- An excessive amount causes problems through adhesions and fibrosis
- Sites: abdominal wall skin (esp. umbilical), bowel wall (see pp. 146–147), pelvic organs
Ovarian endometriotic cysts and endometrioid cystadenomas
- Often do not have a stromal component (so may not fulfil the criteria above)   tufting and stratification
- Many are monoclonal endometrioid cystadenomas   nuclear pleomorphism
- Some show cytological atypia of the lining (= *atypical endometriosis*): —nuclear hyperchromasia
- Atypical endometriosis may be a form of borderline cystadenoma   cytoplasmic eosinophilia
Nodular rectovaginal endometriosis
- These deposits (of unknown aetiology) are usu. admixed with smooth muscle
Metastatic endometriosis
- May explain occurrence of endometrial tissue in pleural (trans-diaphragmatic implantation is also plausible), pulmonary and intracranial sites

Inflammatory Conditions

Acute endometritis
- Microabscesses
- Infiltration and *destruction* of glandular epithelium
- Causes: *Chlamydia spp.*, *Strep./Staph./E.coli*, IUCD, radiation, postpartum/miscarriage
Chronic non-specific endometritis
- Usu. *ab initio*, *Chlamydia spp.*, postpartum, IUCD, adenocarcinoma; may result in DUB
- Gland distortion   } the odd plasma cell, without these
- Stromal fibrosis, spindle cell transformation of stromal cells } features, is insufficient for histodiagnosis
- Plasma cells (usu. >1 per 10× objective) ± others (i.e. a mixed chronic inflam^y infiltrate)
- d/dg atypical hyperplasia *vs.* inflam^y atypia in severe endometritis
Chronic endometritis of specific types
- Xanthomatous (elderly, cervical stenosis)
- Granulomatous: e.g. TB (best seen in the late secretory phase if pre-menopausal) or post ablation
- Focal necrotising endometritis: lymphocytes, PMN and rare Mφ (but no plasma cells) centred on scattered glands with destruction of gland epithelium ± formation of intra-glandular collections
Intra-uterine contraceptive device (IUCD) effects
- Shortening of the secretory phase
- Haemorrhage of the stroma
- Atrophy and fibrosis
- Squamous metaplasia
- Endometritis: acute (intraglandular abscesses and stromal polymorphs) and chronic
- ±Actinomycosis

Endometrial/Uterine Metaplasias

Squamous
- Squamoid morules lack intercellular bridges and keratin; they may have central necrosis
- Squamous metaplasia has intercellular bridges +/ keratin

Mucinous

- Abundant mucin (necessary for diagnosis) and bland nuclei
- If it occurs in hyperplastic endometrium !d/dg low grade mucinous adenocarcinoma

Ciliated

- Whole gland must be ciliated to qualify
- Cytoplasm is more eosinophilic

Clear cell ± hobnail cell

- Glycogenated clear cells (esp. in pregnancy)
- ± Hobnail cells (a reparative change)
- d/dg clear cell carcinoma but metaplasia is favoured by: ⤙ bland nuclei
  normal architecture
  no invasion
  no mass lesion
  ER +ve, p53 −ve (or weak/focal)

Eosinophilic/oncocytic

- May get regenerative-type nuclear atypia
- d/dg oxyphilic endometrioid adenoCA: ➤ lack of neoplastic type nuclear atypia (mitoses, etc.)
  ➤ normal arch., no invasion, no mass lesion

Papillary syncytial

- Syncytium ± PMN infiltrate
- Papillae lack well-developed fibrovascular cores (but some core tissue is possible in florid metaplasia)
- Bland nuclei ± degenerative-type atypia
- Is a reaction to endometrial breakdown (benign or malig.) and may occur on the surface (only) of degenerating parts of endometrioid adenoCA (!do not call it high grade papillary serous carcinoma)
- d/dg papillary serous high grade endometrial adenoCA: ➤ low grade nuclei in metaplasia
  ➤ stromal cores in carcinoma
  ➤ ER −ve, p53 strong diffuse +ve in CA

Stromal metaplasias

- Benign bone/cartilage (! do not call MMMT if this occurs in the stroma of an adenocarcinoma)
- Adipose metaplasia: can occur, but must still raise the possibility of uterine perforat^n if in curettings
- Extramedullary haemopoiesis: investigate for haematological disease if EMH is present in isolation
- Multiple mesenchymal 'metaplasias': consider the possibility of fetal origin

Glial tissue

- May occur as heterotopia or as part of a MMMT (incl. gliosarcoma)

See also 'Glial tissue' (p. 251) and 'Gliomatosis peritonei' (p. 254).

Residual Endometrial Changes Post Endometrial Ablation

- Early (<3 months): necrosis, granulation tissue, inflammation
- Later: scarring and inflam^n (± granulomas)
- Simple cuboidal re-epithelialisation
- Foci of residual unaffected endometrium

FIGO Staging of Corpus Carcinoma (only applies to carcinomas)

I – confined to corpus

   IA – intra-endometrial (no muscle invasion)

   IB – <$\frac{1}{2}$ myometrium ⎱ some pathologists take the *stratum vasculare* as the
   IC – ≥$\frac{1}{2}$ myometrium ⎰ half-way mark when direct measurement is difficult

II – invades cervix but confined to uterus

   IIA – surface/glandular involvement only (see Kadar *et al.* 1982)

   IIB – cervical stroma is invaded

III – locoregional spread

   IIIA – serosa/adnexa/cytology +ve in ascites or washings

   IIIB – vaginal spread (incl. metastasis)

   IIIC – LN mets (obturator/iliac/parametrial/sacral/para-aortic)

IV – *mucosa* of bladder/rectum (IVA) or other LN/distant mets (IVB)

Aspects of Corpus Carcinoma

- FIGO grading (endometrioid types only): solidity (≤5%, >50%), add 1 for G3 nuclei
- Grade 3 nuclei = ↑size, coarsely clumped chromatin and large irregular nucleoli
- Papillary serous carcinoma and CCC are G3 by definition (state 'grade 3 equivalent')
- Distinguish solid adenocarcinoma from squamoid/squamous differentiation; if mixed, grade on the adeno part

- WHO considers squamoid/squamous differentiation in adenocarcinoma to be a variant of endometrioid adenoCA (the older terms of ASC and adenoacanthoma are no longer acceptable)
- Type = dominant type (e.g. must be >50% mucinous to call mucinous) – serous is an exception
- If >10% other type = 'mixed' (but state dominant type)
- Need ≥ 25% serous to call it serous (but always state if there is a serous component, however small)
- 1° uterine serous carcinoma is ≈ always WT1 −ve (cf. d/dg tubal/ovarian/peritoneal 1° which are +ve)
- 1° SmCC requires different chemoRx to other types
- Immuno (all subtypes): vimentin +ve (to some extent) and mCEA −ve (a few are focal membranous +ve)
- Immuno (endometrioid G1 & G2): p16 −ve in >90% of cases, ER or PgR +ve in 85% of cases
- Immuno (other): 10% of CCC are ER +ve; serous CA are p16 strong +ve (90%), ER/PgR +ve (50%)
- Immuno: 'Type 1 CA' (endometrioid G1-G2 or mucinous) are usu. ER +ve, diffuse strong p53 −ve, 'Type 2 CA' (serous, CCC) are usu. ER −ve, diffuse strong p53 +ve (but   vity is not helpful in d/dg)
- d/dg G3 endometrioid vs. glandular variant of serous carcinoma: see immuno above
- d/dg metaplasias vs. the 'type 2 carcinomas' (CCC and serous): see metaplasia section pp. 239–240
- d/dg clear cell squamous areas vs. CCC
- FIGO criteria for squamous differentiation = any 1 of:

① keratin
② intercellular bridges
③ minor criteria (any 3):

sheet-like architecture
sharp cell margins
cytoplasmic eosinophilia
cytoplasmic abundance

Diagnosing myoinvasion
- ! Exclude block from the cornu (cancerised intramural passage of the Fallopian tube)
- ! Exclude cancerisation of adenomyosis or deeply invaginating stratum basalis:
  - ➤ presence of endometrial stroma ± residual benign glands
  - ➤ absence of a PMN inflamed 'granulation tissue' tumour stroma
  - ➤ blunted advancing front (cf. jagged pattern of invasive carcinoma)
  - ➤ grade 1 morphology (a weak criterion)

all these favour
cancerisation
over
myoinvasion

Uterine Smooth Muscle Tumours
- These may contain an adenomatoid tumour of focal stromal metaplasia (esp. adipose)

Cellular leiomyoma/highly cellular leiomyoma
- Def^n: more cellular than myometrium ('cellular') or endometrial stromal tumour ('highly cellular')
- Macro: may be typical or may be yellow +/ soft (±haemorrhage/necrosis)
- Borders may be infiltrative but no other features of malignancy
- d/dg endometrial stromal tumour/sarcoma: artefactual cleft-like spaces, thick muscular vessels, fascicular arch., spindled nuclei, areas that merge with the myometrium (and immuno) all favour leiomyoma
- d/dg leiomyosarcoma: lack of necrosis, pleomorphism and ↑mitoses – ∴ need extensive sampling

Malignant (uterine leiomyosarcoma)
- Malignancy can be confidently diagnosed if all 3 of the following are present:
  - ➤ coagulative tumour cell necrosis (not inflam^y ulceration necrosis or hyaline necrosis)
  - ➤ significant pleomorphism (significant = visible at low power i.e. ×10 objective)
  - ➤ >5/10 hpf mitoses

Smooth muscle tumour of uncertain malignant potential (STUMP) – any of the following:
- Necrosis but minimal pleom.
- Pleom. but without definite tumour necrosis [i.e. simplastic with ?necrosis]

and low mitotic
count (i.e. <5/10hpf)

- Other definitions (e.g. no pleom/necrosis but with mitoses higher than mitotically active leiomyoma)

Other variants of smooth muscle tumour
- Simplastic: defined as ≥5% cells atypical; malignant if necrosis/mitoses
- Mitotically active: defined as having >5/10hpf normal mitoses (upper limit ranges from 9–15/10hpf; if any more than this consider STUMP); malignant if necrosis/pleomorphism
- Epithelioid: malignant if >5/10hpf mitoses even if no necrosis/pleomorphism. Infiltrative margins, necrosis and size >6cm are bad prognostic features. Four variants are:
  - ① leiomyoblastoma (eosinophilic cells)
  - ② clear cell (signet ring)

    ③ trabecular/plexiform (looks epithelial)

    ④ *plexiform tumourlet* (7mm max. Ø, hyaline stroma)

- Benign Metastasising Leiomyoma: a complication of surgery
- Leiomyomatosis: ➤ intravascular: may have a clefted/lobulated outline ± hydropic change
                    ➤ diffuse peritoneal – see *leiomyomatosis peritonei*, p. 254
- Myxoid Leiomyosarcoma: ➤ atypical cells (like myxoid MFH) – not just myxoid stroma
                       ➤ low cellularity results in a low mitotic count (<2/10 hpf)
                       ➤ vascular invasion is usu. seen

Effects of GnRH analogues (e.g. Zoladex®) on leiomyomas

- ↑ Hyalinisation, necrosis, cellularity, vessel wall thickness and mitoses (but usu. <3/50hpf)
- ± Infiltrative borders
- ?↑ Lymphoid infiltrates

Effects of pregnancy and progestagens on leiomyomas

- ↑ Oedema, necrosis, cellularity, mitoses, pleomorphism
- ± Haemorrhage (= *apoplectic leiomyoma* if it is also cellular)

Endometrial Stromal Tumours

Stromal nodule

- A non-invasive (by definition) stromal tumour (∴ requires extensive sampling)
- Some will allow ≤3 blunt extensions into the myometrium, each <3 mm long

(Low grade) stromal sarcoma

- Invades myometrium +/vessels (! 1° extrauterine forms exist but ovarian tumours are usu. mets)

Features common to stromal nodule and low grade sarcoma

- Cells resemble the stromal cells of proliferative endometrium [± rare endometrioid/clear cell glands]
- Arborising small thin-walled vessels (not thick-walled as in leiomyoma/leiomyosarcoma)
- 'Starburst' hyalinisation foci in the stroma ± cystic/myxoid change
- Some divide these into 'cellular' and 'hyaline vascular' subtypes ∝ the relative amount of the above
- ±Sex cord-like elements (some say = ESTSCLE if <50% sex cord-like elements or UTROSCT if >50% while others require UTROSCT to be composed solely of such elements without a 'conspicuous' endometrial stromal component): the elements are usu. sex cord marker +ve (calretinin, Melan A, CD99 [in 60%] and inhibin α), hCaldesmon −ve
- ±Smooth muscle foci (! do not confuse with muscle invasion): If >30% = 'endometrial stromal nodule/sarcoma with smooth muscle differentiation'
- Immuno: CD10 +ve; −ve for oxytocin receptor, hCaldesmon, CD99 (but see UTROSCT above), CD34 and HDAC8; ! upto 40% of cellular leiomyomas and many leiomyosarcomas can be CD10 +ve but this tends to be patchy unlike stromal tumours; strong diffuse desmin +ve favours smooth muscle
- d/dg smooth muscle tumours (*q.v.*): these are usu. oxytocin receptor, hCaldesmon and HDAC8 +ve; inhibin −ve; desmin, CD34 and CD10 ±ve; vimentin, actins and CK do not help because they may be +ve in both
- d/dg hyalinising spindle tumour with giant rosettes (because of the hyaline) – see p. 312
- d/dg PEComa has a nested arch. with cells radiating (*cf.* whorling) around vessels and are HMB45 +ve
- d/dg intravascular leiomyomatosis has clefts, lobulations, fascicular arch. and thick-walled vessels
- d/dg adenosarcoma: in adenosarcoma the glands are more widespread and often dilated

High grade stromal sarcoma and undifferentiated uterine sarcoma

- Definition is not universally agreed but there are usu.: >10/10 hpf mitoses, pleomorphism and necrosis
- High mitotic count alone (in a tumour resembling endometrial stroma) is not sufficient for diagnosis
- Diagnosis requires the exclusion of specific differentiation: smooth/striated muscle, cartilage, carcinoma, etc.
- If there are foci or low grade stromal tumour = 'high grade stromal sarcoma' else = 'undiff uterine sarcoma'

Mixed Müllerian Neoplasia

- Atypical Polypoid Adenomyoma (glandular atypia and squamoid morules ++)
- Adenofibroma: <2/10hpf stromal mitoses and lacks sig. stromal atypia/hypercellularity else = adenosarcoma

- Adenosarcoma: (see also p. 248) – sarcomatous overgrowth (i.e. $\geq 20\%$ of the tumour is glandless sarcoma) suggests a more aggressive course; d/dg adenofibroma, atypical endometriosis, tamoxifen polyp, MMMT, endometrial stromal tumour with epithelial elements, Wilms', etc.
- Carcinosarcoma (MMMT):   ➢ note tumour size and presence/extent of myoinvasion
  -                       ➢ state grade of epithelial component
  -                       ➢ list any heterologous elements

Fallopian Tubes and Broad Ligament

Salpingitis Isthmica Nodosa
- Often bilateral, smooth serosal surface
- Multiple little lumena surrounded by hypertrophic muscle
- Extend to variable depth in tubal wall
- Thought to be a multiple diverticular process $\approx$ adenomyosis

Primary Tubal Tumours (Carcinoma/MMMT/FATWO)
- Can be of any type that occurs in the ovary $\therefore$ strict def^n of tubal $1°$ requires both of the following
  - ① the tumour is macroscopically located within the tube
  - ② tumour in the corpus, cervix or ovary must be absent or different to the tubal tumour

Female Adnexal Tumour of Probable Wolffian Origin (FATWO or TPWO)
- Middle aged, usu. broad ligament/tube but also in ovary; most are asymptomatic, stage I and benign
- Variable size (upto 20 cm $\varnothing$)
- Bland epithelial cells with rare mitoses and prominent BM forming closely packed solid or open tubules that may be variably cystic (lace-like or sieve-like). Diffuse and trabecular arch. also occur
- Variable fibrous stroma $\pm$ lobular arrangements
- Immuno: +ve for broad range CK, vimentin, inhibin-α, S100; $-$ve for EMA
- Malignancy (general): mitoses ++, cytol. atypia, vascular invasion, prom. spindle cell component
- Malignancy (if bland cytology): large size ($>$10cm), capsular breach, $\uparrow$cellularity, peritoneal implants
- d/dg other tubular/glandular neoplasms (sex cord, endometrioid, adenocarcinoma)

Ovaries

Stromal Hyperthecosis and Stromal Hyperplasia
- Clin: $\pm$ androgenic/oestrogenic Sx, $\pm$ endometrial neoplasia, DM, obesity
- Usu. bilateral enlargement, diffuse or nodular (with nodules $<$5mm $\varnothing$)
- Increase in stromal cells
- =Hyperthecosis if it also shows islands of luteinised cells (eosinophilic [Leydig-like] to vacuolated) $\pm$ associated true Leydig cell hyperplasia (at the hilum)
- d/dg stromal luteoma, stromal Leydig cell tumour and luteinised thecoma

Cysts (Non-neoplastic)
- d/dg cystic neoplasia (cystic change is common in any tumour in the ovary – $1°$ or $2°$)
- Endometriotic (see p. 239)
- 'Simple cyst': a cyst with an attenuated/non-discernible lining and no other diagnostic features
- Surface epithelial inclusion cysts (ovarian 'endosalpingiosis') – are more common with age, are small (usu. $<$1cm), usu. superficial and have a simple lining that may be columnar/tubal/endometrioid/ endocervical $\pm$ psammoma bodies, Arias-Stella reaction or (rarely) true dysplasia
- Functional cysts. These include:
  - ➢ *follicle cyst* – a unilocular cyst lined by granulosa cells (inner layer) and theca interna cells (outer layer). If only the thecal cells are luteinised this is called *follicular hyperthecosis*
  - ➢ *theca lutein cyst* – a follicle cyst with both layers luteinised (i.e. have expanded eosinophilic cytoplasm)
  - ➢ *corpus luteum cyst*: yellow wall with smooth lining macroscopically; lined by large luteinised granulosa cells $\pm$ hyaline globules (intra/extracellular), contain bloodied fluid
- *Hyperreactio luteinalis*: assoc^d with $\uparrow\uparrow$hCG; massive enlargement ($\pm$ torsion) of (usu. both) ovaries by multiple theca lutein cysts (may contain amber/haemorrhagic fluid) and oedematous stroma.

- Large solitary luteinised cyst of pregnancy and the puerperium: assoc^d with ↑↑hCG; unilateral cyst (upto ≈20cm) with 1 to many layers of luteinised cells showing Arias-Stella-like pleomorphism

Polycystic ovarian syndrome/disease (PCOS)

- Stein-Leventhal Syndrome: hirsuitism, obesity, 1° infertility, oligomenorrhoea/amenorrhoea
- Effects of ↑ oestrogenism/anovulation on the endometrium (disordered prolif., simple hyperplasia)
- Polycystic ovaries:
  - ➤ peripheral small (1mm–1cm ∅) follicle cysts with follicular hyperthecosis
  - ➤ collagenous fibrosis of the subcapsular stroma
  - ➤ lack of corpora lutea and albicantia (due to the anovulatory cycles)
  - ➤ ± stromal hyperthecosis

FIGO Staging of Ovarian Tumours
- Designed for surface epithelial tumours (incl. borderline) but may be applied to non-epithelial tumours too

I   – confined to ovaries
    IA – one ovary, capsule intact
    IB – both ovaries, capsule intact
    IC – positive cytology in ascites/peritoneal washings or capsular breach

II – pelvic extension (incl. implants)
    IIA – uterus/tubes
    IIB – other pelvic tissues
    IIC – IIA or IIB plus positive cytology in ascites/peritoneal washings

III – peritoneal mets beyond pelvis
    IIIA – microscopic only
    IIIB – macro upto 2cm in max. dimension
    IIIC – >2cm or regional LN mets (obturator/iliac/lateral sacral/para-aortic/inguinal)

IV – distant mets (incl. non-regional LN, liver parenchyma[4] or cytologically +ve pleural effusion)

Serous Tumours

Benign

- Paucity of papillae, simple epithelium, cilia ++, bland cytology, no invasion
- If <10% borderline still call benign but 'with focal low grade atypia'
- *Serous surface papilloma*: ➤ a rare exophytic variant
  - ➤ may be bilateral
  - ➤ papillae may break off into the peritoneal cavity

Borderline ('atypical proliferative')

- Tufting, stratification (usu. >4 layers), mitoses (usu. normal and <4/10hpf), cytol. atypia (usu. <severe)
- Ciliated cells tend to decrease with increasing atypia
- Implants: ➤ invasive (infiltrative architecture)
  - ➤ non-invasive[5] (desmoplastic/non-desmoplastic)
  - ➤ d/dg endosalpingiosis: simple glands (no papillae), non-atypical epithelium ± psammoma bodies (see 'Endosalpingiosis' on p. 254 for more detail)
- ±LN deposits
- ±Microinvasion = single cells +/ small papillaroid/cribriform groups surrounded by clefted spaces, each focus ≤ 10mm^2 area by 2003 WHO criteria[6]. Stromal reaction (desmoplasia, oedema, inflam^n), nests with irreg. outlines/projections or severe cytol. atypia suggest frank invasion (→ more sampling) or *microinvasive serous carcinoma* (implies high grade *cf.* 'borderline tumour with microinvasion')
- *micropapillary serous carcinoma* (= *intraepithelial low grade serous carcinoma*):
  - ➤ non-hierarchical branching (i.e. small fronds come directly off large cores) in ≥5mm^2 in ≥1 section
  - ➤ microinvasion is a bad prognostic but not necessary for diagnosis
  - ➤ stage II tumours may have ↑risk of progression *cf.* other borderline serous tumours

---

[4] liver capsule mets is stage III
[5] well-defined border between implant and underlying tissue; the presence of implant epithelium in the normal septae between adipose lobules is not considered a sign of invasion
[6] used to be <3mm ∅ and some still use '<3-5mm in each of the two largest dimensions on a section'

- d/dg *seromucinous tumours*: these contain a mixture of mucinous (endocervical) and other Müllerian epithelium ± 'indifferent cells' (with eosinophilic cytoplasm). The arch. and behaviour is more like serous *cf.* mucinous tumours and borderline, microinvasive and invasive forms are described

Malignant

- Def^n: diffuse (>10mm^2 area) destructive invasion with desmoplasia
- Complex papillae, solid areas, bad cytology
- Grading = 1, 2, 3 based on solidity ($<5\%$, $>50\%$), nuclear atypia ↑with grade (pleom., mitoses)
- *Psammocarcinoma*:   ➤ low grade nuclei
   ➤ $>75\%$ of tumour has psammoma bodies
   ➤ prognosis $\approx$ borderline
- d/dg 1° peritoneal serous carcinoma (or borderline tumour): see p. 255

Immuno

- +ve: CA-125 ($\approx 50\%$ of 1° thyroid PTC show focal +vity also), CK7, c-kit, S100, EMA
- WT1 diffusely +ve (also in tubal, mesothelial and other lesions – see pp. 16–17)
- −ve: vimentin, mCEA, CK17, CK19

Mucinous Tumours

Benign

- Intestinal/endocervical epithelium; simple acini/flat
- If $<10\%$ borderline still call it benign but 'with focal low grade atypia'
- d/dg dominating mucinous cysts in a teratoma, Brenner's or Sertoli-Leydig tumour

Borderline ('atypical proliferative')

- Intestinal-type (IBMT): bilaterality is unusual (! consider extra-ovarian mets):
   ➤ borderline requires tufting and stratification (<4 layers); ± complex glands; ± thin papillae
   ➤ assoc^d with cellular pseudomyxoma ovarii (PMO) [$\approx$ colloid carcinoma] ± PMP (! d/dg 2°)
   ➤ immuno: CK7 +ve (usu. strong), CK20 +ve (but may be focal/weak)
- Endocervical-type (EBMT): lack goblet or absorptive cells, bilaterality is more common:
   ➤ complex papillae and PMN (± microinvasion). *NB*: most invasive tumours are intestinal type
   ➤ assoc^d with acellular PMO due to rupture of the cyst [$\approx$ extravasat^n mucocoele], not PMP
   ➤ immuno: CK7 +ve, CK20 −ve
- PMO (cellular or acellular) does not have an inflam^y or multinucleated giant cell reaction
- Intraglandular cribriformity and stroma-free papillaroid tufts are accepted as borderline if cytological atypia is not 'marked' ('marked' $\approx$ cytol. changes of high grade dysplasia of colonic adenomas)
- Peritoneal implants: invasive (rare, seen with IBMT) or non-invasive (seen with EBMT ± LN mets)
- ± Microinvasion: stromal invasive focus/foci (see below for definition), each <5mm in max. extent; if there is 'marked' atypia in invasive and adjacent glands then = *microinvasive mucinous carcinoma*

Malignant

- Def^n: *EITHER*: ① (Hart-Norris) no stromal invasion but: stratification >4 layers with moderate to marked atypia (some call this 'mucinous intraglandular neoplasia' if there is also glandular complexity ± papillaroid tufts; others define 'intraepithelial carcinoma' as stratification ≥4 layers *or* marked cytol. atypia)
   OR: ② (WHO) stromal invasion (>5mm in extent by Riopel criteria) defined as any of these:

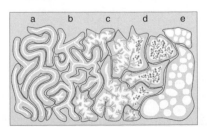

   ➤ 'obvious invasion' i.e. as for a desmoplastic adenocarcinoma elsewhere
   ➤ infiltrative glands/cords/nests/single cells in ovarian or desmoplastic stroma
   ➤ solid glandular formations (>10mm^2 area and ≥3mm in each of 2 linear dimensions by WHO criteria) in one or more of the following 'back-to-back' architectures (i.e. with little/no stroma): complex papillary, glands with 'malignant-appearing' epithelium ± necrotic contents ± complex/serpiginous shapes or cribriform. See Figure 17.1: a) serpiginous, b) complex glands, c) complex true papillary d) irregular glands with necrotic contents, e) cribriform

FIGURE 17.1 Architectures of ovarian mucinous carcinoma

- The presence and extent of stromal invasion may be the single most important prognostic factor
- Assoc[d] with NEC (SmCC or large cell)
- *Mural nodules*: good prognosis (e.g. 'sarcoma-like'/pseudotumour, usu. <5cm ∅) or bad prognosis (e.g. anaplastic/spindle carcinoma or sarcoma – may be very large tumours) or carcinoids (pp. 252–253)
- d/dg metastatic adenoCA: see 'Immuno' below and 'Features Favouring Secondary (Metastatic) Carcinoma', p. 248
- Grade: G1: <5% solid (state whether invasion is present or not)   ⎫ some up the grade by 1
           G2: 5–50% solid, smaller glands, more complexity   ⎬ if there is marked atypia
                and stratification   ⎭
           G3: >50% solid, marked cytological atypia, multinucleated cells common

Immuno
- CA-19.9, mCEA and vimentin +ve; CA-125 −ve in 75%; WT1 −ve; CK17 −ve
- d/dg colorectal CA: ovary is typically CK 7 +ve, may give focal/weak +vity for CK20 and CEA and β-catenin +vity is restricted to the cytoplasm; colorectal is typically CK7 −ve, CK20 and CEA are both diffuse/strongly +ve and β-catenin +vity is nuclear plus cytoplasmic

Endometrioid Tumours

Benign
- Usu. adenofibromas, simple glands (stratification present but mitoses rare)
- Assoc[d] with endometriosis (see also: *atypical endometriosis*, p. 239)
Borderline
- Adenofibroma/cystic; features of endometrial hyperplasia
- Mitoses *usu.* <3/10 hpf
- ± Microinvasion = stromal invasion in an area < 5mm ∅ (but some say < 3mm ∅)
- ± Squamous metaplasia
- Low grade: mainly adenofibromatous with simple hyperplasia and cribriform areas <5mm ∅
- High grade: ➤ adenofibroma or villoglandular papillary cystadenoma
                ➤ complex hyperplasia
                ➤ cribriform areas usu. >5mm ∅
- Confluent epithelial foci >5mm ∅= malignancy

Malignant
- Def[n]: *EITHER*: ① confluent epithelial mass >5mm ∅
  OR: ② destructive stromal invasion more than microinvasion
- Morphology is like endometrioid endometrial carcinoma ± cystic change
- ± Squamous metaplasia → keratin granulomas in peritoneum (! do not mistake for implants)
- Variant: microglandular (d/dg granulosa cell tumour)   ⎫ these sex cord-like variants are EMA +ve,
                                                          ⎬ inhibin −ve unlike true sex cord tumours
- Variant: Sertoliform (trabecular)   ⎭ (EMA −ve, inhibin +ve)

- Variant: oxyphil   ⎫ these show more
- Variant: spindle cell   ⎭ typical foci elsewhere
- Grading: is as for endometrial carcinoma (p. 240)
- d/dg: Sertoli or Sertoli-Leydig tumours: small gland type of endometrioid CA (± luteinised stromal cells) can be misdiagnosed as Sertoli-Leydig. Look for larger gland formations in endometrioid
- d/dg synchronous endometrial and ovarian 1° (esp. if small endometrial 1° with surrounding hyperplasia and stage 1 typical ovarian tumour with adenofibroma or ovarian endometriosis)
- d/dg metastasis to ovary is favoured by: ➤ advanced endometrial 1° tumour that is not myometrial/serosal predominant - the latter suggests an ovarian 1° (! or 1° in adenomyosis)
  See also section on 'Features
  Favouring Secondary
  (Metastatic) Carcinomas', p. 248
                                              ➤ evidence of tubal spread
                                              ➤ lymphatics +ve (1° endometrial CA favours LN mets over peritoneal)
                                              ➤ small ovaries but bilateral involvement

Immuno
- +ve: CA-125, CK7, c-kit; CA-19.9 ±ve; vimentin ±ve; see p. 246 re inhibin and EMA in sex cord tumours
- −ve: CK20, CK17, CK19, WT1

Brenner Tumours and TCC

Benign
- Small solid adenofibromas
- Nests of transitional epithelium ± metaplastic cysts (mucinous/squamous)
- ± Associated teratoma / mucinous tumour / serous tumour

Borderline
- Larger, cystic, papillary/polyp lined by mild-moderately atypical transitional epithelium
- No invasion

Malignant
- Desmoplastic invasive high grade TCC with benign/borderline elements
- If no assoc^d benign/borderline elements = TCC: (more aggressive but also more responsive to Rx)
- ± admixed with other surface epithelial tumours
- Immuno: CK7 and WT1 +ve; uroplakin III, thrombomodulin and CK20 −ve (unlike d/dg urinary TCC)

Clear Cell Tumours

Benign
- Adenofibromas
- Simple glands (not stratified)
- Hobnail cells but no atypia/mitoses

Borderline
- Adenofibroma with focal stratification of slightly atypical cells
- No destructive stromal invasion
- Mitoses <1/10hpf
- If ↑atypia = clear cell carcinoma *in situ*

Malignant (= clear cell carcinoma, CCC)
- Solid macro; micro: tubulocystic and solid patterns (50% have assoc^d endometriosis/atypical endometriosis)
- High grade nuclei in apical location appear partly extruded (= 'hobnail cells')
- Clear cell cytoplasm is rich in glycogen and lipid (± some mucin, usu. at the apical tips ± signet ring cells)
- 25% have hyaline globules (as in YST)
- Oxyphilic variant (d/dg YST, hepatoid carcinoma) – has more typical foci of CCC elsewhere
- Mitotic count may be low but >6/10 hpf is a poor prognostic [There is no good grading system for CCC]
- d/dg YST: ➤ age <30 years favours YST
  - ➤ presence of other YST patterns or germ cell elements favours YST
  - ➤ papillae of CCC are complex with hyalinised stromal cores
  - ➤ papillae of YST are simple with loose stroma containing a central vessel
  - ➤ immuno: EMA +ve, CD15 +ve, AFP −ve favour CCC and *vice versa*[7]
- d/dg juvenile granulosa cell tumour – clinical, also more typical histological features elsewhere
- d/dg metastatic RCC: ➤ RCC has a typical vascular pattern; CCC may have assoc^d endometriosis
  - ➤ RCC is mucin −ve while CCC may have some mucin
  - ➤ LP34 +vity: only 8% of RCC *cf.* 100% of CCC;
  - ➤ RCC favoured by +vity for CD10 and 'RCC MA' and −vity for CK7
  - ➤ CA-125, ER, PgR +ve favour CCC (99% of RCC are ER and PgR −ve)
- d/dg secretory endometrial carcinoma, clear cell malignant melanoma, 2° HCC, etc.

---

[7] ≈ 1 in 5 of CCC are AFP +ve, so you need a panel of immuno plus other features

Typing and Grading Ovarian Surface Epithelial Carcinomas
- WHO requires ≥90% purity to call a tumour by that type – otherwise it is 'mixed' (but mention if <10% of some other type is present – esp. if it is a more malignant subtype)

Universal grading system (Shimizu *et al.*, 1998)
- Analogous to breast cancer grading: each part has a score of 1–3; add scores to determine the grade
- **Predominant architecture:** glandular/tubulocystic = 1, papillary/villoglandular = 2, solid = 3
- **Nuclear pleomorphism:**[8] mild = 1 (∅variation ≤2:1), mod = 2 (upto 4:1), severe = 3 (variation >4:1)
- **Highest mitotic count/10 hpf:** 1 = <10, 2 = 10–24, 3 = ≥25 (field ∅= 0.663 mm, area = 0.345 mm^2)
- Grade 1 = 3–5; 2 = 6–7; 3 = 8–9 (this system applies to all CA types but doesn't work well for CCC)

Mixed Müllerian and Endometrioid Stromal Tumours of the Ovary
- Carcinosarcoma: implants have both elements but LN mets only contain carcinoma. May be a source of glial tissue incl. glioblastoma
- Adenosarcoma: stromal atypia is usu. mild/mod; stromal mitoses usu. >4/10 hpf; pericellular retic; d/dg atypical endometriosis, adenofibroma (p. 242), granulosa cell tumour (p. 249)
- Endometrioid Stromal Tumour: d/dg uterine 1° (∴ hysterectomy indicated)/thecoma (inhibin +ve)

Small Cell Carcinoma of the Hypercalcaemic Type
- Young, bilateral, very aggressive
- Solid with follicles of eosinophil material ± mucinous cysts
- Round to oval/fusiform cells, mitoses ++ (>20/10hpf)
- EMA +ve, inhibin −ve (opposite to *most* juvenile granulosa cell and other sex cord/stromal tumours)
- d/dg SmCC of the pulmonary type and other SBRCT (e.g. DSRCT/lymphoma) – *q.v.*

Small Cell Carcinoma of the Pulmonary Type
- SmCC and other NEC usu. arise adjacent to a mucinous or endometrioid tumour
- d/dg SmCC of the hypercalcaemic type and other SBRCT (e.g. DSRCT/lymphoma) – *q.v.*

Other Carcinomas
- *SCC*: usu. arises in another tumour or is a metastasis from (e.g.) the cervix
- *Hepatoid Carcinoma*: is like HCC in every way
- *Undifferentiated Carcinoma*: is so poorly diff as to defy further classification

Features Favouring Secondary (Metastatic) Carcinoma
- Extensive surface involvement
- Prominent vascular invasion[9], esp. outside the ovary or at the hilum
- Nodular growth pattern (esp. if there is variation in growth pattern between nodules)
- Single cell infiltration, signet ring cells or cells floating in mucin
- Bilaterality (! metastatic mucinous CA may be unilateral and show 'maturation' to low grade cytology)
- Mucinous tumour mets: bilaterality (esp. if with high grade disease but ! pancreatic mets may be bland); small tumour size (<10cm), expansile tumour nodules separated by normal ovarian stroma, lack of typical borderline areas, presence of cellular PMP (appendix 1°) and small glands in clusters haphazardly scattered next to larger areas of tumour. The presence of cystic areas with bland mucinous lining mean nothing. For immuno, see 'Mucinous Tumours' on p. 245
- d/dg non-mucinous colonic CA *vs.* endometrioid CA: dirty garland necrosis and well-formed glands with high grade nuclei favour colonic adenoCA (because with 1° endometrioid carcinoma, nuclear differentiation correlates with glandular differentiation) – as does a CA-125 & CK 7 −ve, CEA & CK20 +ve phenotype. Squamoid differentiation, endometriosis and converse immuno favour endometrioid
- CK7 +ve/CK20 −ve phenotype is *not* strong evidence of ovarian 1° (*cf.* adenocarcinoma of other gynae parts, breast, lung, gastric or pancreaticobiliary origin)

---

[8] also takes into account NCR, chromatin clumping (absent in mild), and nucleolar prominence (inconspicuous in mild, large and eosinophilic in severe). Bizarre cells may be present in severe (only). Use the most pleomorphic part of the tumour where this pleomorphism fills ≥1/2 a ×10 objective field

[9] vascular invasion *alone* is unusual and should alert one to the possibility of intravascular granulosa cells (which may be mitotic) which is thought to be a surgically induced artefact and is benign

Krukenberg tumours

- Younger age group *cf.* 1° ovarian carcinomas. The rare 'primary Krukenberg tumour' = no evidence of extra-ovarian 1° even after 10 year F/U or extensive autopsy with histological sampling
- Marked stromal proliferation (! may mask the tumour cells unless they are specifically sought)
- Epithelial component: signet ring, diffuse mucinous and tubular variants (! d/dg Sertoli-Leydig tumours)
- Immuno: the *epithelial* cells should be −ve for α-inhibin and calretinin, +ve for CK/EMA/mucin, etc.
- ! Lobular breast carcinoma, gastric adenocarcinomas and thyroid PTC can all be CK7 and CA-125 +ve
- d/dg: fibrothecoma, sclerosing stromal tumour, steroid cell tumour with signet ring cells
- d/dg goblet cell carcinoid (1° or 2°)

Sex Cord/Stromal Tumours

Granulosa cell tumours (old term = gynoblastoma)

TABLE 17.2   Adult and juvenile granulosa cell tumours

Adult Granulosa Cell Tumour	Juvenile Granulosa Cell Tumour
small cells, little cytoplasm	larger cells, abundant cytoplasm
can be luteinised	often luteinised
nuclear grooves of the 'coffee-bean' type	no grooves
small nuclei & nucleoli	large vesicular nuclei & nucleoli, focally marked pleomorphism
variable arch.: solid-tubular, insular, trabecular, regular microfollicles containing eosinophil blobs (Call-Exner bodies), macrofollicular (functional cyst-like), parallel arrays of wavey cords ('moiré silk'), diffuse sarcomatoid.	multinodular growth & irregular macrofollicles
mitoses uncommon	mitoses ≈ 6/10 hpf (± abnormal forms)
fibro/thecomatous stroma (if granulosa cells comprise >10% of the tumour area/cellularity = 'granulosa cell tumour', else = 'fibroma/fibrothecoma with minor sex cord elements')	may show cystic spaces lined by hobnail cells (d/dg clear cell carcinoma *q.v.*)

- Immuno/stains: usu. −ve for EMA (but some cases show focal +vity, esp. juvenile ones), +ve for inhibin-α, calretinin, CD99 (membranous), vimentin, ± CK (paranuclear dot); αSMA and S100 are +ve in ≈ 50% of cases. Reticulin is −ve or sparse and packeted (not pericellular)
- d/dg 1° or metastatic CA, NET, glomus tumour, PNET, GIST or adenosarcoma (staining and morphology)
- d/dg fibroma/fibrothecoma with minor sex cord elements (reticulin and % granulosa cells)
- d/dg granulosa cell proliferations (multifocal, small – usu. microscopic unless luteinised – usu. occur in the centre of a *corpus atreticum*, often a Hx of pregnancy), Sertoli-like variants also occur
- d/dg melanoma may look similar in areas (and rarely is α-inhibin +ve) – ! some sex cord/stromal tumours are +ve for Melan A +/ HMB45 (in fact, some consider Melan A to be a sex cord marker)

Sertoli and Leydig tumours (old term = androblastoma)

- For Sertoli, Leydig and Sertoli/Leydig tumour histology and some d/dg see p. 227
- A 'stromal Leydig cell tumour' has true Leydig cell islands (Reinke crystalloid +ve) in amongst fibrothecomatous stroma (see the d/dg of luteinised thecoma in the next section) whereas the rare 'non-hilar Leydig tumour' lacks a fibrothecomatous component
- For sex cord tumour with fibrothecomatous elements, see 'The fibroma...thecoma spectrum'
- d/dg: stromal luteoma, steroid cell tumour NOS, pregnancy luteoma, Sertoli-variant of 'granulosa cell proliferations', SCTAT, gynandroblastoma and gonadoblastoma – see those entities below
- d/dg: prominent mucinous cyst in Sertoli-Leydig *vs.* 1° mucinous tumours
- d/dg: tubule/cord/nest pattern of Sertoli component *vs.* carcinoid, granulosa cell tumours and endometrioid carcinoma (can be very difficult if all endometrioid glands are of the small type)

Gynandroblastoma

- Rare benign virilising tumour ± oestrogenic effects
- Mixture of Sertoli, granulosa, Leydig and thecal cells ± luteinised stromal cells
- At least two of the components should each contribute >10% of the tumour to qualify for diagnosis
- Mitoses are sparse

The fibroma, fibrothecoma, thecofibroma, thecoma spectrum
- Clin.: wide age range, ± associations (Meig, Gorlin, sclerosing peritonitis), ± oestrogenism (∝ amount of thecoma) incl. endometrial neoplasia
- Macro: wide size range, circumscribed firm solid white mass ± yellow areas ± degenerative cysts
- Fibroma cells (spindled, collagen-producing, whorls/storiform) ± a little intracellular lipid
- Thecoma cells (spindled to round, lipidised to eosinophilic [luteinised], nests/sheets)
- ± Sex cord elements (granulosa/Sertoli-like): estimate percentage (if <10% = 'fibrothecoma with minor sex cord elements' else if >10% then = 'sex cord tumour with fibrothecomatous elements')
- Stroma: variably hyaline, calcific, oedematous
- Distinguishing the subtypes:
  - ➤ 'luteinised thecoma' if there are any luteinised cell areas (but see d/dg below)
  - ➤ 'thecoma' if   ☞ there is evidence of steroid production +/
    - ☞ there is an arbitrarily 'sig. proportion' of thecoma (or inhibin-α +ve) cells (some say this proportion should be >50%, otherwise call it 'thecofi-broma'/'fibrothecoma')
- Immuno/stains: vimentin +ve, CK −ve, (inhibin-α +ve in theca cells). Reticulin is pericellular +ve
- Malignancy in fibroma: ➤ soft and fleshy tumour
  - ➤ haemorrhage +/necrosis
  - ➤ ↑cellularity (esp. if with a 'herringbone' or intense storiform pattern)
  - ➤ ='cellular fibroma' if ≤ moderate atypia and ≤3/10 hpf mitoses
  - ➤ ='fibrosarcoma' if ≥ moderate atypia and >3/10 hpf mitoses
- Malignancy in thecoma: ➤ large size (e.g. >20cm ∅)
  - ➤ ↑cellularity
  - ➤ ≥4/10 hpf mitoses
- d/dg fibromatosis (multifocal and infiltrative i.e. it envelops normal follicles and is not circumscribed)
- d/dg 'fibroma-like nodule' is <1cm ∅ by definition (otherwise its a fibroma)
- d/dg massive oedema (infiltrative/diffuse, loose stroma, dilated thin vessels, patchy cellularity – ! may be 2° to lymphatic invasion by metastatic cancer)
- d/dg stromal Leydig cell tumour (has Reinke crystalloids)   } otherwise these tumours can't be
- d/dg steroid cell tumour (has <10% fibromatous elements)   } distinguished from a luteinised thecoma
- d/dg stromal hyperthecosis (usu. bilateral, not a cause of a discrete mass)
- d/dg pregnancy luteoma (usu. bilateral and multiple)
- d/dg sclerosing stromal tumour (*vide infra*): it is a variant of luteinised thecoma
- d/dg other spindle neoplasms (smooth muscle, PNST, 1° ovarian endometrial stromal tumour, etc.)

Sclerosing stromal tumour
- Younger age, benign, androgenic/oestrogenic Sx
- *Cellular lobules* containing a mixture of αSMA +ve myoid cells, fibroma cells and small oval luteinised/vacuolated lipidised cells with *small*, ER/PgR +ve nuclei that may be eccentric.
- d/dg signet ring carcinoma cells – but these contain mucin and have malignant nuclei
- d/dg signet ring stromal tumour: but this is not lobular and lacks lipid and HPC-like vessels
- d/dg luteinised thecoma (*q.v.*) – some consider this a variant of the same entity

Steroid cell tumour NOS (lipid cell tumour NOS)
- Clin: wide age range, virilising (usu.)/local Sx
- Macro: wide size range, solid
- Leydig-like cell areas (± vacuoles but no crystalloids)   } in sheets, columns
- Adrenocortical-like cell areas (incl. vascular sinusoids)   } or nests
- Pleomorphism is mild, nucleoli small and mitoses rare
- Immuno: +ve for vimentin, inhibin-α and steroid enzymes; CK ±ve
- Features of malignancy: size (≥8 cm), necrosis, pleomorphism (≥ moderate), mitoses (≥ 2/10 hpf)
- d/dg: 'NOS' distinguishes this from Leydig cell tumours and stromal luteoma (*q.v.*)
- d/dg luteinised thecoma (fibrothecomatous component more prominent)
- d/dg luteinised granulosa cell tumour (more typical granulosa cell morphology elsewhere)
- d/dg pregnancy luteoma (multiple, bilateral, more mitotic – otherwise very similar histology)
- d/dg lipid-rich Sertoli cell tumour (look for tubules/bilayered cords)
- d/dg RCC/CCC (! some steroid cell tumours contain glycogen – so use other features)
- d/dg metastatic ACC
- d/dg melanoma: ! both may be HMB45 +ve and rare melanomas stain for α-inhibin
- d/dg any hepatoid tumour (e.g. YST, eosinophilic endometrioid/CCC, 1° hepatoid CA, HCC, etc.)

Stromal luteoma

- Oestrogenic Sx in a postmenopausal woman. Benign and small (but must be >5mm ⌀ by definition)
- Eosinophilic polygonal cells with small, central nuclei (Leydig-like) in cords/clusters, ± lipofuscin
- Sparse fibrohyaline stroma
- Accompanied by bilateral stromal hyperthecosis and Leydig cell hyperplasia
- d/dg nodular stromal hyperthecosis (those nodules are ≤5mm ⌀– otherwise indistinguishable)
- d/dg Leydig-cell tumours (Reinke crystalloids; hilar location also favours Leydig cell tumour)
- d/dg Steroid cell tumour NOS (large size, i.e. >3cm, and extension beyond the stromal compartment)

Pregnancy luteoma

- Benign, ± virilising, !may present as a FS for incidental 'tumour' at postpartum sterilisat^n/Caesarian
- Solid masses (≤20cm) ± haemorrhagic foci, often multiple and bilateral with a Hx of pregnancy
- Eosinophilic (luteinised) cells with mitoses ++ (± abnormal forms), ± mild pleomorphism
- ± Colloid follicle-like spaces, ± hyaline globules (intra/extracellularly)
- Packeted reticulin pattern – not single cell
- d/dg steroid cell tumour or luteinised thecoma – but these usu. have non-luteinised foci +/ lipid cell or adrenocorticoid areas and are solitary

Sex cord tumour with annular tubules (SCTAT)

- Solid tubules: parallel lines of small nuclei (usu. with nucleoli) separated by tall clear cytoplasm
- These tubules form annuli around one (simple) or many (complex) hyaline masses which may calcify
- If assoc^d with Peutz-Jeghers then multifocality and Ca^{2+} are common – otherwise they are rare
- May contain granulosa cell tumour-like areas +/ solid lipidised Sertoli cell tumour nest-like areas
- d/dg gonadoblastoma and Sertoli cell tumour (*q.v.*)

Germ Cell Tumours

Glial tissue

- Pure glial tissue without other components (incl. neurons/glands) is a fully mature tissue associated with good prognosis and benign clinical course – even as peritoneal deposits (if glands are present consider the possibility of endometriosis/endosalpingiosis before diagnosing it as other elements)
- Occurs as peritoneal deposits from either mature or immature teratomas (! look for other elements)
- May occur as a monodermal teratoma (a glial-lined cyst)
- May be found in local LN draining teratomas or in other soft tissues (e.g. chest wall/scalp)

Mature teratoma

- May undergo granulomatous resolution (foreign body reaction to spilled keratin in the wall)
- Spilled keratin may cause multiple peritoneal granulomas (! may result in FS for ?neoplasia)
- May contain an angiomatoid/glomeruloid vascular proliferation (! this is not immature tissue)
- 2° malignancy incl. SCC then adenocarcinoma/melanoma. Others (e.g. sarcomas) are rare
- *Struma ovarii* (def^n: thyroid tissue in a teratoma that is EITHER macroscopically obvious OR microscopically predominant):
  - ➢ may be predominantly cystic with attenuated lining (d/dg mucinous/serous tumours)
  - ➢ may show any form of thyroid pathology (diagnostic criteria for follicular CA are uncertain)
  - ➢ ± tubular/Hürthle/clear cell change (d/dg CCC, endometrioid, sex cord tumours)
  - ➢ ± peritoneal implants (see 'Strumosis Peritonei', p. 254)
  - ➢ ± intermingled or adjacent carcinoid (= *strumal carcinoid*). ! Do not diagnose as MTC, even if they are calcitonin/amyloid +ve, because these carcinoids are much less aggressive. They are also usu. CEA −ve and do not have the classical appearance of medullary CA

Immature teratoma

- Def^n: a teratoma with immature elements (! mature elements may predominate)[10]
- Immature elements = any tissue with embryonic (but not fetal) morphology: neural (= primitive neuroepithelium in solid islands, rosettes or tubules – ! not retinal tissue), skeletal muscle, etc.
- 2° malignancies may arise as in testicular MTD (for criteria, see p. 226). Foci of YST are not prognostic if each focus is <3mm ⌀ and there are ≤3 foci in total
- Confluent overgrowth (some say of ≥1cm ⌀) of any single immature tissue = a tumour of that tissue (e.g. RMS, PNET, ependymoma, high grade glioma, etc.)

---

[10] some 'experts' say that a few (upto 4) immature foci (each upto several mm^2 in area) in an otherwise mature teratoma does not worsen prognosis and so should not result in a diagnosis of immature teratoma. This view is not universal and the supporting evidence is limited

- Grade ∝ aggregate area of any immature tissues on any 1 slide using ×4 objective and ×10 eyepiece:

  I   ≤1 field   = low grade: may be followed up

  II   >1 but ≤ 3 fields   = high grade: adjuvant Rx given

  III   >3 fields   = high grade: adjuvant Rx given but worse prognosis

- Implants: ➤ behaviour ∝ their grade ∴ graded separately to main tumour
  - ➤ are benign if purely mature (e.g. glial tissue)
  - ➤ chemoRx induces maturation but this matured stuff may continue to grow (= 'growing teratoma syndrome', more commonly seen with testicular NSGCT)
- d/dg: mature teratoma (sampling), heterologous MMMT (elderly, lack neuroepithelium)

Dysgerminoma

- Histologically identical to non-spermatocytic seminoma (see p. 225)

Yolk sac tumour (YST) and its endodermal sinus variant

- Usu. young and unilateral (± contralateral teratoma), ↑AFP, cut surface may be spongy
- Rare YST in the elderly arise by somatic events in an epithelial CA (usu. endometrioid/mucinous)
- For histology and immuno, see p. 226. Polyvesicular vitelline type is common in the ovary
- d/dg: CCC (see p. 247)
- d/dg: solid YST vs. MTU (rare in ovary): MTU may have ↑hCG, lacks YST patterns, has larger more pleomorphic nuclei with overlapping (solid YST nuclei don't overlap) and is AFP −ve, OCT4 +ve
- d/dg: generally, the variety of patterns and cytologies in any YST help distinguish it from other entities (e.g. hepatoid YST vs. HCC, endometrioid YST vs. endometrial carcinoma, etc.)

Embryonal carcinoma (MTU)

See p. 226.

Choriocarcinoma (ChC)

- For general information, see p. 226 (under MTT) and pp. 65–66
- Unlike in the testis, ovarian ChC need not show a villous/papillary architecture
- d/dg gestational ChC (ovarian ChC has its own vasc. sinusoids and occurs at an older age)
- d/dg ChC-like areas in poorly diff carcinomas

Gonadoblastoma

- Arise in abnormal gonads (e.g. dysgenetic gonad – usu. with some Y chromosome material; or an undescended testis in the male), often bilateral
- Although itself benign, it can give rise to a germ cell malignancy (e.g. dysgerminoma, YST, MTU)
- Macro: ≤ few cm ∅ and solid ± Ca^{2+} (2° germ cell malignancy may dominate the macro and micro)
- *Nests* of sex cord cells (granulosa/Sertoli-like) contain germ cells and Call-Exner-like hyaline blobs
- Luteinised fibrous stroma ± Ca^{2+}
- d/dg mixed germ cell – sex cord stromal tumour (normal gonads, not nested, no blobs)
- d/dg microscopic gonadoblastoma-like foci in normal immature ovaries (fetus/infant)
- d/dg SCTAT/granulosa cell tumour (lack germ cells)

Malignant mixed germ cell tumour

- ≥2 malignant germ cell elements are required for diagnosis – dysgerminoma is usu. one of the them
- Others include: YST, immature teratoma, MTU, ChC, polyembryoma
- Mature teratoma elements may also be present

Polyembryoma

- A form of mixed YST/MTU that is rare on its own (usu. is part of a mixed germ cell tumour)
- Loose mesenchyme contains *embryoid bodies* (= a central bilaminar germ disc of columnar MTU epithelium and flatter endoderm epithelium with an amnion-like cavity over the MTU and a vesicular/reticular YST cavity under the endoderm)
- ± Minor usual-type MTU elements +/ hepatoid differentiation
- d/dg diffuse embryoma is a ≈ 50:50 mix of YST and MTU in curvi-laminar arch., no embryoid bodies

Ovarian Carcinoid

- Usu. occur as a monodermal teratoma but can arise in the wall of mucinous cysts of any origin
- Subtypes (the mucinous types are considered by some to be argyrophil adenocarcinomas – see 'Appendix' on p. 152):
  - ➤ insular: midgut type, solid islands punctured by little glandular acini – d/dg granulosa tumour with Call-Exner bodies
  - ➤ trabecular: hindgut type, bilayered palisaded ribbons – d/dg Sertoli tumour

> well diff mucinous: small nests with goblet cells and cells with red grainy cytoplasm and NE nuclei (see p. 271) ± mucin pools and fibrosis. Mitoses are sparse
> atypical mucinous: crowded/confluent glands, cribriform/microcystic foci
> mucinous with a carcinomatous component: high grade cytology, single signet ring cell invasion, numerous mitoses
> other: mixed trabecular/insular, strumal carcinoid (p. 251)
- d/dg: metastatic carcinoid is favoured by multifocal nodules, bilateral involvement, vasc. invasion ++, peritoneal deposits, evidence of a GI/lung 1° and lack of mucinous cyst/other teratomatous components. See also 'Features Favouring Secondary (Metastatic) Carcinoma', p. 248

Ovarian Lymphoma
- Wide age range, bilaterality and deep LNp without peritoneal spread is suggestive; ± ↑CA-125
- 1° lymphoma is very rare – usu. it is part of a widespread process.
- ≈All are B-cell (see Chapter 10: Lymphoreticular): DLBCL, Burkitt, MZL, FCL
- Micro: diffuse growth sparing native follicle structures ± sclerosis +/ spindling
- d/dg: SmCC/granulosa cell tumour/adenoCA} but lymphoma does not form acinar structures
- d/dg: dysgerminoma/sarcoma/ALL/CGL (granulocytic sarcoma)

Frozen Section of Ovarian Masses
- Take two blocks (or 1 per 10cm ∅) from the thickest/most atypical areas macroscopically
- In the young exclude disseminated germ cell malignancy (usu. dysgerminoma)
- Is it non-neoplastic e.g. functional? (! do not mis-diagnose mitotic theca spindle cells as sarcoma, ! corpus luteum cells can have nucleoli and mitoses, ! pregnancy luteoma may have abnormal mitoses)
- If neoplastic is it epithelial? If so, decide if: > benign (→ no staging/LN dissection)
                                                                 > borderline/malignant (→ staging and LN dissection)
- Can you place in it the epithelial/germ cell/sex cord stromal categories?
- Specific entities e.g. if carcinoid, consider whether 1° or possibly metastatic (*vide supra*) because the latter warrants per-operative examination of the GIT and other ovary

Effects of Drugs on the Female Genital Tract

See also 'Uterine Smooth Muscle Tumours' on p. 242.

Hormone Replacement Therapy (HRT)
- Types: oestrogen only (for the hysterectomised) or combined with a progestagen (continuous [no withdrawal bleeds] or sequential [→ withdrawal bleeds])
- Scant endometrium usu. implies benignity if the endometrial cavity was entered (∴ avoid using the term 'inadequate' in the report)
- Sequential combined HRT: shows prolif. endometrium during the oestrogenic phase and may show: early secretory/prolif./inactive/atrophic histology during the progestagenic phase. The RR of developing atypical hyperplasia/adenocarcinoma is ≈ 2.0
- Continuous combined HRT: shows scant tissue/inactive/prolif./early secretory ± pre-decidual change. No ↑risk of hyperplasia
- AdenoCA developing on combined HRT: usu. low grade and stage and may show mucinous metaplasia
- Combined HRT has no known adverse effect on patients with a PMHx of surgery for endometrial/ovarian carcinoma or SCC of the genital tract
- Oestrogen only HRT has an risk of endometrial hyperplasia/adenoCA (usu. low grade and stage)

Progestagens and Danazol
- Endometrium shows: > atrophy, or
                                  > pre-decidual change with atrophic glands ± subnuclear vacuoles
- ± Arias-Stella reaction

Tamoxifen

Endometrium
- ↑Endometrial thickness (≥1cm)
- Cystic change
- Prolif.-type change/polyps (see under 'Endometrial Polyps' on p. 238)
- Hyperplasia: usu. non-atypical, cystic with focal crowding/branching, stromal fibrosis ± metaplasias
- Endometriosis and adenomyosis may be more florid (and even occur postmenopausally) ± metaplasias
- Adenocarcinoma (any type or grade)
- Mixed-Müllerian neoplasia (controversial): carcinosarcoma/adenosarcoma

Other sites
- Ovarian cysts: pre-menopausal functional cysts; postmenopausal both functional and neoplastic
- Oestrogenic effects on vaginal and cervical epithelium

Gonadotrophins
- Endometrium shows normal/hypersecretory/LPD-like changes (see pp. 236–238)
- Arias-Stella reaction (see p. 237)

Gonadotrophin Releasing Hormone (GnRH = Gonadorelin) Analogues
- Continuous pituitary stimulation exhausts LH and FSH → induces a postmenopausal-like state
- Endometrial atrophy ± glandular-stroma asynchrony
- Atrophy of vaginal and cervical epithelium
- Ovaries show ↓ nõ of follicle cysts and ↓ nõ of *corpora lutea*

Clomiphene
- No progestational effects
- Endometrium is normal or shows LPD-like effect or inactive/weakly prolif. change
- Ovaries show functional follicle cysts

Peritoneal Conditions and Diseases of the Secondary Müllerian System

Gliomatosis Peritonei
- Peritoneal glial deposits from a mature or immature teratoma.
- Benign if purely glial (for more information, see sections on 'Glial tissue' on p. 240 and p. 251 and 'Mixed Müllerian Neoplasia' on p. 248)

Strumosis Peritonei
- Peritoneal thyroid deposits from a teratoma/struma.
- Behaviour can only be judged clinically – benign histology is not reliable

Leiomyomatosis Peritonei
- Multiple, benign, bland fibromuscular nodules usu. <2cm ⌀ in young women (± decidualised cells)
- ! May present as FS during laparotomy (e.g. Caesarian)
- d/dg (all these are usu. >2cm ⌀ ± other associated findings): mets from a uterine 1° (not bland), retroperitoneal leiomyosarcoma (may be bland) or GIST (usu. bland)

Pseudomyxoma Peritonei (PMP)
- Associated with IBMT (and cellular PMO) or mucinous tumours of the GIT (usu. appendix)
- The appendix is ∴ often removed at surgery – it should be all embedded to look for mucinous hyperplasia / neoplasia (see under 'Appendix' on p. 152)
- Acellular mucin should be extensively sampled to look for epithelial cells (for further details and reporting guidelines, see 'PMP' section on p. 375)

Endosalpingiosis
- Ages 12–66 years, associated with ovarian serous tumours (benign, borderline and malignant)
- Smooth-contoured oval glands ± rare blunt papillae with prominent fibrovascular cores
- Contain all cell types of normal Fallopian tube
- No cytological atypia

- Stroma: concentric layers of loose fibrous tissue and lymphocytes
- d/dg endometriosis (different stroma ± siderophages)
- d/dg serous inclusion cysts (lining is flat to cuboidal cells – not proper serous [± except focally])
- d/dg serous borderline tumours of ovary or 1° peritoneum
  - ➤ papillarity, tufting and detached buds are all absent in endosalpingiosis
  - ➤ cytological atypia is trivial to absent in endosalpingiosis
- d/dg adenocarcinoma:
  - ➤ no invasion in endosalpingiosis
  - ➤ simple and regular gland spaces in endosalpingiosis
  - ➤ no cytological atypia in endosalpingiosis
  - ➤ cilia (seen in endosalpingiosis) are rare in adenocarcinoma

Florid Papillary Mesothelial Hyperplasia
- Usu. incidental microscopical finding but rarely seen as nodules of a few mm in max. dimension
- Bland polygonal cells in papillary clusters or sheets with well-defined cytoplasm and minimal cytological atypia ± psammoma bodies (few)
- Small papillae/tubules may extend superficially into the stroma but show the same bland features and the delicate fibrous stroma around these structures is mainly parallel to the surface
- d/dg mesothelioma: extensive proliferation, marked atypia (may be focal), deeper invasion, necrosis
- d/dg borderline serous tumours: columnar cells with less well-defined cytoplasm, serous differentiation (cilia), more anisonucleosis, more papillarity, more psammoma bodies, haphazard arrangement of cell nests

Primary Peritoneal Carcinoma or Borderline Tumours
- May be serous or other types that occur in the ovary ∴ the def^n requires all of the following:
  - ① the ovaries must be of normal size or enlarged only by benign conditions
  - ② any ovarian involvement is either confined to the surface or (if deeper) is $< 5 \times 5$ mm^2
  - ③ any surface involvement (of either ovary) must be less extensive than extra-ovarian involvement

Borderline Serous Tumours of the Peritoneum
- Similar to serous psammocarcinoma but there is no invasion and there is less calcification
- d/dg endosalpingosis, florid papillary mesothelial hyperplasia

Serous Psammocarcinoma of the Peritoneum
- Invasion of stroma or vessels
- Moderate cytological atypia at most
- No cell nests >15 cells in diameter
- Psammoma bodies in ≥75% of the papillae/nests

Bibliography

Agarwal, S. and Singh, U.R. (1992) Immunoreactivity with S100 protein as an indicator of pregnancy. *Indian Journal of Medical Research*, **96**, 24–26.

Al-Nafussi, A. (2006) Histopathological challenges in assessing invasion in squamous, glandular neoplasia of the uterine cervix. *Current Diagnostic Pathology*, **12** (5), 364–393.

Baker, P. and Oliva, E. (2007) Endometrial Stromal tumours of the uterus: a practical approach using conventional morphology and ancillary techniques. *Journal of Clinical Pathology*, **60** (3), 235–243.

Bell, S.W., Kempson, R.L. and Hendrickson, M.R. (1994) Problematic uterine smooth muscle neoplasms. A clinicopathologic study of 213 cases. *American Journal of Surgical Pathology*, **18** (6), 535–558.

Bennett, A.E., Rathore, S. and Rhatigan, R.M. (1999) Focal necrotizing endometritis: a clinicopathologic study of 15 cases. *International Journal of Gynecological Pathology*, **18** (3), 220–225.

Brown, L.J.R. (2003) The diagnosis of cervical glandular intra-epithelial neoplasia, in *Progress in Pathology*, Vol. 6 (eds N. Kirkham and N. Shepherd), Greenwich Medical Media, Ltd, London, pp. 115–144.

Buckley, C.H. and Fox, H. (2002) *Biopsy Pathology of the Endometrium*, 2nd edn, Hodder Arnold, London.

Chu, P.G. and Weiss, L.M. (2002) Keratin expression in human tissues and neoplasms. *Histopathology*, **40** (5), 403–439.

Clement, P.B. and Young, R.H. (2000) *Atlas of Gynecologic Surgical Pathology*, 1st edn, W.B. Saunders Co. Ltd., Philadelphia.

Clement, P.B. and Young, R.H. (eds) (1993) Tumors and Tumorlike Lesions of the Uterine Corpus and Cervix, in *Contemporary Issues in Surgical Pathology Nō.19*, Churchill Livingstone, New York.

Coleman, D.V. and Evans, D.M.D. (1999) *Biopsy Pathology and Cytology of the Cervix*, 2nd edn, Chapman and Hall.

Cotran, R.S., Kumar, V. and Collins, T. (eds) (1999) *Robbins Pathologic Basis of Disease*, 6th edn, W.B. Saunders Co., Philadelphia.

Deen, S., Thomson, A.M. and Al-Nafussi, A. (2006) Histopathological challenges in assessing borderline ovarian tumours. *Current Diagnostic Pathology*, **12** (5), 325–346.

Feeley, K.M. and Wells, M. (2005) Hormone replacement therapy and the endometrium. *Journal of Clinical Pathology*, **54** (6), 435–440.

Feeley, K.M. and Wells, M. (2001) Advances in endometrial pathology, in *Recent Advances in Histopathology*, Vol. 19 (eds D. Lowe and J.C.E. Underwood), Churchill Livingstone, Edinburgh, pp. 17–34.

Ferry, J.A. and Young, R.H. (1997) Malignant lymphoma of the genitourinary tract. *Current Diagnostic Pathology*, **4** (3), 145–169.

Irving, J.A., Carinelli, S. and Prat, J. (2006) Uterine tumors resembling ovarian sex cord tumors are polyphenotypic neoplasms with true sex cord differentiation. *Modern Pathology*, **19** (1), 17–24.

Ismail, S.M. (1999) Drug-induced changes in the female genital tract, in *Recent Advances in Histopathology*, Vol. 18 (eds D.G. Lowe and J.C.E. Underwood), Churchill Livingstone, Edinburgh, pp. 89–107.

Kadar, N.R., Kohorn, E.I., LiVolsi, V.A. and Kapp, D.S. (1982) Histologic variants of cervical involvement by endometrial carcinoma. *Obstetrics and Gynecology*, **59** (1), 85–92.

Kalof, A.N. and Cooper, K. (2007) Our approach to squamous intraepithelial lesions of the uterine cervix. *Journal of Clinical Pathology*, **60** (5), 449–455.

Kalof, A.N., Evans, M.F., Simmons-Arnold, L. *et al.* (2005) p16^{INK4A} immunoexpression and HPV *in situ* hybridization signal pattern: potential markers of high grade cervical intraepithelial neoplasia. *American Journal of Surgical Pathology*, **29** (5), 674–679.

Keen, C.E., Szakacs, S., Okon, E. *et al.* (1999) CA125 and thyroglobulin staining in papillary carcinomas of thyroid and ovarian origin is not completely specific for site of origin. *Histopathology*, **34** (2), 113–117.

Kim, K.R., Peng, R., Ro, J.Y. *et al.* (2004) A diagnostically useful histopathologic feature of endometrial polyp: the long axis of endometrial glands arranged parallel to surface epithelium. *American Journal of Surgical Pathology*, **28** (8), 1057–1062.

Kurman, R.J. (ed) (2002) *Blaustein's Pathology of the Female Genital Tract*, 5th edn, Springer-Verlag, New York.

Lee, K.R. and Scully, R.E. (2000) Mucinous tumors of the ovary: a clinicopathologic study of 196 borderline tumors (of intestinal type) and carcinomas, including an evaluation of 11 cases with 'pseudomyxoma peritonei'. *American Journal of Surgical Pathology*, **24** (11), 1447–1464.

Lloyd, J., Evans, D.J. and Flanagan, A.M. (1999) Extension of extramammary Paget disease of the vulva to the cervix. *Journal of Clinical Pathology*, **52** (7), 538–540.

Lowe, D.G., Buckley, C.H. and Fox, H. (1997) Advances in gynaecological pathology, in *Recent Advances in Histopathology*, Vol. 17 (eds P.P. Anthony, R.N.M. MacSween and D.G. Lowe), Churchill Livingstone, Edinburgh, pp. 113–137.

McCluggage, W.G. (2006) My approach to the interpretation of endometrial biopsies and curettings. *Journal of Clinical Pathology*, **59** (8), 801–812.

McCluggage, W.G. (2005) Immunoreactivity of ovarian juvenile granulosa cell tumours with epithelial membrane antigen. *Histopathology*, **46** (2), 235–236.

McCluggage, W.G. and Wilkinson, N. (2005) Metastatic Neoplasms involving the ovary: a review with an emphasis on morphological and immuno-histochemical features. *Histopathology*, **47** (3), 231–247.

McCluggage, W.G. (2003) Metaplasias in the female genital tract, in *Recent Advances in Histopathology*, Vol. 20 (eds D. Lowe and J.C.E. Underwood), Royal Society of Medicine Press, Ltd, London, pp. 29–52.

McCluggage, W.G. (2000) Recent advances in immunohistochemistry in the diagnosis of ovarian neoplasms. *Journal of Clinical Pathology*, **53** (5), 327–334.

Mikami, Y., Kiyokawa, T., Moriya, T. *et al.* (2005) Immunophenotypic alteration of the stromal component in minimal deviation adenocarcinoma ('adenoma malignum') and endocervical glandular hyperplasia: a study using oestrogen receptor and α-smooth muscle actin double immunostaining. *Histopathology*, **46** (2), 130–136.

Obaidat, N.A., Alsaad, K.O. and Ghazarian, D. (2007) Skin adnexal neoplasms – part 2: An approach to tumours of cutaneous sweat glands. *Journal of Clinical Pathology*, **60** (2), 145–159.

Reid-Nicholson, M., Iyengar, P., Hummer, A.J. *et al.* (2006) Immunophenotypic diversity of endometrial adenocarcinomas: implications for differential diagnosis. *Modern Pathology*, **19** (8), 1091–1100.

Rekha, W., Amita, M., Sudeep, G. *et al.* (2005) Growing teratoma syndrome in germ cell tumour of the ovary: A case report. *Australian and New Zealand Journal of Obstetrics and Gynaecology*, **45** (2), 170–171.

Riopel, M.A., Ronnett, B.M. and Kurman, R.J. (1999) Evaluation of diagnostic criteria and behavior of ovarian intestinal-type mucinous tumors: atypical proliferative (borderline) tumors and intraepithelial, microinvasive, invasive, and metastatic carcinomas. *American Journal of Surgical Pathology*, **23** (6), 617–635.

Rollason, T.P. (1998) Epithelial lesions of the endocervix, in *Progress in Pathology*, Vol. 4 (eds N. Kirkham and N.R. Lemoine), Churchill Livingstone, Edinburgh, pp. 179–199.

Rosai, J. (ed) (2004) *Rosai and Ackerman's Surgical Pathology*, 9th edn, Mosby, Edinburgh.

Scully, R.E., Young, R.H. and Clement, P.B. (1998) Tumors of the ovary, maldeveloped gonads, Fallopian tube and broad ligament, in *Atlas of Tumor Pathology Fascicle Nō 22*, 3rd series, Armed Forces Institute of Pathology, Washington DC.

Shimizu, Y., Kamoi, S., Amada, S. *et al.* (1998) Toward the development of a universal grading system for ovarian epithelial carcinoma. Testing of a proposed system in a series of 461 patients with uniform treatment and follow-up. *Cancer*, **82** (5), 893–901.

Shimizu, Y., Kamoi, S., Amada, S. *et al.* (1998) Toward the development of a universal grading system for ovarian epithelial carcinoma I. Prognostic significance of histopathologic features: problems involved in the architectural grading system. *Gynecologic Oncology*, **70** (1), 2–12.

Sivridis, E., Giatromanolaki, A., Koutlaki, N. *et al.* (2005) Malignant female adnexal tumour of probable Wolffian origin: criteria for malignancy. *Histopathology*, **46** (6), 716–718.

Symmers, W. St. C. (ed) (1978) *Systemic Pathology*, Vol. 4, 2nd edn, Churchill Livingstone, London.

Tavassoli, F.A. and Devilee, P. (eds) (2003) *WHO Classification of Tumours: Pathology & Genetics Tumours of the Breast and Female Genital Organs*, 1st edn, IARC Press, Lyon.

Wells, M. and Wilkinson, N. (1997) Effects of drugs in the endometrium: recent advances. *Current Diagnostic Pathology*, **4** (3), 121–127.

Yanai-Inbar, I. and Scully, R.E. (1987) Relation of ovarian dermoid cysts and immature teratomas: an analysis of 350 cases of immature teratoma and 10 cases of dermoid cyst with microscopic foci of immature tissue. *International Journal of Gynecological Pathology*, **6** (3), 203–12.

Web sites

RCPath, Standards and Minimum Datasets for Reporting Cancers. URL: www.rcpath.org.uk (accessed May 2005).

Working Party of the RCPath and NHSCSP (1999) Histopathology Reporting in Cervical Screening. NHSCSP Publication nō. 10, http://www.cancerscreening.nhs.uk/cervical/publications/nhscsp10.pdf (accessed March 2007).

18. Breast

Ductal Hyperplasia of Usual Type, ADH and DCIS

Criteria for Distinguishing Hyperplasia of Usual Type from ADH or DCIS

TABLE 18.1   HUT or ADH/DCIS?

Ductal Hyperplasia of Usual Type (HUT)	ADH/DCIS
irregularly spaced and overlapping nuclei	non-overlapping nuclei (spacing is regular or irregular)
nuclei get smaller towards centre of the lumen	nuclei don't get much smaller towards the centre
streaming of nuclei between cribriform spaces and along the long axis of the duct	'Roman bridge' perpendicular ordering of nuclei between cribriform spaces
cribriform spaces are irregular	spaces usu. punched out but may be irregular
big spaces peripherally with smaller ones centrally	even-sized spaces throughout the duct
spaces have a fuzzy inner border due to lumenal cells' apical snouts	spaces have a crisp or scalloped inner border
micropapillary variant has 2-cell-types with marked pyknosis of cells at the tuft tips	micropapillary variant has a single cell type (incl. at periphery of duct). The cells are irregularly arranged and hyperchromatic throughout without marked pyknosing towards the tuft tips
ADH is suggested when features of both HUT (e.g. presence of columnar cells) & DCIS occur in the same duct	

Criteria for Distinguishing Atypical Ductal Hyperplasia (ADH) from DCIS
- Either of the following may be accepted as ADH:
① < 2 complete ducts filled with (what would otherwise be called) low grade DCIS (Page)[1]
② < 2 mm of low grade DCIS (Tavassoli)
- But it is DCIS if there is   *either*   ➤ comedo necrosis – regardless of size/nõ of ducts (Lagios)
                                or   ➤ high grade nuclei (AFIP)

Comparative Immunohistochemistry of Hyperplasia of Usual Type (HUT), ADH and DCIS
- HUT: Fodrin +ve; contains a mixture of CK5/6 +ve and CK5/6 −ve cells
- ADH: −ve for Fodrin and Cyclin D1; CK5/6 −ve cells fill the periphery with a compressed central portion of mixed +ve and −ve cells
- Low grade cribriform DCIS: Cyclin D1 +ve; CK5/6 −ve

Ductal Carcinoma in situ (DCIS)
- Cancerisation of lobules is just one form of DCIS and has the same management implications
- Size (= extent of DCIS) and distance to the excision margins are the most important features
- Size determines the risk of recurrence and suitability for conservation (if <3–4 cm) or mastectomy
- 3D reconstruction studies have shown that skip lesions may be present upto 2 cm from main lesion
- EORTC margin status recommendations: >2 cm = 'clear'
  (based on the closest distance of   1–2 cm = 'uncertain'
  DCIS to the margins of a specimen)   <1 cm = 'incomplete' (excision)

  > ! Check if your local surgeons accept this terminology – otherwise just give the measurement

- van Nuys grading of DCIS:
  ➤ high nuclear grade regardless of necrosis (= high grade): may benefit from radioRx
  ➤ other nuclear grade with necrosis (= intermediate): lower disease-free survival *cf.* no necrosis
  ➤ other nuclear grade without necrosis (= low grade): if there is no Ca^{2+}, these may extend more widely than the radiology suggests ($\frac{1}{4}$ of cases occupy >1 quadrant)

---

[1] if exactly two ducts, some call it 'atypical intraductal proliferative lesion' with the understanding that this could be either ADH or DCIS and further investigation or treatment is warranted.

Diagnostic Criteria Handbook in Histopathology: A Surgical Pathology Vade Mecum by Paul J. Tadrous
Copyright © 2007 by John Wiley & Sons, Ltd.

- European (nuclear) grading of DCIS is currently recommended by the NHSBSP and is based on:
    - **cell spacing:**   ☞ high grade: irregular with no palisading over any micropapillae
                            ☞ low grade: regular with central nuclei and palisading over any papillae
    - **nuclear size and pleomorphism:**
        - ☞ high grade: average nuclear size of $>3\times$ the size of an RBC with $\approx 2\times$RBC size variation
        - ☞ low grade: average nuclear size of $<2\times$ the size of an RBC with variation upto $1.5\times$RBC
    - **mitoses**:   high grade: usu. many $\pm$ abnormal forms;   low grade: few mitoses
    - **nucleoli**:   high grade: common $\pm$ multiple;   low grade: inconspicuous nucleoli
    - **chromatin**: high grade: coarse with irregular membrane; low grade: $\approx$ round nuclear membrane
    - intermediate grade is between high and low and encompasses most cases of clear cell/apocrine DCIS
    - grade according to the worst (highest grade) area, not the predominant type.
- Although architecture is usu. not as sig. as grade you should distinguish the following special types:
    - *Micropapillary*: tends to be widespread and multiquadrantic
    - *Apocrine*: only diagnose if severe atypia and comedo necrosis/DCIS architecture
    - *Encysted papillary CIS*: (see p. 264)
- Cystic hypersecretory DCIS (colloid cysts with an attenuated micropapillary $\pm$ cribriform DCIS lining)
- Comedocarcinoma is an old term for comedo DCIS (usu. high grade) and should not be used
- Clinging carcinoma is an old term for flat or micropapillary DCIS (may be low grade) or ADH where the atypical cells/clumps appear partly attached ('clinging') to either the BM or to a columnar layer of non-atypical cells. The term is best avoided. Look for more typical DCIS/ADH elsewhere
- Immuno: ER and PgR +ve in $\approx$ 50%. ER assoc^d with lower grade, non-comedo and lack of c-erbB-2; c-erbB-2 is +ve in $\approx$ 50% and assoc^d with higher grades, comedo and +vity in invasive component
- DCIS is a unifocal ($\pm$ skip lesions) clonal premalignant lesion amenable to prophylactic excision
- LCIS is a risk factor for carcinoma in both breasts so is not locally excised and margin status is not important (but close F/U is)
- d/dg: low grade solid DCIS (E-cadherin +ve, HMW CK $-$ve) differs from LCIS (E-cadherin $-$ve, HMW CK +ve) in showing more cellular cohesion and cytoplasmic basophilia, less uniformity in cell size and arrangement and no intracytoplasmic lumena. ! Mixed ductal-lobular CIS may also occur

Microcalcifications

- Biopsies for μCa^{2+} should be X-rayed:
    - so that the presence of μCa^{2+} can be confirmed in the Bx/slices
    - is the μCa^{2+} representative of that seen on the mammogram?
    - so that the core (or slices) with the μCa^{2+} be identified for possible serials
- State whether μCa^{2+} is associated with benign or carcinomatous elements
- Use polarised light to detect Ca^{2+} oxalate (because weddelite does not stain with H&E)
- μCa^{2+} should be $\geq 100\mu$ in size (per grain or cluster) to be detectable by mammography $-$ if only smaller fragments are present then diagnose as B1 (unless other abnormalities are also present)

Diseases of the Nipple

Paget's Disease of the Nipple
- Assoc^d with underlying DCIS/invasive carcinoma
- Epidermis infiltrated by single/groups of large cells $\pm$ acinar formations, cytoplasm usu. clear
- Lymphocyte exocytosis
- Immuno: intraepidermal tumour cells are +ve for CK7, CAM5.2, CEA, EMA and c-erbB-2; S100 $\pm$ve
- d/dg normal Toker cells: these are CK7 +ve, c-erbB-2 $-$ve and have benign morphology
- d/dg atypical keratinocytes in inflammatory skin conditions
- d/dg melanoma: S100 may be +ve in Paget's but melanomas are CK and c-erbB-2 $-$ve, HMB45 +ve
- d/dg Bowen's disease is HMW CK +ve (unlike Paget's)

'Adenoma of the Nipple' Mass Lesions
- These are a variety of solid, tubular and papillary epithelial proliferations of the main nipple ducts
- Assoc^d with concurrent malignancy in 14% (occurs in the contralateral breast in 2%) or DCIS

- Proliferations and tubules have a 2-cell type (± nuclear hyperchromasia) and a cellular stroma
- ± Pseudoinfiltrative pattern (sclerosing adenosis-like), ± secretory change
- ± Central necrosis (may look like comedocarcinoma – but with benign cytology)
- Extensive sclerosis with entrapment of irregular ducts can simulate malignancy
- May ulcerate and have lots of Toker cells in the overlying epidermis (! do not call Paget's)
- Variant: florid intraduct papillomatosis
- Variant: syringomatous adenoma (like syringoma ± perineural invasion / squamous metaplasia)
- d/dg IDC: two-cell type and lack of pleomorphism or DCIS favour benignity

Mammary Duct Fistula and Duct Ectasia
- Fistula often associated with duct ectasia or sub-areolar abscess (also smoking)
- Fistula usu. has a squamous/granulation tissue lining
- Duct ectasia usu. occurs near the nipple (± discharge) and shows ① dilated benign duct, ② containing lumenal debris and foam cells and ③ surrounding fibrosis and lymphocytes, Mϕ and plasma cells (= plasma cell mastitis if numerous) ± intraepithelial inflam^n / denudation or lumen obliteration ± recanalisation

Invasive Carcinoma

General Aspects, Grading and Receptor Scoring
- *Prognostics:* size, nodal status and type (ductal worse than lobular worse than most special types)
- *Nodal status:*
  - ≤3 nodes +ve = better prognosis; ≥ 4 nodes +ve = worse prognosis
  - internal mammary node +ve = worse prognosis
  - apical node +ve = worse prognosis
  - node −ve: ☞ c-erbB-2 +ve → better response to chemoRx
    - ☞ if tumour <1 cm then (possibly) *no chemoRx* if low grade and young patient
    - ☞ peritumoural vascular invasion is important as a: ◆ surrogate marker of LN status
      - ◆ predictor of local recurrence
- *Grade*: grade all histological types. Give a score from 1–3 for each of these:
  - **tubules** (<10% and >75%): use the average across the whole tumour (for pleom. and mitoses use the growing edge); (for mucinous/cribriform CA count the spaces in the solid sheets as tubule lumena)
  - **pleomorphism**: 1 = little variation from normal ductal cells; 2 = more open nuclei with mod. variation and occ. nucleoli; 3 = vesicular, marked variation, occ. large bizarre forms
  - **mitoses** per 10 hpf at the tumour periphery – extrapolate if tumour too small to cover 10 fields. Cut-offs for scores 1 and 3 depend on field diameter e.g. ≤7, >14 for 0.5 mm Ø ; ≤5, >11 for 0.44 mm Ø and ≤10, >20 for 0.6 mm ∅
  - add the scores to get the grade as follows: grade 1 = 3–5, grade 2 = 6–7, grade 3 = 8–9
- Nottingham Prognostic Index (NPI) = (0.2 × size in cm) + grade + Node_score
  - 'Node_score' = 1 (if no LN are +ve); 2 (if 1–3 LN are +ve); 3 (if >3 LN are +ve)
  - 'size' is the maximum diameter (of the highest grade lesion if there are multiple tumours)
- *DCIS*: The presence of an extensive *in situ* component (i.e. DCIS extending >1 mm beyond the invasive component) predicts likelihood of margin involvement and hence risk of local recurrence. If an extensive *in situ* component is present give two size measurements: ① invasive tumour alone and ② whole tumour (i.e. invasive + adjacent DCIS)
- *c-erbB-2*: Overexpression of HER2 results in membranous staining by immuno, is assoc^d with poor prognosis, high grade and favourable response to chemoRx – anthracyclines as well as trastuzumab (Herceptin®) but resistance to tamoxifen and CMF. An example of indications for HER2 testing by immuno could be any of: ① high grade tumour ② multifocal tumour ③ node positive – but currently most advocate that *all* newly diagnosed breast cancers be tested.

Herceptest™ Score for immunohistochemical assessment of HER2 over-expression:
If <10% cells stain, this is score 0 (= Negative result), if > 10% cells stain then score as:

1+	partial membrane staining, weak	= Negative
2+	complete membrane, weak-moderate	= Borderline requiring confirmation by FISH
3+	complete membrane, strong	= Positive

- *Receptor Status: (only invasive carcinoma is scored – not DCIS, unless specifically requested)*
Nuclear staining may be semiquantitated using the histo-score (H-Score) or Allred's Quick Score:

H-Score: Tumour cell staining intensity is scored $i0$–$i3$ where $i0$ is no staining and $i3$ is staining of equal intensity to normal control cells. Record the % of tumour cells staining at each intensity level.

$$\text{H-score} = 0 \times \%i0 + 1 \times \%i1 + 2 \times \%i2 + 3 \times \%i3 = (0 - 300)$$

The H-score may be interpreted as ≤ 50 = negative, 51–100 = weakly positive (+), 101–200 = moderately positive (++) and >201 = strongly positive (+++).

Quick score: Over the whole tumour on a section assess the proportion of cells showing some staining and score 0–5 thus: 0%, $<1\%$, $<10\%$, $<34\%$, $<67\%$, $\geq 67\%$; then score the average intensity of the positively stained cells as 1–3 (weak, intermediate, strong) or score 0 if no cells stain. Add the proportion and intensity scores to get the Quick Score value (= 0 or 2–8). Interpretation: 0 = negative, 2 = borderline, 3 = weakly positive, 4–8 = positive.

TABLE 18.2 Response to hormone therapy

Receptor	Status	% that respond
ER +ve	PgR +ve	80
ER +ve	PgR −ve	60
ER −ve	PgR +ve	20
ER −ve	PgR −ve	0

Tumours likely to be ER +ve: G1, mucinous, lobular and those with elastotic stroma

Tumours likely to be ER −ve: G3, medullary and those with lymphocytic stroma

Tumours that are positive for PgR may be treated with newer alternatives to tamoxifen

Even borderline/weakly +ve cases may benefit from hormone Rx – hence the need for scoring

Rules for Special/Mixed Types of Carcinoma
- Pure ILC, tubular, invasive cribriform and mucinous carcinomas require $\geq 90\%$ purity ($<10\%$ NST)
- If mixed tubular and cribriform components use 50% to decide if 'tubular' or 'invasive cribriform'
- For 'mixed tubular/ductal' or 'tubular/lobular' 75–90% should be of tubular type
- Otherwise a tumour is of mixed type if 50–89% is of a special type (if $<50\%$, it is adenoCA of NST)

Medullary Carcinoma of the Breast
① syncytial growth pattern of grade 3 cells
② lymphoplasmacytic infiltrate } throughout the whole tumour
③ pushing margins
- DCIS is usu. absent and ER and PgR usu. −ve.
- Called *atypical medullary* if any of the following:
  ➢ scanty lymphoplasmacytic infiltrate
  ➢ microscopically infiltrative pattern at the margin
  ➢ dense areas of fibrosis
  ➢ ductal NST pattern in upto 25% (if $>25\%$ it becomes 'infiltrating ductal CA NST')

Infiltrating Lobular Carcinoma (ILC)
- Classical: ovoid cells with little cytoplasm, eccentric nuclei with little pleomorphism ± cells with 1 or more vacuoles ('private acini') containing a central DPAS +ve mucin droplet (= targetoid cytology, also seen in IDC). These infiltrate in cords, single files and 'Indian files' (= single files but with a gap/stroma between each cell) ± in concentric layers around ducts (= targetoid architecture)
- Alveolar: solid aggregates of ≥ 20 cells
- Solid: sheets (rather than the single files and targetoid arch. of classical lobular): d/dg lymphoma
- Tubulolobular: lobular growth pattern with both single files and *micro*tubules in $>90\%$ of the tumour
- 'Mixed lobular' if: ➢ $\leq 80\%$ of tumour is of one specific subtype
  ➢ pleomorphic lobular (lobular growth pattern with pleomorphic cells)
  ➢ signet ring lobular
  ➢ upto 10% ductal NST ($>10\%$ = 'mixed ductal and lobular carcinoma')
- Cadherins: Lobular neoplasia is associated with loss of E-cadherin membranous staining (less commonly, weak staining with abnormal distribution including cytoplasmic) whereas tubulolobular CA and ductal lesions are often positive. P-cadherin is also absent in $>80\%$ of ILC but also absent in some ductal carcinomas. E-cadherin is present in normal duct epithelium. P-cadherin is only positive in myoepithelium in normal breast tissue – not lumenal cells

Lobular Neoplasia (ALH and LCIS)
- ALH ($\geq$3 cell layers): 1) fewer the 50% acini filled and distended; 2) persistence of lumena; 3) other cell types admixed
- LCIS: >50% acini filled and distended by neoplastic lobular epithelial cells without other cell types. Pagetoid spread up the ducts is more common than in ALH

Tubular Carcinoma
- Architecture: stellate with central elastosis
- Stroma: cellular desmoplastic stroma $\pm$ metachromasia
- Tubules: angulated patent tubules
- Cytology: 1 cell type, apical snouts
- Associations: DCIS low grade cribriform / micropapillary, CCL

> d/dg: compare these features to some benign mimics of cancer: microglandular adenosis, radial scar / CSL and sclerosing adenosis (*vide infra*)

Other Lesions

Columnar cell lesions (CCL)
- CCL are associated with μCa^{2+} and may co-exist with DCIS, tubular carcinoma or lobular neoplasia
- On their own CCL are considered a form of fibrocystic change and Mx is conservative (if no atypia)
- Columnar cells with elongated nuclei and apical snouts (columnar cell change is also called CAPSS)
- Immuno: CK19 +ve, CK5 −ve, ER and PgR strong and diffuse +vity (normal TDLU shows patchy, variable +vity)
- CCL encompass one of the definitions of what used to be called 'blunt duct adenosis'
- CCL are classified as: ➤ columnar cell change: $\leq$ 2 cell layers   ❭ $\pm$ nuclear atypia (roundening
  ➤ columnar cell hyperplasia: > 2 cell layers   ❭ of nuclei and loss of polarity)
- CCL exclude cases with sufficient atypia to warrant a diagnosis of ADH or DCIS

Radial Scar/CSL
- Stellate architecture with central elastosis
- Hypocellular fibrotic stroma
- Elongated tubules, cystic at periphery
- Two cell types, no apical snouts
- $\pm$ HUT/ADH/DCIS (incl. high grade)/lobular neoplasia/invasive carcinoma
- $\pm$ Other fibrocystic changes

Sclerosing Adenosis
- Lobular arch. and central cellularity, may infiltrate nerves and vessel walls (! does not imply malignancy)
- Myoepithelial cells may proliferate
- Elongated tubules with obliterated lumens
- Two cell types, no apical snouts
- $\pm$ Apocrine metaplasia: ? assoc[d] with atypical hyperplasia elsewhere (*Atypical Apocrine Adenosis* is defined as having a three-fold difference in apocrine nuclear size and has $\uparrow$ risk of malignancy)

Microglandular Adenosis (MGA)
- Infiltrative, disorderly architecture
- Stroma: no desmoplasia, may show hyalinisation, no metachromasia
- Small round glands (not elongated tubules)
- One cell type, no apical snouts (but some cases may show some myoepithelial cells)
- No DCIS (*carcinoma ex microglandular adenosis* is very rare)
- $\pm$ Atypical features (usu. seen in recurrence; ? significance): gland budding, nuclear stratificat[n], nucleoli
- Epithelial cells may be S100 +ve in MGA but usu. −ve in tubular carcinoma

Phyllodes Tumours
- Usu. older women and unilateral
- Epithelium: cleft-like, benign $\pm$ hyperplasia/metaplasia (carcinoma is rare)
- Stroma: monoclonal, abundant, cellular $\pm$ giant cells, focal degeneration, focal CD34 & Bcl-2 +vity
- *Benign:*   ➤ >90% of the margin is of the 'pushing' type
  ➤ minimal stromal overgrowth/cellularity/pleom. (an occ. bizarre cell excepted)
  ➤ <10/10 hpf stromal mitoses (each field $\varnothing = 0.44$ mm)

- *Borderline*: features in between benign and malignant
- *Malignant*:   ➢ >50% of the margin is of the 'infiltrative' type
                  ➢ marked stromal overgrowth/cellularity/pleomorphism
                  ➢ >10/10 hpf stromal mitoses (each field $\emptyset = 0.44$ mm)
                  ➢ ± heterologous sarcomas: liposarcoma (most common), osteosarcoma, chondrosarcoma, RMS
                  ➢ p53 +vity (moderate to strong) in stromal cells favours malignancy
                  ➢ c-kit (CD117) +ve sub-epithelial stromal cells (also in 50% of benign phyllodes)
                  ➢ CD10 moderate to strong cytoplasmic +vity in >20% of the stromal cells (usu. sub-epithelial site) in upto 50% of cases (*cf.* <3–5% of cases of fibroadenoma / benign phyllodes).
                  ➢ d/dg spindle cell carcinoma is CD34 –ve (and usu. Bcl-2 –ve)
- Variant: 'intraductal phyllodes'

Lymphoma of the Breast
- Bimodal age distribution: 30s and 60s; axillary LN involved in 30–60% of cases
- Skin fixation, UOQ, inflammatory carcinoma-like [*NB*: 'inflammatory carcinoma' is carcinoma with a clinical appearance of redness ± peau d'orange skin dimpling; histologically it is any carcinoma usu. with widespread vascular invasion but not usually inflamed]
- Associations: ➢ silicone implants (associated with FCL/TCL)
                   ➢ autoimmune and lymphoproliferative disorders
                   ➢ bilateral gynaecomastia in men
- Radiology: hypoechoic on ultrasound and MRI shows multifocal rapid enhancement
- Patterns: ➢ LEL/SIDL[2] (*vs.* d/dg Pagetoid spread/DCIS.)
                   ➢ Indian filing – i.e. dyscohesive single filing (*vs.* d/dg ILC)
                   ➢ angiotropic (*vs.* d/dg DCIS)
- Cytology: usu. DLBCL, esp. immunoblastic (*vs.* d/dg poorly diff. carcinoma)

Pseudolymphoma of the Breast
- Def[n]: some underlying lesion (e.g. hamartoma, FA) with a dense reactive lymphoid infiltrate
- d/dg lymphoepithelioma-like carcinoma

Lymphocytic Lobulitis/Sclerosing Lymphocytic Lobulitis
- Plasma cells, lymphocytes and LEL in an otherwise normal TDLU (some require >100 such leukocytes for diagnosis) – ! the leukocytes may mask a co-existent ILC
- Seen in: DM, other autoimmune conditions, in the 'normal' lobules at the periphery of some cancers and in the 'normal' breast tissue of women at increased genetic risk of breast carcinoma

Sarcomas
- 1°: angiosarcoma is one of the commonest and occurs deep (in the breast parenchyma); sample any sarcoma widely to exclude malignant phyllodes (i.e. look for the epithelial formations)
- 2° (post-radioRx): are usu. high grade; MFH/osteosarcoma are most common with angiosarcoma being one of the rarest 2° sarcomas (it usu. arises in the dermis within the radiation field)
- For details, d/dg and the Stuart-Treves syndrome, see pp. 319–321

Diabetic Mastopathy
① sclerosing lymphocytic lobulitis
② lymphocytic vasculitis
③ stromal keloidal fibrosis and epithelioid fibroblasts
- Early onset, long-standing IDDM (but can rarely also occur in NIDDM)
- Often bilateral, hard, painless masses

Juvenile Papillomatosis (Swiss Cheese Disease / Multiple Peripheral Papillomas)
- Papillomas and hyperplasia with cysts or other prolif. epithelial lesions (including LCIS/DCIS)
- Low level ↑ lifetime risk of malignancy

---

[2] Solid **IntraD**uctal **L**ymphoid proliferation

Intraduct Papilloma (Central Papilloma)
- Must have a well-developed myoepithelial layer for diagnosis
- Features favouring benignity:
  - ➢ apocrine metaplasia
  - ➢ well-developed fibrovascular cores
  - ➢ lack of vertically-oriented elongated lumenal cells
  - ➢ lack of surrounding DCIS
  - ➢ history of discharge rather than a mass
  - ➢ CD44s +ve epithelial cells (myoepithelial +vity is irrelevant)
- ≥ 4 layers = *intraduct papilloma with hyperplasia* (includes solid areas)
- Atypical cells (i.e. non-comedo DCIS morphology) involving $<\frac{1}{3}$ of the papilloma and <3 mm in total = *intraduct papilloma with atypia* (↑ cancer risk)
- If >3 mm focus of atypical cells or if atypia in >90% of the papilloma = DCIS
- if atypia involves $>\frac{1}{3}$ of the papilloma (but <90% and <3 mm total) = DCIS arising in a papilloma

Sclerosing Papilloma and Duct Adenoma
- Sclerotic change within either a central or peripheral papilloma ± entrapped tubules d/dg carcinoma
- When associated with a predominantly solid architecture in a central duct it is called *duct adenoma*

Encysted Papillary CIS (also called Encysted or Intracystic Papillary Carcinoma)
- Usu. larger (2–3 cm) than papillomas (1 mm) and may be central (solitary) or peripheral (multiple)
- Fibrous capsule: may contain entrapped tubules but invasion not diagnosed unless into normal breast
- Must show loss of two-cell type at least focally and may contain areas of DCIS (usu. micropapillary/cribriform subtypes)
- Poorly developed fibrous cores, tall cells, cytological atypia (subtle) and lack of apocrine change
- Cell monotony, atypia and lack of two-cell type are useful predictors of malig. on core Bx (not mitoses)
- Good prognosis if no true invasion and no DCIS outside the fibrous capsule
- d/dg Papillary CIS: this shows CIS in an otherwise typical papilloma and has a less prominent capsule (*cf.* encysted papillary CIS)

Gynaecomastia
- Florid type: periductal oedema and cellular myxoid stroma, ↑ nõ. of ducts
- Fibrous type: hypocellular fibrosis, ↓ nõ. of ducts, hyperplasia is less common
- Ducts are irregularly branching
- Lobules absent (except in a small minority of cases and may be assoc^d with Kleinfelter's syndrome)
- Gynaecomastoid HUT shows slender tufts of cells (not bulbous like micropapillary DCIS)
- Assoc^d with PASH, many drugs, CRF, malnutrition and any cause of oestrogenism (incl. cirrhosis)

Some Lesions to Bear in Mind
- Ductal adenoma (well-circumscribed central papilloma with a solid lobulated arch. ± sclerosis esp. in the central part of the lobules ± sclerosing adenosis-like pseudoinfiltration; has a two-cell type)
- Tubular adenoma (FA variant: sparse stroma and epithelial component consists in packed tubules)
- Mammary hamartoma (including muscular hamartoma and adenolipoma): a mass of haphazardly arranged TDLUs, some dilated (but usu. not hyperplastic) in stroma that usu. contains fat
- Lactational nodules ('lactational adenoma') = any benign lesion (FA, hamartoma, adenosis) that enlarges to form a palpable mass during pregnancy then regresses after lactation and may recur with next pregnancy. Cellular with lactational change (= vacuolated cytoplasm and hobnail morphology) ∴ d/dg carcinoma, esp. on core Bx – clinical Hx, 2-cell type and architecture all help
- Granular cell tumour
- Micropapillary carcinoma: shows 'reversed polarity' i.e. BM forms the 'inner lumen' of little acini-like structures that have a peripheral space around them (= true lumen and apical aspect of cytoplasm)
- Invasive ductal carcinoma with osteoclast-like giant cells
- Small cell carcinoma of the breast – d/dg metastatic SmCC
- Argyrophil carcinoma (Grimelius +ve due to α-lactalbumin with monotonous cellularity may give false impression of carcinoid but these are NE granule −ve and behave as ductal carcinoma NST)
- Matrix-producing, metaplastic and sarcomatoid carcinomas: CK +ve, p63+ve (and CD34 −ve unlike phyllodes, FA and PASH which are all CD34 +ve, Bcl-2 +ve).
- Skin adnexal carcinomas (may be ER and PgR +ve, e.g. mucinous carcinoma). Breast primaries can be AR +ve whereas other sites including skin are usu. negative for androgen receptor
- Metastatic carcinomas (e.g. medullary carcinoma of the thyroid, meningioma, etc.)

- Secretory carcinoma (intra- and extracellular vacuoles of mucin, microacini ± solid/pap apocrine)
- Cystic hypersecretory hyperplasia (colloid cysts with a flat layer of bland cells – d/dg the DCIS equivalent)
- Myofibroblastoma: variably cellular spindle cells (αSMA and desmin +ve) with hyaline collagen bundles d/dg SFT
- Adenomyoepithelioma (counterpart of the epithelial-myoepithelial carcinoma of salivary glands)
- AdCC: ER and PgR usu. −ve; membranous c-kit +ve (in epithelial cells) and αSMA and nuclear p63 ≈ always +ve (in myoepithelial cells); calponin and smooth muscle myosin heavy chain −ve. d/dg invasive cribriform CA (≈ always ER +ve; c-kit and p63 −ve) or collagenous spherulosis (c-kit −ve, calponin and smooth muscle myosin heavy chain +ve – as well as αSMA and p63 +ve)
- PASH (pseudoangiomatous stromal hyperplasia) cells are CD31 −ve (unlike d/dg vascular lesions)
- Angiomatosis (vs. angiosarcoma vs. haemangioma), fibromatosis and nodular fasciitis
- Granulomatous mastitis (idiopathic variety is lobulocentric, non-necrotising and lacks vasculitis)
- Basal-like Carcinoma: a CK14 +ve (± CK5/6, CK17, S100, αSMA; −ve for ER, PgR & HER2) aggressive subtype of G3 IDC ± lung / brain mets. Mitoses +++, tumour necrosis, central scar

Some Pitfalls in Breast Histopathology [3]
- Previous FNA/Bx may cause seeding of cells from papillomas or DCIS – d/dg invasive carcinoma
- Calcium oxalate is birefringent but unstained by H&E so may be missed unless you polarise it
- Gynaecomastoid hyperplasia of usual type (do not mis-diagnose as micropapillary DCIS)
- Apocrine atypia and papillary apocrine change can be misdiagnosed as malignant/DCIS
- Lactational change may occur in postmenopausal or non-pregnant / non-lactating women and men
- Clear cell change: vacuolated clear cells (small nuclei, retain lobular arch. and myoepithelium)
- Sclerosing lesions vs. tubular carcinoma (see specific criteria on p. 262)
- Occ. stromal bizarre giant cells in various lesions do *not* indicate pleomorphism (esp. in phyllodes)
- Stromal/spindle lesions. do levels to look for epithelial component of phyllodes, consider artefact of previous FNA or core Bx track, PNST, myofibroblastoma, metaplastic carcinoma, etc. If still uncertain report as 'spindle cell lesion of uncertain nature, B3'
- Fibroepithelial lesions: if unsure whether phyllodes or FA call it 'fibroepithelial lesion, B3'
- Lymph nodes containing epithelial rests in their capsules – ! do not call these metastases
- Radiation effect: affects stromal and other cells – not just epithelium. Degenerate malignant cells may be missed or dismissed as histiocytes (use CK/CD68 immuno)
- Misdiagnosing clinging carcinoma or post chemoRx DCIS as duct ectasia
- ILC may be dismissed as chronic inflammation or stromal hypercellularity
- Low grade lymphoma may be dismissed as chronic inflam[n] – extensive LEL should raise suspicion
- Lymphocytic lobulitis can co-exist with lobular carcinoma and may mask the cancer cells
- Mucocoele-like lesions: benign ones (e.g. ruptured cyst in fibrocystic change) lack epithelial atypia, DCIS and abundant intracystic epithelium; d/dg neoplastic ones (colloid CA or ruptured cystic hypersecretory DCIS)

NHSBSP Reporting Categories – Core Biopsy
B1   normal tissue, uninterpretable tissue (crush, clot, etc.) and mild abnormalities insufficient to explain the clinical or radiological findings (e.g. fine microcalcifications – i.e. $<100\mu$ per grain or cluster – in involuted lobules is invisible to X-ray)
B2   includes HUT and non-parenchymal lesions such as abscess/fat necrosis
B3   ADH not suspicious for DCIS, papillary lesions not suspicious for encysted papillary carcinoma, lobular neoplasia *in situ* (ALH/LCIS), radial scar/CSL, features suggesting phyllodes
B4   ADH suspicious for DCIS, DCIS in a single incomplete duct space or with apocrine morphology, features of carcinoma but complicated by: crush/fixation artefact, hypocellularity or detached malignant cells in blood clot as the only evidence of atypia
B5   definite carcinoma: DCIS/definite papillary CIS (B5a), invasive (B5b), invasion not assessable (B5c)

Frozen Section Diagnosis (some benign lesions to consider before diagnosing carcinoma)

- Sclerosing lesions: e.g. sclerosing adenosis, papillomatosis, radial scar/CSL, ductal adenoma
- Gland rich-lesions: e.g. microglandular adenosis, mammary hamartoma, nipple adenoma

---

[3] mostly summarised from NHSBSP Publication Nō. 50, 2001

- Atypical cytological alterations: apocrine/lactational/clear cell change; chemo/radioRx effect
- Epithelioid soft tissue lesions: e.g. granular cell tumour, haemangioendothelioma, fat necrosis

Bibliography

Carvalho, S., Silva, A.O., Milanezi, F. et al. (2004) c-KIT and PDGFRA in breast phyllodes tumours: overexpression without mutation. Journal of Clinical Pathology, 57 (10), 1075–1079.

Cotran, R.S., Kumar, V. and Collins, T. (eds) (1999) Robbins Pathologic Basis of Disease, 6th edn, W.B. Saunders Co., Philadelphia.

Douglas-Jones, A.G. (2004) Lymphocytic lobulitis in breast core biopsy: a peritumoural phenomenon. Journal of Pathology, 204 (Suppl.), 20A.

Ellis, I.O., Dowsett, M., Bartlett, J. et al. (2000) Recommendations for HER2 testing in the UK. Journal of Clinical Pathology, 53 (12), 890–892.

Ellis, I.O., Humphreys, S., Michell, M. et al. (2004) Guidelines for breast needle core biopsy handling and reporting in breast screening assessment. Journal of Clinical Pathology, 57 (9), 897–902.

Elston, C.W. and Ellis, I.O. (eds) (1998) The Breast, in Systemic Pathology, Vol. 13, 3rd edn (ed W. St. C. Symmers), Churchill Livingstone, Edinburgh.

Fulford, L.G., Easton, D.F., Reis-Filho, J.S. et al. (2006) Specific morphological features predictive for the basal phenotype in grade 3 invasive ductal carcinoma of breast. Histopathology, 49 (1), 22–34.

Galea, M.H., Blamey, R.W., Elston, C.E. et al. (1992) The Nottingham prognostic index in primary breast cancer. Breast Cancer Research & Treatment, 22 (3), 207–219.

Harvey, J.M., Clark, G.M., Osborne, C.K. et al. (1999) Estrogen receptor status by immunohistochemistry is superior to the ligand-binding assay for predicting response to adjuvant endocrine therapy in breast cancer. Journal of Clinical Oncology, 17 (5), 1474–1481.

Hermsen, B.B.J., von Mensdorff-Pouilly, S., Fabry, H.F.J. et al. (2005) Lobulitis is a frequent finding in prophylactically removed breast tissue from women at hereditary high risk of breast cancer. Journal of Pathology, 206 (2), 220–223.

Ivan, D., Selinko, V., Sahin, A.A. et al. (2004) Accuracy of core needle biopsy diagnosis in assessing papillary breast lesions: histologic predictors of malignancy. Modern Pathology, 17 (2), 165–171.

Mastropasqua, M.G., Maiorano, E., Pruneri, G. et al. (2005) Immunoreactivity for c-kit and p63 as an adjunct in the diagnosis of adenoid cystic carcinoma of the breast. Modern Pathology, 18 (10), 1277–1282.

Millar, E.K.A., Beretov, J., Marr, P. et al. (1999) Malignant phyllodes tumours of the breast display increased stromal p53 protein expression. Histopathology, 34, 491–496.

Mohsin, S.K., Weiss, H., Havighurst, T. et al. (2004) Progesterone receptor by immunohistochemistry and clinical outcome in breast cancer: a validation study. Modern Pathology, 17 (12), 1545–1554.

Moll, R., Mitze, M., Frixen, U.H. et al. (1993) Differential loss of E-cadherin expression in infiltrating ductal and lobular breast carcinomas. American Journal of Pathology, 143 (6), 1731–1742.

Moore, Y. and Lee, A.H.S. (2001) Expression of CD34 and bcl-2 in phyllodes tumours, fibroadenoma and spindle cell lesions of the breast. Histopathology, 38 (1), 62–67.

Narnes, D.M. and Millis, R.R. (1995) Oestrogen receptors: the history, the relevance and the methods of evaluation, in Progress in Pathology, Vol. 2 (eds N. Kirkham and P. Hall), Churchill Livingstone, Edinburgh, pp. 89–114.

NHSBSP/Non-operative Diagnosis Subgroup of the National Co-ordinating Group for Breast Cancer Screening (2001) Guidelines for non-operative diagnostic procedures and reporting in breast cancer screening, 1st edn, NHSBSP Publication Nō. 50. Available online at: http://www.cancerscreening.nhs.uk/breastscreen/publications/nhsbsp50.pdf (accessed August 2007)

NHSBSP (National Health Service Breast Screening Programme)/The Guidelines Working Group of the National Co-ordinating Committee for Breast Pathology (2005) NHSBSP Publication Nō: Pathology Reporting of Breast Disease. A Joint Document Incorporating the Third Edition of the NHS Breast Screening Programme's Guidelines for Pathology Reporting in Breast Cancer Screening and the Second Edition of The Royal College of Pathologists' Minimum Dataset for Breast Cancer Histopathology. NHS Cancer Screening Programme/Royal College of Pathologists, London.

Available online at: http://www.cancerscreening.nhs.uk/breastscreen/publications/nhsbsp58-high-resolution.pdf (accessed August 2007)

Pai, S.A. and Bhat, M.G. (2005) A diabetic breast lump. Journal of the Royal Society of Medicine, 98 (2), 61–62.

Poller, D.N. and Ellis, I.O. (1995) Ductal carcinoma in situ (DCIS) of the breast, in Progress in Pathology, Vol. 2 (eds N. Kirkham and P. Hall), Churchill Livingstone, Edinburgh, pp. 47–87.

Rabban, J.T., Swain, R.S., Zaloudek, C.J. et al. (2006) Immunophenotypic overlap between adenoid cystic carcinoma and collagenous spherulosis of the breast: potential diagnostic pitfalls using myoepithelial markers. Modern Pathology, 19 (10), 1351–1357.

Rasbridge, S.A., Gillet, C.E., Sampson, S.A. et al. (1993) Epithelial (E-) and placental (P-) cadherin cell adhesion molecule expression in breast carcinoma. Journal of Pathology, 169 (2), 245–250.

Reis-Filho, J.S. and Schmitt, F.C. (2002) p63 expression in sarcomatoid/metaplastic carcinomas of the breast. Histopathology, 42 (1), 94–95.

Rosen, P.P. (2001) Rosen's Breast Pathology, 2nd edn, Lippincott Williams & Wilkins, Philadelphia.

Ross, J.S. (2005) Predictive and prognostic molecular markers in breast cancer, in Recent Advances in Histopathology, Vol. 21 (eds M. Pignatelli and J. Underwood), The Royal Society of Medicine Press, London, pp. 31–49.

Shousha, S. (1996) New aspects in the histological diagnosis of breast carcinoma. Seminars in surgical Oncology, 12 (1), 12–25.

Silva, E.G. and Balfour Kraemer, B. (1987) Intraoperative Pathologic Diagnosis. Frozen section and other techniques, 1st edn, Williams & Wilkins, Baltimore.

Tse, G.M.K., Tan, P-H., Ma, T.K.F. et al. (2005) CD44s is useful in the differentiation of benign and malignant papillary lesions of the breast. Journal of Clinical Pathology, 58 (11), 1185–1188.

Tse, G.M.K., Tsang, A.K.H., Putti, T.C. et al. (2005) Stromal CD10 expression in mammary fibroadenomas and phyllodes tumours. Journal of Clinical Pathology, 58 (2), 185–189.

Trendell-Smith, N.J., Peston, D. and Shousha, S. (1999) Adenoid cystic carcinoma of the breast: a tumour commonly devoid of oestrogen receptors and related proteins. Histopathology, 35 (3), 241–248.

19. Endocrine

Thyroid

Normal Histology
- Thin vascular connective tissue septa divide the gland into lobules of 20–40 follicles each
- The more active the follicle: the smaller it is, the taller its epithelium, the paler its colloid
- Hyperactive follicles' colloid may show peripheral scalloping vacuolation (not seen in resin or FS)
- Adult thyroid colloid contain birefringent calcium oxalate crystals ($\uparrow$ with age)
- Parafollicular C cells (present in mid and lower lobes) reside within the follicle BM and number <10 per low power ($\times 10$ objective) field. They are +ve for CgA and CgB (follicular cells are −ve for both)
- Sanderson polsters: collections of small follicles form a focal bulge into larger ones and the epithelium overlying the bulge is more columnar – ! do not confuse for papillae
- TFTs (! ranges vary by lab, age and gender): TSH (0.4–5.7 mIU/l); free T_4 (8–24 pM/l); free T_3 (2.5–7 pM/l); total T_3 (1.1–3nM/l)

Multinodular Goitre (MNG)
- Called '*endemic goitre*' if present in >10% of the population
- Such functional goitres go through stages from *parenchymatous goitre* (nodular hyperplasia), through *colloid goitre* (inactive areas filled with colloid) to typical *multinodular goitre* with a mixed pattern and evidence of haemorrhage and fibrosis
- A *dominant nodule* may have a true capsule (= '*adenomatoid nodule*') and some are monoclonal $\therefore$ any encapsulated nodule, even in the background of a MNG, should be managed as an adenoma
- Rare PTC-like nuclei may be found but do not indicate PTC unless they form clusters or are concentrated in a particular nodule [*NB:* nuclear clearing alone can be due to biotin-rich nuclei]
- d/dg: dyshormonogenetic goitre and diffuse sclerosing follicular and macrofollicular variants of PTC

Graves' Disease

Untreated
- Microfollicles and larger follicles (collapsed, stellate outline/papillaroid infoldings) with little colloid
- Columnar follicular epithelial cells and prominent colloid scalloping
- Minor lymphoid infiltrate $\pm$ germinal centres
Treated
- Iodine: $\quad \triangleright$ accumulation of colloid that is more eosinophilic (*cf.* untreated)
  $\quad\quad\quad \triangleright$ the tall epithelium shrinks to become cuboidal
- Anti-thyroid drugs: exaggerated hyperplasia with $\uparrow$ microfollicles

Hashimoto's Thyroiditis (and d/dg incl. Lymphocytic Thyroiditides)
- Diffuse involvement (may be nodular) with parenchymal destruction
- Lobular architecture is exaggerated with hyaline septal fibrosis and chronic inflam[n]
- Intense interlobular lymphoplasmacytic infiltrate with 2° follicles
- Intralobular lymphoplasmacytic infiltrate $\pm$ IELs
- In diffuse areas T and B cells occur in equal nõs and B-cells have a normal $\kappa{:}\lambda$ ratio
- Some follicles appear hyperactive/hyperplastic
- Oxyphil (Askanazy, Hürthle cell) change
- Small follicles and solid islands of Hürthle cells with mitoses (! d/dg Hürthle cell neoplasm)
- Focal PTC-like nuclei are common and not grounds for diagnosing PTC unless arch. is also typical
- Juvenile variant (= *Lymphocytic Thyroiditis*) has less oxyphil change, parenchymal loss and fibrosis
- Sclerosing variant has $\approx$33% of parenchyma replaced by broad fibrous bands that separate more typical Hashimoto areas $\pm$ squamous metaplasia – confined to thyroid capsule (unlike some d/dg)
- Sequelae: lymphoma, sclerosing MEC with eosinophilia, sequestration ($\rightarrow$ 'lateral aberrant thyroid')
- d/dg sclerosing Hashimoto's *vs.* the following (*q.v.*): diffuse sclerosing variant of PTC, Riedel's thyroiditis, sclerosing MEC with eosinophilia and primary myxoedema

Diagnostic Criteria Handbook in Histopathology: A Surgical Pathology Vade Mecum by Paul J. Tadrous
Copyright © 2007 by John Wiley & Sons, Ltd.

- d/dg *Focal Lymphocytic Thyroiditis (= Focal Chronic Thyroiditis)*:
  - ➢ this is focal, silent and may be assoc[d] with other autoimmune disorders or PTC
  - ➢ parenchymal loss, germinal centres and oxyphil change are rare
  - ➢ the infiltrate is predominantly subcapsular and septal (not intralobular)
- d/dg in general: lymphoma, radiation change, LN metastasis of PTC – esp. on FS (*q.v.*)

Riedel's Thyroiditis (Woody Struma / Ligneous Thyroiditis)
- Rare, may be part of multifocal fibrosclerosis, clin. d/dg carcinoma
- Dense ('keloidal') fibrosis replaces parenchyma obliterating lobular architecture
- Extends beyond thyroid capsule to encase surrounding structures
- Focal lymphoplasmacytic infiltrate (reversed κ:λ ratio and no germinal centres – *cf.* d/dg Hashimoto's)
- Sclerosing phlebitis
- d/dg fibrous reaction surrounding an adenoma that is usu. degenerate/cystic
- d/dg: sclerosing Hashimoto's, paucicellular variant of anaplastic CA, sclerosing PTC, 1° myxoedema

Primary Atrophic Thyroiditis (Primary Myxoedema)
- Hyaline fibrous tissue replaces parenchyma but lobularity may still be discerned (unlike Riedel's)
- The few remaining follicles are small with oxyphil change/squamous metaplasia
- Minor chronic inflammatory foci (follicles are rare)

de Quervain's Subacute Giant Cell Thyroiditis (and d/dg Granulomatous Thyroiditides)
- Young, viral/URTI prodrome, ± hyperthyroidism with painful goitre, self limited ∴ Bx is rare
- Early: focal follicle epithelial cell damage and PMN infiltration
- Later: ➢ mixed inflam[y] cell infiltrate: lymphocytes, plasma cells, Mφ, eosinophils, PMN
  - ➢ intralobular *and* interlobular fibrous collagen deposition (characteristic)
  - ➢ multinucleate giant cells (esp. around colloid)
  - ➢ mononuclear cells form a multilayered lining to some follicles
- Uninvolved parts of the gland show inactive features (flattened epithelium, eosinophil colloid, etc.)
- d/dg: in granulomatous thyroiditides due to TB, sarcoid or fungi – the granulomas may be well formed and not centred on the colloid of a follicle

Radiation-induced Changes
- The cytological features (see p. 368) are too bizarre for the relatively normal architecture and may not be widespread
- Stromal fibrosis and atrophy of follicular epithelium may occur (esp. if previously euthyroid)
- Prominent Hürthle cell change ± lymphocyte-rich inflam[n] (d/dg Hashimoto)
- Adenomatoid proliferations may be prominent in previously thyrotoxic patients
- PTC (aggressive follicular/solid variants) may arise years after radiation exposure

Dyshormonogenetic Goitre
- Multinodular hyperplasia with highly cellular/adenomatoid nodules of varied cytoarchitecture
- Small follicles (esp. in between the nodules) with scant colloid (the lack of normal thyroid tissue in between the nodules helps distinguish this from d/dg parenchymatous MNG)
- Follicles have plump cells with pleomorphism and mitoses (!d/dg neoplasm)
- 'Endocrine-type' atypia is also seen (random, sporadic, *pronounced* nuclear pleom. but no mitoses)
- 'Streaming' and extension of follicles outside the capsule ± pseudovascular invasion (! d/dg neoplasm)
- d/dg follicular CA (true vascular invasion, multiple nodules usu. have the same cytoarchitecture)
- d/dg radio-iodine-treated goitre (may look the same, use CPC)

Follicular Adenoma
- Typically solitary and encapsulated but the capsule is thin and some may lack a capsule
- Has an expansile growth pattern but lacks capsular or vascular invasion (else = carcinoma)
- Does not infiltrate between follicles (embed all if <3 cm ∅ else take ≥ 10 blocks of the interface)
- Adenoma (*vs.* dominant nodule in MNG) is more likely if the background is not multi-nodular
- Histotype (colloid, microfollicular (= '*fetal adenoma*'), solid, trabecular, mixed) is clinically irrelevant
- '*Atypical adenoma*' has marked nuclear atypia and mitotic activity without invasion

- Hürthle cell variant (i.e. >75% of the tumour cells are Hürthle cells – old name = '*Hürthle cell adenoma*') can show marked atypia and mitoses +/ haemorrhage and necrosis and papillae may be present (but not nuclear changes of PTC)
- Clear cell variants exist (but ! exclude d/dg metastatic RCC)
- Immuno: +ve for thyroglobulin, TTF-1 (nuclear stain[1])
- ! d/dg PTC (due to pseudopapillary areas occurring within degenerative changes) – but any nuclear clearing in follicular adenoma is not accompanied by nuclear membrane accentuation and any CK19 +vity is focal (*cf.* diffuse in PTC)
- d/dg follicular variant of PTC: diagnosis is made on unequivocal PTC nuclear changes. If these are equivocal/focal some diagnose 'well-differentiated tumour of uncertain malignant potential' or, if there is minimal capsular invasion, 'well-differentiated carcinoma of uncertain malignant potential'

Follicular Carcinoma
- Microfollicular, macrofollicular, solid, trabecular and pseudopapillary forms
- Hürthle cell variant[2] (i.e. >75% of the tumour are Hürthle cells) is more likely to metastasise to LN
- Immuno: thyroglobulin +ve, calcitonin −ve, galectin-3 +ve[3], HBME1 ±ve
- Ki-67 LI >5% is a poor prognostic
- d/dg follicular variant of PTC: see 'Follicular Adenoma', above; and 'Variants of PTC', below
- d/dg metastatic carcinoma esp. clear cell variant *vs.* RCC

Widely invasive type
- *EITHER*: ① naked eye invasion *OR* ② extensive vasc. invasion by microscopy (e.g. >5 vessels)

Minimally invasive type
- Microscopic evidence of either of the following two:

① capsular invasion:
  ➤ tumour cells must penetrate the entire *original* capsule (! a neocapsule may form around an invasive tongue, ! epithelium trapped in the capsule [circumferentially disposed +/ not connected to the main tumour mass] is not invasion)
  ➤ blunt-ended breaks in the capsule at invasion site (*cf.* sharp ends of d/dg FNA puncture artefact)
  ➤ a true invasive tongue is usu. mushroom-shaped
  ➤ some say that *equivocal* capsular invasion alone (with adequate sampling and without vascular invasion) equates to 'follicular tumour of uncertain malignant potential' while others will diagnose carcinoma on only partial invasion into the capsule
  ➤ d/dg FNA track artefact (pseudo capsular invasion):
    ☞ needle track: haemorrhage, granulation tissue, siderophages ± cholesterol crystals
    ☞ cells escape from capsule in linear fashion (not mushroom)
    ☞ breaks in capsule have sharp ends if caused by an FNA needle

② vascular invasion:
  ➤ requires intracapsular or extratumoural vessels only – not tumour cells in intratumoural vessels
  ➤ requires intralumenal tumour mass covered by endothelium (CD31/CD34) ± attached to wall
  ➤ d/dg endothelial hyperplasia in capsular vessels (pseudo vascular invasion) – ! but do levels because this is assoc[d] with true vascular invasion elsewhere

Papillary Carcinoma (PTC)
- Def[n]: ① evidence of follicular epithelial cell differentiation (incl. follicles and/or papillae)

	② nuclear features:	➤ enlargement
	(demonstration of	➤ irregular outline (usu. with thickened membrane)
	invasion is not necessary)	➤ deep grooves, pseudoinclusions
		➤ pallor, 'ground glass' chromatin ('Orphan Annie eyes')
- Typical features also include:		➤ nuclear overlapping/crowding
		➤ nuclear elongation
		➤ peripheral nucleoli
		➤ squamous differentiation

---

[1] ∴ must block biotin well because thyroid cells are rich in endogenous biotin.
[2] *NB*: it is outdated to diagnose an entity as 'Hürthle cell carcinoma', instead we now speak of Hürthle cell variants of other tumours e.g. follicular adenoma, follicular CA, PTC, poorly diff. CA, etc.
[3] galectin-3 is not entirely specific for malignancy but if positivity is *widespread* and *strong* it may be taken as supportive evidence of malignancy.

- The typical nuclear features may be (multi)focal but if only minor changes are seen in a non-invasive follicular arch. tumour, some call it 'follicular tumour of uncertain malignant potential'
- Architecture:
  - ➢ usu. infiltrative/stellate but can be encapsulated[4]
  - ➢ both follicles (usu. elongated) and papillae (with fibrovascular cores) are present
  - ➢ inspissated colloid may be seen
  - ➢ follicles blend into papillary areas
  - ➢ multinucleated histiocytes in lumena of follicles – high specificity for PTC
  - ➢ ± cribriform or trabecular areas
  - ➢ trabeculae have elongated nuclei polarised perpendicular to their long axis
- Stroma:
  - ➢ hyaline sclerotic/desmoplastic
  - ➢ calcification ± psammoma bodies (proper lamellated bodies *cf.* d/dg the calcified concretions seen in the follicle lumena in some non-neoplastic conditions)
- Immuno: +ve: CK19 (+ve in ≈ all cases so −vity is useful for exclusion but >50% of benign thyroids are also +ve), HBME1, CK7, pan-CK and 34βE12, RET, thyroglobulin (not squamoid areas), CD15, galectin-3, [LP34, CA-125 and CEA are +ve in ≈ 50% of cases], *vide infra* for EMA and AB
- Immuno: −ve: Calcitonin, CgA, CK20
- Prognostics ∝ age, size, stage
- d/dg artefactual nuclear clearing occurring in follicular lesions due to poor fixation:
  - ➢ transition is gradual without clear demarcation and it is worst in the centre of the lesion
  - ➢ other nuclear features (enlargement, crowding, irregular membrane, etc.) are not seen
- d/dg true papillae of PTC *vs.* Sanderson polsters/hyperplastic papillae:
  - ➢ fibrovascular core favours PTC
  - ➢ nuclear features of PTC favour PTC
  - ➢ psammoma bodies favour PTC papillae (although polsters may rarely show calcification)
  - ➢ strong +ve staining of the tips of the papillae with AB and EMA favour PTC papillae as non-neoplastic ones give weak/negative staining
- d/dg multifocal pap lesions without psammoma bodies: consider the tumour of Gardner's syndrome

Variants of PTC
- Typical follicular:
  - ➢ usu. encapsulated and often composed of small follicles ∴ d/dg fetal adenoma
  - ➢ must be follicular throughout – if mixed follicular/PTC, call it usual type PTC
- Diffuse follicular: variably-sized follicles incl. large ones, lacks a capsule ∴ d/dg colloid goitre – scrutinise for PTC features
- Macrofollicular: >50% large follicles ± capsule ∴ d/dg colloid goitre – scrutinise for PTC features (best seen in the smaller follicles)
- Solid: tight islands of cells with PTC nuclei separated by variable-thickness fibrous bands ± focal follicular/papillary areas
- Encapsulated
- PTC with lipomatous stroma
- PTC with exuberant nodular fasciitis-like stroma (assoc[d] with breast phyllodes)
- Diffuse sclerosing PTC:
  - ➢ clinical, serology and low power histology look like d/dg thyroiditis
  - ➢ look for papillae, psammoma bodies, nuclear features of PTC
- Tall cell PTC:
  - ➢ >30% of tumour cells have a height:width ratio >2
  - ➢ eosinophilic granular cytoplasm and PTC features
  - ➢ immuno: CD15 +ve, EMA +ve
  - ➢ d/dg Warthin's tumour-like PTC: tall-cell PTC lacks a dense lymphoid stroma
  - ➢ d/dg columnar cell variant of poorly diff thyroid carcinoma (which is not a PTC)
    - ☞ columnar cells are often taller than PTC tall cells
    - ☞ cytoplasm does not have the eosinophilic granular quality
    - ☞ nuclei are pseudostratified and chromatin-rich (unlike PTC)
- Warthin's tumour-like: papillary Hürthle cell tumour with PTC nuclei and lymphoid stroma
- Oxyphilic (Hürthle cell) – must see PTC nuclear changes, not just papillae
- Cribriform morular PTC (similar to FAP-associated thyroid carcinoma *q.v.*)
- Trabecular (d/dg HTT, *vide infra*)
- De-differentiated PTC: definite PTC with areas of poorly diff/anaplastic carcinoma
- Microcarcinoma: is defined by the WHO as <1cm ∅

---

[4] with *encapsulated* lesions it is best to err on the side of a follicular adenoma unless morphological criteria for PTC are very strong.

- Occult PTC: is one diagnosed as a result of tumour effects (usu. LN mets) where the 1° is not clinically apparent – usu. because they are small (but not necessarily microcarcinoma)
- Latent PTC: is one that is discovered without it causing any clinical effects (e.g. in thyroidectomy for goitre or at PM) – usu. small but not necessarily microcarcinoma. It needs no additional Rx

Hyalinising Trabecular Tumour (HTT/HTA/Paraganglioid Tumour/PLAT)
- Encapsulated (malignancy defined by capsular +/ vascular invasion as for follicular adenoma)
- Nests and trabeculae of elongated cells with hyalinising matrix ± calcification/psammoma bodies
- Lightly eosinophilic cytoplasm ± perinuclear halo and 5μ perinuclear giant yellow lysosomes
- Nuclear features: grooves, inclusions, fine chromatin
- Small cystic spaces +ve for thyroglobulin
- Immuno: Ki-67 (granular cytoplasmic and membranous positivity), usu. −ve for 34βE12 and CK7/19
- d/dg MTC: the nuclear features and long trabeculae are unusual for MTC – but always do immuno
- d/dg HTT-like foci: these occur in follicular adenomas and hyperplastic nodules
- d/dg trabecular PTC: any focus of typical PTC should trump the diagnosis of HTT

Medullary Carcinoma (MTC)
- Consider familial form if: multifocal/bilateral and background C-cell hyperplasia ± S100 +ve sustentacular cells
- Well circumscribed ± capsule
- Nuclei: NE nucleus (i.e. evenly-distributed fine grainy chromatin and absent/inconspicuous nucleoli)
- Few mitoses (>1/25hpf is a worse prognostic) – but can see more in some variants e.g. small cell MTC
- Cytoplasm: fine azurophilic granules (i.e. red on MGG, but the eosinophilia is not obvious on H&E)
- Many cell forms/variants: round, spindle, polygonal, binucleate, oxyphilic, squamoid, clear, signet ring (± mucin and +ve for CEA), small or large (anaplastic) + isolated tumour giant cells
- Tendency to cell dyscohesion
- Stroma: amyloid (± Ca^{2+}, ± giant cells), fibrous bands, prominent microvascularity
- Arch.: lobular/'zellballen'/solid/trabecular/cords ± central necrosis, follicular, papillary
- Immuno/stains: granular cytoplasmic CgA and Grimelius +vity, calcitonin (strong, diffuse +vity is a good prognostic), CEA +ve (unlike the calcitonin +ve strumal carcinoids of the ovary), S100 +ve sustentacular cells in the paraganglioid variant, CK +ve (unlike paragangliomas)
- d/dg: metastatic carcinoid or lobular breast carcinoma, any 1° thyroid tumour, angiosarcoma: MTC should be diagnosable by looking for the nuclear and stromal features and foci of more typical MTC elsewhere ± immuno/stains
- d/dg SmCC vs. small cell MTC: difficult, small cell MTC is also aggressive and often calcitonin −ve. CEA +vity may help (favours MTC)
- d/dg anaplastic carcinoma thyroid: a relatively low mitotic count should suggest MTC, look for foci with more typical features/immuno
- d/dg medullary adenoma: bland encapsulated lesions lacking amyloid are called adenoma by some but these may still metastasise and many do not accept the existence of a benign counterpart of MTC
- d/dg C-cell hyperplasia: vide infra
- d/dg mixed MTC and follicular or MTC and PTC: vide infra

C-Cell Hyperplasia
- C-cell hyperplasia occurs in MEN 2 (± cytological atypia) and also adjacent to non-MTC neoplasms, in Hashimoto's thyroiditis, in hypergastrinaemic and hypercalcaemic states
- Diffuse type: EITHER >50 cells per low power field OR groups >20 cells across
- Nodular type: the follicle is replaced by C-cells
- Immuno: collagen IV may be useful to delineate the BM
- d/dg MTC: hyperplasias are contained within the follicle BM (must show a single, complete, continuous surrounding of BM without breaks or foci of reduplication – else = MTC)
- d/dg nodular hyperplasia vs.:
  - ➢ cross section of an MTC tumour embolus in thin-walled vessel or intrathyroid 'metastasis'
  - ➢ palpation thyroiditis (focal follicles are partly/filled with histiocytes ± lymphocytes/plasma cells/giant cells)
  - ➢ tangential shave of a normal follicle
  - ➢ islands of squamous metaplasia, parathyroid tissue, ultimobranchial body/thymic rests

Differentiated Carcinoma of Intermediate Type (Mixed Medullary and Follicular Carcinoma)
- Follicular and cribriform areas are intermingled with C-cells or solid C-cell islands
- WHO criteria: must have ① thyroglobulin +ve follicular areas; *and* ② calcitonin +ve MTC areas
- d/dg entrapped benign follicles in an invasive MTC
- d/dg collision tumour (follicular CA and MTC or PTC and MTC) – may be impossible to distinguish
- d/dg aberrant calcitonin expression in an otherwise typical follicular carcinoma[5]
- d/dg thyroglobulin +ve MTC – may have a better prog. *cf.* usual-type MTC (? radio-iodine sensitive)

Poorly Differentiated Thyroid Carcinoma
- Def[n]: CA with differentiation in between well diff (follicular CA, PTC, MTC) and undiff (anaplastic CA)
- Insular carcinoma, columnar cell carcinoma and other (less-well characterised) types exist

Insular carcinoma
- Arch.: large, tightly-packed solid islands ± extensive necrosis ± stromal sclerosis, islands are often separated by loose vascular stroma (*cf.* dense fibrous bands)
- Cells: relatively uniform (*cf.* anaplastic carcinoma), ↑NCR, variable mitotic rate, vesicular hyperchromatic nuclei, small nucleoli
- Foci of better diff areas (follicular, PTC, MTC) or worse (anaplastic CA – carries a worse prognosis)
- Minor foci of insular CA in a PTC/follicular CA should be mentioned but does not alter the diagnosis
- Immuno: +ve for thyroglobulin (focal) and Bcl-2 (most cases), −ve for calcitonin
- d/dg anaplastic carcinoma: Bcl-2 +vity and lack of pleomorphism favour insular carcinoma
- d/dg CASTLE but CASTLE has prominent nucleoli, CD5 +vity and ≈ no necrosis

Columnar cell carcinoma
- Arch.: solid, glandular, cribriform, pap.; *EITHER* a) frankly invasive (worse prognosis);
  OR b) encapsulated (± microinvasion of capsule or vessels)
- Columnar cells have hyperchromatic, elongated, pseudostratified nuclei ± cytoplasmic vacuoles
- d/dg metastatic colorectal/endometrioid carcinoma: histologically very similar
- d/dg PTC (tall cell and cribriform morular variants – *q.v.*)

Undifferentiated Thyroid Carcinoma (Anaplastic Carcinoma)
- Usual type has epithelioid, spindle and giant cells with significant nuclear pleomorphism, mitoses ++, vascular invasion and inflam[y] cells (incl. PMN). d/dg sarcomas
- 1° SCC (and ASC) are considered variants of anaplastic due to their aggressive course ∴ exclude the d/dg before making this diagnosis (i.e. 2° SCC, benign squamous lesions, CASTLE)
- Paucicellular variant has spindle cells with milder pleomorphism concentrated at the periphery with a central paucicellular expanse of sclerosis-like necrosis containing ghost vessels
  - ➢ d/dg Riedel's thyroiditis: look for vascular invasion, necrosis, cellular periphery and mets
  - ➢ d/dg myofibroblastic lesions: because this anaplastic CA variant may be +ve for MSA
- Other variants incl.: 'carcinosarcoma' (= metaplastic CA with heterologous elements), angiomatoid (see d/dg angiosarcoma on p. 321), lymphoepithelial (see d/dg CASTLE) and anaplastic CA with osteoclast-like giant cells
- Small cell variant: outmoded – instead classify as SmCC, insular CA, MTC, lymphoma, HX, etc.
- Immuno: ±ve (useful if +ve) for CK, CEA (esp. in SCC), vimentin, FVIIIRA (focal), EMA; −ve for calcitonin and thyroglobulin

FAP-associated Thyroid Carcinoma
- F ≫ M, may be multifocal in FAP
- Cribriform areas (empty follicles), trabeculae of columnar cells, squamoid morules, spindle elements
- Nuclear features of PTC only focally, biotinylated nuclear inclusions
- d/dg tall cell PTC, cribriform morular PTC (use CPC), columnar cell carcinoma, HTT, etc.

Thyroid Tumours Resembling Thymic Tumours

SETTLE (Spindle and epithelioid tumour with thymus-like elements)
- Youths, indolent but may metastasise (esp. to lung/kidney)
- Arch. is lobular (cellular masses separated by thick sclerotic fibrous septae)

---

[5] generally, a single aberrant immuno result should never change the diagnosis if there are no other corroborating features.

- Bland cytology with rare mitoses (*cf.* d/dg synovial sarcoma where mitoses are more common)
- Spindle cell elements (fascicles/storiform) predominate and merge with epithelial elements
- Epithelial elements (papillary/tubular/trabeculae/sheets) may contain HC-like structures
- Mucus/respiratory epithelium may form cysts (unlike in d/dg synovial sarcoma)
- No immature lymphocytes (generally, lymphocytes are scant) unlike in d/dg intrathyroidal thymoma
- Immuno: ➢ CK +ve (both spindle and epithelioid cells)
  - ➢ spindle cells are +ve for MSA, αSMA and CD99
  - ➢ CD5, calcitonin and thyroglobulin are all −ve
- d/dg: anaplastic thyroid CA, immature teratoma, synovial sarcoma (esp. *vs.* extrathyroidal SETTLE)

CASTLE (Carcinoma showing thymus-like elements, Intrathyroidal thymic carcinoma)

- Middle-aged, indolent, local complications, mets are rare
- Arch: lobular/insular with fibrous septae, extrathyroidal spread is common
- Histology: squamoid thymic CA (see p. 96) ± adjacent thymic rests
- Immuno: −ve for thyroid/C-cell markers, CD5 +ve, Bcl-2 +ve
- d/dg: lymphoepithelial variant of anaplastic thyroid CA (but that is CD5 −ve and not lobular)
- d/dg: 1°/2° thyroid SCC, FDC sarcoma, lymphoma and insular carcinoma of the thyroid (*q.v.*)

Mucin-containing Tumours

- 1° adenosquamous carcinoma (has an aggressive course in the thyroid)
- Mucinous carcinoma (! exclude d/dg metastatic origin)
- Amphicrine variant of MTC may secrete mucin and have signet-ring-like cells
- MEC: epidermoid component may contain pearls. Thyroglobulin +vity may be seen
- Sclerosing MEC with eosinophilia:
  - ➢ usu. arises in background of Hashimoto's
  - ➢ both mucoid and epidermoid components show nests and cords
  - ➢ the background shows a diffuse sclerotic stroma containing eosinophils and other inflam[y] cells
  - ➢ immuno: thyroglobulin is usu. −ve
  - ➢ d/dg: NSHL, sclerosing Hashimoto's, PTC with squamoid metaplasia, SCC

Lymphomas

- ± Background of thyroiditis and may also involve local LN or 'home' to the GIT
- usu. DLBCL or MALToma (incl. plasma cell predominant variant). Histol. is similar to elsewhere
- d/dg florid Hashimoto's: CD43 +vity, confluent sheets of B-cells and florid LEL favour lymphoma

Some Pitfalls in Thyroid Tumour Diagnosis

- Don't call PTC: ➢ a cyst (cystic PTC)
  - ➢ a colloid goitre (diffuse follicular PTC, macrofollicular PTC)
  - ➢ a thyroiditis (diffuse sclerosing variant)
- Don't call anaplastic carcinoma Riedel's thyroiditis (paucicellular variant)
- Don't call MTC a PTC or follicular carcinoma: NE nuclei, calcitonin, CgA +ve; thyroglobulin −ve

Frozen Section Histology and Per-operative Cytology in Thyroid Diagnosis

- Concomitant imprint cytology can give complementary information (esp. in PTC and MTC)
- Distinguish thyroid from parathyroid (thyroid has birefringent oxalate crystals ± C-cells and has larger, more variably-sized follicles with denser colloid *cf.* parathyroid. Imprint cytology also helps)
- ! Beware separated nodules of thyroid that may be misidentified by the surgeon as 'LN' – such seques-tration (= 'lateral aberrant thyroid') may occur in MNG or Hashimoto's – do not misdiagnose as LN metastasis.
- Distinguish LN metastasis from fibrous Hashimoto's (look for a LN sinus architecture) – in fibrous Hashimoto's the fibrosis can mimic a LN capsule or desmoplasia, the lymphoid follicles can mimic LN follicles and the atypical Hürthle cells can mimic metastatic carcinoma deposits.
- Distinguish Riedel's thyroiditis from desmoplastic carcinomas
- 'Orphan Annie eye' nuclei/nuclear inclusions do not show on FS (∴ do imprint cytology)
- Distinguish calcified amyloid deposits of MTC from psammoma bodies of PTC
- Defer to paraffin if ?lymphoma or ?metastatic carcinoma from elsewhere (e.g. colon, lung, breast)
- FS should not be used on a 1° tumour to distinguish follicular adenoma *vs.* follicular carcinoma

Parathyroid

Normal Histology
- Dark chief cells (functional, minority cell type, pale eosinophilic cytoplasm with tiny or absent lipid droplets), transitional chief cells, light chief cells (resting, water clear cytoplasm and paranuclear lipid droplets). The cytoplasm contains argyrophil granules and they may form follicles with colloid-like material (+ve for PTH ± amyloid but no oxalate crystals – d/dg thyroid follicles)
- Immuno: +ve for CgA and PTH; −ve for CEA, CgB and thyroglobulin (*cf.* thyroid follicle and C-cells)
- Oxyphil cells (inactive oncocytes) ↑ with age and may form nodules in the elderly (if large, the only difference to functional oxyphil adenoma may be EM evidence of protein synthesis in adenomas)
- Adipocytes ↑ with age to 40's and are ∝ to nutritional state. Fat constitutes 10–50% of gland volume
- Normal plasma total $[Ca^{2+}]$ = 2.1–2.6 mM/l with [PTH] = 0.1–0.9 ng/ml

Frozen Section
- Record the position of the gland (left upper, left lower, etc.)
- Record the trimmed weight ($\approx$ 30 – 40mg per normal gland; ≥60mg is abnormal provided ≥3 other normal glands can be identified)
- Weigh and examine any trimmings in case these too are parathyroid (or thymus – *vide infra*)
- Confirm that it is parathyroid tissue (d/dg thyroid, LN, thymus, adipose, brown fat)
- State if any of the surrounding tissue is thymic (this indicates that the gland is a lower one)
- Distinguishing adenoma *vs.* hyperplasia is not important at FS but missing a carcinoma is disastrous
- A fat stain for intracytoplasmic lipid globules may be useful in d/dg normal *vs.* abnormal tissue:
    - ➤ Sudan IV and oil red O stain lipid positively, toluidine blue/methylene blue are −ve stains
    - ➤ normal/atrophic chief cells have large globules (upto $\approx$ size of nucleus)
    - ➤ hyperplastic/neoplastic chief cells have absent lipid or sparse small globules
- d/dg pure oxyphil parathyroid adenoma *cf.* thyroid Hürthle cell neoplasm (may be impossible)
- d/dg microfollicular parathyroid adenoma *cf.* thyroid follicular neoplasm (may be impossible)

Features Favouring Adenoma Over Hyperplasia
- No single feature is absolute or present in every case (adenomas can mimic hyperplasia and vice versa)
- One enlarged gland with ≥3 normal ones identified – strong evidence whatever the histology[6] (*NB*: in hyperplasia the enlargement of all glands may be asymmetrical; double adenomas may rarely occur)
- Excess weight: if ≫1g it's more likely to be an adenoma
- Thin capsule separating it from a rim of uninvolved gland (but a capsule may be incomplete/absent)
- Rim of uninvolved gland (lipid stains may help): may be absent, atrophic, normal or hyperplastic
- Absence of adipocytes (but occasional scattered adipocytes are often present in adenomas)
- Single diffuse growth (*cf.* multinodularity typical of hyperplasia)

Other features of adenomas
- Cell type: chief or oxyphil (may be elongated) or, rarely, spindle cells. Lymphocytes may be admixed
- Degenerative changes: cystic, myxoid, Ca^{2+}, haemorrhage; subsequent fibrosis may entrap tumour cells, usu. with haemosiderin (! d/dg do not misdiagnose as capsular invasion implying parathyroid CA)
- Mitoses are sparse to absent (Ki-67 LI is usu. <3%)
- 'Endocrine-type' atypia foci occur (esp. adjacent to haemorrhage or in oxyphil cells) but are not mitotic
- d/dg: rare papillary and follicular variants may cause confusion with thyroid neoplasia

Other features of hyperplasia
- 1° hyperplasia may be chief cell (nodular/diffuse, $\approx$ 2° hyperplasias) or water-clear cell (diffuse)
- Chief cell type: may have other cell types sparsely admixed. May have a 'dominant nodule'
- Water-clear cell type: very rare variant, large clear cells (not the same as pale chief cells), looks like low grade RCC (*NB*: RCC and pulm. SCC are the commonest causes of ectopic hyperparathyroidism)
- Mitoses are *usu.* absent in 1° hyperplasia but may be seen in 2° hyperplasias (e.g. in CRF, etc.)

Parathyroid Carcinoma
- Clin: usu. ↑↑ PTH, ↑↑ $[Ca^{2+}]$ (common cause of death), pre-op tumour palpable, per-op 'stuck down'
- Thick hyaline fibrous capsule and internal broad fibrous bands enclosing nodules (may be expansile)
- Arch.: sheets, trabeculae and rosettes are said to be typical (but any may occur in adenomas too)

---

[6] the need to identify ≥3 normal glands is because some people have <4 glands in total so their normal total gland mass is concentrated in fewer (but bigger) normal glands.

- Invasion of adjacent structures (e.g. thyroid) or distant mets are definitive evidence of malignancy
- Invasion of vessels or capsule (! d/dg scarring in an adenoma – use follicular thyroid CA criteria)
- Cells are monotonous but may have frequent prominent nucleoli +/ ↑NCR or be spindled
- Pleomorphism may be generalised or focal (with mitoses, unlike d/dg 'endocrine-type' atypia)
- ± Coagulative tumour cell necrosis
- Mitoses and Ki-67 LI may be very low but if high (>5/10hpf and >5%) or abnormal favour carcinoma over adenoma
- If absolute criteria are lacking (local invasion and mets) and other criteria are equivocal the terms *atypical adenoma* or *parathyroid tumour of uncertain malignant potential* may be used
- Immuno: nuclear +vity for p105 (pRb) favours carcinoma over adenoma (−vity means nothing)
- d/dg pseudoinfiltrative pattern of parathyroid tissue implants from previous surgery (use CPC)
- d/dg pseudoinfiltrative pattern of clear cells in the wall of a benign parathyroid cyst
- d/dg metastatic tumours (esp. clear cell types)

Adrenal

Normal Histology
- Capsule varies in thickness and may be focally absent (→ fusion of adrenal with kidney/liver)
- Fetal cortex is an ≈ homogeneous mass of eosinophilic hepatocyte-like cells, a more basophilic rim of developing definitive cortex appears after birth and the adult form is established by late teens
- The outer *zona glomerulosa* (ZG) is only focally present (if continuous it is considered hyperplasia)
- *Zona fasciculata* (ZF): large cells with abundant lipidised cytoplasm (? a storage zone)
- *Zona reticularis* (ZR): smaller, lipid poor, eosinophilic, compact cells, the inner ones showing lipofuscin ± apoptoses
- An invaginated sheath of cortex invests the central vein and may develop pathology (nodules, etc.)
- Medulla is only present in the head and body and consists in ill-defined nests of polygonal/elongated chromaffin +ve NE phaeochromocytes, (larger, more basophilic and less-well defined *cf.* cortex cells) with coarse and marginating chromatin and focal 'endocrine-type' atypia. Sustentacular and ganglion cells are also present. Eosinophilic globules may be seen in the phaeochromocytes and ganglion cells
- Normal plasma ACTH = 3–15 pM/l with peak cortisol of 700 (a.m.) and 280 (p.m.) nmol/l

Cortical Hyperplasia due to ACTH
- ACTH source may be pituitary (Cushing's/stress) or ectopic (usu. NET of bronchus, thyroid, thymus, pancreas or adrenal medulla)
- Bilateral ↑ cortical thickness with relative ↓ZF and ↑ZR
- Diffuse hyperplasia is more common than multi-nodular hyperplasia
- d/dg multi-nodular diseases of the cortex with ↓/normal plasma ACTH levels:
  - ➤ incidental nodules: unencapsulated, multiple, tiny/upto few cm, ZF-like or ZR-like cells
  - ➤ macronodular hyperplasia without ACTH secretion: distorting nodules of ZF-like cells
  - ➤ PPNAD: familial Cushing's ± Carney complex, pigmented nodules with small clear cells

Cortical Neoplasia – Adrenocortical Adenoma and Adrenocortical Carcinoma (ACC)
- Well-circ. with pseudocapsule, usu. single, orange/yellow/mottled cut surface, may be pigmented
- Adjacent cortex may be normal, atrophic or hyperplastic
- ± Spironolactone bodies in tumour/adjacent cortical cells (if Rx with aldosterone inhibitors for Conn's):
  - ➤ large eosinophilic round inclusions in ZG or peripheral ZF cells
  - ➤ whorled/spiral/'scroll-like' with surrounding clear halo
- Cells: usu. ZF-like but ZG-like (esp. in Conn's) and oncocytic or ZR-like foci occur with focal 'endocrine-type' atypia. Pure oncocytomas may be very large even though benign
- Arch.: alveolar and trabecular architectures are more common in benign tumours (*cf.* solid/diffuse)

Features favouring malignancy
- Clin. risk factors: childhood, large size (esp. if > 1 kg or non-functioning), sex hormone production
- In the absence of mets or gross local invasion (e.g. of the IVC), must use a multiparameter approach and CPC to give an estimate of malignancy risk (i.e. metastatic potential)
- Some diagnose malignancy if there is the simultaneous finding of: ① ↑ mitotic count (>5/50hpf with a 0.47 mm field ⌀) ② abnormal mitoses, and ③ venous invasion. Other risk factors are:
  - ➤ locally recurrent tumours (these all eventually metastasised in Hough's series)
  - ➤ tumour divided into lobules by broad fibrous bands ('broad' means >1 hpf wide)

- ➢ confluent areas of tumour necrosis, esp. if extensive ('extensive' means ≥ 2 contiguous hpf)
- ➢ a solid/diffuse cell architecture (= patternless sheets in >33% of the tumour; non-diffuse is defined as >67% showing patterned architectures e.g. alveolar, broad trabecular, etc.)
- ➢ vascular/sinusoidal invasion (defined as tumour cells in vessel lumen)
- ➢ ↑ proliferation (mitotic count of >20/50 hpf or >10/100 hpf or >10/10 hpf or Ki-67 LI >3% have all been quoted with a 20/50 hpf mitotic count used as the cut-off between low grade and high grade carcinomas in one system)
- ➢ nuclear grade III or IV (by Fuhrman grading) – although some claim pleom. is unhelpful
- ➢ capsular invasion (defined as cell nests/cords into or through the capsule, some also require a stromal reaction): on its own this is unhelpful unless there is invasion of adjacent organs
- ➢ a low proportion (Weiss suggests ≤25%) of clear (lipidised ZF-like) cells
- ➢ immuno +vity for MMP-2 favours malignancy (and worse prog. if >20% of cells are +ve)

- If a spindle/sarcomatoid component is prominent some diagnose *adrenocortical carcinosarcoma*
- Some diagnose 'adrenocortical tumour of uncertain malignant potential' if the above features are equivocal or sparse (e.g. only 2 or 3 features present)
- d/dg ACC *vs.* RCC *vs.* HCC is decided on CPC, EM and immuno (see table 19.1)
- d/dg phaeochromocytoma: ACC may have a few lipidised cells, an alveolar pattern and be +ve for NSE, synaptophysin and CD56 (± ↑ catecholamines clinically) but is −ve for CgA. Phaeochromocytoma may be +ve for ACTH and have some lipidised cells but is −ve for the D11 cortical Ab by immuno. ACC is further favoured by +vity for inhibin-α and Melan-A

TABLE 19.1 Immuno of adrenocortical *vs* conventional renal cell and hepatocellular carcinomas

Antibody	ACC	RCC	HCC
D11	+ve	−ve	−ve
Melan-A (A103)	+ve	−ve	−ve
inhibin-α	+ve (focal)	−ve	−ve
EMA	−ve	+ve	−ve (in ≈ 75%)
vimentin	±ve	+ve	usu.−ve
CK (AE1/3 or CAM 5.2)	−ve	+ve	±ve
α₁AT	−ve	±ve	±ve
AFP	−ve	−ve	±ve
pCEA	usu. −ve	−ve	+ve (canalicular)
CD10	−ve	+ve	+ve (canalicular)
Hep Par 1	−ve	−ve	+ve

Phaeochromocytoma (Adrenal Medullary Chromaffin Paraganglioma, Chromaffinoma)
- Macro: well-circ. (not encapsulated) and brown (hence 'phaeo') ± degenerative changes. Multiple, bilateral tumours occur as a continuum of the background multinodular medullary hyperplasia in MEN 2
- Arch.: zellballen/trabecular/solid with peripheral S100 (+/ GFAP) +ve sustentacular cells
- Cells: polygonal/spindle, granular eosinophilic cytoplasm (± focal lipidisation) with basophilic granules, NE nuclei and 'endocrine-type' atypia, ± intranuclear cytoplasmic inclusions, ± cytoplasmic DPAS +ve globules (the latter are also rarely seen in adrenocortical neoplasms)
- Mitoses are usu. sparse (≤1/20 hpf)
- Stroma: delicate rich vascularity, alveolar reticulin pattern, hyalinisation, (± amyloid in a minority)
- Immuno/stains: chromaffin +ve (diffuse and granular cytoplasmic browning), +ve for CgA and other NE markers ± various NE peptides (incl. ACTH, PP or VIP [→ WDHA]), CK −ve
- Variants: ① composite phaeochromocytoma is one with a neural tumour component (neuroblastoma, ganglioneuroblastoma, MPNST, *etc.*) ② pigmented phaeochromocytoma is black with melanin-like pigment granules in cells ③ extra-adrenal phaeochromocytoma (1° sites include bladder, peri-renal, coeliac axis, heart)
- Malignancy (= mets via blood or LN) risk factors: confluent necrosis, local invasion ++, ↑ prolifⁿ (≥ 3 mitoses/20 hpf) and lack of globules or sustentacular cells. [*Note:* no phaeo is definitely benign]
- d/dg: metastatic tumour, adrenocortical neoplasia (*vide supra*)
- d/dg nodular hyperplasia in MEN 2 (some use an arbitrary size threshold of >1cm ∅ = neoplastic)

Some Other Tumours
- Lipoma and Myelolipoma: mature adipose ± haemopoietic marrow may form a benign mass lesion or occur as 'heterologous' foci in adrenocortical tumours

- Malignant melanoma can arise as a 1° adrenal tumour (as well as mets)
- Metastases: esp. from lung or kidney, because these may be confused for 1° adrenal tumours

For neural tumours of the adrenal medulla (neuroblastoma, etc.), see p. 59

Pituitary

Normal Histology
- The anterior pituitary has a paraganglioid architecture with cell balls of trophs surrounded by S100 +ve folliculostellate cells. Occasional small thyroid-like follicles may form
- Reticulin is packeted
- Lateral wings are rich in somatotroph acidophils (! simulate the pure cell population of an adenoma)
- Transdifferentiation and single cells expressing >1 hormone occur (as do plurihormonal adenomas)
- The *pars intermedia* may show small columnar-lined clefts ± cystic change and squamous metaplasia (! d/dg craniopharyngioma or Rathke's cleft cyst)
- The border of anterior and posterior hypophysis is blurred (! the basophil trophs appear to invade it)
- Pituitary stalk axons have eosinophilic swellings (Herring bodies) ± granular cell islands (tumourlets)
- The neurohypophysis contains axons and altered spindly glial cells (pituicytes) ± salivary acini rests
- Normal upper limit of prolactin = 600 mIU/l in serum (25 ng/ml in plasma) for non-pregnant females and 450 mIU/l (20 ng/ml) in males; can be around 5000 mIU/l (210 ng/ml) near term in pregnancy tailing off with lactation

Stains and Interpretation of Staining Patterns
- H&E (PAS Orange G for acidophil/basophil/chromophobe is outdated, capricious and not useful)
- Retic: shows expanded packets in hyperplasia and is typically weak/absent (vascular only) in neoplasia
- Immuno: ➤ 1° panel: CK, PRL, GH, ACTH, α-subunit (of the glycoprotein hormones)
  - ➤ 2° panel if α-subunit is +ve: β-subunits (of TSH, FSH and LH)
  - ➤ SF-1 (nuclear stain: +ve in gonadotroph adenomas incl. silent ones)
  - ➤ Pit-1 (nuclear stain: +ve in somatotroph, lactotroph and thyrotroph adenomas)
  - ➤ hCG (for craniopharyngioma)
  - ➤ GFAP (for granular cell tumour and gliomas)
- Problems with immuno interpretation can occur due to:
  - ➤ trapped normal cells (! do not misdiagnose as a plurihormonal adenoma)
  - ➤ overstaining by ACTH (high background – d/dg adenoma) and the normal grouping of ACTH +ve cells (d/dg hyperplasia)
  - ➤ pure populations of GH cells (in the lateral wings of the pituitary) simulating adenoma
  - ➤ cross-reactivity between FSH and LH β-subunits
  - ➤ secretory exhaustion: patients with ↑↑serum hormone levels may show −ve immuno because little hormone is left in the cells (but ISH for hormone mRNA should be +ve)
  - ➤ over-interpretation of PRL due to PRL cell hyperplasia and Hx of hyperprolactinaemia that may be due to pituitary stalk compression from any tumour/lesion.
- ∴ Use the pattern of hormone staining (see Figure 19.1) and H&E, retic and CPC:

Non-Neoplastic Conditions
- Radiation-induced changes
- Hypophysitis: lymphocytic (usu. autoimmune), CMV and granulomatous (incl. sarcoid)
- Infarction/apoplexy (haemorrhagic necrosis) post pregnancy (Sheehan) or within a tumour (is one cause of the empty sella syndrome; hydrocephalic pressure-induced pituitary atrophy being another)

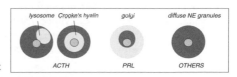

FIGURE 19.1   Immuno of some pituitary hormones

Pituitary Adenomas and Carcinoma

Nomenclature
- Aggressive adenoma = invasive adenoma: adenoma with local invasion
- Carcinoma requires distant mets to the leptomeninges, spinal cord, vertebrae, liver, etc., is very rare and is usu. +ve for PRL, ACTH or GH. They may over-express p53 (unlike non-atypical adenomas)
- Atypical adenoma: adenomas with ↑ proliferation (e.g. Ki-67 LI >4%) – not universally accepted
- Microadenoma: adenoma <10mm in maximum dimension (macroadenoma ≥ 10mm) by radiology

- Plurihormonal adenoma: the same cells (or separate neoplastic populations) express >1 hormone. There is no minimum % criteria as long as all populations are neoplastic (not entrapped cells)
- Silent adenoma: does not produce hormonal effects but may contain hormone products by immuno
- Null cell adenoma: a silent adenoma which is not immunoreactive for hormonal peptides and lacks EM features of specific trophs

Grading
- This is actually a form of radiological staging and not performed by the pathologist
  1. non-invasive microadenoma confined below the sella diaphragm
  2. non-invasive microadenoma all or partly above the sella diaphragm
  3. invasion of (but confined to) the bony *sella turcica*
  4. invasion of other local structures

General histology
- The acinar pattern of reticulin is diminished or lost (but retic is retained around the blood vessels)
- Arch.: large irregular cell nests, trabeculae, solid, papillary and rosette formations may all occur
- Cells are usu. larger than normal (but may be smaller) ± variable pleomorphism/hyperchromasia, mitoses may be abundant – none of these features are predictive of malignancy
- Tumour necrosis (d/dg apoplexy which may also occur) is a bad sign but does not imply malignancy
- Bromocriptine Rx → fibrosis, small cell size ± haemorrhage; somatostatin Rx → fibrosis

Subtypes
- Corticotroph (ACTH): Tumour cells are typically PAS +ve even when not basophilic. Functioning adenomas cause Crooke's hyalin (perinuclear CK, CAM5.2 +ve) to deposit in surrounding *non-neoplastic* ACTH cells (takes 6 months of hypercortisolaemia to develop and upto 1 year to clear) – if absent consider hyperplasia (*cf.* adenoma) or silent corticotroph adenoma (which is more likely to be aggressive). Crooke's adenoma is a rare variant where the tumour cells have Crooke's hyalin
- Somatotroph (GH)/Mammosomatotroph (GH + PRL): Pit-1 +ve. Rarely β-TSH +ve. Paranuclear rounded CAM5.2 +ve blobs (= eosinophilic 'fibrous bodies' which may indent the nucleus) are said to be pathognomonic. ***Sparsely granulated forms*** have chromophobic cells with weak/−ve GH staining (± Golgi pattern) and well-formed fibrous bodies. ***Densely granulated forms*** have eosinophilic cells, dense diffuse cytoplasmic GH staining ± weak perinuclear CK ± α-subunit +vity.
- Lactotroph/Mammotroph (PRL): Pit-1 +ve. May show psammoma bodies or amyloid. Sparsely granulated: chromophobes with paranuclear PRL staining only. Densely granulated: eosinophilic cells with diffuse cytoplasmic PRL. Always exclude 2° ↑ PRL due to hypophysitis/other tumour
- Gonadotroph (LH/FSH): solid nests with peripheral palisades of polarised cells; nuclear SF-1 +ve
- Rarer adenomas (all Pit-1 +ve): Thyrotroph; Acidophil stem cell (oncocytes, PRL, GH, fibrous bodies); Silent subtype 3 (fibrosis, vascularity, plurihormonal: GH, β-TSH, PRL, etc., local bone invasion, EM helps)
- Oncocytoma: null-type, +ve for PTAH and synaptophysin, −ve for DPAS, CD68, S100 and GFAP; d/dg granular cell tumour (shows the opposite staining reactions) or acidophil stem cell adenoma

Differential diagnoses
- Hyperplasia is reticulin +ve (expanded packets) and has a mixed (albeit skewed) cell population
- Metastatic carcinoma
- Craniopharyngioma and Rathke's cleft cysts (see p. 184)
- Granular cell tumour (see oncocytoma in list above) – also d/dg HX or (normal) granular cell tumourlets
- Normal anatomical/physiological variants and artefacts of staining (*vide supra*)
- Mixed adenoma with gangliocytoma (of the neurohypophysis) – very rare

Other Tumours
- Pituicytoma: astrocytoma of the neurohypophysis with elongated cells and fasciculation: GFAP +ve
- Meningioma and rare local tumours: germ cell tumours, chordoma, etc.
- Metastatic carcinoma, granular cell tumour, HX and Rathke's pouch lesions are discussed above

Frozen Section / Per-Operative Assessment
- FS is best avoided (the small amount of tissue can be damaged by freezing) – use imprint cytology
- Decide if it is pituitary tissue: adenomas show a monomorphous population of small cells ± 2° structures (papillae, psammoma bodies, etc.) but it may not be possible (or necessary) to make this diagnosis at this time

- Exclude metastatic carcinoma/granular cell tumour and consider a glial, meningeal or neural lesion (! remember the normal neurohypophysis)/hypophysitis ± granulomas/Rathke's pouch/cleft lesions

Carcinoid Tumours

- See other chapters (e.g. pp. 93–94, pp. 139–140, p. 152 and pp. 252–253) for definitions of special types of carcinoid. For endocrine pancreas, see pp. 178–179.
- Grading :
  1. ≈ usual-type carcinoid
     a. small nests/trabeculae, palisaded round cells, uniform nuclei with ≈ absent nucleoli and no mitoses
     b. significant solid areas, non-aligned cells ± spindle forms, anisonucleosis, visible nucleoli and mitoses sparse but normal
  2. ≈ atypical carcinoid ⎫ See pp. 93–94 and pp. 139–140.
  3. ≈ malignant carcinoid ⎬ *NB*: avoid the term 'malignant carcinoid' ⎭ because all grades may be malignant
- Features correlated with aggressive behaviour in general (specific tumours may have other features):
  ➢ higher grade (incl. nuclear grade e.g. prominent nucleoli) and local invasiveness
  ➢ large size
  ➢ coagulative tumour cell necrosis
  ➢ vascular invasion
  ➢ ↑ proliferation (mitotic count and Ki-67 LI)

Paraganglioma

- Arch.: zellballen (+ / trabeculae in abdominal ones) surrounded by retic (but individual cells are not)
- The cell balls are surrounded by fine capillaries ± stromal haemorrhage/hyaline
- Cells have moderate cytoplasm (± eosinophilic globules in abdominal paragangliomas)
- Nuclei may show eosinophilic pseudoinclusions, 'endocrine-type' atypia and more irregular/vesicular chromatin ± distinct nucleoli (*cf.* d/dg carcinoids)
- Abdominal paragangliomas may look like phaeochromocytoma (p. 276)
- Gangliocytic paraganglioma: see p. 179
- Chemodectomas are paragangliomas of carotid, aortic, Zukerkandl and jugulotympanic bodies
- Immuno: CgA (± other NE Ags) +ve, CK and αSMA −ve, sustentacular cell +vity for S100 or GFAP
- Malignancy: ? few/no sustentacular cells, ? mets/vasc. invas[n], ? necrosis/mitoses: none are definite
- d/dg MTC, myxopapillary ependymoma, paraganglioid carcinoid, PLAT, melanoma, laryngeal NEC: presence of sustentacular cells and absence of CK favour paraganglioma
- d/dg glomus tumour[7]: αSMA −ve, CgA +ve, sustentacular cell +ve, rich stromal *micro*vasculature and lack of pericellular reticulin all favour paraganglioma
- d/dg *glomus coccygeum*: this is a normal structure (see p. 286 under the d/dg of 'Glomus Tumour')

Familial/Multiple Endocrine Pathology Syndromes

Multiple Endocrine Adenopathy/Neoplasia (MEA/MEN)
- Most are AD but some (esp. MEN 2b) arise as spontaneous mutations with no FHx
- MEN 1: (Wermer, all the 'P's) – parathyroid, pancreaticoduodenal (PP, ZE, etc.), pituitary (PRL, etc.), ± adrenocortical proliferations
- MEN 2: MTC and phaeochromocytoma and
  a) parathyroid (Sipple)
  b) mucosal neuromas and GIT ganglioneuromas (MTC is aggressive; also called MEN 3)

---

[7] *NB*: some normal paraganglia are termed glomi (e.g. *glomus jugulare, glomus caroticum*, etc.) and their cells are called glomus type 1 (= chief) and 2 (= sustentacular) cells. This has resulted in some of their paragangliomas also bearing the term 'glomus' e.g. 'glomus jugulare tumour'. All this can cause terminological confusion with true glomus tumours (which are not paragangliomas) – see p. 285

Familial MTC
- Does not have the other features of MEN

Carney Complex / Syndrome
- Myxomas (skin and heart)
- Lentigines (skin)
- Melanotic Schwannomas
- Adrenal, pituitary and thyroid neoplasms and Sertoli cell tumours

> Not to be confused with Carncy *triad*:
> ① epithelioid GIST
> ② pulmonary chondroma
> ③ non-adrenal paraganglioma

Bibliography

Al-Brahim, N.Y.Y. and Asa, S.L. (2006) My approach to the pathology of the pituitary. *Journal of Clinical Pathology*, **59** (12), 1245–1253.

Andersen, C.E. and McLaren, K. (2003) Best practice in thyroid pathology. *Journal of Clinical Pathology*, **56** (6), 401–405.

Asa, S.L., Puy, L.A., Lew, A.M. *et al.* (1993) Cell type-specific expression of the pituitary transcription activator Pit-1 in the human pituitary and pituitary adenomas. *Journal of Clinical Endocrinology and Metabolism*, **77** (5), 1275–1280.

Baloch, Z.W. and LiVolsi, V.A. (2007) Our approach to follicular-patterned lesions of the thyroid. *Journal of Clinical Pathology*, **60** (3), 244–250.

Baloch, Z.W. and LiVolsi, V.A. (2000) Newly described tumours of the thyroid. *Current Diagnostic Pathology*, **6** (3), 151–164.

Bishop, P.W. (2002) An immunohistochemical vade mecum. *Current Diagnostic Pathology* **8** (2), 123–127. Available online at: http://www.e-immunohistochemistry.info (accessed March 2007).

Biswas, S. and Rodeck, C.H. (1976) Plasma prolactin levels during pregnancy. *British Journal of Obstetrics and Gynaecology*, **83** (9), 683–687.

Damiani, S., Fratamico, F., Lapertosa, G. *et al.* (1991) Alcian blue and epithelial membrane antigen are useful markers in differentiating benign from malignant papillae in thyroid lesions. *Virchows Archiv A Pathological Anatomy and Histopathology*, **419** (2), 131–135.

Chau, P. and Chan, J.K.C. (2003) Fine-needle-aspiration-induced histologic changes. *Current Diagnostic Pathology*, **9** (2), 77–147.

Gaffey, M.J., Traweek, S.T., Mills, S.E. *et al.* (1992) Cytokeratin expression in adrenocortical neoplasia: an immunohistochemical and biochemical study with implications for the differential diagnosis of adrenocortical, hepatocellular, and renal cell carcinoma. *Human Pathology*, **23** (2), 144–153.

Hough, A.J., Hollifield, J.W., Page, D.L. *et al.* (1979) Prognostic factors in adrenocortical tumours. *American Journal of Clinical Pathology*, **72** (3), 390–399.

Johnson, S.J., Sheffield, E.A. and McNicol, A.M. (2005) Examination of parathyroid gland specimens. *Journal of Clinical Pathology*, **58** (4), 338–342.

LiVolsi, V.A. and DeLellis, R.A. (1993) *Pathology of the Parathyroid and Thyroid Glands*, 1st edn, Williams & Wilkins, Baltimore.

Matias-Guiu, X. (1999) Mixed medullary and follicular carcinoma of the thyroid gland. *American Journal of Pathology*, **155** (5), 1413–1418.

McNicol, A.M. (2003) Criteria for diagnosis of follicular thyroid neoplasms and related conditions, in *Recent Advances in Histopathology*, Vol. 20 (eds D. Lowe and J.C.E Underwood), Royal Society of Medicine Press Ltd, London.

McNicol, A.M. (2001) Disorders of the anterior lobe of the pituitary, in *Recent Advances in Histopathology*, Vol. 19 (eds D. Lowe and J.C.E Underwood), Churchill Livingstone, Edinburgh.

McNicol, A.M. (2000) Diseases of the adrenal cortex. *Current Diagnostic Pathology*, **6** (3), 171–180.

Ng, W-K. (2003) Radiation-associated changes in tissues and tumours. *Current Diagnostic Pathology*, **9** (2), 124–136.

Rindi, G., Azzoni, C., La Rosa, S. *et al.* (1999) ECL cell tumor and poorly differentiated endocrine carcinoma of the stomach: prognostic evaluation by pathological analysis. *Gastroenterology*, **116** (3), 532–542.

Silva, E.G. and Balfour Kraemer, B. (1987) *Intraoperative Pathologic Diagnosis. Frozen section and other techniques*, 1st edn, Williams & Wilkins, Baltimore.

Sobrinho-Simões, M. and Fonseca, E. (1994) Recently described tumours of the thyroid, in *Recent Advances in Histopathology*, Vol. 16 (eds P.P. Anthony, R.N.M MacSween and D.G. Lowe), Churchill Livingstone, Edinburgh, pp. 213–229.

Sobrinho-Simões, M., Magalhães, I., Fonseca, E. *et al.* (2005) Diagnostic pitfalls in thyroid pathology. *Current Diagnostic Pathology*, **11** (1), 52–59.

Stephenson, T.J. (1997) Criteria for malignancy in endocrine tumours, in *Recent Advances in Histopathology*, Vol. 17 (eds P.P. Anthony, R.N.M MacSween and D.G. Lowe DG), Churchill Livingstone, Edinburgh, pp. 93–111.

Sternberg, S.S. (ed) (1997) *Histology for Pathologists*, 2nd edn, Lippincott Williams & Wilkins, Philadelphia.

Symmers, W. St. C. (ed) (1978) *Systemic Pathology*, Vol. 4, 2nd edn, Churchill Livingstone, London.

Weiss, L.M. (1984) Comparative histologic study of 43 metastasizing and nonmetastasizing adrenocortical tumours. *American Journal of Surgical Pathology*, **8** (3), 163–169.

Web site

RCPath, Standards and Datasets for Reporting Cancers. www.rcpath.org.uk (accessed July 2006).

20. Skin

Normal

- Possesses adnexal structures (unlike squamous mucosae[1]) and structure varies with site
- Epidermis: contains many S100 +ve basal melanocytes, many CD1a +ve Langerhans dendritic cells scattered throughout and a few CD20 +ve suprabasal Merkel cells. Toker cells (CK7 +ve) are present in the nipple epidermis and should not be mis-diagnosed as Paget's disease. The *stratum corneum* is thickest in thick skin (palms and soles) where it may display a lower *stratum lucidum*
- Dermis: the superficial *papillary dermis* is loose (areolar) connective tissue with vertical components constituting the dermal papillae and investments extending down the adnexa as *adventitial dermis*. It contains the superficial vascular plexus in its deepest part. The *reticular dermis* is less cellular dense collagenous tissue with thick collagen bundles parallel to the skin surface and contains the deep capillary plexus in its deepest part. Elastic fibres are normally present throughout and ↑with age
- Mast cells are more numerous in distal (glove and stocking) sites than proximal and have been measured in adults at 108/mm^2 distally and 77/mm^2 proximally (≈ 21/hpf and 15/hpf respectively) and there is an overlap in counts between normals and patients with mastocytosis
- Glabrous skin occurs near the transition to the mucosae of internal tracts (e.g. labia minora, penile shaft and outer layer of foreskin, perianal region, nipples, eyelids and lips) and is recognised by the presence of sebaceous glands that secrete directly onto the epidermis (rather than into hair shafts)
- For normal hair histology see the section on 'Hair and Alopecia', p. 295

Painful Lumps in the Skin / Subcutis

- **Traumatic neuroma**
- **Eccrine spiradenoma**
- **Angiolipoma** (if multiple and symmetrical consider Dercum's *adiposis dolorosa*)
- **Blue rubber bleb naevus** (a syndromic vascular naevus)
- **Angioleiomyoma**
- **Glomus tumour**
- **Schwannoma** (incl. granular cell tumour)
- **Pilomatrixoma**
- **Endometriosis**
- **Neurofibroma**
- **Dermatofibroma**

> Traditionally, this group is composed of lumps that are associated with spontaneous pain – even if sporadic – not just tenderness.

Lesions Affecting the Palms / Soles

- Dishidrotic eczema (pompholyx): tense intraepidermal bullae, spongiosis, mild inflammation
- Friction / heat blister: intraepidermal clear fluid bullae without inflammation
- Volar psoriasis
- 2° syphilis
- *Erythema multiforme* (bullous form may show the Nikolsky sign i.e. the blister can be shifted)
- *Keratoderma blenorrhagicum* (psoriasis-like pustular histology)
- *Epidermolysis keratosis palmaris et plantaris*
- Scabies / dermatophytes
- Arsenic / tar keratosis (looks like a flat SK – it is not usually dysplastic)
- Tumours: eccrine poroma (! not BCC), acral melanocytic naevi / melanoma, verrucae, etc.

---

[1] with the exception of sebaceous lobules in some mucosae e.g. Fordyce spots in the cheeks, lips and tongue (not to be confused with angiokeratoma of Fordyce or Fox-Fordyce disease)

Diagnostic Criteria Handbook in Histopathology: A Surgical Pathology Vade Mecum by Paul J. Tadrous
Copyright © 2007 by John Wiley & Sons, Ltd.

Epidermal Lesions (Squamous and Basal Cell)

Pseudoepitheliomatous Hyperplasia (PEH)
- Shows maturation from basaloid to squamous cells (unlike most invasive SCC)
- Occurs: ➤ at the edge of chronic ulcers
  - ➤ with extramammary Paget's disease
  - ➤ with granular cell tumours
  - ➤ with T-cell lymphomas (d/dg lymphoepithelial carcinoma in the nasopharynx)
  - ➤ in the wall of thymic cysts

The Borst-Jadassohn Phenomenon
- Clonal BCP
- Clonal Bowen's
- Hidroacanthoma simplex, eccrine poroma
- Epidermodysplasia verruciformis
- d/dg metastasis (e.g. of bronchial SmCC to the skin[2])

Epidermolysis
- Seen in viral warts, congenital ichthyoses, linear epidermal naevus, BCP, epidermolytic acanthoma, at the edge of SCC and in other lesions (! do not confuse with acantholysis)
- Epidermal perinuclear halos, hypergranulosis and large granules

Epidermal Cyst (and related entities)
- Epidermal cyst = ① retention cyst of pilosebaceous infundibulum or ② epidermal implantation cyst
- No rete ridges or dermal papillae in retention type (else consider d/dg dermoid / implantation / pigmented hair cyst)
- If partly trichilemmal keratinisation = infundibular cyst; if all trichilemmal = trichilemmal cyst
- If retention-type and <1mm ∅ = milium (d/dg miliarium [clin. 'prickly heat' / 'sweat rash'] = inflammatory retention cyst of sweat duct). Do not confuse any of these with colloid milium (p. 300).
- If multiple on scalp and face consider Gardner's syndrome
- d/dg epidermoid cyst (dermoid): these don't just have a proper epidermis-like lining (as epidermal cysts must have) but also a proper dermis-like investment (rete, adnexa, etc.). A traumatic epidermal implantation cyst may have rete (= implantation dermoid)
- d/dg see sections on 'Vellus hair cyst' (p. 295) and 'Dilated pore of Winer' (p. 292)

Acanthoma
- The term cannot be used unqualified (otherwise consider d/dg *prurigo nodularis*)
- Types: clear cell, large cell, epidermolytic and the following:
- Pilar sheath acanthoma: keratin-filled endophytic basaloid proliferation replaces hair follicle
- Warty dyskeratoma (solitary KF): endophytic and crateriform with acantholysis, dyskeratosis and laminated keratin. The base shows dermal villi / papillae lined by a single layer of basal cells
- Keratoacanthoma: histologically indistinguishable from well-diff SCC

Seborrhoeic Keratosis (SK, Basal Cell Papilloma)
- A hyperkeratotic, exophytic, papillomatous growth with a mixture of squamous and basaloid cells
- Typically show a 'stuck on' exophytic appearance when the slide is viewed without magnification
- In *acanthotic SK* the basaloid cells predominate, in others (e.g. *hyperkeratotic SK*) the squamous cells do
- Horn cysts are usu. orthokeratotic (but mixed and parakeratotic forms occur[3])
- Basaloid cells in solid, reticulated ('*adenoid SK*') or Borst-Jadassohn ('*clonal SK*') configurations

Flat SK (incl. the clinical lesions called 'stucco keratosis')
- Papillomatosis and 'church spire' hyperkeratosis. Squamous cells usu. outnumber basaloid ones
- d/dg linear epidermal naevus, flat viral wart and acrokeratosis verruciformis of Hopf – only clinical features can distinguish between these

---

[2] unlike 1° NEC of the skin (Merkel cell) which *usually* spares the epidermis with a Grenz zone
[3] pure parakeratotic forms are known as 'squamous pearls' and are most commonly seen in SCC

Pigmented SK
- Pigmented basaloid keratinocytes

Melanotic SK (Melanoacanthoma)
- Intermingled pigmented dendritic melanocytes ++, non-pigmented basaloid keratinocytes
- Horn cysts are few / absent

Irritated SK
- SK with a host response and squamous eddies[4] ± regression / acantholysis

Inverted follicular keratosis
- Endophytic ± exophytic component
- Bulbous downgrowths, squamous eddies ++, mitoses ++
- Stromal inflammation
- d/dg keratoacanthoma, BCC (but the typical BCC stroma is absent), viral wart

Plantar Wart (Verruca Plantaris, Myrmecia Wart)
- HPV 1, sole/palms/ungual, painful (unless *mosaic* type i.e. multiple ≈ confluent warts)
- Childhood form resolves (months), adult becomes chronic ± progression to verrucous carcinoma
- Arch.: crateriform parakeratotic plug and myrmecial downgrowths ± cysts lined by warty epithelium
- No exophytic component (but the keratin may rise above the surface)
- Prominent koilocytosis
- Active growth phase: large eosinophil and basophil keratohyaline granules and eosinophilic intranuclear inclusions (d/dg molluscum contagiosum inclusions)

Plane Wart (Verruca Plana)
- HPV 2 / 5, women and children, face/shin/dorsum, Köbner phenomenon (i.e. occurs at sites of trauma)
- Not much papillomatosis – and parakeratosis is not a feature
- Koilocytosis and basket-weave hyperkeratosis
- Dyskeratosis, perivascular chronic inflammation ± RBC extravasation

Epidermodysplasia Verruciformis (EV)
- HPV 5 / 8, familial (rare and pre-malignant), sporadic (HIV-assoc[d] EV-like lesions – multiple)
- Like a large cell acanthoma but with cytological atypia and prominent keratohyaline granules
- Large cells are clearer and may form suprabasal Borst-Jadassohn-like nests

Clear Cell Acanthoma (of Degos)
- Raised moist red lesion on (usu.) legs of older adults
- Exophytic smooth proliferation of pale (not large) keratinocytes (glycogen ++, melanin −ve)
- Intermingled occ. intraepidermal PMN
- Well-demarcated from normal epidermis and adnexal structures spared
- d/dg large cell acanthoma (*vide infra*) and hidroacanthoma simplex (p. 292)

Actinic Keratosis (AK)
- Sun-exposed skin
- Dermis: solar elastosis of collagen ± telangiectasia and inflammation
- Basal epidermal dysplasia with adnexal sparing (→ alternating ortho and parakeratosis)

Large cell acanthoma
- Epidermal plaque with (polyploid) cells 2× normal size, normal NCR and basket-weave orthokeratin
- Rete pegs broader / flatter / absent
- d/dg EV / EV-like lesions / verruca plana} but these all have warty changes of the granular layer

Bowenoid actinic keratosis (*vs.* Bowen's disease)
- Clinical features and distribution help in making the distinction
- Bowen's disease involves the adnexal structures (Bowenoid AK does not)
- Bowenoid AK dysplasia may not be uniformly full-thickness (! but true Bowen's may not be full-thickness at its periphery)

---

[4] unlike horn cysts or pearls, eddies are non-keratinising (not even parakeratinising)

Naevus Sebaceus of Jadassohn (incl. Organoid Naevus)
- Present from birth, usu. on head (± local trauma); epidermal and sebaceous features ↑ with age
- ↓ Nõ of terminal hair follicles in subcutis (abortive hair microcysts may be seen)
- Epidermal hyperplasia: verrucous (= organoid naevus, d/dg linear epidermal naevus) or trichoblastic basaloid proliferations (d/dg BCC)
- Variably ↑nõ of sebaceous lobules (may show cystic spaces and may directly connect to epidermis)
- ± Other adnexal elements: apocrine / eccrine glands, smooth muscle straps, etc.
- ± Neoplasia e.g. syringocystadenoma papilliferum, BCC (true BCC is uncommon *cf.* d/dg trichoblastic basaloid proliferations)

Basal Cell Carcinoma (BCC)
- Has characteristic stroma (with amyloid in 50%): myxoid, desmoplastic or keloidal
- Metastatic risk ∝ size, depth of invasion and PMHx of RadioRx or immunosuppression
- May be surrounded by AK change ∴ do levels if this is all you see on a punch Bx for '?BCC'
- Immuno of basaloid cells: +ve for Bcl-2 ($\approx$ all cells), CD10, Ki-67 (>20%); −ve for CD34, CK20, CK15, Ber-EP4 is at least focally +ve (*cf.* −ve in pure SCC)
- Immuno of stroma: +ve for stromelysin 3, −ve for CD34
- d/dg: eccrine poroma (esp. on palms/soles – where true BCC almost never occurs)
- d/dg trichoepithelioma or its sclerosing variant (= sclerosing epithelial hamartoma, esp. if in children)
- d/dg basaloid proliferations (above DF, fibrous papule, myxomas or naevus sebaceus of Jadassohn – ! but true BCC may co-occur with these): lack infiltrative arch., are restricted to stimulus lesion, may contain CK20 +ve Merkel cells; mitoses and p53 +ve cells are rare
- d/dg sebaceous tumours *vs.* clear cell BCC
- d/dg AdCC or eccrine tumours *vs.* adenoid BCC
- d/dg basaloid follicular hamartoma has altered stroma but lacks mitoses, apoptoses and retraction clefts

Variants
- Fibroepithelioma of Pinkus (slender reticulate strands) d/dg eccrine syringofibroadenoma / adenoid SK
- Adenoid (acid mucin, mucin not seen within the cells and the cells don't show secretory morphology)
- Metatypical: BCC merges into squamoid / spindled morphology ± squamous pearls but no well-demarcated foci of typical SCC (otherwise = basisquamous carcinoma, esp. if unusually infiltrative)
- Superficial 'multicentric' and morphoeic types (↑ risk of local recurrence, d/dg desmoplastic trichoepithelioma)
- BCC with trichilemmal differentiation (incl. keratin whorls/plugs without other squamoid features)
- Others: micronodular, cystic (± haemorrhage or acid mucin), signet ring, myoepithelial, pigmented (= melanin), clear cell (and true sebaceous differentiation), BCC with monster cells (no prog. implication), etc.

Squamous Cell Carcinoma (SCC)
- Def^{n}: a tumour of squamous differentiation with invasion

SCC variants
- Rhabdoid SCC, acantholytic SCC (*vide infra*), verrucous SCC (*vide infra*)
- Spindle cell SCC (previous trauma/radioRx, CK and vimentin +ve, desmosomes on EM)
- Papillary SCC: an exophytic pedunculated papilloma with obvious cytological atypia and mitoses in the squamotransitional lining (± superficial clear cell change); keratin pearls and frank invasion may be absent. d/dg verrucous Bowen's is not an exophytic papilloma
- Keratoacanthoma-like SCC (some pathologists do not believe keratoacanthoma can be diagnosed morphologically, so when the morphological features of a keratoacanthoma are seen the lesion is diagnosed as 'a well diff keratoacanthoma-like SCC' with a statement about excision).

Grading SCC
- Broders' Grade:

I	>75% differentiated	≡ 'well differentiated'	The amount of 'differentiation' in
II	25–75% diff	≡ 'moderately diff'	this grading system is, by convention,
III	<25% diff	≡ 'poorly diff'	taken to mean the amount of
IV	no differentiation	≡ 'undifferentiated'	keratinisation.

- Some dermatopathologists prefer a 'grading' based on the depth of invasion:
  - ➤ high grade: invades beyond the level of the eccrine glands
  - ➤ low grade: does not invade beyond the level of the eccrine glands

Differential diagnoses
- Pseudoepitheliomatous hyperplasia: SCC is characterised by abrupt maturation (keratinisation) i.e. without the progressive maturation from a basal layer that is typical of PEH
- Inverted follicular keratosis (irritated BCP with squamous eddies)
- Metatypical BCC
- Melanoma (spindle type)
- Proliferating pilar tumour is circumscribed, has trichilemmal keratinisation, a basal layer, hyaline basement membrane, rare mitoses and mild or absent atypia ± a simple pilar cyst component

Acantholytic SCC (Carcinoma Segregans)
- Esp. head and neck or recurrent SCC after radioRx
- Pseudoglandular spaces (d/dg ASC / MEC – but SCC has hyaluronic acid not neutral mucin)
- Hypertrophied and acantholytic sweat ducts
- Pseudoangiosarcomatous pattern – d/dg.
  - ➤ not multifocal
  - ➤ focally there is better SCC differentiated areas
  - ➤ attachment to epidermis
  - ➤ EM shows desmosomes not Weibel-Palade bodies

Verrucous Carcinoma
- Sole (cuniculatum), genitoperineal (Bushke-Lowenstein), mouth (florid papilloma): mid-aged men
- Complications: sinuses and bony destruction; mets are rare
- Arise within a viral wart
- Exophytic component: hyperkeratotic papillary ± parakeratosis
- Endophytic component:
  - ➤ deep bulbous keratinised processes (often beyond eccrine glands and into subcutis)
  - ➤ keratin and necrosis → sinuses
  - ➤ intercellular bridges and glassy cytoplasm
  - ➤ intraepithelial abscesses
  - ➤ dense peritumoural chronic inflammation
- d/dg
  - ➤ viral wart: if superficial / fragmented can't distinguish ∴ repeat with deeper biopsy
  - ➤ keratoacanthoma: history (smooth hemispherical papule) and depth (not beyond eccrine)
  - ➤ conventional SCC: ☞ if any foci of cytological malignancy, it is not verrucous carcinoma
  - ☞ if there are filiform projections at the base, it is not verrucous carcinoma

Soft Tissue and Histiocytic Lesions

Angiokeratoma Circumscriptum
- Solitary: an isolated occurrence
- Multiple: fingers (angiokeratoma of Mibelli), scrotum (of Fordyce), widespread (Fabry disease)
- Papillary dermis: blood capillary ectasia surrounded by and closely applied to the rete peg basal layer
- Superficially: acanthosis and hyperkeratosis; deeper: no deep component
- d/dg: verrucous haemangioma (has a deep component); lymphangioma circumscriptum (no blood)

Myofibromatous Lesions
- These include: dermatomyofibroma, adult myofibroma and myofibromatosis

Glomus Tumours
- Tumours of thermoregulatory 'myoid' vascular wall cells; any body site (but painful if superficial)
- There are 3 components: ① glomus cells, ② smooth muscle and ③ angiomatoid vessels
- Glomus cells: monotonous, round, pale cytoplasm (PAS-enhancing rim +ve for pericellular reticulin and collagen IV) with central round nuclei; stroma may be hyaline ± myxoid with many nerve twigs
- Variant: solid – glomus cells predominate in a nested / organoid pattern
- Variant: glomangioma (angiomatoid vessels with a peripheral 'lining' or islands of glomus cells)
- Variant: glomangiomyoma – components ② and ③ are prominent
- Variant: infiltrating glomus tumour – has ↑ risk of local recurrence
- Malignancy (glomangiosarcoma): mitoses and ↑cellularity and cytol. atypia / frankly sarcomatous areas

- Immuno (glomus cells): +ve for αSMA, MSA, ± desmin; −ve for CK, S100, CgA, calretinin, inhibin
- d/dg: haemangioma, AVM, HPC, naevus, acrospiroma, carcinoid, paraganglioma (p. 279)
- d/dg myopericytoma / glomangiopericytoma / myofibromatosis: features in between glomus and HPC
- d/dg *glomus coccygeum*: this is a normal macroscopic structure (several mm ⌀) just anterior to the tip of the coccyx and may have satellite foci. Knowledge of its existence and CPC avoid misdiagnosis

Fibrous Papule of the Face (Nose)

- ① dilated blood vessels, ② fibrosis and ③ large fibroblasts
- May have an overlying basaloid epidermal proliferation (! not d/dg BCC)

Infantile Digital Fibromatosis

- Low power: non-specific mass of proliferating cellular fibrous tissue
- High power: eosinophilic globules in the cytoplasm of the plump spindle myofibroblast cells
- Eosinophilic globules are also seen in the stromal cells of fibroepithelial tumour of the breast

Histiocytoses

CLASS I histiocytoses: Langerhans cell / histiocytosis X (HX)
See pp. 57–58.
CLASS II Histiocytoses: non-Langerhans / indeterminate cell and macrophage
- Xanthogranuloma (Juvenile / Adult) (see p. 325):
  - contains a mixture of histiocytes from the whole spectrum of the Zelger morphological sub-types: vacuolated, xanthematised, scalloped, oncocytic and spindled
  - xanthematised (Touton) giant cells are classic but other type occur
  - has admixed chronic inflam[y] cells (may have eos. ++ → d/dg HX but in xanthogranuloma histiocytes are S100 −ve, CD1a −ve, CD68 strongly +ve)
  - spindle cell variant (esp. in juvenile) → d/dg fibroblastic soft tissue lesions
  - d/dg dermatofibroma: storiform areas, haemosiderin, sparse foci of lipidisation, epidermal changes, prominent vasculature and stromal monster giant cells favour DF, also CPC
- Reticulohistiocytoma (FXIIIa +ve)
- Multicentric reticulohistiocytosis (FXIIIa −ve)
- Xanthomas / xanthelasmas
- *Xanthoma disseminatum*: d/dg HX, but xanthoma disseminatum has:
  - good prognosis (unless respiratory tract involved)
  - *giant cells* are common
  - scattered eosinophils
  - spindle and scalloped multinucleate histiocytes which are S100 −ve, CD1a −ve, FXIIIa +ve and CD68 very strongly +ve (*cf.* only weak staining in HX)
- Rosai-Dorfman disease
- Other rare conditions (e.g. Erdheim-Chester disease, benign cephalic histiocytosis, etc.)
- d/dg reactive histiocytic lesions:
  - epithelioid / foreign-body histiocyte reactions
  - necrobiosis-associated granulomas (e.g. GA, rheumatoid nodules, necrobiosis lipoidica)
  - necrotic / necrobiotic xanthogranuloma (assoc[d] with haematological disease)
  - haemophagocytic syndrome-associated infiltrates
CLASS III histiocytoses: malignant histiocytoses
- Rare, CD68 +ve, exclude other tumours / lymphomas: refer to specialist texts

DF, DFSP, Kaposi sarcoma, Desmoids, Juvenile Xanthogranuloma, Atypical Fibroxanthoma (AFX), Vascular and Other Soft Tissue Lesions
See Chapter 21: Soft Tissues.

Melanocytic Lesions

Pagetoid Melanocytosis (PM)
- Malignant melanoma
- Spitz / Reed naevus
- Naevi of: palms, soles, vulva, genital skin, infants
- Recurrent / traumatised naevus ('pseudomelanoma')

- If present in dysplastic naevus, it is limited to the lower half of the epidermis
- No benign lesion has lateral extension of the PM
- No benign lesion has cytological atypia of the Pagetoid cells (! unless recent UV exposure)
- PM is not seen in ordinary naevi
- d/dg epithelial (true Paget's, Bowen's, Pagetoid AK, 2° CA, adnexal CA) or lymphohistiocytic cells

Mitoses in Benign Melanocytic Lesions
- If you find one, search for others
- An isolated normal mitotic figure may occur in:
  - ➤ any benign naevus if of normal form and there are no other atypical features
  - ➤ recurrent / traumatised naevus
  - ➤ the clonal component of a clonal naevus

Regression in a Melanocytic Lesion
1. Chronic inflammation (usu. lymphohistiocytic)
2. Vascular proliferation, vascular ectasia
3. Lamellar fibrosis parallel to the epidermis
4. Melanophages
- d/dg stromal features of atypical naevi: evidence of melanocyte destruction/loss favours regression

Ephelis
- Normal epidermis
- ↑ Pigmentation, normal numbers of melanocytes
- d/dg *café au lait* spots: these may have big pigment granules (giant melanosomes) unlike ephelides

Becker's Pigmented Hairy Epidermal Naevus
- Nearly normal skin: accentuated normal epidermal ridge pattern
- Mild ↑ melanocytes and pigmentation
- Very mild chronic inflammatory infiltrate

Blue Naevi
- Ito (claviculoscapulohumeral) and Ota (ophthalmomaxillary) naevi are blue naevus variants
- d/dg melanoma: because blue naevi may go deep with a rounded margin and asymmetric pigment
- d/dg pigmented NF: difficult – Wagner-Meissner bodies and assoc^d NF-1 favour NF

Common blue naevus
- Dendritic cells with fine melanin granules ⎫ two cell
- Melanophages with coarse melanin granules ⎬ types

Cellular blue naevus
- Dendritic cells (pigmented)
- Balls and bundles of small non-pigmented spindle cells with uniform oval nuclei
- *Atypical cellular blue naevus*: bizarre (e.g. giant) cells ± nuclear pleom. (but sparse mitoses and no necrosis)

Combined blue naevus
- Blue naevus cells (! do not mistake for the deep pigmentation seen in melanoma)
- Ordinary naevus cells

Malignant blue naevus
- ↑ Mitoses, necrosis and pleom. (incl. nuclear atypia and macronucleoli): d/dg metastatic melanoma

Recurrent Naevus (Pseudomelanoma)
- Usu. after shave Bx but can also occur after trauma (traumatised naevus)
- Examine the previous Bx to rule out an atypical melanocytic lesion or melanoma
- ↑ Epidermal melanocytes ⎫
- Single cells and nests ⎬ Only in the region of the dermal scar
- Variable pigmentation ⎪
- Random cytological atypia ⎭
- An isolated normal mitosis may be seen
- Residual benign naevus beneath dermal scar
- ! Do not confuse the dermal scarring with the fibrosis of a regression reaction to melanoma

Neurotised Intradermal Melanocytic Naevus vs. Solitary Circumscribed Neuroma
- Neuroma has a partial EMA +ve capsule and shows scattered neurofilament +ve axons admixed in it
- Neuroma has artefactual peripheral clefts, fascicular arch. ± ancient change / PEH

Halo Naevus (of Sutton)
- Usu. symmetrical
- Random 'degenerative' atypia
- Mitoses are rare (and superficial)
- Heavy mononuclear infiltrate throughout the lesion but esp. at the periphery
- No expansile nests
- Downward maturation

Clonal Naevus
- Discrete aggregates of epithelioid melanocytes are present in the upper half of a usual naevus:
  - contain dusty pigment and surrounded by melanophages
  - an isolated normal mitosis may be present (if more, think melanoma)
  - aggregates are not infiltrative or expansile (*cf.* melanoma)
  - mild cytological atypia with small nucleoli (if bigger nucleoli, think melanoma)
- d/dg melanoma arising in a naevus (do levels and look for the above features)
- d/dg deep penetrating naevus (but the clonal component is superficial in clonal naevus)

Atypical Nodular Proliferations in a Congenital Naevus
- Big congenital naevus with a nodule
- Expansile dermal nests
- Uniform cytological atypia
- Mitotic figures are rare
- There are areas of transition between the nodule and the surrounding naevus

Naevus of Acral / Genital Skin (Flexural Naevus)
- Usu. <1cm ∅ and histologically circumscribed
- Architectural atypia (often papillomatosis in genital ones)
- Nests: variable size/shape (esp. vertical ovals) with cohesive cells and retraction cleft around the nest
- Mild random cytological atypia
- Occasional single cells rise in the epidermis (Pagetoid) – but usu. limited to centre of the lesion
- Genital / Flexural: occ. dermal mitoses – d/dg melanoma (but melanoma usu. occurs in the elderly)
- Acral Naevi: a junctional shoulder (i.e. junctional component overshoots) and dermal fibrosis are typical
  - d/dg dysplastic naevus: no lamellar fibrosis or lentiginous component
  - d/dg melanoma: melanoma is favoured by:
    - irregular acanthosis
    - widespread PM
    - dermal component atypia / mitoses

Infantile Naevus / Neonatal Naevus
- Pagetoid melanocytosis
- Mild cytological atypia
- An occasional dermal mitosis
- d/dg melanoma: melanoma is expansile with more atypia and mitoses throughout the lesion ± necrosis with lack of downward maturation

Lentigo Simplex
- ± Familial syndromes, not actinic, no malig. potential, genital ones may be large and variegated
- Rete ridge elongation (or broad acanthosis in genital ones)
- ↑ Numbers of melanocytes (not atypical)
- ↑ Pigmentation

Lentigo Senilis (Actinic Lentigo)
- Elderly, actinic distribution, multiple, reticulated black ink spot variant may be worrying clinically
- Bud-like rete elongation ± rete fusion
- Hyperkeratosis incl. keratin cysts (i.e. BCP-like)

- Normal numbers (or slight ↑) of melanocytes (not atypical) } with skip lesions in the reticulated
- ↑ Pigmentation } black ink spot variant

Lentigo Maligna
- *Atypical* melanocytes: ↑ cytoplasmic vacuolation and irregular hyperchromatic angulated nucleus
- Basal palisading of these melanocytes ± parallel spindle nests
- Adnexal epithelium is involved
- Actinic damage ± epidermal atrophy
- Chronic dermal inflammation assoc[d] with (multifocal) invasion (d/dg spindle SCC / DFSP)
- Invasive foci are of the spindle cell desmoplastic type ± neurotropism (= *Desmoplastic Melanoma*)
- d/dg *de novo* intraepidermal epithelioid melanocytic dysplasia (a melanoma precursor) only shows a non-confluent lentiginous proliferation of atypical epithelioid melanocytes (± variable PM) without nests or naevus and of insufficient density to be called *in situ* melanoma (Rx is complete excision)

Dysplastic Naevus
- ≥4mm, flat and variegated
- Asymmetrical with 'shouldering' (i.e. the junctional component overshoots) if compound
- Nested and lentiginous hyperplasia
- 'Random' cytological atypia
- Intracellular pigment may be of the fine 'dusty' type
- Delicate, elongated rete and horizontal rete bridging by spindly cells (rete fusion is usu. <3 pegs)
- Lamellar fibroplasia of the papillary dermis
- Vascular and lymphocytic dermal reaction
- Features raising suspicion of melanoma (see also the sections on melanoma on pp. 290–291):
  - ➢ uniform cytological atypia / *regions* where all cells show atypia (i.e. not random individual cells)
  - ➢ extensive confluent rete peg bridging (≥3 pegs)
  - ➢ Pagetoid 'buckshot' spread (dyscohesive, atypical melanocytes infiltrate the epidermis) esp. if extending higher than the mid-epidermis

Grading dysplastic naevi
- Refers to the cytological atypia (not architecture)
- *Mild*: nucleus ≈ same size as a keratinocyte's, hyperchromatic chromatin, inconspicuous nucleolus
- *Moderate*: nuclear size varies upto 2× the size of a keratinocyte nucleus, vesicular / hyperchromatic chromatin, inconspicuous nucleolus
- *Severe*: nuclear size varies >2× keratinocyte, vesicular, prominent nucleolus, abundant cytoplasm
- 'High grade' (= moderate-severe) should be re-excised if it reaches the margins (or is <5 mm clear if dysplasia is severe)

Spitz Naevus

Typical Spitz naevus
- Flesh-coloured dome-shaped papule (<1cm) in children/adolescents (clinical d/dg haemangioma)
- Usu. compound (epithelioid type has small nests, spindle type has whorled vertical nests)
- Epithelioid cells: with nuclei larger than a keratinocyte nucleus and with *round* nucleoli
- Spindle cells: plump cells with smooth-contoured, oval nuclei and small nucleoli
- Upward migration of melanocytes (PM) may occur centrally in a symmetrical lesion
- Eosinophilic globules near the dermoepidermal junction
- ± Telangiectasia, oedema, epidermal hyperplasia
- Variants: pigmented (Reed), intradermal, intraepidermal, desmoplastic, atypical / malignant
- d/dg melanoma:
  - ➢ symmetrical and sharp lateral demarcation
  - ➢ downward maturation and irregular contours at the base
  - ➢ retraction clefts, adnexal involvement, superficial pigment
  - ➢ mitoses and Pagetoid spread are rare
  - ➢ immuno: see 'Immunohistochemistry in melanocytic lesions', p. 291

NB: malignant Spitz is considered a variant of melanoma (*q.v.*)

Desmoplastic Spitz naevus
- Symmetrical
- Maturation
- Perineural 'invasion'

Intraepidermal Spitz naevus
- Mimics melanoma *in situ*
- Individual cell upward migration (PM) – not reaching the highest layers
- Mitoses are rare
- Cells appear moulded

Pigmented Spindle and Epithelioid Cell Naevus of Reed (Spitz Variant)
- Symmetrical, pigmented, dome-shaped lesion on the thigh of a young woman
- Predominantly junctional
- Mitoses in nests
- Upward migration of individual melanocytes (PM), not reaching stratum corneum
- Transepidermal elimination of pigment and *groups of pigmented melanocytes*
- The above results in a 'raining down' pattern

Deep Penetrating Naevus (DPN) = Plexiform Spindle Cell Naevus
- Young, M=F, limbs>face>upper trunk, deeply pigmented / blue, <1cm ∅
- Symmetrical, wedge-shaped, tip may reach subcutis ± octopus-like down-growing 'tentacles' of cells
- Often part of a compound naevus with a normal (and usu. small) junctional component
- Heavily pigmented cells, uniform mild atypia, ± intranuclear cytoplasmic inclusions
- Maturation takes the form of increased horizontal spindling of cells deeper in the lesion
- Mitoses rare (but may be deep)
- No Pagetoid spread
- Not a true blue naevus as the DPN cells are not dendritic (difficult to demonstrate on LM)

Features in Melanocytic Lesions that should raise the suspicion for Malignant Melanoma
- No one feature is diagnostic of malignant melanoma
- Some melanomas (e.g. neurotropic, spindle cell, desmoplastic) usu. show exceptions to these rules
- Asymmetry of the lesion
- Lack of downward maturation (! but small cell melanoma shows maturation in the form of little nests, and there are melanomas with paradoxical maturation – deep pigment, ↑mitoses, ↑Ki-67 and HMB45 with lack of zonation all help here in that they favour melanoma)
- Deep pigmentation (! but hypermelanotic naevi have melanin throughout – with benign cytology)
- A pushing, well-defined margin at the base / large nests at the base
- Uniform chronic inflammatory response at the base
- Non-traumatic ulceration (i.e. without scale crust, haemorrhage and parakeratosis)
- Pagetoid 'buckshot' melanocytosis esp. if involving adnexal epithelium or extending beyond the dermal component
- Upper dermal fibroplasia (in superficial melanomas) or more widespread fibrosis
- Widespread cytological atypia
- 'Powdery' / 'dusty' intracellular pigment (*cf.* more coarse granules)
- Mitoses esp. in dermal component and esp. deeper down
- Expansile dermal nests (i.e. displace and compress surrounding structures)
- Dyscohesion of melanocytes in dermal nests
- Dermal nests which are different from surrounding nests may indicate transformation: the difference may be pigmented *vs.* non-pigmented or a small cell nest
- Areas of regression

Desmoplastic vs. Neurotropic vs. Spindle Cell Melanoma
- Similar clinical: elderly, head and neck predominant
- Immuno: +ve for S100 (but may be focal), NSE (upto 95% of cases) and vimentin
- Immuno: HMB45, MUM1 and Melan-A are usu. −ve (but if +ve, it helps)
- Desmoplastic:
  - ➤ bulky mass
  - ➤ associated with lentigo maligna but can arise *de novo*
  - ➤ patchy lymphoid infiltrate, going deep
  - ➤ uniform spindle cells with mitoses (even in hypocellular variants)
  - ➤ haphazard, storiform, fascicular arrangement with fibrosis
  - ➤ pigment scarce to absent

        ➤ d/dg dermatofibroma, fibromatosis, desmoplastic naevus
        ➤ d/dg scar: ! scars may contain scattered mildly atypical S100 +ve spindle cells (? regenerating Schwann cells) that are −ve for HMB45 and (usu.) Melan-A

- Spindle:
  - ➤ like desmoplastic melanoma but with pleomorphic cytology
  - ➤ *pleomorphic spindle cell melanoma has worse prognosis*
  - ➤ d/dg AFX, spindle cell carcinoma, MPNST, mucosal melanomas (the latter often have a spindle morphology but are more likely to be +ve for HMB45 and Melan-A)
- Neurotropic:
  - ➤ fascicular growth
  - ➤ pleomorphic cells are present but rare
  - ➤ infiltrates into and around nerve bundles (*cf.* d/dg desmoplastic Spitz naevus)
  - ➤ d/dg neurofibroma, malignant Schwannoma, desmoplastic naevus

Other Melanoma Variants
- Signet ring melanoma: d/dg signet ring carcinoma
- Balloon cell melanoma: d/dg clear cell carcinoma / RCC
- Rhabdoid melanoma
- Malignant blue naevus is a dermal growth ∴ d/dg metastatic melanoma / cellular blue naevus
- Malignant Spitz naevus
- Naevoid melanoma (= minimal deviation melanoma): symmetrical, cytologically homogeneous and minimal stromal reaction

Radial / Horizontal Growth Phase Melanoma (HGP)
- An *in situ* component is present
- Microinvasion (single cells / small aggregates) of the papillary dermis
- Nests of melanoma in the dermis are smaller than those in the epidermis and are not expansile
- Mitoses in the dermal component are very rare to absent
- Often regression or brisk lymphocytic response is seen
- Usu. restricted to Clark level II and <1mm Breslow thick

Vertical Growth Phase Melanoma (VGP)
- Def^n: ≥ 1 dermal nest / cluster *of melanoma cells* 'of suitable size' (often interpreted to mean larger than the largest intraepidermal nest). The nest is often expansile, compressing surrounding structures
- Pleomorphism, apoptoses and mitoses in the dermal nest(s) help to identify them as VGP melanoma
- Regression is usu. absent and lymphocytic response less than HGP
- Often >1mm thick (if into Clark level III or deeper then it is usu. in the VGP)

Immunohistochemistry in Melanocytic Lesions
- HMB45 is   −ve in the dermal component of *typical* benign naevi (but junctional nests are +ve)
              +ve in a zonal manner in Spitz (most superficially, less deep), DPN, cellular blue naevi
              +ve in malignant melanocytes (not zonal but may be patchy)
- Cyclin D1 (Bcl-1, PRAD1): as for HMB45
- Ki-67 (MIB1): as for HMB45 (Spitz naevi average at 5%, melanomas usu. $\gg$9%)[5]
- Melan-A is +ve in non-neurotised melanocytes (benign and malig., dermal and epidermal, 1° and mets)
- S100 and MUM1 are more sensitive *cf.* HMB45 in melanomas
- p53 is −ve in benign naevi (incl. Spitz) but +ve in most nodular melanomas
- For more on HMB45, Melan-A and S100, see pp. 15–16

Clark Levels (Staging)
I   intraepidermal / junctional
II   in papillary dermis but not filling it
III   filling papillary dermis
IV   into reticular dermis
V   into subcutis

---

[5] ! do not count +ve intralesional lymphocytes

Adnexal Tumours

Sweat Gland Differentiation (General)
- Apocrine: eosinophil cytoplasm, basal nuclei; −ve for ER, PgR, Bcl-2; ±ve for GCDFP15, AR
- Eccrine: ±ve for ER, PgR, Bcl-2; acrosyringium is +ve for CK14
- Both: +ve for EMA, CEA, LMW CK
- 'Apoeccrine' glands are mammary-like glands in the skin (esp. anogenital and axilla)

Features favouring a Tricho . . . over a BCC
- Infolding of the stroma into the nests of cells (e.g. papillary mesenchymal bodies)
- Eosinophilic collagenous cuticle surrounding the cell nests
- Cleavage of collagen between cell nests (*cf.* cleavage between cell nests and collagen in BCC)
- Presence of nucleoli
- Well-circ. organoid architecture (and lack of an infiltrative architecture *overall*)
- Absence of a connection to the epidermis (but a connection may be seen in some tricho. . .)
- Immuno: CD34 and CD10 +ve stroma (−ve in basaloid cells), CK20 & CK15 focally +ve, Bcl-2 only seen in peripheral basal cells (not diffuse), low Ki-67 LI (sparse cells only, ≪20%), stromelysin 3 −ve stroma

Trichoadenoma, Trichofolliculoma, Dilated Pore of Winer, Pilar Sheath Acanthoma
- Trichoadenoma has multiple scattered keratotic cysts in a fibrotic stroma
- Winer's pore is a patulous keratotic plug surrounded by variable hair sheath acanthosis (clin: 'black-head')
- Pilar sheath acanthoma (face, upper lip) is like Winer's pore but has a more florid, irregular and complex proliferation of the surrounding epithelium with focal follicular differentiation
- Trichofolliculoma (usu. head) has a central region containing tufts of hair shafts surrounded by a radiation of secondary and tertiary follicular structures

Proliferating Pilar Tumour / Cyst
- Non-invasive lobules of squamous epithelium showing maturation ± basal palisading
- Lobules surrounded by thick BM layer
- Keratinisation is trichilemmal (i.e. not lamellar and without a granular cell layer) ± focal epidermoid
- Squamous buds/pearls ± desmoplasia within the confines of the circumscribed tumour *is not* SCC
- Criteria for malignancy (otherwise ! do NOT call it d/dg SCC):
  - ➢ size (>5cm ∅), location (not on scalp), ulceration, rapid growth
  - ➢ marked pleomorphism (! but CIS may be seen)
  - ➢ necrosis, mitoses ++ (esp. if abnormal forms), local invasion

Hidroacanthoma Simplex (Intraepidermal Poroma)
- Borst-Jadassohn phenomenon of small clear bland cells

Eccrine Poroma
- Connected to the epidermis (else = *dermal duct tumour*)
- 1 cell type – unlike spiradenoma / cylindroma (d/dg)
- ± Lumena (stain +ve with CEA)
- Not palisaded and may occur on palms and soles – unlike BCC (!d/dg)
- Malignancy (= *porocarcinoma*): pleomorphism, invasion, necrosis ± spindle cells, squamous diff^n and melanocytic infiltration (! d/dg melanoma); verrucous Bowenoid variant doesn't have benign ducts in it *cf.* d/dg Bowen's (−ve for CEA, CK7 and S100, unlike porocarcinoma) and Paget's (larger, PAS +ve cells)

Dermal Cylindroma
- Not connected to the epidermis
- 'Jigsaw' nodules with prominent BM peripherally ± spherulosis
- Two cell types (as for eccrine spiradenoma *q.v.* – but the dark outer cells may be more palisaded)
- Intermediate tumours (between cylindroma / spiradenoma) also occur = *spiradenocylindroma*

Eccrine Spiradenoma
- Not connected to epidermis
- Well-circumscribed / encapsulated nodule
- Interlocking cords ± ductule formation
- Prominent BM material, stromal vascular ectasia, ± lymphocytic infiltrate
- Two cell types: dark nuclei (outer), open nuclei with even chromatin (inner): both have scant cytoplasm
- Mitoses ≈ 1/10 hpf

Malignancy in Cylindroma and Eccrine Spiradenoma
- Infiltrative growth   ⎫ You often get a frankly malignant component
- Pleomorphism ± necrosis   ⎬ next to a well-formed benign component.
- Mitotic count and size are less important

Syringoma
- Head and neck (eyelid) / any site
- Occurs in the superficial half of the dermis and is circumscribed, occ. connection to the epidermis
- Dense fibrotic stroma
- Small cysts (1 to many layers ± keratin) with 'comma' tails; nests also present
- Small bland nuclei ± clear cell change (if pleom. and mitoses consider d/dg syringoid eccrine carcinoma)
- Immuno: EMA in basal layer, CEA in inner layer of cells in the cysts. ER and PgR –ve
- ! d/dg microcystic adnexal carcinoma (*vide infra*) and desmoplastic trichoepithelioma (may keratinise)

Microcystic Adnexal Carcinoma ('Malignant Syringoma')
- *Not* circumscribed, may extend into deep dermis / subcutis and beyond
- Stromal fibrosis and perineural invasion are helpful features
- Multiple little keratocysts and tubules with ILC/SmCC-like infiltrative streams of cells
- Bland nuclei, NCR not markedly raised, mitoses scarce} these help in d/dg morphoeic BCC
- Immuno: CK7 +ve (like d/dg metastatic breast carcinoma)
- d/dg syringoma: confined to upper dermis and *circumscribed*
- d/dg desmoplastic trichoepithelioma is confined to upper dermis, has more organoid nests, is CK7 –ve

Hidradenoma Papilliferum
- Benign, sporadic, adults, F≫M, perineum (rarely nipple, eyelid, external auditory meatus)
- Mid-dermal cyst (± epidermal link) variably filled with papillary / trabecular / tubulocystic fronds
- Non-inflam^y fibrovascular 'capsule' continuous with the internal stroma (of the papillae, etc.)
- Double lining (inner apocrine, outer cuboidal myoepithelium) but outer cyst wall may be squamous
- Overlying epidermis is ≈ normal and underlying dermis is also ≈ normal (*cf.* d/dg syringocystadenoma)

Syringocystadenoma Papilliferum (SCAP)
- Head (rarely proximal limbs/chest), often part of naevus sebaceus, CIS/malignancy is documented
- Mid-dermal cystic invagination from surface showing variable papillary / villiform fronds
- Plasma cell-rich stroma (many IgA) is typical (and useful in d/dg hidradenoma papilliferum)
- Cell lining is the same as in hidradenoma ± multilayered areas with eccrine-like ductules
- Verrucous hyperplasia of overlying epidermis ± dilated eccrine/apocrine acini in underlying dermis
- CIS / malignancy: nuclear pleom., mitoses ++, disordered arch. and loss of CK5/6 +ve basal cells

Apocrine Carcinoma
- Rare, scalp/axilla/perineum, exclude 1° breast IDC before diagnosis, grade as for breast carcinoma
- Asymmetric, infiltrative, IDC-like tumour (incl. variants e.g. cribriform) and focal decapitation secretion
- Immuno: ±ve for receptors (oestrogen, progesterone and androgen), GCDFP15 and S100
- d/dg metastatic CA: decapitation secretion, focal benign apocrine lesion and attachment to hair follicle
- d/dg tubular apocrine adenoma: carcinoma ducts lack myoepithelium, adenoma has two-cell type

Pilomatrixoma (Calcifying Epithelioma of Malherbe)
- Ghost cell stratified epithelium (no stainable nuclei)
- Basaloid cell islands (if prominent with lobulation and few ghosts = 'proliferating pilomatricoma')
- Variable Ca^{2+} and giant cells (may be numerous)

Pilomatrix Carcinoma (Malignant Pilomatrixoma)
- Large size (e.g. >4cm)
- Predominantly basaloid cells
- Infiltrative growth (invasion of vessels, nerve [perineural] or bone is diagnostic of malignancy)
- *Abnormal* mitoses (high mitotic rate *per se* can be seen in young benign lesions)

Chondroid Syringoma (Mixed Tumour of the Skin)
- Head and neck of the elderly (malignant ones are more often on the extremities)
- Well-circumscribed and intradermal
- Stroma (typical stroma may be absent): myxoid, chondroid, osteoid, fibrous, fat; ± myoepithelial differentiation
- Epithelium: ➢ single cells
                 ➢ solid cords
                 ➢ tubules (two-cell type – outer myoepithelial, inner epithelial)
                 ➢ keratin cysts ± collagenous spherulosis
- Variants: ① 'eccrine': simple tubules with simple cuboidal lining (1 layer)
              ② 'apocrine': complex tubules with ≥ two-cell thick apocrine lining ± pilosebaceous areas

Malignancy in Chondroid Syringoma (Malignant Mixed Tumour)
- Infiltrative growth ± satellite tumour nodules
- Marked pleomorphism
- Tumour necrosis
- *Abnormal* mitoses / excessive mitoses

> If there are no proven metastases, some call this *atypical chondroid syringoma*.

Sebaceous Lesions: Hyperplasia, Adenoma, Epithelioma (= Sebaceoma) and Carcinoma
- All may be associated with Muir-Torre syndrome and the neoplasms may show squamoid differentiation
- All have outer mitotic basaloid cells (without palisading/clefting *cf.* d/dg BCC with sebaceous differentiation) and inner cells showing multiple vacuoles indenting a central nucleus. All but carcinoma are well-circumscribed
- Hyperplasia: ↑nõ (≥5) of normal lobules with a single or double basal layer; they extend more superficially than normal and connect to a single central dilated infundibular duct (+ surrounding inflammation and fibrosis in the extensive lesions of rhinophyma)
- Adenoma: ↑nõ of lobules with multiple layers of basal cells (that comprise <50% of the lobule cells)
- Sebaceoma: ↑nõ of lobules, more irregular in size and arrangement with ≈50% or more basal cells
- Carcinoma: mostly basal cells, irregular arrangement and size of lobules with asymmetry and invasive arch. and pleomorphic multivacuolated cells in the centre of some lobules; eyelid ones may show Pagetoid spread into conjunctiva and are more often fatal via systemic mets

Merkel Cell Carcinoma (Trabecular Carcinoma, Primary NEC of the Skin)
- Assoc^d with: overlying squamous cell atypia / Bowen's / concomitant SCC / Pagetoid (Pautrioid) spread
- Trabecular / organoid / medullary patterns and glandular differentiation may all occur, usu. with a Grenz zone
- Most cases have an intermediate cell size (i.e. ⌀ between 2 to 3 times that of a mature lymphocyte)
- Monotonous oval nuclei, even chromatin, small nucleoli
- Mitoses ++ (mitotic count >10 per one hpf or a Ki-67 LI of >50% is a poor prognostic)
- Vascular stroma
- Lack of a band-like lymphoid infiltrate at the tumour-stroma junction is a poor prognostic
- Divergent differentiation is rare: RMS, AFX-like, leiomyosarcoma and lymphoepithelioma are all reported
- Immuno:
    ➢ +ve: paranuclear dot-like with all these: AE1/AE3, CAM5.2, MNF116, ± neurofilament
    ➢ +ve: CgA, synaptophysin, NSE, EMA, BerEp4, Fli-1 (in 90%), CD99 (50%), c-kit (75%)
    ➢ +ve: CK20 (unlike other SmCC except salivary gland), CD56, nuclear TdT (50%)
    ➢ −ve: CEA, HMW CK, CK7, LCA, CD3/20/34, TTF-1; S100 is +ve in $\frac{1}{3}$ of cases
- d/dg metastatic SmCC bronchus: bronchial SmCC is CK20 −ve, Ck7 +ve

Hair and Alopecia

Normal Hair
- The bulb of a growing hair (anagen) is in the subcutis (for the scalp) or deep dermis (elsewhere)
- The bulb of a resting hair (telogen) is at the level of the bulge (insertion point of arrector pili)
- The transition from anagen to telogen is called catagen
- During its catagen ascent, the bulb leaves behind a fibrous band marking its route called a follicular stela (or streamer)
- Normally about 85%, 3% and 12% of hairs are in anagen, catagen and telogen respectively
- Hair shaft: contains medulla, cortex and outer cuticle. The cuticle is thickened in catagen hairs and the shaft has a stellate cross-section in telogen. Vellus hairs lack coarse pigment granules and medulla
- Terminal:vellus ratio $\approx$ 7:1
- Anagen:(telogen + catagen) ratio $\approx$ 14:1   } data from Whiting, 2001

Alopecia Areata / Alopecia Totalis / Alopecia Universalis
- Clin.: non-scarring patchy scalp (areata), total scalp (totalis) or whole body (universalis) hair loss
- Bx: transversely sectioned punch Bx is more sensitive (*cf.* vertical sections), esp. in the inactive phases, as it allows quantitative counts of various types of hair follicles (to calculate ratios)
- Active phase: hair bulbs and stelae show 'swarm of bees' lymphocytic infiltrate ($\pm$ Mϕ and eos.) with exocytosis $\pm$ apoptoses and pigmentary incontinence
- Inactive phase:
  - $\succ$ inflammation subsides
  - $\succ$ pigmentary incontinence in the hair bulbs and stelae remain
  - $\succ$ $\uparrow$ vellus, catagen and telogen hairs (and stelae)
  - $\succ$ $\downarrow$ anagen hairs
  - $\succ$ $\pm$ 'nanagen' follicles (= irregular eosinophilic transformation of telogen/catagen shaft keratin)
- Terminal:vellus ratio $\approx$ 1.5:1 to 0.6:1 according to severity
- Anagen:(telogen + catagen) ratio $\approx$ 2:1 to 2.3:1
- Absolute loss of follicles is rare but if it occurs and is severe the prognosis for hair recovery is poor
- d/dg: tinea capitis (PMN), 2° syphilis (plasma cells), scarring alopecias (pseudopelade of Brocq, LE), mechanical alopecias (e.g. trichotillomania) and congenital/familial alopecias (no inflam[n]), androgenic alopecia and telogen effluvium
- The data in this section is based on Whiting, 2001 *q.v.* for illustrations and details

Scarring Alopecias
Primary (Pseudopelade of Brocq = Alopecia cicatrisata)
- Brief early phase: mononuclear cells in and around pilosebaceous unit sparing its lower $\frac{1}{3}$, the epidermis and sweat glands (the epidermis remains normal throughout *cf.* lichen planopilaris)
- Late: fibroelastic cords replace pilosebaceous units and arrector pili may insert into them
- d/dg atrophic (late) lichen planopilaris – this is not limited to the scalp (while pseudopelade is)
Secondary
- Causes incl.: DLE, morphoea, lichen planopilaris, post-neoplastic scarring
- *Folliculitis decalvans* has intrafollicular pustules and the surrounding infiltrate has PMN and plasma cells early on with scarring later $\pm$ granulation tissue and foreign body giant cell granulomatous reaction to hair keratin (d/dg acne folliculitis keloidalis, acne conglobata, pilonidal sinus, pseudopelade)

Trichotillomania
- $\uparrow\uparrow$ In catagen hairs (and any anagen follicles are usu. empty) with no (or mild non-specific) inflam[n]
- Pigment casts (clumps of pigment in the follicular canal)
- Trichomalacia (twisted / distorted hairs in the follicular canal)

Vellus Hair Cyst (Eruptive Vellus Hair Cyst) and Differential Diagnoses
- Multiple dermal cysts; sporadic or inherited (AD)
- A dermal squamous retention cyst containing vellus hair shafts $\pm$ a small follicle attached to the wall
- Mostly epidermoid keratinisation $\pm$ focal trichilemmal keratinisation
- d/dg epidermal cyst: no vellus hairs (see p. 282 for more)
- d/dg steatocystoma multiplex: multiple sebaceous lobules abut the undulating wall; no granular layer
- d/dg pigmented hair cyst: pigmented hair shafts with medullae, $\pm$ rete ridges / dermal papillae

Inflammatory and Lymphoproliferative

Spongiotic Dermatitis (SD)
- Clinically 'eczema' of various causes; eosinophils ++ in contact dermatitis, atopy and drugs
- Acute: spongiosis (intercellular oedema) ++, lymphocyte exocytosis, superficial perivascular lymphoid infiltrate
- Subacute: parakeratosis, acanthosis, papillomatosis, mixed chronic inflam^y infiltrate, less spongiosis
- Chronic: minimal / no spongiosis, upper dermal fibrosis, more acanthosis and papillomatosis
- Example lesions showing SD include:
  - ➢ eczemas (exogenous and endogenous) = acute and subacute SD
  - ➢ lichen simplex chronicus and nodular prurigo (variants of chronic SD)
  - ➢ stasis dermatitis (band-like prominent vessels in pap. dermis, fibrosis, haemosiderin [that extends sig. deeper than the papillary dermis unlike d/dg pigmented purpuric dermatoses], ± ulceration, PEH). A severe form (called acroangiodermatitis) may be confused for KS clinically
  - ➢ psoriasiform dermatoses (psoriasiform acanthosis = ① rete ridge acanthosis, ② parakeratosis, ③ lack of a granular layer) e.g. psoriasis (may show Köbner phenomenon), seborrhoeic dermatitis, pityriasis rubra pilaris, 2° syphilis (*vide infra*)
  - ➢ pityriasis rubra pilaris: parakeratin shoulders aside orthokerat plugged follicles
  - ➢ psoriasis vulgaris: suprapapillary thinning of epidermis with spongiform pustules of Kogoj becoming Munro microabscesses above the granular layer, papillae clubbed with ↑vascularity, PMN encrusted parakeratin – d/dg MF, dermatophytes, 2° syphilis
  - ➢ dermatophytoses (PMN ± psoriasiform acanthosis)
  - ➢ pityriasis rosea (with RBC extravasation in the papillary dermis and parakeratotic mounds)
  - ➢ lichen striatus (with vacuolar interface change)
- d/dg mycosis fungoides:
  - ➢ MF intraepidermal lymphocytes are numerous, large, cerebriform and form collections (Pautrier microabscesses) but spongiosis is minimal / absent (! do not confuse peri-lymphocyte halos with spongiosis)
  - ➢ SD exocytotic lymphocytes may be large and reactive ('activated') and spongiosis may be minimal in the more chronic forms ∴ interpret with caution

Syphilis (2° and 3°)
- Clin.: variable macules/papules, guttate psoriasis-like lesions, anogenital condylomata lata, alopecia
- Epidermis: psoriasiform acanthosis, spongiosis, exocytosis, PMN (± psoriasis-like spongiform pustules / microabscesses), ± dyskeratosis, ± basal vacuolation
- Papillary dermis: oedema, mixed chronic inflam^n + variable nõ. of plasma cells (may be lymphocyte / Mɸ predominant or even granulomatous in later stages and 3° syphilis)
- Deeper dermis: perivascular (± periadnexal) mixed chronic inflam^n + variable nõ. of plasma cells
- Vessels: endothelial swelling and proliferation (± a PMN vascular reaction in early stages)
- Warthin-Starry: spirochaetes best seen in epidermis (but −ve in upto 70% of cases)
- d/dg dermatophyte, pityriasis rosea, psoriasis, etc.

Nodular Prurigo (Prurigo Nodularis)
- = Nodular lichen simplex chronicus due to any cause of chronic itch/scratch ∴ features of the 1° cause may be superimposed
- Early: ➢ orthokeratotic hyperkeratosis and irregular acanthosis
  - ➢ changes involve acral portions of adnexa to variable degree
- Later: ➢ papillomatosis and PEH-like downgrowths
  - ➢ papillary dermis: vertical collagen fibrosis, perivascular lymphohistiocytic infiltrate, plump endothelial vessels and stellate fibroblasts
  - ➢ polymorphs of all types may be present (e.g. eos. in atopy)
  - ➢ deeper dermal fibrosis and mucin
  - ➢ ± nerve trunk hypertrophy and nerve twig proliferation

Seborrhoeic Dermatitis
- Early: ➢ basket-weave hyperkeratosis with lymphocyte exocytosis and dyskeratosis
  - ➢ superficial perivascular lymphohistiocytic infiltrate
  - ➢ papillary dermal vessel dilatation ± RBC extravasation

- Later:
  - ➤ parakeratosis, irregular psoriasiform acanthosis, PMN, keratin follicular plugging
  - ➤ inflam^y infiltrate extends down to mid dermis
  - ➤ dermal PMN and nuclear dust (but no frank LCV)
- Late:
  - ➤ hyperkeratosis with epidermal atrophy and follicular plugs
  - ➤ ↓ dermal inflam^n

Lymphocyte Predominant Patchy Deep / Mid Dermal Infiltrates
- Jessner's: dermis and superficial subcutis, diffuse ± perivascular / periadnexal; few histiocytes / plasma cells
- Polymorphous light eruption: ≈ exclusively lymphocytes, ± spongiosis ± papillary dermal oedema
- Leukaemic infiltrates tend to have a diffuse predominant (*cf.* perivascular/adnexal) pattern
- Others: LE, lymphoma, PLEVA, pernio (p. 300), lymphocytic hyperplasia (*lymphocytoma cutis*), insect bite (this usu. has eos. ± plasma cells), gyrate erythemas (tight perivascular infiltrates ± vessel wall infiltration d/dg lymphocytic vasculitis) e.g. *erythema chronicum migrans / erythema annulare centrifugum*

Incontinentia Pigmenti
- F>M but ?X-linked
- eosinophil spongiosis in a newborn / few-month-old

Interface Dermatitis
Vacuolar interface change / dermatitis
- Basal keratinocyte cytoplasmic vacuolation
- ± Paucicellular lymphoid infiltrate around the DEJ ± pigmentary incontinence
- Example lesions: LE, dermatomyositis, PLEVA, TEN / GVHD, erythema multiforme, fixed drug eruption, 2° syphilis
- Vacuolar change may overlap / co-exist with lichenoid interface dermatitis
Lichenoid interface dermatitis
- Basal keratinocyte necrosis (colloid Civatte bodies, irregular BM contour, lymphocyte exocytosis, pigmentary incontinence)
- Band-like lymphocytic infiltrate
- Example lesions: LP, lichenoid drug eruptions, lichen nitidus, conditions with vacuolar change

Erythema Multiforme Group
- Group includes: erythema multiforme minor (EMM), Stevens-Johnson (= EMM + mucosal lesions), TEN (Lyell's syndrome) and fixed drug eruption (FDE). The distinction between them is clinical
- Due to drugs (esp. TEN/Stevens-Johnson), other causes (esp. EMM) e.g. post infect^n (esp. HSV)
- Bullous, macular, papular, targetoid lesions (incl. palms) ± mucosal erosions ± scarring, ± sloughing
- Epidermis:
  - ➤ vacuolar interface change, lymphocyte exocytosis, spongiosis, orthokeratotic hyperkeratosis
  - | ± Nikolsky sign | ➤ dyskeratoses → confluent → subepidermal bulla with a coagulative necrotic roof
- Dermis: superficial perivascular lymphohistiocytic infiltrate (often sparse in TEN), oedema, RBC extravasation (no vasculitis), ± pigmentary incontinence
- FDE: dermal infiltrate is denser and extends deeper (± eos.); ± more pigmentary incontinence
- d/dg: GVHD: can be impossible on a single Bx. See p. 306 for more guidance

Lupus Erythematosus
- Clin.: spectrum varying from CDLE (skin, but no visceral involvement, ANA uncommon) to SLE (viscera ± no skin involvement, ANA common); CDLE usu. involves ① sun-exposed skin with ② scaly erythematous patches and ③ scarring (incl. permanent hair loss)
- Epidermis:
  - ➤ atrophic ± dyskeratoses and squamoid phenotypic change of the stratum basale
  - ➤ vacuolar interface change (and subepidermal clefting in the rare *bullous LE*)
  - ➤ thickened (>1 basal cell nuclear ∅) and tortuous BM (↑ with age and immune complex deposition)
  - ➤ hyperkeratosis and plugging ('tin-tack' *cf.* the 'flask' shapes typical of LP)
- Dermis:
  - ➤ lymphocyte predominant (± plasma cells) infiltrate: patchy (esp. periadnexal), DEJ and interstitial
  - ➤ upper dermal acid mucin, oedema ± light RBC extravasation
- Subcutis:
  - ➤ ± lupus panniculitis (p. 303)

- Direct IF: granular IgG at DEJ (= *lupus band*) seen in:
    - ➤ clinically involved skin   in CDLE / SLE
    - ➤ clinically normal sun-exposed skin   in SLE
    - ➤ clinically normal non-sun-exposed   in SLE of ↑↑ activity and greater risk of renal disease
- Immuno EM: deposits just deep to the *lamina densa*
- Variants: ➤ bullous LE (DEJ clefting, dapsone sensitivity ± dermal tip PMN) d/dg DH
    - ➤ verrucous LE (papillomatoid or crateriform ± lower dyskeratoses ++) d/dg: LP, hypertrophic AK, keratoacanthoma or SCC
    - ➤ SCLE and neonatal LE (more DEJ changes, dermal oedema ± fibrinoid, less inflam^n)
    - ➤ tumid LE (dermal-only form) d/dg other lymphocyte predominant patchy infiltrates (see p. 297)
- d/dg: LP (*vide infra* but ! a true overlap syndrome occurs), drugs, other patchy lymphocyte predominant infiltrates

Pityriasis Lichenoides et Varioliformis Acuta (PLEVA, Mucha-Habermann Disease)
- Wedge-shaped infiltrate (thin end of wedge is deep), predominantly lymphocytic
- Dermal (incl. perivascular) ± epidermal haemorrhage
- Vacuolar interface change and exocytosis
- No large cells (*cf.* d/dg LyP / lymphoma)

Pityriasis Lichenoides Chronica (PLC)
- As for PLEVA but with parakeratosis ± haemorrhage and no necrosis / vacuolar change / exocytosis

Lichen Planus (LP)
- Young adults, self limited, ± Köbner phenomenon (i.e. occurs at / along sites of trauma)
- Epidermis: orthokeratotic hyperkeratosis, wedge of hypergranulosis, variable acanthosis and atrophy
- DEJ: saw-toothed lichenoid inflammation ± clefting / blood bullae (saw-toothing less common in mucosae)
- Dermis: almost pure lymphocytic infiltrate (plasma cells are rare in cutaneous LP but can be seen with mucosal LP or drugs)
- Variant: lichen planopilaris = pilar infundibulum LP with phagocytosed naked hair shaft fragments; the infiltrate often reaches the lower 1/3 of the follicle and surrounding dermis (*cf.* d/dg early pseudopelade of Brocq)
- Variant: lichen planus pemphogoides and bullous LP: d/dg pemphigoid
- d/dg lichenoid drug eruption: eruption has parakeratosis and a mixed dermal infiltrate (esp. eos. ± plasma cells), the infiltrate may extend deeper and around vessels and apoptoses may be high in the epidermis
- d/dg *lichen planus-like keratosis*: has parakeratosis and a mixed dermal infiltrate (esp. plasma cells and eos.) and is a solitary lesion on the upper body of adults ± adjacent actinic damage / AK or SK
- d/dg LE: LP has 'saw-toothing' and lacks dermal mucin, thick BM, deep infiltrates, prominent vacuolar interface change, uniform atrophy and multinucleated keratinocytes with > 2 nuclei
- d/dg erythema multiforme group: in these, the infiltrate may reach the mid epidermis (unlike LP)

Lichen Nitidus
- Little (1–2mm) papules on arms, abdomen, shaft of penis
- Granulomatous lichenoid inflammation expanding one dermal papilla (or a couple of papillae)

Necrobiotic Conditions
- Necrobiotic collagen is intensely eosinophil, swollen, homogeneous (and granular in places)

Necrobiosis lipoidica
- Sandwiched necrobiotic transformation of lower dermal collagen (may affect full skin thickness)
- Superficial and deep perivascular chronic inflam^y cell infiltrate (plasma cells are characteristic)
- Plasma cells, palisaded Mφ, lymphocytes ± lipid in necrobiotic collagen
- Granulomatous variant has sarcoid-like naked granulomas
- In older fibrotic lesions the necrobiosis is less prominent or concentrated and may be hard to detect
- d/dg granuloma annulare: necrobiosis lipoidica has less dermal mucin and more perivascular plasma cells
- d/dg septal panniculitis (because necrobiosis lipoidica may extend into the septa of the subcutis)

Granuloma annulare (GA)
- Plasma cells, palisaded Mφ and lymphocytes around necrobiotic collagen
- Dermal mucin +ve; giant cells are rare
- Variants: perforating (superficial), subcutaneous, diffuse (seen in DM)

Rheumatoid nodule
- Like GA but larger and deeper
- Usu. only found in seropositive cases of RhA (∴ check CPC before diagnosing it)

Paraprotein-associated xanthogranuloma with necrobiosis
- Xanthogranulomatous inflammation separated by necrobiotic collagen
- May extend deep (clin d/dg incl. Weber-Christian disease)

Urticaria
- Clinically 'hives'
- Perivascular oedema (easiest to see in superficial vessels *cf.* deep)
- Telangiectasia (incl. ↑ lymphatic channels)
- Later get a sparse perivascular inflam^y cell infiltrate (eos. ± PMN early → mononuclear later)

Urticarial Vasculitis
- Like urticaria but with evidence of vasculitis
- Subtle vasculitis (leukocytoclasia and fibrinoid change)
- d/dg: consider CTD esp. LE, RhA

Cuteneous Mastocytosis
- Incl.: urticaria pigmentosa, maculopapular and diffuse cutaneous mastocytosis, solitary mastocytoma
- Infantile: lightly pigmented macules, regress; Adult: more pigment ± telangiectasia, no spontaneous regression, systemic involvement common. May present as bullous lesions
- Epidermis: ↑pigmentation of the basal layer
- Papillary dermis: mast cells (some spindled) may form sheets / nodules / perivasc. cuffs ± eosinophils
- Nodular lesions may extend to subcutis (typically in solitary mastocytoma)
- Superficial lymphohistiocytic infiltrate (esp. adults)
- Variant: bullous mastocytosis – subepidermal split with festooning

Actinic Reticuloid
- Chronic photodermatitis of elderly men. Reversible. Pruritic, thick, red skin (d/dg MF)
- Multinucleated stellate myofibroblasts (may be worrying) ± granulomatous inflam^n
- Actinic damage and mixed, deep dermal infiltrate incl. eosinophils.
- Lymphocytes may be atypical (d/dg MF)
- Psoriasiform acanthosis, little epidermotropism, ± Pautrioid collections (d/dg MF)

Lymphomatoid Papulosis (LyP)
- Clin.: M>F, 30s, continuing eruption of self-healing ulcerating papules
- Histology looks like a lymphoma:
  - dense infiltrate of atypical lymphocytes that are: ← lichenoid superficially / perivascular deeply / wedge-shaped rarely
  - epidermal ulceration / necrosis
  - vascular endothelial proliferation
- Willemze type: A) large cells, moderate-abundant cytoplasm, RS-like (CD30 +ve), mixed cellularity
  - B) more monomorphic Sézary/MF-like cells with occasional large cells
  - C) like A but anaplastic lymphoma histol. (sheets of large cells, less mixed cellularity)

Granuloma Faciale
- Dense (band-like and perifollicular) superficial mixed inflam^y cell infiltrate with Grenz (clear) zone
- Nuclear dust
- One of the 'fibrosing vasculitis' group (includes erythema elevatum diutinum – EED)
- d/dg *erythema elevatum diutinum*: EED has more PMN and dust (i.e. a frank LCV is more obvious), has less of a Grenz zone and is dapsone sensitive
- d/dg isolated fibrosing vasculitis: this may be present without either granuloma faciale or EED

Pernio (Chilblains)
- Papillary dermal oedema and superficial and deep lymphocytic vasculitis 2° to cold exposure

Lupus Pernio
- Sarcoid of the skin of the face
- d/dg acne rosacea (= granulomatous reaction around vellus hair follicle infundibulae)

Sweet Syndrome (Acute Febrile Neutrophilic Dermatosis)
- Clin.: red plaques ± pustules assoc[d] with resp. infection, pregnancy, AML, other cancers, etc.
- Papillary dermal oedema (± vesiculation)
- Band of reticular dermal PMN with leukocytoclasia ± RBC extravasat[n] but no frank vessel damage
- Later mononuclear cells become more numerous
- d/dg: pyoderma gangrenosum, cellulitis, dermis near abscess/folliculitis, granulomatous vasculitides

Pustules in the Skin
- Intraepidermal: subcorneal pustular dermatosis, bullous impetigo, drugs, psoriasis, HSV / VZV
- Intradermal: pustular contact dermatitis, *pustulosis palmaris et plantaris, pemphigus vegetans*

Caseation in the Skin
- *Lupus miliaris disseminatus facei* – caseating dermal granulomas (may be assoc[d] with TB)
- Bazin disease – calves of adolescent girls with a positive tuberculin test
- TB (! d/dg granulomatous rosacea may have necrotising or sarcoidal granulomas focally as a reaction to sebaceous material)

Deposits in the Skin

Amyloid
- *Lichen amyloidosus:* itchy, raised rash, rare in Caucasians; epidermal hyperplasia, mild chronic inflam[n] ± pigmentary incontinence, amorphous small amyloid globules in the papillary dermis, ± basal vacuolar change, ± dyskeratoses; d/dg: lichen simplex chronicus, colloid milium, hyalinoses
- Macular amyloidosis is similar to *lichen amyloidosus* but without epidermal hyperplasia
- 1° localised nodular amyloidosis: larger masses in the dermis or around vessels
Colloid milium
- Clin: sporadic (elderly, actinic) or familial (young, hyalinosis); 1–2mm semi-translucent papules
- Rounded cracked hyaline masses in the superficial dermis, may stain like amyloid (d/dg is clinical)
Calcium
- Calcinosis cutis: amorphous mass of calcific material ± giant cell reaction at periphery. Look for underlying CTD / other cause of dystrophic Ca^{2+} before calling it 'idiopathic'. *Idiopathic scrotal calcinosis* is a subtype that may show the remnants of an epidermal cyst lining in serial sections
- Calciphylaxis: serious necrotising lesion of dermis and subcutis usu. assoc[d] with ↑PTH/CRF and caused by fibroblastic endarterial occlusion of small and medium-sized vessels with Ca^{2+} in their walls
Elastic
- Elastic globules (blue autofluorescence in UV light) may be a normal finding in some circumstances
- Actinic elastosis (may have a giant cell response = annular elastolytic giant cell granuloma)
Hyalinoses / metabolic disorders
- Pattern may be globular, vascular, or extensive dermal deposits of a variety of materials e.g. familial amyloid, Russell and colloid bodies, colloid milia, fibrinoid, cryoglobulins, BM material (porphyrias)
- Massive cutaneous hyalinosis: deep dermal and subcutis nodules composed of monoclonal κ light chains but not in amyloid form
- Juvenile hyaline fibromatosis: d/dg keloid in children
- Gout: uric acid deposits (may dissolve out of sections)
- Dermal mucins: myxoedema, LE, scleroedema, etc.

Cutaneous Leishmaniasis
- May see an ulcerating granulomatous lesion extending deeply (± fibrinoid necrosis)
- ± Little double-dots in the macrophages (esp. on Giemsa – see Chapter 23: Infection and Immunity)

Morphoea / PSS
- Early: endothelial swelling and a lymphoplasmacytic infiltrate (perivascular, peri-eccrine and at dermo-subcutis junction) with horizontal fibroplasia of mid and deep dermis
- Later: scarring (loss of rete) and adnexal atrophy, no mucin, pilosebaceous units are usu. absent
- In late stages inflam^n is sparse but may persist at the periphery of the lesion / around eccrine coils
- May affect subcutis (as a sclerotic septal panniculitis)
- d/dg scleroedema, scleromyxoedema / lichen myxoedematosus (*vide infra*)
- d/dg lichen sclerosus: band-like infiltrate, epidermal basal lamina damage, site (see p. 215)
- d/dg scarring (traumatic): consider the history, cellularity $\pm$ haemosiderin / foamy Mϕ

Eosinophilic fasciitis (Shulman's syndrome)
- Clin. diagnosis: PB eosinophilia, skin lesions (spare the face) $\pm$ pain. Also seen with the L-tryptophan eosinophilia-myalgia syndrome. *Morphoea profunda* is clinicopathological overlap (usu. ANA +ve)
- Mixed chronic inflam^n of the deep fascia $\pm$ skeletal muscle
- May expand the intralobular septa of subcutis and involve the deep dermis
- Variable eosinophils (may be absent, not required for diagnosis) and plasma cells (esp. perivascular)

Scleromyxoedema / Papular Mucinosis (Lichen Myxoedematosus)
- Scleromyxoedema has papules and confluences while papular mucinosis has only papules
- Assoc^d with paraprotein / monoclonal gammopathy
- Mucin in upper third of the dermis
- ↑ Mast cells and fibroblasts

Scleroedema (= Scleredema)
- Clin.: adults, upper back, non-pitting woody thick skin; post URT infection / assoc^d with DM
- ↑ Collagen (hypocellular) of normal pattern and with interspersed mucin (subtle) $\pm$ trapped adipocytes
- d/dg morphoea / PSS: scleroedema has mucin and no scarring (rete flattening, adnexal atrophy)
- d/dg nuchal-type fibroma: same histology but more localised; esp. on back of neck $\pm$ Gardner's

Leukocytoclastic Vasculitis (LCV)
- Clinically 'palpable purpura' in dependent areas (limbs / buttocks); associated with ⟨ Malignancy / Autoimmune disease / Infection / Drugs/viruses
- Immune complex mediated acute vasculitis of dermal venules
- PMN in vessel wall and karyorrhexis $\pm$ RBC extravasation / haemosiderin
- Usu. no systemic vasculitis *except* with Henoch-Schönlein purpura (= arthralgia, GI bleeds, GN)
- Direct IF: IgG and C3 in vessel wall, but immuno may be −ve in old lesions (> 24h)
- Thrombosis and fibrinoid necrosis (*NB*: seborrhoeic dermatitis can give leukocytoclasia without these)
- Anetoderma (= macular atrophy: loss of elastin in upper and mid dermis) may have LCV early on but more typically shows a mild mononuclear infiltrate.   medium-sized vessels also involved
- Also get a small vessel vasculitis in PAN and Wegener's but: ⟨ subcutis as well as dermis involved
- Other causes incl. EED and HSV (for more information, see p. 71)

Lymphocytic Vasculitis
- Def^n: perivascular / intramural lymphocytes and extravasation of erythrocytes
- Pigmented purpuric dermatoses e.g. lichen aureus (that has a band-like infiltrate, Grenz zone and $\approx$ normal epidermis) and others (which have a perivascular infiltrate, spongiosis and exocytosis): these all have superficial / papillary dermal haemosiderin (*cf.* d/dg stasis dermatitis)
- Toxic erythema (clin. rash assoc^d with pregnancy, food, drugs, viruses, etc.)
- Rickettsial or viral exanthem (viruses can also result in LCV, e.g. around an HSV blister)
- Pernio, PLEVA and PLC (see p. 300 and p. 298)
- Drug eruption, CTD and Behçet's (can all also result in LCV)
- Sclerosing vasculitides: isolated, EED and granuloma faciale (see p. 299)
- *Pyoderma gangrenosum*: a non-specific chronic ulcer with PMN predominating in the dermis but mononuclear/granulomatous inflam^n may predominate deeply (into the subcutis). Any vasculitis is often 2°. May begin as coalescence of folliculitis. Occurs isolated or with various systemic diseases

Parapsoriasis
- Large plaque parapsoriasis = early (patch stage) MF:
    - ➤ papillary dermal oedema and psoriasiform acanthosis
    - ➤ atypical lymphocytes in papillary dermis and epidermis (without spongiosis)
- Small plaque parapsoriasis = chronic superficial dermatitis (a mild psoriasiform eczema *without* a thinned suprapapillary plate, PMN exocytosis, prominent papillary dermal capillaries or ↑mitoses)

Pagetoid Reticulosis
- Strictly epidermal MF
- Solitary lesion (= Woringer-Kolopp disease), otherwise it's probably not Pagetoid reticulosis
- T-cells are usu. CD30 +ve, CD4/8/neither +ve, γδ ±ve
- Excellent prognosis

Primary Cutaneous CD30 +ve Large T-cell Lymphoma
- Def^n: ① large cells should comprise ≥30% of the neoplastic population
             ② ≥75% of the large cells must be CD30 +ve
             ③ exclude systemic disease by CPC
- Not children   (i.e. rare in children)
- Not EMA   (i.e. usu. EMA −ve)
- Not ALK   (i.e. usu. ALK t(2;5) −ve)
- The tumour is usu. localised but upto 10% cases have nodal involvement
- A solitary, non-regressing lesion resembling LyP (A or B) on histology is called 'Anaplastic lymphoma, LyP-like' – it is considered a 'borderline lesion'
- Pseudoepitheliomatous hyperplasia may be florid (! d/dg SCC)

Other CD30 Positive Infiltrates
- Transformed tumour stage MF (a bad prognostic)
- LyP of Willemze type A
- 2° CD30 +ve ALCL (ALK and EMA +ve and clinical LNp)
- HL in the skin

B-Cell and Other Lymphomas
- d/dg reactive hyperplasia (e.g. insect bite, *Borrelia burgdorferi*, post vaccination / injection / acupuncture, hypersensitivity to heavy metals, idiopathic): Lymphomas may show destruction of adnexa and a deep-predominant pattern of infiltration (a weak feature); lymphocyte morphology, immuno and CPC also help. (For more on skin lymphomas and d/dg hyperplasia, see p. 110)

Follicular Mucinosis
- Children: benign, lymphocytes and eosinophils
- Adults: mycosis fungoides, cerebriform lymphocytes

Borderline Lesions (Borderline Cutaneous T-cell Proliferations)
- LyP of Willemze type C
- LyP-like ALCL (i.e. anaplastic lymphoma, LyP-like subtype thereof)

Pannus Adiposus

Panniculitis
- Any cause may show fat necrosis, Ca^{2+} and lipogranulomatous inflam^n and some may ulcerate
- There is variable overlap in the site of the inflam^n between septal and lobular types ∝ the stage of disease

Weber-Christian disease
- Clin: relapsing febrile nodular panniculitis – it is a diagnosis of exclusion (see d/dg)
- Mixed inflam^n but PMN and lobular predominant panniculitis without abscess formation
- Later: microcysts of free fat may develop and may discharge to the surface; may get dense fibrosis
- d/dg: LE, $α_1AT↓$, cold/trauma/factitial or histiocytic cytophagic panniculitis, other specific cause

Septal panniculitis
- *Erythema nodosum*: PMN and lymphocytic inflam^n expand septa → granulomatous inflam^n → fibrosis
- α-1-antitrypsin deficiency: PMN inflam^n and dissolution of collagen → adipose lobules 'float' in pus
- Sclerotic types: deep morphoea, eosinophilic fasciitis and ischaemic liposclerosis
- d/dg deep extension of necrobiotic diseases, infections or vasculitis

Lobular panniculitis
- Pancreatic panniculitis: basophilic ring adipocytes (anucleate) and calcification
- Lupus panniculitis: basophilic ring adipocytes, lymphocytic + plasma cell inflam^n, septal mucin ± overlying lupus
- Granulomatous vasculitis: nodular vasculitis = *erythema induratum* (if evidence of TB = Bazin's)
- PAN (PMN and fibrinoid necrosis in vessels) / calciphylaxis (calcification of small vessels)
- Subcutaneous fat necrosis of the newborn child / sclerema neonatorum } *vide infra*

Mixed lobular / septal panniculitis
- Cold/trauma-induced (incl. factitial) panniculitis: ± PMN, haemorrhage, Ca^{2+}, foreign/faecal matter
- Infection: direct mycobacterial infection, gummatous syphilis
- Abnormal cell infiltrates: Rosai-Dorfman disease, TCL (panniculitis-like, angiocentric, etc, − p. 114), histiocytic cytophagic panniculitis (= haemorrhagic panniculitis with haemophagocytic syndrome: may see 'bean bag cells' = Mφ with engulfed lymphocytes, RBC and other cell fragments)
- Granulomatous, other: Crohn's, sarcoid (d/dg WG, Churg-Strauss syndrome, etc.)

Sclerema Neonatorum
- Clin.: lardaceous sick baby, fatal, IEM
- Needle clefts containing crystals but no or minimal inflammation / fat necrosis
- Widened septa

Subcutaneous Fat Necrosis of the New Born
- Clin.: nodules on cheeks, buttocks, rest of body. Good health, benign, ? birth trauma related
- Needle clefts, basophilic fat necrosis, giant cell inflammation, focal calcium deposits

Blistering Diseases

Overview Mnemonic
- **Pemphi**(gus/goid)
- **Ery**thema multiforme (see p. 297)
- **Herpeti**formis (DH) *et al.* (linear IgA disease and chronic bullous dermatosis)
- **Epi**dermolysis bullosa acquisita / congenita
- **Porphy**rias
- Some others (HSV / VZV, pompholyx / pustular disorders, bullous variants e.g. of LP, LE, etc.)

The Pemphigus Group
- Acantholysis → intraepidermal blisters; may involve adnexal epithelium, ± Nikolsky sign
- Direct IF (on *peri*lesional skin): IgG ± C3 in intercellular spaces
- Indirect IF[6] shows circulating Ab to keratinocyte surface glycoproteins (e.g. desmoglein 1 in foliaceous or desmoglein 3 in vulgaris); disease severity ∝ titre (∴ used for monitoring)

Pemphigus vulgaris
- Clin.: middle-aged onwards; blister and erosions at mucocutaneous junctions and intertriginous areas
- May be extensive and life threatening if not Rx (currently with steroids / immunosuppression)
- Suprabasal split → rounded cavity cells and 'tombstone' appearance of remaining basal cells
- Early: spongiosis of lower epidermis (± eos.); late: mixed dermal chronic inflam^n
- Healing results in >1 layer of cells beneath the split/erosion and epidermal downgrowths ('villi')

Pemphigus vegetans
- Neumann type starts as pemphigus vulgaris, Hallopeau type starts as suprabasal acantholytic clefts
- In both types the lesions heal with verrucous epidermal hyperplasia with pronounced villi
- Intraepidermal eosinophils and eosinophil abscesses

---

[6] the patient's serum is applied to a section of monkey oesophagus or normal human skin (from a donor) then labelled with fluorescent anti-human Ig to reveal any Ig in the patient's serum that may have bound to the tissue

Pemphigus foliaceous
- Younger (patients), better (prognosis) and higher (split – at stratum granulosum) *cf.* vulgaris

Pemphigus erythematosus
- Clin.: mild form of foliaceous resembling LE but localised to the head and neck; ± MG and thymoma
- Direct IF: intercellular deposits and a Lupus band

Benign familial chronic pemphigus (Hailey-Hailey disease)
- Clin.: AD, 20–30 years, intertriginous areas affected
- Micro: epidermis shows 'dilapidated brick wall' acantholysis, IF is −ve

Differential diagnosis of pemphigus
- Actinic / post radioRx acantholysis
- Darier's disease = multiple keratosis follicularis (KF) – see p. 282 under 'Acanthoma'
- Warty dyskeratoma = solitary KF – see p. 282 under 'Acanthoma'
- Grover's disease (transient acantholytic dermatosis): small areas of acantholysis (!∴ do levels) that may resemble Darier's, SD, pemphigus or Hailey-Hailey disease
- Subcorneal pustular dermatosis (SPD): pustules (± spongiform ∴ d/dg psoriasis), ± acantholysis
- IgA pemphigus is an SPD subtype with direct IF showing intercellular IgA (not IgG)
- Bullous impetigo (no acanthosis *cf.* d/dg SPD, a Gram stain may show bugs)
- Older lesions of dermatitis herpetiformis (DH) (d/dg IgA pemphigus)
- Scabies (scabies may produce circulating bullous *pemphigoid* Ags) – diagnosis requires finding the mite, eggs/shells or faeces in the burrow which is mostly intracorneal (→ intraepidermal at the end)
- Viruses: HSV / VZV (blister/pustule ± inclusions ± underlying LCV) or pox (± pilosebaceous units)
- Acantholytic SCC (*vs.* vegetans which lacks atypia and shows eosinophil abscesses)
- Psoriasis (*vs.* foliaceous but this is more of a clinical similarity *cf.* histological)
- Paraneoplastic acantholysis: esp. seen with NHL / CLL / Castleman / thymoma / sarcomas this shows +ve indirect IF on rat bladder (unlike the pemphigus group)
- Necrolytic erythemas: shows d/dg psoriasis-like spongiform pustules and parakeratosis with intracellular oedema just below the stratum granulosum. Examples are: necrolytic acral erythema (HCV), acrodermatitis enteropathica (AR Zn deficiency), pellagra (deficiency of niacin / tryptophan), necrolytic migratory erythema (glucagonoma)
- Incontinentia pigmenti (p. 297) and drug-induced pemphigus can be distinguished by CPC

The Pemphigoids
Bullous pemphigoid
- Clin.: elderly; steroid responsive, large, tense bullae distributed: —⟨ Widespread / Oral (and other) mucosae / Limbs / Flexors
- Subepidermal split and dermal eosinophils
- Direct IF: IgG and C3 at the DEJ at the *lamina lucida* – take Bx from a small new lesion
- Indirect IF: circulating IgG ➢ to an extracellular glycoprotein in the BM zone of the DEJ
  ➢ to an intracellular keratinocyte hemidesmosome (70–100%)
  ➢ severity NOT ∝ titre

Cicatricial pemphigoid
- Clin.: chronic, scarring mucosal disease (esp. oral / oesophageal / conjunctival)
- Direct IF: linear IgG in the DEJ
- Indirect IF: rarely shows circulating Ig (only 10% of cases)

Differential diagnosis of pemphigoid
- Herpes gestationis, DH, chronic bullous dermatosis   } *vide infra*
- EBA: use the salt split skin test (see p. 305, under EBA) or the alcohol-fixed indirect IF test (pemphigoid antigenicity is destroyed but EBA is preserved)
- Bullous variants of: lichen planus, amyloidosis, mastocytosis, drug/arthropod reaction and LE

Herpes Gestationis (Pemphigoid Gestationis)
- Clin.: itchy, vesicular eruption; pregnancy / puerperium; recurs; ± miscarriage
- Subepidermal split (due to basal cell necrosis) and eosinophils ++
- Direct IF: linear C3 at the DEJ at the *lamina lucida* (in 100% of cases)
- Indirect IF: circulating IgG (herpes gestationis factor, HGF)
- HGF fixes C3 at the DEJ in normal human skin *in vitro*

Dermatitis Herpetiformis
- Clin.: chronic, young adults, widespread groups of itchy (dapsone sensitive) papules and vesicles, usu. symmetrical, gluten sensitive jejunopathy (75%) but only a minority have malabsorption clinically
- Associations: HLA B8, DR3 and DQw2
- Subepidermal split with PMN and oedema in dermal papillae tips, the PMN may form microabscesses
- Older lesions show acantholysis, eosinophils, vasculitis → d/dg pemphigus (esp. IgA pemphigus)
- Direct IF: granular IgA (includes J-chain ∴ is dimeric and possibly from gut)
- Indirect IF: no circulating Abs – but serology is usu. +ve for IgA-class anti-tTG Abs
- Immuno EM: deposits just below the *lamina densa* (at the anchoring fibrils)

Linear IgA Disease (Adult Type) and Chronic Bullous Dermatosis of Childhood – see Table 20.1

TABLE 20.1   Linear IgA disease or chronic bullous dermatosis?

Feature	Linear IgA Disease (Adult Type)	Chronic Bullous Dermatosis of Childhood
clinical	idiopathic / drug-induced	self limiting (usu. gone by age 8)
histology	similar to DH	similar to DH
assoc^{n}s	low incidence of HLA B8 & gluten sensitivity	assoc^d with HLA B8 but not gluten sensitivity
direct IF	linear IgA	linear IgA
indirect IF	no circulating Ab	circulating Ig common

Epidermolysis Bullosa Acquisita (EBA)
- Clin.: adults, trauma → blisters on wrists, fingers, feet
- Associations: **A**utoimmune disease / amyloid; **B**owel disease (CIBD); **C**ancers
- Subepidermal split: non-inflam^y with festooning (d/dg porphyria) or inflam^y (d/dg DH, pemphigoid)
- Direct IF: linear IgG and C3 at DEJ (Bx non-blistered skin – e.g. peri-lesional – else ↑false −ve)
- Indirect IF: circulating Ig is uncommon (only 25% of cases)
- Immuno EM: deposits just below the *lamina densa* (Abs target type VII collagen)
- d/dg bullous pemphigoid (do split skin test): apply patient's serum to normal skin split with 1M NaCl then label with anti-human IgG labelled Ab. In pemphigoid IgG binds to the epidermal part of the split skin. In EBA it binds to the dermal part. (See also the alcohol-fixed indirect IF test, p. 304)

The Porphyrias
- Clin.: photosensitive cutaneous disease in all types (except acute intermittent porphyria)
- Accumulation of PAS +ve material (= type IV collagen) around dermal blood vessels and DEJ
- Non-inflam^y split at DEJ, dermal papillae project into cavity (i.e. 'festooning') ± actinic damage
- Direct IF: IgG passively entrapped within the PAS +ve material (i.e. *not* immune-mediated)

RadioRx (Effects of Ionising Radiation)

Acute Radiation Effects (up to 6 months post exposure)
- Clin.: epilation / erythema → radiodermatitis (erythema, inflam^n, dry desquamation) → radiation burn (wet desquamation, vesicles, ulceration); the extent of these changes will depend on the dose
- Epidermis: spongiosis, intraepidermal ± DEJ vesicles → confluent epidermal necrosis and ulceration with upper dermal fibrin deposition (≈ second degree thermal burn)
- ↓ Mitoses, loss of hair shafts, follicular keratin plugs
- Swelling of epithelial and endothelial cells with ↑ apoptoses
- Upper dermal oedema, capillary dilatation, arteriolar fibrin thrombi, ↑melanin pigment
- Mixed *diffuse* dermal inflam^n (incl. PMN and eos.) ± exocytosis

Chronic Radiation Effects
- Clin.: poikiloderma (due to thin epidermis variable melanocyte enzyme activity and capillary ectasia)
- Epidermis: variably atrophic with flattening of rete pegs ± dyskeratosis, basal/sub-basal vacuolation
- Atypia of basal keratinocytes ± melanocytes (! some report occasional atypical mitoses)
- Papillary and reticular dermis replaced by irregular hyaline fibrosis (pale on H&E) with fibrillary interstitial fibrinoid and prominent elastosis (can go deep and incl. subcutis – unlike d/dg solar elastosis)
- Atypical fibroblasts: plump, angular, amphophil cytoplasm, vesicular nuclei ± binucleate forms
- Dermal capillary ectasia, anisochromasia of plump endothelial cells, arteriolar hyaline, endarteritis obliterans of larger vessels (usu. scant) and fibrinoid necrosis (usu. 2° – e.g. near ulcers)

- Chronic ulcers have a fibrinopurulent base but little or no granulation tissue
- ± Pigmentary incontinence, ± siderophages (but not dermal inflam^n unless 2° pathology is present)
- Patchy destruction of pilosebaceous units → bulbous scars near plugged infudibula / arrector pili

Radiation Atypias and Neoplasia
- Benign cytomegaly may occur at any time in any cell type: NCR is normal, irreg. nuclear membrane (not thickened), cytoplasmic +/ nuclear vacuolation, multinucleation, bizarre shapes, irreg. staining
- Epidermal dysplasia (AK-like) occurs after some years and SCC after 15–20 years (on average)
- Atypical vascular lesions (similar to those described in the breast – see p. 320) and d/dg angiosarcoma: both may be multiple and occur after 1–20 years (average 3 years for benign, 6 years for malig.)
- Hobnail haemangioma-like vascular lesions (confined to dermis – unlike angiosarcoma):
  - ➤ wedge-shaped 'proliferations' (but no mitoses and Ki-67 is −ve) – thin end of wedge is deep
  - ➤ dilated (usu. empty) vascular spaces superficially, more slit-like deeper
  - ➤ plump ± hyperchromatic endothelium (but no multilayering or other angiosarcoma-like atypia)
  - ➤ ± small papillaroid intralumenal stromal projections (d/dg Dabska's tumour in children – but that is often subcutaneous with a lymphoid infiltrate and dilated channels with florid tuftings [the adult equivalent is reteform haemangioendothelioma – this has flatter branching spaces])

Immunodeficiency

Graft vs. Host Disease (GVHD)
- Clin.: skin changes, hepatic dysfunction and diarrhoea
- Aetiology: congenital (maternal lymphocytes) / acquired (post BMTx, liver, SI, lung and kidney Tx)
- Acute graft *vs.* host skin reaction (GVHR) starts in the 1st 3 months post Tx and is important because it precedes hepatic and GIT involvement (early Rx gives best chance of survival):
  - ➤ papillary dermis: ☞ sparse lymphocytic infiltrate and exocytosis (otherwise the changes could be due to radiation)
    - ☞ RBC extravasation and siderophages (but no true vasculitis)
    - ☞ Civatte bodies (are not, in themselves, diagnostic of lichenoid change)
    - ☞ ± PMN and eosinophils
  - ➤ epidermis:
    - Grade 1: vacuolar interface change – starts at deep tips of rete ridges and hair follicles
    - Grade 2: dyskeratosis ± satellite cell necrosis (= 'satellitosis' – lymphocytes partly surround an apoptotic cell)
    - Grade 3: sub-epidermal clefting (due to coalescence of necrotic keratinocytes)
    - Grade 4: complete sloughing (loss) of necrotic epidermis
  - ➤ d/dg: viral exanthem, fungal infection, chemo/radioRx effect ∴ use CPC and exclude specific pathogens by appropriate stains
  - ➤ d/dg: TEN (and other members of the erythema multiforme group):
    - ☞ can be impossible to differentiate (need CPC ± serial [in time] Bx with immuno)
    - ☞ PMN favour GVHR
    - ☞ pilosebaceous involvement favours GVHR (eccrine occurs in both)
  - ➤ immuno: ☞ NK cells (CD16, CD56) in the epidermis favour GVHR over TEN
    - ☞ T-cell:Mϕ ratio: ◆ purely Mϕ favours lymphocyte depleted GVHR over TEN
      - ◆ mixed, Mϕ predominant or 1:1 favours TEN over GVHR
      - ◆ mixed, T-cell predominant favours GVHR over TEN
- Chronic: (usu. after 100 days)
  - ➤ early lichenoid stage: like LP (may also occur in acute GVHR, either way it's a bad prognostic)
  - ➤ late sclerotic stage: epidermal atrophy and ↑ pigment, thickened dermis, loss of adnexa

HIV / AIDS and the Skin
- Acute HIV exanthem (micro: just a perivascular lymphohistiocytic infiltrate)
- Eosinophilic folliculitis:
  - ➤ pruritic reaction to infundibular Ag, may indicate advanced HIV (low CD4 count)
  - ➤ early: lymphocytes and eos. in sebaceous duct / infundibular region → mixed exocytosis and spongiosis
  - ➤ later: florid perifollicular inflam^n → fibrosis

- (Staphylococcal) folliculitis
- Seborrhoeic dermatitis ($\pm$ dyskeratosis, leukocytoclasia and plasma cells in HIV)
- Psoriasis
- LP (hypertrophic)
- Photosensitivity (chronic actinic dermatitis, photosensitive granuloma annulare, hyperpigmentation)
- HIV interface dermatitis: vacuolar degeneration ++, no eosinophils / neutrophils
- KS: prognosis $\propto$ HIV disease activity and level of immunosuppression (see pp. 322–323)
- T-cell lymphomas (*cf.* EBV-related DLBCL elsewhere); MF is rare $\therefore$ consider CD8 +ve mimic
- Opportunistic infections (often occur with a low CD4 count – <150 cells/μl):
    - oesophageal candidiasis; cutaneous Histoplasma, Cryptococcus and Candida (the commonest)
    - CMV, giant and verrucous molluscum, persistent herpes (HSV and VZV have the same histology)
    - atypical mycobacteria
- Oral hairy leukoplakia: prognosis is poor if CD4 count is >300 (see p. 133)
- Bacillary angiomatosis (more often multiple *cf.* d/dg pyogenic granuloma – see p. 319)
- Nodular / Norwegan scabies (! d/dg resemble pseudolymphoma): see p. 304 (under 'Differential diagnosis of pemphigus') and p. 349
- Drug eruptions: photosensitive / lichenoid with eosinophils / erythema multiforme group
- Immune Reconstitution Disease Syndrome (IRDS – due to HAART) – CMV and erosive HSV

Bibliography

Alsaad, K.O., Obaidat, N.A. and Ghazarian, D. (2007) Skin adnexal neoplasms – part 1: An approach to tumours of the pilosebaceous unit. *Journal of Clinical Pathology*, **60** (2), 129–144.

Azorin, D., Rodriguez-Peralto, J.L., Garcia-Garcia, E. *et al.* (2003) Cutaneous papillary squamous carcinoma. Report of three new cases and review of the literature. *Virchows Arch*, **442** (3), 298–301.

Bittencourt, A.L., Monteiro, D.A. and De Pretto, O.J. (2007) Infiltrating giant cellular blue naevus. *Journal of Clinical Pathology*, **60** (1), 82–84.

Brenn, T. and Fletcher, C.D.M. (2005) Radiation-associated cutaneous atypical vascular lesions and angiosarcoma. Clinicopathologic analysis of 42 cases. *American Journal of Surgical Pathology*, **29** (8), 983–996.

Busam, K.J. and Barnhill, R.L. (1995) The spectrum of Spitz tumours, in *Progress in Pathology*, Vol. 2 (eds N. Kirkham and P. Hall), Churchill Livingstone, Edinburgh, pp. 31–46.

Busam, K.J., Chen, Y.T., Old, L.J. *et al.* (1998) Expression of Melan-A (MART1) in benign melanocytic naevi and primary cutaneous malignant melanoma. *American Journal of Surgical Pathology*, **22** (8), 976–982.

Cerroni, L., Gatter, K. and Kerl, H. (2004) *An Illustrated Guide to Skin Lymphomas*, 2nd edn, Blackwell Publishing Ltd., Oxford.

Chorny, J.A. and Barr, R.J. (2002) S100-positive spindle cells in scars a diagnostic pitfall in the re-excision of desmoplastic melanoma. *American Journal of Dermatopathology*, **24** (4), 309–312.

Cook, M. (2003) Cutaneous malignant melanoma. *Royal College of Pathologists: Education in Pathology*, **123**, 26–27.

Cerio, R. (ed) (2001) *Dermatopathology*, Springer-Verlag, Berlin.

Culpepper, K.S., Granter, S.R. and McKee, P.H. (2004) My approach to atypical melanocytic lesions. *Journal of Clinical Pathology*, **57** (11), 1121–1131.

Ding, X., Diaz, L.A., Fairley, J.A. *et al.* (1991) The anti-desmoglein 1 autoantibodies in pemphigus vulgaris sera are pathogenic. *Journal of Investigative Dermatology*, **112** (5), 739–743.

Elder, D., Elenitsas, R., Jaworsk, C. *et al.* (1997) *Lever's Histopathology of the Skin*, 8th edn, Lippincott-Raven, Philadelphia.

Elder, D., Elenitsas, R., Johnson, B. Jr. *et al.* (1999) *Synopsis and Atlas of Lever's Histopathology of the Skin*, 1st edn, Lippincott Williams & Wilkin, Philadelphia.

Fajardo, L.F. and Berthrong, M. (1981) Radiation injury in surgical pathology Part III. Salivary glands, pancreas and skin. *American Journal of Surgical Pathology*, **5** (3), 279–296.

Farthing, P.M., Bouquot, J.E. and Speight, P.M. (2006) Problems and pitfalls in oral mucosal pathology. *Current Diagnostic Pathology*, **12** (1), 66–74.

Francis, N. (2003) Immunosuppression-related cutaneous disease. *Royal College of Pathologists: Education in Pathology*, **123**, 31–32.

Goodlad, J.R. and Hollowood, K. (2001) Primary cutaneous B-cell lymphoma. *Current Diagnostic Pathology*, **7** (1), 33–44.

Janssens, A.S., Heide, R., den Hollander, J.C. *et al.* (2005) Mast cell distribution in normal adult skin. *Journal of Clinical Pathology*, **58** (3), 285–289.

Junqueira, L.C., Carneiro, J. and Long, J.A. (1986) *Basic Histology*, 5th edn, Appleton-Century-Crofts (Prentice-Hall), Norwalk, CT.

Kohler, S., Hendrickson, M.R., Chao, N.J. *et al.* (1997) Value of skin biopsies in assessing prognosis and progression of acute graft-versus-host disease. *American Journal of Surgical Pathology*, **21** (9), 988–996.

Lombart, B., Monteagudo, C., López-Guerrero, J.A. *et al.* (2005) Clinicopathological and immunohistochemical analysis of 20 cases of Merkel cell carcinoma in search of prognostic markers. *Histopathology*, **46** (6), 622–634.

MacKie, R.M. (1996) *Skin Cancer*, 2nd edn, Martin Dunitz, Ltd., London.

MacLennan, K.A. and Diebold, J. (1998) Anaplastic large cell lymphoma. *Current Diagnostic Pathology*, **5** (4), 165–173.

McGovern, V.J. (1976) *Malignant Melanoma: Clinical & Histological Diagnosis*, John Wiley & Sons, New York.

McKee, P.H. (1997) Diagnosis of autoimmune-mediated acquired sub-epidermal blisters: variation on a theme. *Current Diagnostic Pathology*, **4** (1), 10–19.

McKee, P.H., Calonje, E. and Granter, S.R. (eds) (2005) *Pathology of the Skin with Clinical Correlations*, 3rd edn, Elsevier Mosby, Philadelphia.

McMenamin, M.E. and Sweeney, E.C. (1997) Psoriasis and eczema. *Current Diagnostic Pathology*, **4** (1), 20–27.

Mooi, W.J. (2001) The expanding spectrum of cutaneous blue naevi. *Current Diagnostic Pathology*, **7** (1), 56–58.

Mooney, E.E. and Shea, C.R. (1997) Cutaneous vasculitis. *Current Diagnostic Pathology*, **4** (1), 1–9.

Ng, W-K. (2003) Radiation-associated changes in tissues and tumours. *Current Diagnostic Pathology*, **9** (2), 124–136.

Obaidat, N.A., Alsaad, K.O. and Ghazarian, D. (2007) Skin adnexal neoplasms – part 2: An approach to tumours of cutaneous sweat glands. *Journal of Clinical Pathology*, **60** (2), 145–159.

Orosz, Z. (1999) Melan-A/Mart-1 expression in various melanocytic lesions and in non-melanocytic soft tissue tumours. *Histopathology*, **34** (6), 517–525.

Parker, F. (1988) The structure and function of skin, in *Cecil Textbook of Medicine*, 18th edn (eds J.B. Wyngaarden and L.H. Smith Jr.), W.B. Saunders Company, Philadelphia, pp. 2300–2306.

Ramdial, P.K. (2000) Selected topics in HIV-associated skin pathology. *Current Diagnostic Pathology*, **6** (2), 113–124.

Robson, A. (2003) Inflammatory dermatoses. *Royal College of Pathologists: Education in Pathology*, **123**, 31.

Skelton, H.G. 3rd, Smith, K.J., Barrett, T.L. *et al.* (1991) HMB-45 staining in benign and malignant melanocytic lesions. A reflection of cellular activation. *American Journal of Surgical Pathology*, **13** (6), 543–550.

Stevens, A. and Dalziel, K. (1998) The histopathology of drug rashes. *Current Diagnostic Pathology*, **5** (3), 138–149.

Sundram, U., Harvell, J.D., Rouse, R.V. *et al.* (2003) Expression of the B-cell proliferation marker MUM1 by melanocytic lesions and comparison with S100, gp100 (HMB45), and MelanA. *Modern Pathology*, **16** (8), 802–810.

Kadar, N.R., Kohorn, E.I., LiVolsi, V.A. and Kapp, D.S. (2007) TdT expression in Merkel cell carcinoma: potential diagnostic pitfall with blastic hematological malignancies and expanded immunohistochemical analysis. *Modern Pathology*, **20** (11), 1113–1120.

Symmers, W. St. C. (ed) (1980) *Systemic Pathology*, Vol. 6, 2nd edn, Churchill Livingstone, Edinburgh.

Trejo, O., Reed, J.A. and Prieto, V.G. (2002) Atypical cells in human cutaneous re-excision scars for melanoma express p75NGFR, C56/N-CAM and GAP-43: evidence of early Schwann cell differentiation. *Journal of Cutaneous Pathology*, **29** (7), 397–406.

Ueki, H. and Yaoita, H. (eds) (1989) *A Colour Atlas of Dermatoimmunohistology*, Wolfe Medical Publications, Ltd., London.

Urmacher, C.D. (1997) Normal Skin, in *Histology for Pathologists*, 2nd edn (ed S.S. Sternberg), Lippincott Williams & Wilkins, Philadelphia, pp. 25–45.

Wechsler, J. (2001) Reactive and neoplastic histiocytic skin disorders, in *Progress in Pathology*, Vol. 5 (eds N. Kirkham and N.R. Lemoine), Greenwich Medical Media, Ltd, London, pp. 27–43.

Weedon, D. (2002) *Skin Pathology*, 2nd edn, Churchill Livingstone, London.

Weiss, S.W. and Goldblum, J.R. (eds) (2001) *Enzinger and Weiss' Soft Tissue Tumors*, 4th edn, Mosby, St Louis.

Whiting, D.A. (2001) The histopathology of alopecia areata in vertical and horizontal sections. *Dermatologic Therapy*, **14** (4), 297–305.

Willemze, R. and Meijer, C.J.L.M. (1998) Classification of cutaneous lymphomas: crosstalk between pathologist and clinician. *Current Diagnostic Pathology*, **5** (1), 23–33.

Web sites

Royal College of Pathologists (2002) Standards and minimum datasets for reporting common cancers: Minimum dataset for the histopathological reporting of common skin cancers, 1st edn, www.rcpath.org.uk (accessed May 2005).

21. Soft Tissues

Muscle

Smooth Muscle Tumours (Non-Uterine)
- Usu. well-circ., eosinophilic spindle cells with cigar-shaped nuclei ± terminal paranuclear vacuole
- Immuno: must be at least focally +ve for desmin and αSMA; CK ±ve (in 30%), S100 ±ve (uncommon)
- Variants include: inflammatory (lymphocytes ++), epithelioid (d/dg melanoma)
- d/dg low grade myofibroblastic sarcoma: infiltrative, pale spindle cells, tapered nuclei, no vacuole
- d/dg: melanoma (esp. if S100 is +ve), synovial sarcoma or metastatic CA (esp. if EMA or CK is +ve)

Criteria for malignancy
① In vulval skin: malignant if >2 of: infiltrative, >5cm ∅, ≥5/10 hpf mitoses, > mild atypia; (if only 1 or 2 of these then = 'atypical' and if also coagulative tumour cell necrosis this raises the suspicion of malignancy)

② In somatic soft tissues, scrotal skin or arising from main vessels:
- Mitotic activity is most sig. but size, cellularity, atypia and necrosis also correlate with behaviour
- Benign if amitotic (such leiomyomas also tend to have hyaline, myxoid and calcific areas)
- Nuclear atypia is only acceptable as ancient change if the tumour is *both* hypocellular *and* amitotic

③ In the retroperitoneum – classification by mitotic count:
- 0 / 50 hpf = 'leiomyoma' but may recur. Upgrade to 'potentially malignant' if there is *any* cytol. atypia
- 1–4 / 50 hpf = 'potentially malignant' even more so if large size/cellular/cytol. atypia or necrosis
- ≥5 / 50 hpf = leiomyosarcoma

Exceptions
- Retroperitoneal tumours in old women that resemble uterine leiomyomas and are usu. ER / PgR +ve may have mitotic activity (<10/50 hpf) but are still benign (! d/dg GIST if attached to rectum)
- Dermal (incl. nipple) pilar-type smooth muscle tumours are infiltrative but thought not to have metastatic potential whatever the histology – but any tumour involving the subcutis or well-circumscribed dermal tumours should be treated as for tumours in 'somatic soft tissues' – see ② , above

Myositis Ossificans
- Usu. young, ± Hx of trauma, rapid growth; if multiple consider *myositis / fibrodysplasia ossificans progressiva* (AD, skeletal anomalies, poor prognosis)
- Radiol.: well circ., outer calcific shell, close to bone but not attached to it (= 'air gap' sign)
- Histology: zonation (reversed *cf.* d/dg fracture callus and parosteal osteosarcoma):
  - soft centre: mitotic nodular fasciitis-like proliferation ± remnants of skeletal muscle (the background is loose and vascular *cf.* the dense fibrogenic spindle cell areas in parosteal osteosarcoma)
  - mid-zone: osteoid reams ± chondroid
  - outer shell: maturation to trabecular lamellar bone (! immature lesions lack a shell)

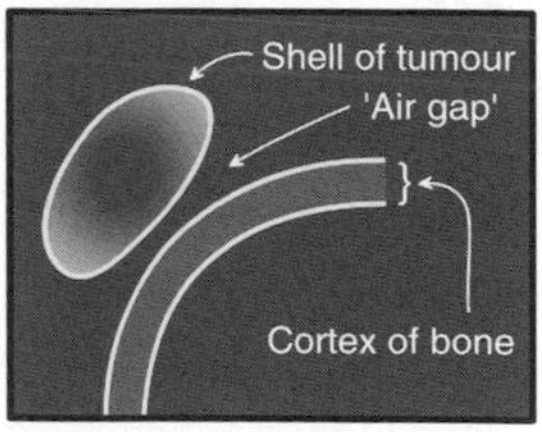

FIGURE 21.1   Air gap sign

- Also occurs in mesentery ('*intra-abdominal myositis ossificans*') and subcutis (*panniculitis ossificans*)
- d/dg soft tissue sarcoma: CPC (incl. radiol.), zonation and lack of cytol. atypia help (nucleoli may be prominent in myositis ossificans and zonation poorly developed but mitoses should not be atypical)
- d/dg osteosarcoma (esp. parosteal, high grade surface and extraskeletal). See p. 337

Rhabdomyosarcoma (RMS)
- For histology, see p. 58 (*NB*: in adults prognosis does *not* correlate well with histotype)
- d/dg 'heterologous elements' in some other tumour (esp. in adults)
- d/dg *mixed mesenchymoma* = any combination of ≥2 of ① osteosarcoma, ② RMS or ③ liposarcoma – without MPNST but regardless of any undiff., MFH or fibrosarcoma elements
- d/dg *malignant Triton tumour* = MPNST with admixed RMS elements

Diagnostic Criteria Handbook in Histopathology: A Surgical Pathology Vade Mecum by Paul J. Tadrous
Copyright © 2007 by John Wiley & Sons, Ltd.

Other Muscle-related Lesions
- *Intramuscular myxoma* (circumscribed, bland, hypocellular and ≈ avascular)
- See sections below for *proliferative myositis, intramuscular lipoma, hibernoma, haemangioma, angiomatosis* and *lipoblastomatosis*
- For *rhabdomyoma* see p. 79 and p. 233

Myofibroblast / Fibroblast

Myofibroblast Immunocytochemistry
- +ve for vimentin and αSMA ± desmin, ± smooth muscle myosin
- Many myofibroblastic *lesions* are CD68 +ve (= 'fibrohistiocytic' differentiation)
- CD117 (cytoplasmic blob +vity, not the membranous accentuation of GIST), CD171 −ve

General Points on (Myo)Fibroblastic Lesions
- Post-op spindle cell nodule, nodular fasciitis and myositis ossificans: have many spindle myofibroblasts
- Proliferative fasciitis / myositis and ischaemic fasciitis: have spindle and ganglion-like myofibroblasts
- Spindle myofibroblasts: abundant eosinophilic fibrillary cytoplasm
- Ganglion-like myofibroblasts: abundant basophil cytoplasm, vesicular nucleus, prominent nucleolus
- d/dg collagenous fibroma *vs.* 'burnt out' fasciitis: fibroma has stellate cells and collagen but few mitoses and is not spontaneously regressing

Post-Operative Spindle Cell Nodule
- Clin.: tumour-like mass in vagina/endometrium/prostatic urethra/bladder 5 weeks–3 months post-op
- Macro: oedematous, ulcerating, infiltrative borders
- Micro: plump fibroblasts with large nucleoli, myxoid stroma, chronic inflam^y infiltrate and upto 25/10hpf mitoses
- d/dg: sarcomas: but post-op nodule cells are not hyperchromatic and have no abnormal mitoses
- Immuno: myofibroblastic (vimentin, desmin and αSMA +ve) ± CK (d/dg spindle cell carcinoma)
- Related entity: *pseudosarcomatous fibromyxoid tumour* of the GU tract (no assoc^d trauma / surgery)

Inflammatory Myofibroblastic Tumour and Inflammatory Pseudotumour
- Synonyms/variants: inflammatory myofibroblastic tumour, plasma cell granuloma, fibroxanthoma (depending on the relative prominence of fibroblasts, plasma cells and foamy Mφ respectively)
- Often discussed as a group but inflam^y myofibroblatic tumour has prom. myofibroblasts with some atypia and ALK-1 +vity and is a true neoplasm while the other variants (inflam^y pseudotumours) are either reactive or autoimmune (some may be part of IgG4-related disease, esp. if plasma cell granuloma type)
- Sites: lung, peritoneum, skin (d/dg angiolymphoid hyperplasia with eosinophilia), stomach, orbit (as part of multifocal fibrosclerosis), bladder, peripheral liver (fibrohistiocytic), perihilar liver (plasma cell granuloma)
- Macro: several cm, well-circ., not encapsulated. In hollow organs it is polypoid ± ulceration
- Plump active fibroblasts ± focal atypia, lymphocytes, plasma cells, Mφ, foamy Mφ
- Variable mitotic rate
- No well-structured collagenisation pattern ± hypocellular stroma ± necrosis ± calcification
- Immuno: myofibroblastic (vimentin, αSMA, ± CK, ± CD68), may be ALK +ve, CD34 is usu. −ve
- Malignancy (= *inflammatory fibrosarcoma*):
  - ➤ is determined by behaviour rather than histology but often shows widespread pleomorphism (but even bland cases may metastasise ∴ some regard all cases as low grade malignant)
  - ➤ behaviour correlates with site: intra-abdominal ones may recur or metastasise; lower GU and lung sites rarely recur or metastasise (*NB*: calcifying fibrous pseudotumour is benign)
  - ➤ other poor prognostics: ganglion-like cells, aneuploidy, p53 +vity
- d/dg SFT: some regard *calcifying fibrous pseudotumour* (has marked hyaline, Ca^{2+} ± psammoma bodies) as a variant of inflammatory myofibroblastic tumour. See SFT section, p. 324
- d/dg spindle cell carcinoma (esp. if CK +ve) or carcinosarcoma (esp. if polypoid in hollow organ)
- d/dg: other sarcoma: inflam^y component, ALK +vity and lack of *abnormal* mitoses
- d/dg other (ALK +vity helps): histiocytoma, plasmacytoma, myofibroblastoma

Nodular Fasciitis
- Rapid ↑, young adult, subcutaneous, intramuscular, *cranial fasciitis* (esp. in children <2 years old), breast, parotid, retroperitoneum and bladder
- Small (<5 cm) with infiltrative margin
- Spindle / stellate ('tissue culture') myofibroblasts with mitoses ± osteoclast-like giant cells
- Myxoid / collagenous matrix ± microcysts ± bone (= *fasciitis ossificans*)
- Microhaemorrhages and sparse lymphocytic infiltrate

Proliferative Fasciitis / Myositis
- Rare, older age (*cf.* nodular fasciitis), rapid ↑mass in subcutis / muscle
- Mixture: plump spindle cells and ganglion-like cells
- Myxoid / collagenous stroma
- Proliferative myositis separates – but does not destroy – muscle fibres

Ischaemic Fasciitis (Atypical Decubital Fibroplasia)
- Elderly, tissue overlying bony prominences
- Larger (≈ upto 8cm), centred on subcutis but can extend deeper
- Lobular architecture with zones (outer to inner): vascular fibroblastic tissue with ganglion-like cells, myxohyaline tissue and central fibrinoid necrosis
- Immuno: CD68 commonly +ve, some are also CD34 +ve

Sclerosing Peritonitis (Sclerosing Encapsulating Peritonitis) (reactive)
- Encases small bowel (visceral peritoneum)
- Fibrosis is not structured (*cf.* mesothelioma)
- Associations: ➤ idiopathic (adolescent girls)
                  ➤ practolol
                  ➤ CAPD (risk increases with duration of therapy)
                  ➤ Le Veen shunt (peritoneal cavity to systemic vein shunt, done to relieve ascites)
                  ➤ fibrothecoma of the ovary (! do not misdiagnose as metastatic thecoma)

Retroperitoneal Fibrosis (reactive)
- Associations: idiopathic, drugs, autoimmune, infective, aortic aneurysm atheroma leak, post radioRx
- Sclerosing phlebitis (fibrous obliteration of small to medium-sized veins) – do an EVG
- Mixed inflammatory infiltrate incl. eosinophils and may show IgG4 +ve plasma cells (and ↑serum IgG4)
- Starts at lower aorta and extends to involve ureters and mesenteric arteries
- Assoc[d] with a similar fibro-phlebitis in other organs as *multifocal fibrosclerosis*:
  - ➤ idiopathic mediastinal fibrosis
  - ➤ Riedel's thyroiditis
  - ➤ primary sclerosing cholangitis
  - ➤ inflammatory pseudotumour of the orbit
  - ➤ ? also autoimmune pancreatitis, bilateral Küttner's tumour and other IgG4 disorders – see p. 175
- d/dg lymphoma, schistosomiasis, sarcoid, malakoplakia, TB

Fibromatosis (true neoplasm)
① Extra-abdominal (breast, limb girdles, palmoplantar [Dupuytren], knuckle pad, penis [Peyronie])
② Abdominal wall (F≫M, usu. occurs after pregnancy)
③ Intra-abdominal desmoid (± FAP, ± keloidal variant d/dg juvenile hyaline fibromatosis)
- Variable cellularity / collagenisation ± myxoid areas (knuckle pads may show just bland fibrosis)
- No well-structured collagenisation pattern (*cf.* storiform, patternless, herring bone, etc.)
- Mixture of slender nuclei and plump vesicular nuclei; indistinct cytoplasm
- Perivascular serum lakes containing mast cells
- Lymphoid infiltrate / follicles at infiltrative margins
- d/dg low grade myofibroblastic sarcoma: this is uniformly hypercellular with variable / focal pleomorphism and infiltration of skeletal muscle (d/dg proliferative myositis/smooth muscle tumours)
- d/dg fibroma of tendon sheath is circumscribed with slit-like vessels

- d/dg: nuclear β-catenin +vity (seen in most fibromatoses at many sites usu. with some cytoplasmic staining) is absent or only cytoplasmic in many morphologically similar lesions incl. low grade fibromyxoid sarcoma, myofibrosarcoma, leiomyosarcoma, fibrosarcoma, inflammatory myxohyaline tumour, nodular fasciitis, myofibroma(tosis) and scars

Plexiform Fibrohistiocytic Tumour (low grade malignancy)
- Child/adolescent/young adult; F>M; subcutaneous lesion on the extremities (usually)
- Multiple nodules of histiocytoid cells ± foamy Mϕ ± multinucleated cells ± central necrosis
- Nodules separated by fibromatosis-like spindle cell stroma
- Immuno: ±ve for CD68 and αSMA; −ve for S100, FXIIIa, CK, desmin
- d/dg GCT of soft tissue, plexiform NF, granuloma, cellular neurothekeoma, fibrous hamartoma

Fibrosarcoma
- Sites as for MFH; also: enlarging painful swelling on metaphysis of long bone / pelvic flat bone
- Spindled fibroblasts in fascicles and a herring-bone pattern (rather than storiform)
- Variable collagen (*cf.* much collagen in MFH)
- Giant cells are uncommon (*cf.* more common in MFH)
- Grading: the less the collagen and the more the cytological atypia – the higher the grade
- Immuno: this is a diagnosis of exclusion – it should be −ve for S100, CK, EMA and desmin
- Variant: *hyalinising spindle tumour with giant rosettes* has hyaline nodules 'rosetted' by spindle cells
- d/dg: as for MFH (p, 325) – exclude these before making the diagnosis
- d/dg desmoid: this is less cellular, more collagenous, less mitotic (<10/10hpf) and without cytol. atypia and may show nuclear β-catenin +vity

Myxofibrosarcoma
- Clin: older adults, limbs, $\frac{2}{3}$ of cases are subcutaneous – the rest deeper, metastasises to LNs
- Arch.: multinodular with incomplete septa
- >5–10% (some say ≥50%) of the tumour must be myxoid for diagnosis
- Hypocellular areas contain curvilinear vessels surrounded by atypical spindle / stellate cells / inflam^n
- Pseudolipoblasts (contain acid mucin)
- Grade: ➢ low: hypocellular with few mitoses
          ➢ intermediate: more infiltrative, more mitoses, more cellular with upto moderate atypia
          ➢ high: = 'myxoid MFH' (but this terminology is outmoded now)
- d/dg inflammatory myxohyaline tumour: hands, solid fibrous areas, mixed inflam^n and virocytes

Low Grade Fibromyxoid Sarcoma
- Clin.: younger adults, deep to deep fascia, thighs / anywhere
- Bland spindle cells in a whorled arrangement in variably dense / myxoid background
- Very few vessels or mitoses
- Variant: hyaline nodules surrounded by partly radial ovoid spindle cells (S100 and CD57 ±ve) = '*hyalinising spindle cell tumour with giant rosettes*' and may result in indolent lung mets
- Immuno: vimentin +ve. Negative for actin, desmin, CD34, S100

Myofibroblastoma of the Breast
- Well-circumscribed ± central fat entrapment ± chondroid metaplasia
- Variably cellular spindle cells with hyaline collagen bundles – looks like spindle cell areas of spindle cell lipoma
- d/dg SFT (but myofibroblastoma is αSMA and desmin +ve)

Palisaded Myofibroblastoma (Intranodal Haemorrhagic Spindle Cell Tumour with Amianthoid Fibres)
- Usu. inguinal nodes
- Straight fascicles of spindle cells with bland cytology (*cf.* curved fascicles in KS)
- Interstitial haemorrhage (*cf.* intra-slit blood in KS)
- Spindle cells palisade around interspersed stellate collagen bundles (amianthoid fibres)
- Immuno/stains: spindle cells are αSMA +ve, CD34 −ve and no DPAS +ve globules (*cf.* KS)

Adipose

Lipoma, Fibrolipoma, Angiolipoma
- The lesions are usu. encapsulated and the cells have uniform vacuoles of mature fat
- Any lipoma may have focal degenerative (e.g. myxoid) or metaplastic (bone/cartilage) changes
- *Fibrolipoma* is diagnosed if there is a prominent fibrous component
- *Typical angiolipoma*: ↑vascularity (usu. at the periphery) ± fibrin thrombi
- *Cellular angiolipoma:* ➢ subcutaneous
  ➢ overgrowth of vascular component (venular pericytes and endothelium)
  ➢ d/dg: ☞ KS but cellular angiolipoma is / has: ◀── deeper
  ☞ atypical vascular lesions of the breast ◁ circumscribed
  ☞ intravascular haemangioma ◁ fibrin thrombi
  ☞ angiomatosis of skin and soft tissues ◁ mature fat

Intramuscular Lipoma
- Usu. paraspinal, unencapsulated and locally recurrent
- Mature adipose tissue infiltrates and separates muscle fibres
- Vessels are sparse and of capillary type only
- d/dg skeletal muscle may also be involved by lipoblastomatosis, angiomatosis and hibernoma (*q.v.*)
- d/dg intramuscular haemangioma (has many vessels and of different types)
- d/dg muscular dystrophies: lipoma is localised and dystrophic fibre changes are absent

Spindle Cell Lipoma
- Transecting bands of cellular collagen with streaming bland spindle cells and wavy nuclei (S100 −ve)
- Refractile eosinophilic wavy collagen fibres
- May be almost entirely spindle cell (i.e. little fat)
- Immuno of spindle cells: CD34 and Bcl-2 +ve; vimentin +ve, −ve for S100 and αSMA
- d/dg: ➢ deep neurofibroma / histiocytoma but – more cellular than NF, not storiform like BFH
  ➢ liposarcoma but: ☞ no nuclear atypia in spindle cells
  ☞ no liposarcoma-type capillary network
  ☞ no lipoblasts

Pleomorphic Lipoma
- *Superficial*, on back / neck of old men (as for spindle cell lipoma)
- Fibroadipose background with small spindle cells (immuno same as for spindle cell lipoma)
- Occ. lipoblasts (rare)
- Very large 'floret' cells (eosinophilic cytoplasm, peripheral wreath-like nuclear lobes)
- Circumscribed and encapsulated
- Vascularity *not* prominent

Atypical Lipoma
- Superficial by definition (= well diff liposarcoma if deep / retroperitoneal / spermatic cord)
- Easily recognised as a fatty lesion (i.e. lipoma-like – otherwise ! see d/dg spindle cell liposarcoma)
- Cellular fibrous septa with occ. pleomorphic / hyperchromatic / multinucleated cells
- Classic lipoblasts may be present usu. hugging the septa (not required for diagnosis, however, an abnormal chromosome 12 marker chromosome is nearly always present)
- Variably-sized adipocytes ± 'heterologous elements' (smooth muscle, rhabdomyoblasts, bone)
- Mimicked encapsulation (i.e. well-circumscribed but may show focal infiltration microscopically)
- May recur but don't metastasise unless they dedifferentiate (the risk of dedifferentiation correlates with cellularity, mitotic rate and multiple local recurrences)

Chondroid Lipoma
- Well circumscribed (± encapsulated), superficial or deep location incl. intramuscular, (F>M)
- ① mature adipose tissue, ② chondroblast-like cells (eosinophilic round cells with hyperchromatic nuclei), ③ multivacuolated lipoblasts (often in cords/clusters and of variable size – unlike liposarcoma lipoblasts)
- Chondromyxoid matrix (not well-defined areas of hyaline cartilage as in d/dg *liposarcoma with chondromatous differentiation*)

- d/dg myxoid liposarcoma: lipoma lacks the vascular pattern
- d/dg myxoid chondrosarcoma and soft tissue chondroma (these do not show adipose differentiation)

Lipoblastoma
- Extremities of young boys (> girls) < 3 years old
- Fibromyxoid septa divide fat into lobules
- Lipoblast development gradient (vacuolated spindles → larger vacuolated cells → mature fat)
- d/dg liposarcoma but: no typical capillary network and liposarcoma is *extremely* rare in children (<10)

Hibernoma
- Young adults and *usu.* superficial and found in the distribution of normal 'brown fat' (e.g. interscapular)
- Lobulated architecture
- ① multivacuolated cells with central, bland, round nuclei, ② mature adipocytes, and ③ lipoblasts

Angiomyolipoma (Angioleiomyolipoma)
- Kidney, liver, spleen, intra LN (!not mets), deep soft tissues; multifocal and bilateral if assoc^d with TS
- Well-circ. but not encapsulated, may show renal vein invasion
- Islands of smooth muscle spindle cells ± a minor component of polygonal epithelioid cells usu. around vessels (epithelioid variant has >50% sheets of *poorly cohesive* epithelioid cells with variably granular/rhabdoid/oncocytoid/clear cytoplasm plus short spindle cells)
- Mature adipose element ± rare lipoblast-like cells (!d/dg liposarcoma)
- Vascular element (eccentric lumen, abnormally thick walls and peripheral radiating muscle)
- May be pleomorphic and sparsely mitotic but is benign (except for the epithelioid variant)
- Immuno of spindle/muscle cells: Melan-A and HMB45 +ve (PEComa), S100 and epithelial Ags −ve
- d/dg myolipoma (= lipoleiomyoma): bland cytology and no mitoses, abnormal vessels or HMB45
- d/dg epithelial tumours (esp. oncocytoma or CCC) *vs.* the epithelioid variant: CPC, cellular cohesiveness and immuno

Other Adipose-Containing Tumours
- Thymolipoma: mediastinum: well-circumscribed lipoma with admixed thymic tissue
- Myelolipoma (adrenal medulla / breast / liver): lipoma with admixed red bone marrow
- Myolipoma = Lipoleiomyoma (soft tissues, cervix, uterus, ovary): variable adipose in a leiomyoma

Liposarcoma

Myxoid and round cell liposarcoma
- Myxoid background may manifest as lymphangioma-like pools (! d/dg)
- Uniform small cells (*cf.* myxoid MFH) without nucleoli (but a round cell component is usu. present)
- Chicken-wire capillary network (*cf.* thicker vessels in MFH)
- Round cell variant: ➤ sheets of round cells with eosinophilic cytoplasm containing fine vacuoles
  (worst prognosis)   ➤ nucleoli are present
                        ➤ high mitotic rate
                        ➤ lipoblasts are essential for diagnosis of this variant
- The % of round cell morphology determines the grade and nomenclature of the lesion thus:
- Grade: I – hypocellular (0–4% round cell component = 'myxoid liposarcoma')
       II – cellular (5–24% = mixed 'myxoid/round cell liposarcoma')
       III – *EITHER* ≥25% round cell (= 'round cell liposarcoma') *OR* presence of a pleomorphic component

Pleomorphic liposarcoma (and dedifferentiated liposarcoma)
- A pleomorphic liposarcoma may be: *EITHER* MFH-like but with lipid vacuoles
                            OR round cell-like but with bizarre multivacuolated giant cells
- Lipoblasts are essential for diagnosis
- >5/10 hpf mitoses are required to diagnose *dedifferentiated liposarcoma* and this must be a dimorphic neoplasm (distinct well-diff and dedifferentiated components) – not a continuum
- Immuno: S100 −ve
- d/dg mixed mesenchymoma (see RMS d/dg on p. 309 and MPNST on p. 316)

Well-differentiated liposarcoma
- Histologically (and karyotypically) the same as atypical lipoma (*q.v.*) but in a deep location
- Vascularity is not prominent
- Variants incl.: Spindle cell, Lipoma-like, Inflammatory and Sclerosing
- *Spindle cell liposarcoma:*
    - like spindle cell lipoma (incl. site[1]) but without the highly eosinophilic refractile collagen bundles
    - spindle cells are hyperchromatic (although otherwise bland and neuroid)
    - ± lipoblasts (but not essential for diagnosis)
    - immuno: only focally CD34 +ve (*cf.* strong and diffuse +vity in d/dg spindle cell lipoma, NF, DFSP and epithelioid sarcoma)

Neural

Schwannoma
- Clin.: middle-aged, painless, pressure Sx ± NF-2
- Sites: PNS > CNS, deep > superficial (except plexiform and SEMS), solitary > multiple[2]
- Macro: well-circumscribed, nerve at edge ± cystic degeneration
- Micro: ➤ capsule, nerve at edge, dimorphic: ① cellular Antoni A (palisades and Verocay bodies)
                                                ② loose myxoid Antoni B
          ➤ wavy / comma nuclei, rare mitoses, occ. mast cells, thick-walled vessels and hyaline areas
- d/dg includes smooth muscle tumours that may show marked Verocay body-like palisading

Variants
- Cellular: ↑cellularity, scattered mitoses, retains a capsule (helpful in d/dg), usu. no Verocay bodies
- Plexiform: dermis, usu. <3 cm, not assoc[d] with NF-1 or NF-2, multiple dyscohesive encapsulated nodules of Antoni A tissue, d/dg plexiform NF (see p. 316 under 'Neurofibroma')
- Granular cell: vesicular nuclei with nucleoli, rare mitoses, necrosis and spindle areas, sustentacular cells give a deeper DPAS stain than the granular tumour cells (the granularity is due to lysosomes)
- Ancient: shows scattered degenerative nuclear pleomorphism with hyperchromasia – the tumour must be *both* hypocellular *and* amitotic to accept these anomalies as ancient change
    - ➤ d/dg PHAT but this has cellular foci of many pleomorphic cells that are S100 and CD31 −ve (and CD34 +ve in 50%) and there are mitoses (but usu. < 1 / 50 hpf)
- Melanotic (= psammomatous Schwannoma):
    - ➤ assoc[d] with Carney syndrome / complex (! not Carney triad or NF-1)
    - ➤ features favouring melanotic Schwannoma over d/dg metastatic melanoma:
        1. psammoma bodies
        2. lesser degree of nuclear pleomorphism and mitoses
        3. cells have a syncytial appearance
        4. EM: abundant cytoplasmic membrane folds of external lamina
        5. EM: melanosomes – all normal (pleomorphic ones favour malignant melanoma)
        6. immuno is not helpful (both are S100 and HMB45 +ve)
- Glandular: focal glandular differentiation is case-report rare (it usually occurs in malignant PNST)
- Pseudoglandular: entrapped normal glandular structures
- Pacinian: an encapsulated tumour with Pacinian-like structures with concentric onion-skin lamellae (old name = Pacinian NF); d/dg digital Pacinian neuroma = a hyperplastic mix of normal Pacinian corpuscles + nerves without a capsule (it is painful and occurs on the fingers)
- Others: fascicular (a congenital hamartoma), intraneural, Schwannomatosis

Superficial Epithelioid Malignant Schwannoma (SEMS)
- A dermal tumour that infiltrates nerves
- Epithelioid and spindle cells grow in nests and fascicles separated by fibrous tissue
- No epidermal component (else = *neurotropic melanoma*)
- Focally there is classical neural differentiation

---

[1] hence this is an exception to the rule that subcutaneous fat tumours are benign (*NB*: some consider all atypical lipomatous tumours to be biologically identical, the benignity of the superficial ones results purely from the fact that they are more amenable to complete excision so avoid the local recurrences that increase the risk of the dedifferentiation which results in metastases)
[2] 'multiple' includes bilateral acoustic neuroma and plexiform Schwannoma

Neurofibroma (NF)
- Clin.: young adult ± type 1 neurofibromatosis (NF-1); sites: any / skin / subcutis
- Macro: solitary nodule / diffuse thickening / plexiform
- Unencapsulated (infiltrative – ! except some solitary NFs), nerves run through it
- Monomorphic with more cells superficially (Schwann cells, perineural cells and fibroblasts)
- Variably myxoid to collagenous background with wavy fibres ('shredded carrot') and mast cells
- No mitoses or <1/20hpf (some take any mitoses in a deep/diffuse NF as a sign of malignancy)
- ± Tactoid bodies = Meissner-like corpuscles with transversely stacked lamellae
- Immuno: S100 +ve only in the Schwann cells (≈ 50% of the cells *cf.* ≈ 100% in Schwannoma)
- d/dg solitary circumscribed neuroma: has an EMA +ve capsule and contains peripherin +ve axons

Variants
- Pigmented: occ. cells contain melanin (d/dg blue naevus can be difficult)
- Granular cell: DPAS +ve
- Bizarre: ancient change (see p. 315 under 'Schwannoma' for definition)
- Epithelioid: ! H&E is almost identical to the rare S100 −ve, EMA +ve *perineural cell tumour*
- Plexiform: (assoc^d with NF-1) contains a plexiform arrangement of nerves with intact perineurium ∴ d/dg plexiform Schwannoma (also d/dg plexiform fibrohistiocytic tumour). Features favouring plexiform NF are :
  1. myxoid tissue around a nerve (in the perineural space)
  2. a diffuse component of typical NF tissue outside the nerves
  3. larger size i.e. >3cm (∴ a diagnosis of NF-1 should not be made on micro alone)
  4. usu. deeper location (but can also occur in the dermis)

Neurofibromatosis
- Central (NF-2) has bilateral: acoustic neuromas, meningiomas, astrocytoma, optic nerve glioma, etc.
- Peripheral (NF-1) = von Recklinghausen's disease:
  ➢ clin. defined by any 2 of 7 criteria e.g.: *café au lait* spots and neurofibroma (incl. plexiform) or bilateral optic gliomas and Lisch nodules or deep (e.g. GIT) ganglioneuromas and CNS tumours
  ➢ for NF-1 vasculopathy, see p. 73; for phaeochromocytoma, see p. 276
  ➢ malignancy and divergent differentiation are more likely in NF-1-associated neurofibromas

Malignant Peripheral Nerve Sheath Tumour (MPNST)
- Clin.: sporadic, post irradiation, assoc^d with NF-1; occ. pain / paraesthesiae or asymptomatic
- Sites: peripheral extremities, central trunk, head and neck, retroperitoneum (esp. glandular variant)
- Macro: the tumour may be assoc^d with a nerve
- Alternating hyper / hypocellular areas
- Cells run in fascicles (*cf.* haphazard in neurofibroma)
- Significant atypia in hypercellular areas
- Classic features of neural differentiation are seen in the *hypocellular* areas
- Nerve-like whorls, tactoid bodies, thick vessels
- Mitoses > 1/20 hpf
- Fibrosarcoma-like, MFH-like +/ epithelioid areas
- Divergent differentiation (poorer prog.): RMS (= malig. Triton tumour[3]), osteosarcoma, chondrosarcoma, glandular
- d/dg mixed mesenchymoma: but this excludes tumours with an MPNST component, by convention

Neuroblastoma / Ganglioneuroblastoma / Ganglioneuroma / PNET
See p. 59.

Neurothekeoma
See pp. 317–318.

---

[3] a *benign Triton tumour* = the rare *neuromuscular hamartoma* composed of normal nerves + skeletal muscle

Morton's Neuroma
- Fibrous thickening of nerve (perineurium, epineurium and endoneurium) with loss of axons
- Endarterial fibrous thickening of arteries ± thrombosis
- Schwann cell proliferation
- Fibrosis of surrounding soft tissues

Amputation Neuroma (Traumatic Neuroma, Post-Traumatic Pseudoneuroma)
- May occur in the viscera after surgery / trauma; may cause Sx after cholecystectomy
- Disorderly outgrowth of peripheral nerve components around damaged nerve (broken perineurium)
- Schwann cells, fibroblasts and nerve fibres in a dense fibrous matrix ± myxoid change
- Usu. there is no well-defined perineurial enclosure (see d/dg mucosal neuroma below)

Mucosal Neuroma
- Usu. multiple, assoc[d] with MTC and phaeochromocytoma in MEN 2b
- Submucosal / mucosal / dermal location at mucocutaneous junction, eyelid, tongue, GIT
- Endoneural haphazard proliferation of nerve fibres (perineurial capsules are EMA +ve)
- d/dg solitary circumscribed neuroma: has a partial perineurial capsule but usu. occurs on facial skin; it has no association with NF-1 or 2 but d/dg includes NF, Schwannoma, traumatic neuroma and naevi
- d/dg traumatic neuroma: mucosal neuroma ➢ has intact perineuria (EMA +ve)
  ➢ has loose fibrous stroma (not dense fibrosis)

Vascular

General Features of Endothelial Differentiation
- Erythrocytes in slit-like spaces lined by tumour cells
- Intracytoplasmic sharp vacuoles (separated by thin septa if multiple) preferably containing RBC
- Positivity for CD31 (most sensitive and specific, linear membranous +vity – but also gives granular membranous +vity in Mφ found in any tumour), CD34, FVIIIRA, (Ulex is no good and stains some CA)
- EM: Weibel-Palade bodies (= rod-shaped microtubulated bodies *cf.* d/dg melanosomes)

Angiomyofibroblastoma
- Well-circumscribed, small (usu. <3 cm ∅)
- Myxohyaline matrix ± fat (*lipomatous variant*). Only partly myxoid (*cf.* aggressive angiomyxoma)
- Many small, thin-walled vessels
- Stromal cells: epithelioid / spindle, concentrated around vessels, multinucleated forms
- Immuno: ER and PgR +ve, desmin +ve (usu. αSMA −ve), S100 −ve

Aggressive Angiomyxoma
- Infiltrative, big (usu. >10 cm ∅), locally recurrent, usu. in vulva/perineum or deep soft tissues
- Uniformly myxoid with uniform cellularity (stellate and spindle)
- Thin *and* thick-walled vessels ± hyaline change
- Delicate smooth muscle bundles esp. around vessels
- Immuno: vimentin, desmin, MSA and αSMA +ve; S100, CEA, CK −ve

Superficial Angiomyxoma (= Cutaneous Myxoma)
- Infiltrative, usu. <4 cm ∅, multilobulated, dermis / subcutis, locally recurrent
- ± Carney complex[4] (= Carney syndrome): cutaneous and cardiac myxomas, spotty skin pigmentation, endocrine overactivity, AD inheritance
- Myxoid with stellate / spindle cells, occ. mitoses, PMN
- Thin-walled vessels in an arborising pattern (myxoid liposarcoma-like)
- Entrapped hyperplastic epithelial component (epidermal cyst-like or squamous/basaloid strands)
- Immuno: desmin −ve, S100 −ve
- d/dg: (see also 'Lesions in the differential diagnosis of 'Myxoma' ', pp. 326–327)

---

[4] Not to be confused with the Carney triad (assoc[d] with NF-1): ① epithelioid GIST, ② pulmonary chondroma and ③ non-adrenal paraganglioma

> ➢ aggressive angiomyxoma: is larger, involves deeper structures and has a different vascular pattern
> ➢ focal cutaneous mucinosis: lacks lobular architecture, PMN and epithelial structures
> ➢ cutaneous myxoid cyst (= digital myxoid cyst): localised to the fingers
> ➢ neurothekeoma[5]: more prominent lobularity, plump S100 +ve cells
> ➢ myxoid neurofibroma: wavey, buckled nuclei, S100 +ve
> ➢ myxoid liposarcoma: deeper, scattered lipoblasts, S100 +ve
> ➢ myxofibrosarcoma: greater nuclear atypia, hyperchromasia, cells line curvilinear vessels
> ➢ superficial myofibroblastoma ($\approx$ angiomyofibroblastoma without the 'angio' features)

Epithelioid Haemangioma (Histiocytoid Haemangioma, Angiolymphoid hyperplasia with eosinophilia)

- Clin: F>M, young adults, soft tissue lesions (head and neck) $\pm$ lymphadenopathy and PB eosinophilia
- Circumscribed subcutaneous / dermal nodule, intravascular forms also occur
- Vague nodular arch. of vessels with surrounding lympho-eosinophil infiltrate (may be florid to absent)
- Epithelioid endothelium ($\pm$ 'tombstone' arrangement, $\pm$ vacuoles) but pleomorphism and mitoses are not a feature – not all vessels show these features
- Immuno: +ve for CD31, CD34, FVIIIRA; −ve for HHV8, EMA, CK
- d/dg pyogenic granuloma: although these may be epithelioid they are exophytic, lack the typical inflammatory stroma and can show mitoses in both endothelium and stromal cells

Kimura's Disease

- Clin: M≫F, Asian, lymphadenopathy and eosinophilia $\pm$ soft tissue lesions (subcutis, head and neck)
- Dense lymphoid infiltrate and giant cells, ($\pm$ nuclear debris, polykarya, eosinophilic matrix)
- Eosinophils $\pm$ eosinophilic abscesses
- Sclerosis (a late feature)
- The lymphoid infiltrate dominates the vascular proliferation (that does not have epithelioid features)

Cellular Haemangioma (Infantile Haemangioma)

- An immature form of capillary haemangioma with GLUT1 +ve endothelium seen in children – see p. 57
- Lobular growth pattern
- May be apparently solid but actually has compact lumena (do a reticulin)
- More mature capillaries may form towards the periphery
- Abundance of pericytes (MSA +ve)
- May show small whorls but rarely any fascicles
- Mitotic activity (++) and mild atypia may be present
- d/dg angiosarcoma: angiosarcoma is very rare in children and looks like the adult ones

Spindle Cell Haemangioendothelioma (= Spindle Cell Haemangioma)

- Benign, usu. young adult, distal extremities (rare in viscera), 50% are multiple and usu. found in a single anatomical distribution, assoc^d with Maffucci, lymphangiomatosis and Klippel-Trenaunay (but not HIV)
- Well-circumscribed (50% are within a muscular vein)
- Cavernous spaces ($\pm$ pseudopapillae or phleboliths)
- Spindle component forming short fascicles and irregularly branching and ramifying narrow spaces (*cf.* KS)
- Bland cells with rare / no mitoses
- No DPAS +ve globules (*cf.* KS)
- Focal 'pseudoadipocyte' areas composed of groups of vacuolated endothelial cells (not seen in KS)
- Thick-walled AVM-like vessels in the periphery or within the lesion
- Immuno: CD31 and CD34 are confined to cells lining the vascular channels but not the rest of the spindle cells; some of the spindle cells are actin +/ desmin +ve

---

[5] Not to be confused with '*cellular neurothekeoma*' which has little/no myxoid, is S100 −ve and +ve for αSMA, NSE and NKI-C3 (= CD63, a melanoma marker). It is predom. dermal *cf.* d/dg plexiform fibrohistiocytic tumour

Tufted Angioma (Angioblastoma of Nakagawa)
- Capillary lobules with pericytes
- 'Cannon ball' 'buckshot' distribution in the dermis and subcutis
- Crescentic 'semilunar' spaces (? lymphatic) surround the lobules
- There is no significant spindle population
- Stains: reticulin shows a 'vasoformative' pattern (i.e. tubules)

Intramuscular Haemangioma (= Intramuscular Angioma [if lymphatics are present])
- Clin.: may be painful, usu. restricted to one site or muscle group
- Vessels ++, of all types and in various proportions (capillary, cavernous, arterial, venous ± lymphatic)
- Mature adipose tissue may be a prominent component
- d/dg intramuscular lipoma: angioma is too vascular for a lipoma and contains a variety of vessel types
- d/dg angiomatosis of soft tissues: angiomatosis clinically affects >1 site or muscle group

Angiomatosis (Bacillary)
- Clin.: assoc[d] with AIDS/post Tx; sites: dermal / oral / aural polyp, liver / spleen peliotic lesions
- Lobular growth, rounded capillary channels, plump endothelial cells   } (*cf.* d/dg KS)
- PMN in clumps *throughout* (not just near an ulcerated surface as in d/dg pyogenic granuloma)
- Interstitial granular amphophil debris (= Warthin-Starry +ve bacteria *Bartonella henselae* +/ *quintana*)

Angiomatosis (of Soft Tissues)
- Clin.: child/adolescent, limbs, involves any depth from dermis to bone, large contiguous areas
- Mature fat surrounds proliferating vessels
- Subtypes: ① irregular veins with incomplete muscle; cavernous and capillary vessels
                   ② small capillaries only and sparse feeder vessels
- d/dg AVM: no arteries in angiomatosis
- d/dg intramuscular haemangioma: *vide supra*

Angiomatosis (of Lung Septa)
- Assoc[d] with pulmonary veno-occlusive disease (VOD) – see p. 88

Angiomatosis (of Lymph Nodes = Vascular Transformation of LN Sinuses)
- A reactive sinus vessel proliferation 2° to lymphovenous obstruction
- Spindled proliferation with maturation
- Maturation takes the form of capillary ectasia – usu. most marked at the periphery of the LN
- Arch. is preserved and it lacks well-formed fascicles (*cf.* d/dg KS)

Angiomatosis (of Breast)
- Clin.: large (present as a mass), locally recurrent but not pre-malignant and do not metastasise
- Diffuse involvement of the interlobular stroma (spares the TDLU – unlike d/dg angiosarcoma)
- Variably dilated channels (mixture of empty and blood-filled) that do not get smaller at the periphery
- Channels may anastomose but endothelium is flattened and not atypical (*cf.* angiosarcoma)
- d/dg angiosarcoma shows:
  - endothelial atypia (hyperchromasia / tufting / mitoses / nucleoli) ± high grade areas (solid foci, necrosis)
  - destructive invasion (e.g. it infiltrates and overruns the TDLUs)
  - a more heterogeneous density of channels throughout the lesion
  - maturation towards the periphery (calibre of vascular spaces decreases down to capillary ∅)
- d/dg AVM: angiomatosis has no significant smooth muscle component
- d/dg PASH: PASH is lined by CD34 (not CD31) +ve and Bcl-2 +ve stromal cells, not endothelium
- d/dg perilobular haemangioma: this may have focal atypia and anastomoses but is well circumscribed and does not show destructive invasion (it is called 'haemangiomatosis' if multiple)
- d/dg atypical haemangioma (*vide infra*)
- d/dg atypical vascular lesions post radioRx (*vide infra*)

Atypical Haemangioma (of the Breast)
- Small (<2cm ∅), benign lesions with vaguely lobular arch., stromal mast cells and organising thrombi
- ± Feeder vessels nearby / within the lesions
- Atypia = anastomosing channels, local 'invasive' margins (not encapsulated) and focal endothelial hyperchromasia / hyperplasia (usu. in regions of organising thrombi)
- Subtypes: cavernous, compact capillary (d/dg pyogenic granuloma), combined, capillary budding (has some solid spindle areas – d/dg KS)
- d/dg angiosarcoma: no destructive invasion, solid areas, necrosis, blood lakes or large tumours ≫2cm
- d/dg angiolipoma: angiolipoma vessels are concentrated at the periphery of a fat lobule

Atypical Vascular Lesions post RadioRx (of the Breast)
- Small benign lumps (usu. < 1cm ∅) confined to dermis (or to a fibrous nodule if parenchymal – rare)
- Well-circ. but not encapsulated and variable stromal chronic inflam^y cell infiltrate (lymphocytes and plasma cells)
- Empty, angulated, variably-sized channels, some of which may anastomose ± dissect collagen
- Spaced-out, plump single (rarely focal 2) layered endothelium ± hyperchromasia but no other atypia
- d/dg angiosarcoma: unlike angiosarcoma, these are small, lack diffuse skin change / 'bruise-like' discoloration clinically and lack invasion, blood lakes or significant cytological atypia (tufting, mitoses, nucleoli)

Pleomorphic Hyalinising Angiectatic Tumour (PHAT)
- A low grade malignancy with an aptly descriptive name (for immuno see Schwannoma, ancient, d/dg)
- Also ± perivascular fibrin, perilesional lymphocytes, Ca^{2+}, Fe and intranuclear cytoplasmic inclusions
- d/dg: ancient Schwannoma, simplastic haemangioma, MFH (the latter is more mitotic)

Stuart-Treves Syndrome (Stuart-Treves Lymphangiosarcoma)
- Occurs in lymphoedematous arms following axillary radioRx for breast carcinoma
- Solid, epithelioid and papillary endothelial formations
- Unlike post radioRx angiosarcoma, it occurs *outside* the radiation field

Angiosarcoma
- Clin.: blue/black ('bruise-like'), affects any tissue, liver, skin (e.g. face and scalp of the elderly), breast (can be bilateral and usu. deep in the breast if 1° or affects the breast skin if 2° to radioRx)
- Macro: haemorrhagic and often several cm in size
- Destructive infiltration by anastomosing angular channels with atypical endothelium (hyperchromatic, ± tufting / mitoses / nucleoli) ± extravasation 'blood lakes' in higher grades
- Better differentiated at periphery of lesion (i.e. the channels get smaller and have lower grade histology)
- Grade according to worst area (only useful for breast lesions):   Mitoses
    - Grade 1: upto 2 layers, tufting, dissecting and anastomosing channels
    - Grade 2: papillary and solid spindle cell areas
    - Grade 3: mostly solid, necrosis
- Variants: haemorrhagic (blood lakes ++), epithelioid, granular and sclerosing
- Immuno: ➤ +ve for CD31, CD34, FVIIIRA, vimentin
    - ➤ −ve for Melan-A, HMB45, ALK, CEA, thyroglobulin, Hep Par 1, HMW CK
    - ➤ ±ve for LMW CK (CAM5.2 is +ve in ≈ 33% of cases), S100 (≈ 8%), c-kit (≈ 50%)
- d/dg benign vascular lesions in general, but these:
    - ➤ are usu. < 2cm in max. ∅
    - ➤ may have a nearby muscular vessel (but some epithelioid angiosarcomas also have a feeder vessel)
    - ➤ may have smooth muscle in the walls of the vascular channels (but some angiomatoses don't)
    - ➤ spaces are not anastomosing (but this is a weak feature with many exceptions – *vide supra*)
- d/dg specific entities:
    - ➤ Kaposi sarcoma *vs.* solid (spindle cell) angiosarcoma: angiosarcoma has dissecting, ramified channels and significant cytological atypia whereas KS has minimal atypia (except the African endemic form) and curved fascicles with simple channels. CPC is also helpful
    - ➤ sinusoidal haemangioma: sieve-like back-to-back dilated vessels ± hyperchromasia, no invasion
    - ➤ atypical vascular lesions post radioRx (*vide supra*)

➤ grade 1–2 angiosarcoma occurring in infancy (in liver, spleen, lungs or bone) is called '*infantile haemangioendothelioma*' but some use this term to be synonymous with cellular haemangioma in the skin or Kaposiform haemangioendothelioma (described on p. 322)

➤ angiomatoid variant of anaplastic thyroid carcinoma may have anastomosing channels containing blood and +vity for FVIIIRA and vimentin ∴ look for focal better diff tumour foci and use CPC

➤ haemorrhagic angiosarcoma *vs.* choriocarcinoma

➤ sclerosing angiosarcoma *vs.* fibromatosis / other sarcoma (cells arranged in branching bilayered strands favour angiosarcoma)

➤ angiomatosis, haemangiomatosis and atypical haemangiomas (pp. 319–320)

➤ carcinoma, anaplastic lymphoma and melanoma *vs.* epithelioid angiosarcoma (*vide infra*)

➤ Masson's tumour: this is usu. entirely intravascular and is a hyaline papillary form of organising thrombus with single-layered, non-atypical endothelium. However, it may arise secondarily in any other 1° vascular lesion.

➤ reactive angioendotheliomatosis: loose irregular lobules of non-atypical capillaries (usu.) in the dermis

➤ benign lymphangioendothelioma: dissects the dermal collagen but has empty channels and no endothelial atypia

Epithelioid Angiosarcoma
- Clin.: older adults (M≫F), skin, deep soft tissue (incl. muscle – an otherwise rare site for angiosarcoma)
- An origin from the edge of a larger vessel may be seen (a feeder vessel)
- Solid sheets of large epithelioid cells (vesicular nucleus and large eosinophilic nucleolus)
- Small foci of more typical angiosarcoma (if more extensive call it 'angiosarcoma with epithelioid areas')
- Mitoses ++, ± necrosis, haemorrhage
- Vacuoles (containing occ. RBC, not mucin)
- Vasoformative (tubular) reticulin pattern
- Immuno: CD31 +ve, ± LMW CK +ve (HMW CK −ve), ± focal EMA +ve (but usu. −ve): see 'Angiosarcoma', above, for more
- d/dg all epithelioid malignant neoplasms (incl. mesothelioma): endothelial immuno ± EM, RBC vacuoles and retic pattern are the most helpful distinguishing features
- d/dg epithelioid haemangioendothelioma: angiosarcoma does not have the centrifugal architecture of haemangioendothelioma, for other features in the d/dg *vide infra*

Epithelioid Haemangioendothelioma
- Adult, multicentric (except in soft tissues), arises from medium-sized vein/artery; may metastasise
- *Cords* / sheets of polygonal cells in myxohyaline stroma ± plump spindle cell fascicles
- Eosinophilic hyaline cytoplasm, inconspicuous nucleoli
- Cytoplasmic vacuoles (more evident that in epithelioid angiosarcoma)
- Vasoformative (tubular) reticulin pattern (smaller and more broken-up *cf.* epithelioid angiosarcoma)
- Low mitotic count (≤2/10hpf)
- Immuno: CD31 +ve ± αSMA +ve, CK +ve (but CEA and EMA −ve)
- Malignant change: focally solid and more pleomorphic, but mitoses are still few
- d/dg: carcinoma (esp. sclerosing cholangiocarcinoma): different immuno, vacuoles contain RBC not mucin, also carcinomas have worse cytology
- d/dg epithelioid sarcoma: but epithelioid sarcoma has a sheet-like growth pattern, is −ve for CD31 and FVIIIRA, is +ve for EMA, CK and CD34 and does not have RBC in its cytoplasmic vacuoles
- d/dg KS but the spindle cells are plumper than KS and have eosinophilic hyaline cytoplasm
- d/dg epithelioid angiosarcoma: haemangioendothelioma has cords, fewer solid areas, more obvious vacuoles,↓ mitoses, smaller cells, small nucleoli, more myxohyaline stroma and a centrifugal growth pattern around a central vessel
- d/dg intravascular bronchioalveolar tumour – it is the same tumour, but in the lungs
- d/dg myxoid chondrosarcoma

Haemangiopericytoma (HPC)
- Clin.: age ≈ 40 years (d/dg synovial sarcoma occurs younger), assoc[d] with Castleman's disease
- Sites: thigh, retroperitoneum, head and neck, trunk (d/dg synovial sarcoma prefers the extremities)
- Stubby spindle cells with scant cytoplasm and oval nuclei with dispersed chromatin

- Open vascular spaces, some bifid or 'staghorn'
- Immuno: +ve for CD34, vimentin, ± focal actin (but usu. −ve); −ve for CD31, CK, S100
- Diagnosis of exclusion:
  - ➢ must have an HPC pattern and single cell reticulin *everywhere*
  - ➢ must be negative for muscle, nerve sheath and epithelial markers
- 'Benign' variant: no necrosis or pleom. and low mitotic count ($< 1/20$ hpf) – but some still metastasise
- Signs of aggression: necrosis, trabecular arch., mitoses, pleomorphism, vascular invasion
- d/dg:
  - ➢ synovial sarcoma: has an epithelial component (or nested reticulin if monophasic)
  - ➢ HPC-like tumour, sinonasal: site, more rounded cells, no pleomorphism, mitoses rare
  - ➢ glomus tumour: organoid features and αSMA +ve
  - ➢ myopericytoma / myofibromatosis: MSA +ve cells are orientated around the vascular channels
  - ➢ haemangiopericytic meningioma shows focal transition to benign meningioma (but meningeal HPC exists)
  - ➢ solitary fibrous tumour: shows other growth patterns
  - ➢ thymoma, type A: other features of thymoma are present (see pp. 95–96)
  - ➢ clear cell sugar tumour: clear (PAS +ve) cells and positive for CD34, S100, HMB45
  - ➢ mesenchymal chondrosarcoma: focal cartilage islands
  - ➢ RMS or liposarcoma (because HPC may have focal myxoid areas or alveolar architecture)

Intimal Sarcoma
- Large vessels of adults (e.g. aorta, pulm. arteries and venae cavae), embolic effects, poor prog.
- A spindle sarcoma arising from the intima
- Immuno: vimentin +ve but other markers are variable / −ve

Kaposiform Haemangioendothelioma
- Clin.: usu. infants / children, no HIV, die from a consumptive coagulopathy (Kaserbach-Merritt)
- Site: deep soft tissues (esp. peripancreatic retroperitoneum), skin in older patients
- Infiltrative *lobular* growth pattern (lobules may be large ∴ not obvious on core Bx)
- Criss-crossing curved to straight fascicles (shorter *cf.* KS and simpler than spindle cell haemangioma)
- DPAS +ve globules may be present
- Microthrombi are common
- Well-formed capillary areas may be present
- Short narrow vascular spaces lined by attenuated slender cells with dark nuclei (like normal endothelium) are interspersed among the spindle cells (not seen in KS)
- Pericytes (MSA +ve) are present to abundant (*cf.* KS)
- d/dg KS – *vide infra*, also KS is *nodular* (not lobular) and is rare in deep soft tissues and in infants
- d/dg angiosarcoma – haemangioendothelioma lacks a dissecting pattern or cytological atypia

Kaposi Sarcoma (KS)
- Multifocal, skin / visceral sites, HIV, HHV8 (nuclear positivity by immuno)
- Early lesions are polyclonal later becoming monoclonal
- Three main stages: Patch ($\approx$ 'granulation tissue like' histology), Plaque, Nodule
- Nodular (i.e. expansile with altered stroma peripherally – oedema / fibrosis with concentric collagen)
- Criss-crossing, curved, fascicles of spindle cells
- Simple slit-like spaces (appear reteform / sponge-like if cut transversely), spaces contain RBC
- Minimal cytological atypia
- DPAS +ve hyaline globules (intra and extracellularly)
- Interspersed lymphoplasmacytic infiltrate and haemosiderin
- CD34 +ve spindle cells (all tumour cells are +ve *cf.* spindle cell haemangioma)
- Pericytes (MSA +ve) are sparse or absent
- Well-developed capillaries may be present (esp. at the periphery or in the *angiomatous variant*)
- Lymphangiomatous variant KS (dilated empty channels) lacks endothelial multilayering / atypia (*cf.* d/dg angiosarcoma) or focal smooth muscle (*cf.* benign lymphangioendothelioma) and has stromal spindle cells and plasma cells / inflam[n] unlike those differentials
- Skin KS may have a collarette of epidermis mimicking d/dg pyogenic granuloma
- d/dg microvenular haemangioma: unlike KS this well-circ lesion with sclerotic collagen has many branching small vessels, pericytes, invasion of the arrector pili and lacks a KS-like inflam[y] component
- d/dg KS may be clinically confused for acroangiodermatitis (an exaggerated form of stasis dermatitis)
- For other d/dg see the features of the other vascular entities described above.

TABLE 21.1   The 5 main clinical forms of KS

① Classical (Kaposi, 1872)
• **W**esterners / **E**astern European Jews
• **I**ndolent
• **E**lderly males
• **L**ower leg lesions
• **D**ie from other causes
• **A**ssoc^d with tumours esp. lymphomas

② Endemic
• **S**ub-Saharan Africa
• **M**ales
• **A**ggressive lower leg lesions / **C**lassical-like / **S**ystemic

③ Lymphadenopathic
• **R**apidly fatal
• **A**frican children
• **W**idespread LNp, no skin lesions

④ Tx-Associated
• **L**ong-term immunosuppression
• **A**ggressive *cf.* classical
• **F**atal in 30%
• **S**kin and systemic involvement

⑤ AIDS-Associated
• **M**ale homosexuals
• **D**ie from other complications of AIDS
• **M**ultiple purple patches/plaques (usu. on upper body, palate and viscera)

Miscellaneous

Synovial Sarcoma
• Extremities of young adults / chest wall, chemosensitive (esp. in children), cytogenetics: t(X;18)
• Stromal changes: fibrosis, hyaline, Ca^{2+}, mast cells, haemangiopericytoma-like vessels
• Biphasic   ➤ short, stubby, spindle cells closely compacted together with pericellular reticulin
    ➤ nuclei: ovoid, open chromatin ± nuclear overlapping
    ➤ epithelial: 1. elongated glands, +ve for mucicarmine / DPAS
        2. small nests (show up as packeted reticulin *cf.* pericellular)
    ➤ haemangiopericytomatous architecture
    ➤ herring bone / alternating hyper and hypocellular areas
• Monophasic: ➤ more common (×2) and usu. spindle type but may be epithelial
    ➤ reticulin packets (sufficient to make the diagnosis if the clinical fits)
    ➤ EM: may show microvilli-lined spaces as evidence of epithelial differentiation
• Synovioblastic synovial sarcoma: poor prognosis variant, ↑cellular, pleomorphic spindle cells, rhabdoid cells / small blue round cells, mitoses ++, ± necrosis
• Calcifying synovial sarcoma: good prognosis variant, has calcification ++
• Grading: Low: > 50% glandular, <15 mitoses /10 hpf → low risk   (100% 3YS)
    High: < 50% glandular, > 15 mitoses/10 hpf → high risk   (40% 3YS)
• Prognostics: metastasis-free survival is better with the SYT-SSX2 translocation *cf.* SYT-SSX1
• Immuno: triad ① Bcl-2 +ve, ② EMA (EMA and CK are at least focally +ve in spindle and epithelial cells) and ③ CD99 ±ve (membranous, in the spindle cells); S100 ±ve; −ve for CD34, desmin, MSA
• d/dg: HPC, fibrosarcoma, MPNST, mesenchymal chondrosarcoma, leiomyosarcoma, KS

Alveolar Soft Part Sarcoma
• Clin.: young, thigh (or head and neck in children); slow malignant course with late metastases
• Nests of uniform cells with central dyscohesion ± rhabdoid / clear cell change ± solid foci
• Large eosinophilic cells with large nucleoli; ± AB and DPAS +ve cytoplasmic basophilic crystalloids
• Mitoses and pleomorphism are only focal but haemorrhage and necrosis may be prominent
• Peritumoural vascular invasion
• Immuno: nuclear *TFE3* +vity is ≈ specific (! but also +ve in granular cell tumours and some childhood RCC); desmin, MSA, NSE and S100 are all ±ve; −ve for CgA, synaptophysin, HMB45, Melan A, CK, EMA
• d/dg RCC / melanoma (more pleomorphic), malig. granular cell tumour, paraganglioma, PEComa, ACC

Clear Cell Sarcoma of Tendon and Aponeuroses (Malignant Melanoma of Soft Parts)
• Clin.: young, ankle / foot
• Fascicular and nested (retic) infiltration by clear cells with vesicular nuclei and prominent nucleoli

- Wreath-like giant cells / melanin
- Immuno: +ve for S100, HMB45, NSE
- d/dg superficial CCSTA *vs.* cutaneous melanoma: lack of junctional activity in overlying skin
- d/dg epithelioid MPNST: CCSTA is HMB45 +ve and has t(12;22)

Epithelioid Sarcoma
- Clin.: young, hand / wrist, extensive local spread ± mets to scalp, LN, lung
- Commonest sarcoma of hand and forearm (followed by alveolar RMS and synovial sarcoma)
- Subcutis / deeper, attached to tendon / aponeurosis
- Nodules / multinodular conglomerates of epithelioid cells (± myoid/spindle cells), pleomorphism is mild, ± intracytoplasmic vacuoles and cleft-like spaces (d/dg vascular lesion), ± rhabdoid inclusions
- Granuloma-like: bland tumour cells with central hyaline or necrosis and peripheral lymphocytes
- Stroma is dense collagenous (incl. intercellular collagen) ± chondroid / osteoid
- Immuno +ve for: CK (e.g. AE1/AE3), vimentin and EMA +ve; CD34 ±ve
- Immuno −ve for: CD31, CD68, S100, FVIIIRA, CEA
- d/dg granulomas, vascular neoplasm, RMS, rhabdoid tumour, epithelioid Spitz: immuno may help
- d/dg carcinoma: CD34 +vity is rare in carcinomas and there is no epidermal component (*cf.* 1° SCC)
- Worse prognosis if >5cm or proximal variant (esp. perineum / pelvis)
- *Proximal variant:* ➢ sheet-like growth of larger cells with vesicular nuclei, no necrosis
  - ➢ more pleomorphism (carcinoma-like) and rhabdoid inclusions
  - ➢ d/dg extra-renal rhabdoid tumour (*vide infra*) / carcinoma

Extra-Renal Rhabdoid Tumour
- Clin.: young, aggressive (? related to solid / proximal variant epithelioid sarcoma)
- Round epithelioid cells, vesicular nuclei and prominent nucleoli, hyaline globular (rhabdoid) inclusions
- Immuno: +ve for CK, vimentin and EMA (like RCC and epithelioid sarcoma)
- d/dg rhabdoid differentiation in other tumours

Solitary Fibrous Tumour (Localised Fibrous Tumour)
- Mesothelial or 1° soft tissue (interstitial dendritic cell origin – like spindle cell lipoma)
- Well-circumscribed but not usu. encapsulated – may entrap adjacent structures
- A variety of patterns is characteristic: ① patternless pattern: parallel 'ropey' collagen
  - ② wavey neuroid
  - ③ storiform / herring bone
  - ④ haemangiopericytomatous
- Stromal degenerations (myxoid, hyaline, etc.): useful in d/dg synovial sarcoma
- ± Amianthoid fibres (as in palisaded myofibroblastoma, p. 312)
- Immuno: ➢ +ve for the triad of CD34, CD99, Bcl-2; vimentin +ve, (c-kit ±ve)
  - ➢ −ve for S100, CK, αSMA, desmin, FXIIIa, collagen IV, (CD34 in high grade malig. SFT)
  - ➢ *NB*: CD34 and vimentin are characteristic of the interstitial dendritic cell
- Variant: *calcifying fibrous pseudotumour:* ➢ SFT which has 'burnt out' (i.e. no spindle cells)
  - ➢ collagen and psammoma bodies may be present
- d/dg: adenofibroma, synovial sarcoma (see p. 94), NF, Schwannoma, MFH, fibrosarcoma, HPC
- Malignancy: ➢ infiltrative margins (! not just entrapment)
  - ➢ hypercellularity
  - ➢ pleomorphism
  - ➢ necrosis
  - ➢ mitoses >4/10 hpf

Malignant SFTs have 2–50% of nuclei +ve for p53 (*cf.* ≤1% in benign) and a Ki-67 LI of 1-45% (*cf.* ≤2% in benign)

- Grading malignant SFT (*NB*: intermediate grade shows features in between high and low):
  - ➢ low grade: predom. pushing border and elongated bland nuclei; they show obvious SFT patterns and collagen and p53/Ki-67 are at the low end of the malignant range. CD34 is usu. +ve
  - ➢ high grade: extensively infiltrative with plump, pleomorphic, hyperchromatic nuclei; SFT patterns and collagen are not well developed and p53/Ki-67 are at the upper end; CD34 is often −ve

Juvenile Xanthogranuloma
- Multinucleated GC (esp. Touton type – peripheral vacuoles surround a ring of nuclei)
- Does not infiltrate the epidermis
- May infiltrate muscle and deep structures
- May have lots of eosinophils (d/dg HX – do immuno to see if histiocytes are of the Langerhans type)
- Immuno: non-X histiocytes are +ve for CD68, α_1AT, lysozyme and CD31 and −ve for CD1a and S100

Malignant Fibrous Histiocytoma (MFH)
- Sites: soft tissues (extremities/retroperitoneum) / bone (30% are 2° to Paget's/radiation/cartilage tumours)
- Variants:
  - ➤ **M**yxoid (most 'myxoid MFH' are now regarded as high grade myxofibrosarcoma)
  - ➤ **A**ngiomatoid (youths, indolent, termed *angiomatoid fibrous histiocytoma* by the WHO)
  - ➤ **G**iant cell MFH has many osteoclast-like (i.e. bland) giant cells
  - ➤ **I**nflammatory (retroperitoneal, big xanthomatoid cells / virocytes, PMN, d/dg CA mets)
  - ➤ **C**ommon type (Storiform Pleomorphic) focally seen in all variants except angiomatoid
  - ➤ **S**kin (= AFX): slow growing, locally recurrent, mets uncommon
- Storiform pattern (i.e. variably curved bundles of spindle cells radiating from a central hub)
- Variably pleomorphic spindle cells and 'malignant histiocyte'-like cells, ± multinucleated tumour cells
- Usu. much collagen, lipid-laden Mϕ, ± osteoclast-like giant cells
- Immuno: MFH is a diagnosis of exclusion, MSA and CD68 may be +ve but a definitive immunophenotype should result in classification of the lesion as a poorly diff sarcoma of that type
- Angiomatoid type: nodular, subcutaneous and usu. have a rich lymphoplasmacytic component (∴ d/dg LN), blood spaces lack endothelium, relatively bland eosinophilic spindle cells ± haemorrhage (d/dg KS), few mitoses; immuno ±ve for CD68, desmin and MSA (= HHF-35, not αSMA)
- d/dg: fibrosarcoma, MPNST, monophasic synovial sarcoma, spindled metastasis (esp. in bone e.g. from carcinoma of the bronchus, kidney or anaplastic thyroid carcinoma)
- d/dg: many cases of storiform pleomorphic MFH may be poorly differentiated versions of liposarcoma (better prognosis), RMS (worse prognosis) or leiomyosarcoma
- d/dg: many cases of 'giant cell MFH' may be giant cell rich osteosarcomas or leiomyosarcomas
- d/dg: see also 'Some Soft Tissue Lesions with a Storiform Pattern', p. 327

Atypical fibroxanthoma (AFX)
- Skin (esp. head and neck), circumscribed, ± collarette, actinic background, usu. lacks a Grenz zone
- Highly pleomorphic cells (or non-pleom. variant), mitoses ++ (incl. atypical ones), various patterns
- Adnexa may be entrapped but usu. not infiltrated (an infiltrative deep margin goes against a diagnosis of AFX)
- Necrosis, vascular or perineural invasion or deep subcutaneous spread suggest a more malignant sarcoma
- Immuno: αSMA ±ve, CD68 ±ve, −ve for pan CK and S100
- d/dg melanoma, leiomyosarcoma and sarcomatoid SCC must all be excluded before making the diagnosis
- d/dg atypical DF: this is not UV-related, has a background typical of a DF and is FXIIIa +ve

Dermatofibrosarcoma Protruberans (DFSP)
- Dermal, extends into subcutis with cells parallel to the surface to surround adipocytes ('lace-like')
- Arch: asymmetrical, storiform pattern throughout, ± Grenz zone
- Bland spindle cells, mitoses uncommon (usu. <5/10 hpf)
- Overlying epidermis is thinned / ulcerated
- Immuno: CD34 +ve, FXIIIa −ve, p53 +ve, αSMA −ve
- Variant: Bednar: heavily melanin pigmented dendritic cells throughout (*cf.* haemosiderin in DF)
- Variant: fibrosarcomatous (>5% of tumour shows ↑mitoses, fascicular architecture and cytological atypia ± CD34 +vity)
- Variant: giant cell fibroblastoma (young, superficial, uni and multinucleated cells line pseudovasc. spaces)
- Variants: myxoid, diffuse, fascicular, sclerotic, atrophic (d/dg DF), DFSP-MFH (aggressive)
- d/dg AFX: DFSP has bland cytology and few mitoses (except aggressive variants)
- d/dg DF: ➤ epidermal changes in DF (not seen in DFSP)

TABLE 21.2 Immuno of DF *vs.* DFSP

	FXIIIa	CD34
DF	+ve	−ve
DFSP	−ve	+ve

> ➤ admixed foam cells, multinucleated giant cells and inflam^y cells favour DF
> ➤ pattern and extent of subcutis involvement
> ➤ DF is more symmetrical, only focally storiform and contains birefringent collagen

Dermatofibroma / Benign Fibrous Histiocytoma (DF / BFH)
- Dermal, ± minimal extension into subcutis as radiating spikes perpendicular to the surface
- Bland spindle cells, mitoses are uncommon
- Overlying epidermis: acanthosis ± BCP-like pattern or basaloid proliferations resembling BCC
- Junction with normal dermis shows infiltration of spindle cells around hyalinised collagen bundles
- Foamy Mφ (called BFH when these are prominent), giant cells, inflam^y cells ± haemosiderin
- Immuno: CD34 −ve, FXIIIa +ve (but may be −ve towards the centre of sclerotic lesions), αSMA ±ve, p53 −ve
- Variant: cellular (may reach into the superficial subcutis and have small central necrotic foci)
- Variant: aneurysmal (may evolve into a haemosiderotic DF or 'sclerosing haemangioma'):
  > ➤ cellular DF with blood-filled spaces (d/dg KS), mitoses may reach upto 10/10 hpf
  > ➤ immuno: desmin +ve (other muscle markers −ve)
  > ➤ d/dg haemangioma: ☞ the blood spaces are not endothelial-lined in DF
  > ☞ characteristic DF peri-collagen infiltration at the periphery
- Variant: atypical DF ('with monster cells') has sparse mitoses and no necrosis; d/dg AFX (*q.v.*)
- Variant: subcutaneous (well-circumscribed, monomorphic, ± vasc. invasion, CD34 ±ve)
- Variants: keloidal (d/dg juvenile hyaline fibromatosis), lipidised, epithelioid, DF with true BCC, etc.
- d/dg DFSP (see under DFSP) / scar / keloid / stasis change in lower leg
- d/dg storiform collagenoma (collagen ++, fibroblasts are rare, similar lesions occur in Cowden's syndrome)
- d/dg basaloid epidermal changes can be confused for BCC if the underlying DF is not recognised
- d/dg pleomorphic fibroma is hypocellular (unlike atypical DF) with haphazard collagen and some very atypical cells – but mitoses are rare; there is no actinic association

Perivascular Epithelioid Cell Tumour (PEComa)
- May be benign or malignant and occur at ≈ any site; exclude tuberose sclerosis clinically
- Macro: well circ. lobulated solid white fleshy tumour ± fibrous bands (contain hyalinised vessels)
- Epithelioid and spindled components (one may predominate), clear or eosinophilic cytoplasm, nuclei are bland or focally pleom. ± eosinophilic intranuclear inclusions or prominent nucleoli but usu. amitotic if benign); rich sinusoid-like microvasculature ± extravasated RBC; variable hyalinisation
- Stains: PAS +ve, DPAS −ve
- Immuno: +ve for HMB45 (usu. strong, diffuse) ± actins and desmin (usu. in spindled areas) ± CD68, ± CD10, c-kit (membranous, but usu. <50% of cells stain). Melan-A and CD34 may be patchy +ve or −ve. CK, vimentin, S100, calretinin, CD31 and AFP are all −ve.
- EM: cytoplasmic membrane-bound vesicles containing variably dense granular material 350–750 nm ⌀, glycogen and some features of smooth muscle ± cytoplasmic rhomboid crystals. No melanosomes or premelanosomes
- Features correlated with malignancy: haemorrhage / necrosis, local invasion, nuclear pleomorphism (esp. in epithelioid cells), only one cell type (esp. if myomatous) and mitoses ++
- d/dg: melanoma (should be S100 +ve), GIST (not usu. pleomorphic and HMB45 is −ve), uterine stromal tumour or epithelioid leiomyosarcoma (lack strong diffuse HMB45), rhabdoid tumour (HMB45 −ve, CK and desmin +ve in epithelioid cells, typical EM), other clear cell sarcomas (*q.v.*)

Lesions in the differential diagnosis of 'Myxoma'
- It helps to know: ① age, sex, site; ② is it totally myxoid or cellular with myxoid areas (the latter suggests a myxoid variant – *vide infra*); ③ if totally myxoid what is the vascular density / pattern?
- Cardiac myxomas (see p. 79)
- Superficial angiomyxoma (see pp. 317–318 and see all the entities in the d/dg list under that entry)
- Chordoma and soft tissue myxopapillary ependymoma (see pp. 184) – esp. if near the sacrum
- Cellular myxoma (low grade myxoid neoplasm with recurrent potential) has pseudolipoblasts
- Myxoma of the jaw: spindle/stellate cells with intermeshing branched processes ± odontogenic epithelium
- Myxolipoma (is a myxoid variant of spindle cell lipoma)

- Angiomyxoma of deep soft tissues (similar histology to aggressive angiomyxoma of the vulva - *q.v.*)
- Juxta-articular myxoma: d/dg low grade myxofibrosarcoma may be difficult (CPC, esp. site, helps)
- Intramuscular myxoma: sparse vasculature (focally increased), pseudolipoblasts ± muciphages
- Ganglion cyst (may have cellular myxoid foci outside the cyst wall – ! do not over-interpret)
- Nerve sheath myxoma (= a myxoid PNST)
- Ossifying fibromyxoid tumour: extremities, late middle-age, variable atypia, thick acellular 'capsule'
- Low grade fibromyxoid sarcoma: ! d/dg nodular fasciitis. See p. 311
- Myxofibrosarcoma: WHO requires ≥50% of the tumour to have the typical highly vascular stroma with curvilinear vessels; grading ∝ mitotic count, presence of solid cellular areas and necrosis
- d/dg myxoid variant of otherwise cellular tumours:
    - ➢ DFSP, MPNST, GIST, MFH, etc.
    - ➢ chondrosarcoma: has hyaluronidase resistant myxoid (unlike most other myxoid lesions), ! S100 is often −ve
    - ➢ liposarcoma, synovial sarcoma, leiomyosarcoma

Sarcomas 2° to Radiation Exposure
- Most occur ≥2 years post exposure (some use this as a defining requirement)
- Osteosarcoma, angiosarcoma, MFH, fibrosarcoma, chondrosarcoma, synovial sarcoma, mesothelioma, MPNST
- (Fibromatoses, carcinomas, haematolymphoid and CNS neoplasms also occur post radiation)

Some Soft Tissue Lesions with a Storiform Pattern (at least focally)
- Mycobacterial pseudotumour
- DF, DFSP, SFT, MFH / AFX, ovarian fibroma, metaphyseal fibrous defect / non-ossifying fibroma
- Sarcomatoid mesothelioma and carcinoma, malignant meningioma (d/dg 1° intracranial SFT)
- GIST, smooth muscle tumours, vascular tumours, FDC sarcoma, spindle/desmoplastic melanoma

Sarcomas that may be Positive for Cytokeratins
- PNST
- Epithelioid sarcoma
- Angiosarcoma (and epithelioid haemangioendothelioma)
- Rhabdoid tumour
- Leiomyosarcoma (esp. of deep soft tissues)
- Synovial sarcoma (focal groups)

Sarcomas that Metastasise to Lymph Nodes
- Synovial sarcoma
- MFH
- Myxofibrosarcoma
- Epithelioid sarcoma

Tumours which Commonly Mimic Spindle Sarcomas
- Spindle cell SCC, sarcomatoid RCC, anaplastic thyroid carcinoma
- Sarcomatoid mesothelioma
- Melanoma
- Fasciitides, myositis ossificans, myofibroblastic proliferations and pseudotumours

Grading of Soft Tissue Sarcomas
- The NCI and FNCLCC are the most common systems (for details, see Graadt van Roggen, 2001)
- Grade ∝ tumour type, mitotic count and % necrosis (only valid if no prior chemoRx/radioRx)
- Form many tumours, the type alone defines the grade; examples from the NCI system are:
G1 = infantile fibrosarcoma, well-diff/myxoid liposarcoma, epithelioid haemangioendothelioma, MPNST with <6/10 hpf mitoses
G2 = any non-G3 tumour with necrosis at <15%
G3 = RMS, ASPS, mesenchymal chondrosarcoma, Ewing/PNET, any other sarcoma with >15% necrosis

Bibliography

Abdulkader, M., Abercrombie, J., McCulloch, T.A. *et al.* (2005) Colonic angiomyolipoma with a monotypic expression and a predominant epithelioid component. *Journal of Clinical Pathology*, **58** (10), 1107–1109.

Bhattacharya, B., Dilworth, H.P., Lacobuzio-Donahue, C. *et al.* (2005) Nuclear β-catenin expression distinguishes deep fibromatosis from other benign and malignant fibroblastic and myofibroblastic lesions, *Americal Journal of Surgical Pathology*, **29** (5), 653–659.

Billings, S.D. and Hood, A.F. (2000) Epithelioid sarcoma arising on the nose of a child: a case report and review of the literature. *Journal of Cutaneous Pathology*, **27** (4), 186–190.

Chan, J.K.C. (1997) Vascular tumours with a prominent spindle cell component. *Current Diagnostic Pathology*, **4** (2), 76–90.

Day, D.D., Jass, J.R., Price, A.B. *et al.* (2003) *Morson & Dawson's Gastrointestinal Pathology*. 4th edn, Blackwell Science, Ltd, UK.

Evert, M., Wardelmann, E., Nestler, G. *et al.* (2005) Abdominopelvic epithelioid cell sarcoma (malignant PEComa) mimicking gastrointestinal stromal tumour of the rectum. *Histopathology*, **46** (1), 115–117.

Fineberg, S. and Rosen, P.P. (1994) Cutaneous angiosarcoma and atypical vascular lesions of the skin and breast after radiation therapy for breast carcinoma. *American Journal of Clinical Pathology*, **102** (6), 757–763.

Fletcher, C.D.M., Beham, A., Bekir, S. *et al.* (1991) Epithelioid angiosarcoma of deep soft tissue: A distinctive tumor readily mistaken for an epithelioid neoplasm. *American Journal of Surgical Pathology*, **15** (10), 915–924.

Folpe, A.L. and Deyrup, A.T. (2006) Alveolar soft-part sarcoma: a review an update. *Journal of Clinical Pathology*, **59** (11), 1127–1132.

Ganesan, R., McCluggage, W.G., Hirschowitz, L. *et al.* (2005) Superficial myofibroblastoma of the lower female genital tract: report of a series including tumours with a vulval location. *Histopathology*, **46** (2), 137–143.

Ghadially, F.N. (1998) *Diagnostic Ultrastructural Pathology*, 2nd edn, Butterworth-Heinemann, Boston.

Graadt van Roggen, J.F., Lim, T.K. and Hogendoorn, P.C.W. (2005) The histopathological differential diagnosis of mesenchymal tumours of the skin. *Current Diagnostic Pathology*, **11** (6), 371–389.

Graadt van Roggen, J.F. (2001) The histopathological grading of soft tissue tumours: current concepts. *Current Diagnostic Pathology*, **7** (1), 1–7.

Guillou, L. and Fletcher, C.D.M. (1997) Newer entities in soft tissue tumours. *Current Diagnostic Pathology*, **4** (4), 210–221.

Hahn, H.P. and Fletcher, C.D.M. (2005) The role of cytogenetics and molecular genetics in soft tissue tumour diagnosis—a realistic appraisal. *Current Diagnostic Pathology*, **11** (6), 361–370.

Harris, M. (2001) Myofibroblastic proliferations mimicking soft tissue sarcoma, in *Recent Advances in Histopathology*, Vol. 19 (eds D. Lowe and J.C.E. Underwood), Churchill Livingstone, Edinburgh, pp. 83–98.

Hoda, S.A., Cranor, M.L. and Rosen, P.P. (1992) Hemangiomas of the breast with atypical histological features. Further analysis of histological subtypes confirming their benign character. *American Journal of Surgical Pathology*, **16** (6), 553–560.

Holloway, P., Kay, E. and Leader, M. (2005) Myxoid tumours: A guide to the morphological and immunohistochemical assessment of soft tissue myxoid lesions encountered in general surgical pathology. *Current Diagnostic Pathology*, **11** (6), 411–425.

Hornick, J.L. and Fletcher, C.D.M. (2003) Criteria for malignancy in non-visceral smooth muscle tumors. *Annals of Diagnostic Pathology*, **7** (1), 60–66.

Martignoni, G., Pea, M., Bonetti, F. *et al.* (1998) Carcinoma-like monotypic epithelioid angiomyolipoma in patients without evidence of tuberose sclerosis: A clinicopathologic and genetic study. *American Journal of Surgical Pathology*, **22** (6), 663–672.

McKenney, J.K., Weiss, S.W. and Folpe, A.L. (2001) CD31 Expression in Intratumoral Macrophages: A Potential Diagnostic Pitfall. *American Journal of Surgical Pathology*, **25** (9), 1167–1173.

Middleton, L.P., Duray, P.H. and Merino, M.J. (1998) The histological spectrum of hemangiopericytoma: application of immunohistochemical analysis including proliferative markers to facilitate diagnosis and predict prognosis. *Human Pathology*, **29** (6), 636–40.

Morrow, M., Berger, D. and Thelmo, W. (1998) Diffuse cystic angiomatosis of the breast. *Cancer*, **62** (11), 2392–2396.

Morson, B.C. (ed) (1987) Alimentary Tract, in *Systemic Pathology*, Vol. 3, 3rd edn (ed W. St C. Symmers), Churchill Livingstone, Edinburgh.

Ng, W-K. (2003) Radiation-associated changes in tissues and tumours. *Current Diagnostic Pathology*, **9** (2), 124–136.

Pea, M., Martignoni, G., Zamboni, G. *et al.* (1996) Perivascular epithelioid cell. *American Journal of Surgical Pathology*, **20** (9), 1149–1155.

Ramachandra, S., Hollowood, K., Bisceglia, M. *et al.* (1995) Inflammatory pseudotumour of soft tissues: a clinicopathological and immunohisto-chemical analysis of 18 cases. *Histopathology*, **27** (4), 313–323.

Schrüch, W., Seemayer, T.A. and Gabbiani, G. (1998) The myofibroblast a quarter of a century after its discovery. *American Journal of Surgical Pathology*, **22** (2), 141–147.

Rosen, P.P. (1985) Vascular tumors of the breast III. Angiomatosis. *American Journal of Surgical Pathology*, **9** (9), 652–658.

Suster, S., Nascimento, A.G., Miettinen, M. *et al.* (1995) Solitary fibrous tumour of soft tissue. A clinicopathologic and immunohistochemical study of 12 cases. *American Journal of Surgical Pathology*, **19** (11), 1257–1266.

Weiss, S.W. and Goldblum, J.R. (eds) (2001) *Enzinger and Weiss' Soft Tissue Tumors*, 4th edn, Mosby, St Louis.

Yokoi, T., Tsuzuki, T., Yatabe, Y. *et al.* (1998) Solitary fibrous tumour: significance of p53 and CD34 immunoreactivity in its malignant transformation. *Histopathology*, **32** (5), 423–432.

Zamboni, G., Pea, M., Martignoni, G. *et al.* (1996) Clear cell "sugar" tumour of the pancreas. *American Journal of Surgical Pathology*, **20** (6), 722–730.

Zen, Y., Fujii, T., Sato, Y. *et al.* (2007) Pathological classification of hepatic inflammatory pseudotumor with respect to IgG4-related disease. *Modern Pathology*, **20** (8), 884–894.

22. Osteoarticular

Normal

- *Woven bone*: closely packed and irregularly orientated large lacunae with plump osteoblasts. Matrix collagen is haphazardly arranged (woven) so only faint criss-crossing lines are seen by polarisation (no lamellae). Architecture is trabecular or spiculated
- *Lamellar bone*: lacunae are smaller, spindle shaped, more regularly spaced out and have their long axes parallel to the lamellae. The matrix collagen lies in parallel bundles giving lamellae (bright and dark lines). Architecture is trabecular (= cancellous/spongy bone) [lamellae lie parallel to the long axis of the trabeculae] or compact (cortical bone) [with circumferential lamellae]. If lamellar bone is thick enough to be vascularised, concentric lamellae surround the vessels (Haversian systems)
- *Morphometry of mineralisation* (requires undecalcified tissue ± Goldner's or von Kossa-stain):
  - ➢ *calcification front (= mineralisation front)*, the line of *active* mineralisation between osteoid and mineralised bone, can be labelled by pulses of tetracyclines (→ crisp thin line of yellow autofluorescence) and occupies ≈ 40–60% – or more – of normal trabecular surface
  - ➢ *osteoid* covers ≤ 20% of the trabecular surface (and is <5% of trabecular volume) at a thickness of ≤4 bright lamellae by polarisation. Increased with any cause of ↑ turnover
- *Hyaline cartilage:*
  - ➢ chondrocytes occur in (artefactual) lacunae surrounded by a basophilic, MPS-rich zone of matrix (the *territorial zone*) separated from each other by the eosinophilic interterritorial matrix
  - ➢ chondrocytes are round or angulated cells with a single small nucleus and are not mitotically active in mature cartilage. Exceptions: articular cartilage of small tubular bones and children
  - ➢ articular cartilage collagen and chondrocytes are parallel to the surface in the superficial *lamina splendens* (zone I), irregularly arranged in the transitional zone (II) and form vertical columns in the deep zone (III) separated from the calcified zone (IV) by the *tide mark* (wavey calcified line)
  - ➢ epiphyseal growth plate (= *physis*) shows endochondral ossification: small chondrocytes, in vertical columns, have a prolif. zone towards the epiphyseal end of the plate and hypertrophy towards the diaphysis as they mature. Mineralisation occurs in these hypertrophic foci

Non-neoplastic Bone Disease

Osteomalacia and Rickets
- Causes: ↓ vitamin D$_3$ (dietary, solar) or hypophosphataemia (renal, parathyroid, paraneoplastic)
- Osteoid: ↑ volume, ↑ thickness and ↑ surface coverage (usu. to > 35% of trabecular surface area)
- Calcification front: ↓ coverage, irregular and blurred line by tetracycline labelling
- ↑ Osteoblastic activity
- Thickened epiphyseal cartilage with defective mineralisation (extension of cartilage into underlying bone)
- ± Changes of (2°) hyperparathyroid bone disease (see OFC below)
- d/dg non-lethal AD forms of hypophosphatasia: like osteomalacia but has ↓ nõs of osteoblasts
- d/dg aluminium toxicity: in this, the calcification front is sharp and stains red with aurinitricarboxylic acid; there is also ↓ osteoblastic activity

Hyperparathyroidism: Osteitis Fibrosa Cystica (OFC)
- Sites: widespread incl. tubular bones of hands/feet, clavicle, mandible, cranium and others
- Dissecting resorption by ↑ nõs of osteoclasts ± woven bone (osteoclasts have fewer nuclei and are not limited to the trabecular surface *cf.* d/dg the early, lytic, phase of Paget's disease)
- ↑ Osteoblastic activity
- Fibrous replacement of bone marrow (usu. paratrabecular *cf.* d/dg myelofibrosis)
- ± Crystal arthropathies (gout and pseudogout)
- Multiple lytic lesions (these are the '*cystica*' in OFC): degenerative cystic spaces and brown tumours

Diagnostic Criteria Handbook in Histopathology: A Surgical Pathology Vade Mecum by Paul J. Tadrous
Copyright © 2007 by John Wiley & Sons, Ltd.

Brown tumour of hyperparathyroidism
- Lobular arch., active fibrous tissue septa ± woven bone, vessels, haemorrhage and haemosiderin
- Irregularly distributed multinucleated osteoclasts (may cluster around haemorrhage)
- d/dg other giant cell-rich lesions in bone with ≈ identical histology (giant cell reparative granuloma, GC reaction of hands + feet, GC epulis and solid variant ABC) requires CPC (incl. serum PTH levels)
- d/dg GC tumour of bone: multiple lesions favour brown tumour. For histological differences see p. 335

Renal Osteodystrophy
① OFC
② Osteomalacia
③ Osteosclerosis (due to woven bone ++): radiologically may be seen as a 'rugger jersey spine'

Osteoporosis
- Def^n: osteopaenia (difficult to diagnose by histology) of sufficient severity to cause pathological fracture
- The cortex and weight-bearing trabeculae are least affected
- Trabeculae appear thinned and separated ± ↑ surface osteoclasts (subtle)
- Transient, juxta-articular, osteoporosis may show ↑ marrow vascularity ± fat necrosis

Osteonecrosis (Avascular Necrosis, Bone Infarct)
- Days: necrotic marrow → granulomas (reaction to dead marrow/bone fragments), pyknosis and coagulative necrosis, dystrophic calcification and dissolution/saponification of the adipose tissue
- Weeks–months: empty lacunae, bone matrix shows paucity of staining or ↑ basophilia
- Periphery: ➢ viable new bone is laid down around necrotic fragments
  ➢ fibrous and granulation tissue (eventually calcifies → well-defined rim on radiol)

Osteomyelitis
- Clin., radiol. and macro.: may simulate d/dg Ewing's sarcoma or HX
- Reactive woven bone and fibrosis ↑ with time to form a chronic (Brodie's) abscess
- Osteonecrosis is most abundant in the earliest/acute phases
- PMN pus may be found at any stage + other inflam^y cells

Paget's Disease of Bone (Osteitis Deformans)
- A myxovirus infection of osteoclasts in (usu. Anglo-Saxon) people of late middle-age
- Affects single or multiple bones (axial skeleton > peripheral)
- Radiol: early lesions are lytic (flame-shaped in long bones, *osteoporosis circumscripta* in cranium)
- *Early*:
  ➢ large osteoclasts ++ with ↑ nõ of nuclei } resorption is not dissecting
  ➢ ↑ osteoblast activity → woven bone } and osteoclasts are more nucleated
  ➢ marrow is hypervascular and fibrotic } cf. d/dg OFC
- *Late*:
  ➢ jigsaw mosaic of lamellar bone with crenated cement lines replaces trabeculae and cortex
  ➢ both cortex and trabeculae are thicker and irregular with loss of corticomedullary differentiation (also seen on radiology)
  ➢ marrow is fibrosed; osteoblastic and osteoclastic activity subsides
- Paget's sarcoma: a sarcoma developing 2° to Paget's – usu. osteosarcoma (or fibrosarcoma/MFH/chondrosarcoma/other) usu. in long bones, pelvis or skull

Achondroplasia
- The normal columns of chondrocytes in the epiphyseal growth plate are disrupted and shortened
- Mineralisation occurs in the vicinity of hypertrophic chondrocytes but very few of these are formed

Osteopetrosis (Marble Bone Disease of Albers-Schönberg)
- Severe forms result in cytopenic immunodeficiency, anaemia and leukoerythroblastic PB
- ≈ Solid, heavy bones with expanded diaphyses criss-crossed with vertical and transverse streaks
- Dense meshwork of irregular trabeculae composed of bone and cartilage
- Osteoclasts may be numerous (though functionally ineffective)
- Marrow space is reduced and fibrotic

Osteogenesis Imperfecta (Brittle Bone Disease)
- Growth plate fragmentation → bone ends filled with cartilage nodules (radiol: 'bag of popcorn')
- Woven bone +/ thin lamellae (lamellae occur in the less severe forms)
- Crowding of osteocytes and osteoblasts
- ± Osteoporosis

Multinucleated Giant Cell Rich Lesions *(in General – not just osteoarticular)*

- Any anaplastic carcinoma, sarcoma, melanoma, etc. may have giant cells (to be distinguished from the osteoclast-like giant cells present in variants of certain tumours e.g. IDC of breast, pancreas, anaplastic carcinoma of thyroid and peripherally in clear cell chondrosarcoma)
- Inflammatory and granulomatous conditions with multinucleated giant cells derived from macrophages (e.g. xanthogranuloma of the ovary, foreign body reactions, etc.)
- Reaction to intraosseous haemorrhage (incl. haemophiliac pseudotumour)
- Stromal giant cells may occur in: the testis (? age-related), the lower female genital tract (e.g. in fibroepithelial polyps), fibroadenoma (can be bizarre), other breast lesions or interlobular breast stroma, the anus, bladder and nose
- Surrounding stromal emphysematous spaces (e.g. pneumatosis intestinalis, emphysematous colpitis/emphysematous vaginitis)
- Syncytiotrophoblastic differentiation
- HX (esp. Hand-Schüller-Christian disease)
- Juvenile xanthogranuloma (classically Touton-type giant cells)
- Alveolar RMS (typically 'wreath-like' giant cells) and pleomorphic RMS
- Giant cell arteritis
- Giant cell myocarditis
- Giant cell carcinoma of the lung
- Giant cell interstitial pneumonitis
- Anaplastic large cell lymphoma
- Multinucleated FDC (Warthin-Finkeldey type) in reactive (esp. viral) lymphoid proliferations
- Giant cell hepatitis
- Giant cell hepatocellular carcinoma
- Giant cell glioblastoma (grade IV)
- Sub-ependymal giant cell astrocytoma (grade II)
- Uterine carcinosarcoma (epithelial giant cells)
- Giant cell pseudosarcomatous mural nodule in ovarian mucinous cystadenoma
- Phyllodes tumour of the breast
- Metaplastic carcinoma of the breast
- Annular elastolytic giant cell granuloma (skin)
- Lymphomatoid papulosis (LyP)
- Melanocytic naevi ('mulberry cells' – a sign of benignity)
- Atypical fibroxanthoma (AFX)
- Giant cell (de Quervain's) thyroiditis
- ABC and ABC-like lesions/lesions with ABC-like foci within them e.g.:
  - ➤ osteoblastoma, chondroblastoma and chondromyxoid fibroma
  - ➤ giant cell tumours of bone/tendon sheath/PVNS
  - ➤ fibrous dysplasia
  - ➤ mesenchymal hamartoma
  - ➤ giant cell reparative granuloma (is ≈ identical to solid variant ABC) – p. 333
  - ➤ rarely, malignant tumours (e.g. clear cell chondrosarcoma)
- Giant cell epulis (= peripheral giant cell reparative granuloma) – occurs in gums, not jaw bones
- Giant cell reaction of the hands and feet
- Brown tumour of hyperparathyroidism (see p. 330)
- Giant cell reparative granuloma (central): jaw bones ('soap bubble' lucency without periosteal breach/reaction and with tooth displacement but not resorption), irregular distribution of GC (esp. around haemorrhage), vascular stroma with fibrous mononuclear cells producing collagen, metaplastic bone or woven bone with osteoblast rimming, focal haemorrhage (ABC-like) ± Jaffe-Campanacci syndrome: For d/dg see the section on 'Brown tumour of hyperparathyroidism', p. 330

- Chondroblastoma
- Chondromyxoid fibroma
- Metaphyseal fibrous defect and non-ossifying fibroma
- Solitary bone cyst (simple/unicameral/multicameral/latent bone cyst)
- Osteoblastoma
- Osteoclast-rich leiomyosarcoma: like osteoclast-rich osteosarcoma but lacks osteoid/bone
- Osteoclast-rich osteosarcoma: cytological atypia, atypical mitoses, osteoid/bone
- Giant cell tumour of bone (and GCT of soft tissues)
- Giant cell tumour of tendon sheath/PVNS: lipid foamy Mφ ± sparse GC. Like NOF but in synovium
- Benign fibrous histiocytoma (BFH)
- Giant cell fibroblastoma (DFSP variant with pseudovascular spaces lined by multinucleated cells)
- Giant cell MFH
- Giant cell reticulohistiocytoma/reticulohistiocytosis (typically 'ground glass' type giant cells)
- Giant cell angiofibroma (≈ a cross between SFT and giant cell fibroblastoma)
- Pleomorphic lipoma/liposarcoma (typically 'floret-like' giant cells)
- Proliferative fasciitis/myositis and ischaemic fasciitis: ganglion-like multinucleated cells
- Very many other things

Bone Tumours and Tumour-Like Lesions

General Features in the Differential Diagnosis
- Is the tumour producing osteoid or collagen? Osteoid forms branching microtrabeculated structures that surround individual cells and EM shows matrix vesicles. Collagen is laid down in parallel bands/bundles and does not completely surround the cells (see Figure 22.1).
- Immuno/stains do not help distinguish benign *vs.* malignant bone-forming lesions as all osteogenic cells have a similar phenotype and all may show +vity for alkaline phosphatase (ALP)
- Reactive soft tissue lesions: have a Hx of trauma, grow rapidly, show many mitoses (of normal morphology), have tissue culture-type myofibroblasts and some attempt at zonal maturation

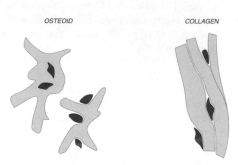

FIGURE 22.1   Osteoid and collagen

- Reactive bone shows:
  - ➢ osteoblastic rimming (single layer continuous lining of active osteoblasts)
  - ➢ maturation of osteocytes i.e. the surface osteoblasts become smaller when surrounded by osteoid to become internal osteocytes)
  - ➢ an attempt at orderly architecture of trabeculae (esp. arches/arcades)
- Malignant bone shows:
  - ➢ a suggestive clinical and radiological context
  - ➢ no rimming and no osteoclast maturation (lacy osteoid surrounds large malignant osteoblasts that look the same as those on the surface)
  - ➢ disorderly architecture of trabeculae and no maturation to a bony shell
  - ➢ invasion into and around pre-existing trabeculae of the medulla (called 'permeation' in the literature = 'invasion' or 'infiltration' in this chapter)

Metastatic Tumours
- Usu. multiple (but may appear solitary in early stages)
- Usu. carcinomas (esp. the 5 'B's: **b**reast, **b**ronchus, **b**idney, **b**yroid and **b**rostate)
- Usu. lytic but sclerotic ones (e.g. prostate and breast) result in ↑↑ serum ALP (unlike d/dg myeloma)
- Usu. in sites of haemopoietic marrow (rare in the distal limb bones): may → leukoerythroblastic PB
- ! May be adjacent to/mixed in with fracture callus (due to pathological fractures)

Fracture Callus
- Shows features of reactive bone (*vide supra*) ± variable amounts of necrotic bone
- Mixed chondro-osseous tissue and cartilage that is proliferative and cellular and matures (hypertrophies) before ossifying (i.e. looks like endochondral ossification in a normal epiphyseal growth plate)

- Zonation (superficial to deep): proliferating fibroblasts (± 'tissue culture'-like) → primitive bone and cartilage → maturing woven bone. (this zonation is reversed in d/dg *myositis ossificans*)
- Marrow spaces are vascular with proliferative fibroblasts that decrease in cellularity with time
- ! Do not miss metastatic carcinoma cells or HX within fracture callus (is the fracture explained?)
- d/dg PTFOL in the rib: but that lesion lacks osteoblastic rimming
- d/dg sarcoma (more likely to be a problem with early callus lesions that are cellular with very little bone and in callus that 'infiltrates' skeletal muscle adjacent to the fracture site):
  - ➢ chondrosarcoma: endochondral-type maturing ossification is not seen in chondrosarcoma
  - ➢ osteosarcoma: callus lacks atypia (of cells and mitoses), soft-tissue tumour necrosis and features of malignant bone (see p. 332). The 'marrow spaces' in osteosarcoma may be filled with malig. cells

Myositis Ossificans
See d/dg under Osteosarcoma (p. 337); see also p. 309.

Bizarre Parosteal Osteochondromatous Proliferation (BPOP)
- Usu. under the periosteum in the tubular bones of the hands and feet (rarely other limb bones)
- Marrow spaces are packed with spindle ± 'tissue culture'-like cells
- Irregular islands of basophilic chondroid showing irregular (but endochondral-type) ossification
- Highly cellular and irregular cartilage cap with plump nuclei and binucleate forms
- d/dg subungual exostosis is a similar condition but affects the *distal* phalanges (unlike BPOP)
- d/dg osteosarcoma: wrong site and no cytological atypia in the spindle cells
- d/dg chondrosarcoma *ex* ecchondroma: wrong site and no continuity of marrow space with underlying bone

Cysts in Bone

Solitary bone cyst (simple / unicameral / multicameral / latent bone cyst)
- Radiol: lucent cyst abuts the diaphyseal surface of the physis in children but may grow away from it to become detached in the diaphysis (= latent cyst). Cortical thinning → pathological fracture
- Macro: trabeculated lining; may be unilocular (unicameral) or have dividing septa (= multicameral)
- Uncomplicated: fibrous lining with no or clear fluid contents ± fibrin deposits (may mineralise)
- ± Osteoclasts (i.e. giant cells), haemosiderin, foamy Mφ, granulation tissue and fracture callus
- 2° sarcomatous change is case-report-rare
- d/dg ABC (esp. in any bridging septa)
- d/dg cementoma (due to the mineralising fibrinoid)

Aneurysmal bone cyst (ABC)
- Radiol: lytic, eccentric 'blowout' lesions; macro: partly solid with cavernous blood-filled spaces
- Cellular mitotic fibrous tissue, giant cells, haemosiderin but no necrosis unless pathological #
- Woven bone (parallel to septa) ± calcified chondroid 'blue bone' (a useful feature if present)
- d/dg must exclude an underlying lesion (see 'Giant Cell Rich Lesions', pp. 331–332)
- d/dg: solid ABC *vs.* GCT of bone: ABC contains woven bone/chondroid, has an irreg. distribution of giant cells, the mononuclear cells are spindled (fibrous tissue) and the site may be unusual for GCT
- d/dg telangiectatic osteosarcoma (has cytological atypia, abnormal mitoses ± tumour necrosis) and low grade osteosarcoma (are *less* cellular/mitotic)
- d/dg giant cell reparative granuloma: ABC is a related entity ∴ use CPC
- d/dg solitary bone cyst: may be impossible by histology esp. in complicated multicameral cases

Other cysts
- Epidermoid, intraosseous ganglion (called subchondral cyst if below joint cartilage), hydatid, etc.

Mesenchymal Hamartoma of the Lateral Chest Wall (Mesenchymoma) in Infants
- Like osteo/chondroblastoma plus lobules of cartilage
- mitoses, haemorrhage, vasc. spaces ± ABC-like areas
- d/dg: osteosarcoma has features of malignancy (p. 332) and has different site and age distribution
- d/dg mesenchymal chondrosarcoma (p. 339)

Eosinophil Granuloma (Histiocytosis X)
- Radiol: well-defined lytic lesion in a child ± periosteal reaction (d/dg osteomyelitis/Ewing's)
- Histology of HX (see pp. 57–58)
- d/dg osteomyelitis: Langerhans cells and unusual sites (e.g. skull) favour HX

Metaphyseal Fibrous Defect (Non-Ossifying Fibroma, Fibrous Cortical Defect or just 'Fibroma')
- Radiol: eccentric, scalloped lesion in the cortex (MFD) or cortex and medulla (NOF) of a youth. Regress
- ± Jaffe-Campanacci syndrome: ① polyostotic NOF, ② skin pigmentat^n, ③ endocrine/mental defects (may also have giant cell reparative granuloma(s) of the jaws); d/dg NF-1 may also show ① and ②
- Fibrosis (cellular, proliferative, ± storiform but no cytological atypia), haemosiderin ± siderophages
- Lipid foamy cell nests ± cholesterol clefts (called *xanthofibroma*[1] if prominent)
- d/dg GCT: NOF osteoclast giant cells are fewer and less nucleate and it doesn't extend to joint surface
- d/dg *periosteal desmoid* of the distal femur: ≈ NOF but less cellular. Requires no Rx – ! do not confuse with d/dg *desmoplastic fibroma* (a locally aggressive *intraosseous desmoid* tumour that lacks giant cells and osseous metaplasia and shows spindle collagenous fascicles without the cytological atypia, hypercellularity and ↑ mitoses of *fibrosarcoma* or *leiomyosarcoma* – see Chapter 21: Soft Tissues)
- d/dg metastatic RCC *vs.* foam cell nests
- d/dg: BFH (rare): similar histology but bigger tumour in older patients ± at site not typical for NOF
- d/dg xanthomatous PTFOL: xanthofibroma has giant cells and lacks woven-to-lamellar zonation

Fibrous Dysplasia (FD)
- Radiol: well-defined 'ground glass' lesion typically in ribs, long bones, skull of a child/young adult
- ± Albright's syndrome = ① **p**olyostotic FD, ② **p**atchy **p**igmentation and ③ **p**recocious **p**uberty
- Woven bone (in 'lobster claw', 'Chinese character' or psammoma-body-like configurations)
- The bone is metaplastic i.e. directly formed from fibrous tissue (no surface osteoblasts)
- The fibrous tissue has a 'patternless pattern' (± focal storiform areas) of bland stubby spindle cells
- Nodules of cartilage ± myxoid foci (! do not misdiagnose as d/dg chondromyxoid fibroma)
- d/dg parosteal osteosarcoma (*q.v.*): if the lesion is *on* the bone (*cf. in* it) consider parosteal osteosarcoma
- d/dg fibrous dysplasia-like osteosarcoma (*q.v.*): this shows infiltration around pre-existent normal trabeculae
- d/dg osteofibrous dysplasia and adamantinoma (*q.v.*)

Osteofibrous Dysplasia (Ossifying Fibroma)
- Infiltrates cortex of long bones in children (usu. ≤10 years old)
- Osteoblast-formed (± rimmed) bone at the periphery, metaplastic bone at centre
- More aggressive *cf.* FD (may be a variant of adamantinoma – they share similar sites and radiol.)
- Immuno: may have single CK +ve cells ∴ this alone is insufficient to diagnose d/dg adamantinoma
- d/dg adamantinoma: always search for epithelial strands and nests if an adult presents with FD or osteofibrous dysplasia

Post-traumatic Fibro-osseous Lesion (PTFOL) of the Rib
- Zonally maturing lace-like bone (woven centrally, lamellar peripherally), osteoblasts are few/absent
- Stroma is bland, amitotic and vascular ± central sheet of xanthomatous cells
- d/dg: FD (lacks woven-to-lamellar zonation, xanthoma cells are not in sheets and trabeculae have typical slender shapes – *vide supra*)
- d/dg osteoid osteoma: this has osteoblast rimming – not seen in PTFOL

Osteoma
- A hamartomatoid/reactive *out*growth of bland lamellar bone that may be cortical +/ cancellous
- Usu. in the skull, jaws, sinuses and may be part of Gardner's syndrome. They are very rare
- d/dg *bone island* is an *intramedullary* focus of cortical-type bone (called *osteopoikilosis* if multiple)
- d/dg reactive osteosclerosis: can be indistinguishable microscopically

Osteoid Osteoma
- Clin.: pain relieved by aspirin; radiol: lucent 'nidus' ± surrounding sclerosis (d/dg Brodie's abscess)
- Macro: nidus is red and granular and usu. <1.5cm ∅; specimen radiographs may help locate it
- Nidus: irregular, cellular (usu. small) trabeculae of osteoid, variable mineralisation to woven bone, focal osteoblastic rimming ± crenated (Pagetoid) cement lines. No cartilage (unless fracture callus).
- Other: surrounding osteosclerosis (thick trabeculae/cortex); RhA-like inflam^y synovitis (if near a joint)
- d/dg osteoblastoma: if histology overlaps, use arbitrary size cut-off (>1.5 cm ∅ = osteoblastoma)
- d/dg osteosarcoma (see 'Osteoblastoma Family of Lesions', below)

---

[1] xanthomatous change in bone is ≈ always a 2° change ∴ if you want to call something a 'xanthoma' look for the underlying lesion e.g. NOF, BFH, ABC, simple cyst, or whatever

Osteoblastoma Family of Lesions
- *cf.* osteoid osteoma these are larger (usu. >2cm), more often axial and don't have the typical radiol.
- At the margin it merges with the non-lesional bone – but does not infiltrate into its marrow spaces
- d/dg usual-type osteosarcoma:
    - ➢ lack of invasiveness (into surrounding bone or soft tissues)
    - ➢ lack of cartilage (unless related to fracture callus)
    - ➢ rim of osteosclerosis, when present, favours osteoblastoma
    - ➢ solid sheets of cells (without matrix) favours malignancy

Benign osteoblastoma
- *cf.* osteoid osteoma these have a more open trabecular pattern and are more vascular
- The surrounding bone is normal or only slightly sclerotic

Pseudomalignant osteoblastoma
- Plump osteoblasts with ancient change (large nuclei with smudged, Arias-Stella-like, chromatin)

Aggressive osteoblastoma (= Malignant osteoblastoma)
- Large (epithelioid) osteoblasts, ↑ cellularity, ↑ mitoses, ↑ peripheral osteosclerosis, basophilic spicules
- ABC-like foci are more likely. They are locally recurrent but not metastatic

Osteoblastoma-like osteosarcoma
- Like osteoblastoma but infiltrates adjacent pre-existing normal bone trabeculae. Mets occur

Adamantinoma
- Usu. in the upper tibia of a young adult. Blood and lymphatic mets may occur eventually
- Osteofibrous dysplasia-like with islands/strands of epithelium (occ. spindled), keratin is unusual
- Epithelium may have peripheral palisading and central stellate reticulum (like ameloblastoma)
- d/dg metastasis: site (mets are rare distal to elbow/knee), epithelium not dysplastic or keratinising

Giant Cell Tumour of Bone (and Giant Cell Tumour of Soft Tissues)
- Spans epiphyseal line to include epiphysis; rare in immature skeleton; ≈ never centred in diaphysis
- GCT in the jaw or tubular bones of hands and feet and multiple GCT can happen, but is very rare (think d/dg brown tumour of ↑ PTH [p. 330] or GC reparative granuloma [p. 331])
- Uniform distribution of giant cells – but giant cells may be sparse
- Ovoid bland mononuclear cells have similar nuclei to giant cells and mitoses (not atypical): these are the neoplastic cells (= inactive osteoblasts), they recruit and activate the osteoclast giant cells
- Immuno: mononuclear cells are vimentin and α_1AT +ve, S100 −ve
- Stroma: vascular ± vasc. invasion (! does not imply malignancy), ± haemorrhage, necrosis and foam cells
- Typically, no collagen (or other matrix) is produced by tumour cells: these typical features must be seen in substantial areas of a tumour to call it GCT, however there may be foci of osteoid or fibrogenesis and NOF-like areas with spindled mononuclear cells can be seen – esp. at the periphery
- Cartilage (non-callus) suggests d/dg chondroblastoma (if well diff) or osteosarcoma (if chondroid)
- Variant: *GCT of soft tissues* (same histology but rare, occurs in elderly and is centred in soft tissues)
- Grade ∝ nõ of mitoses and nõ of giant cells but is not considered clinically useful
- Metastasis of a typical GCT (i.e. the mets also look like typical GCT):
    - ➢ this is called 'metastatic GCT' (*not* 'malignant GCT' – *vide infra*)
    - ➢ if multiple mets consider mis-diagnosis (e.g. it may be a GC-rich osteosarcoma)
- Malignancy in a GCT = a frank high grade sarcoma (usu. osteosarcoma, fibrosarcoma or MFH) arising:
    - ➢ in a typical GCT at 1st presentation (= '1° malignant GCT'), or
    - ➢ as a recurrence after surgery/radiotherapy
- d/dg osteosarcoma can be difficult unless: there is cytological atypia, it arises in the immature skeleton, it does not span the epiphysis, there is malignant bone and typical radiol., it shows soft tissue infiltration (*NB* benign GCT may extend into soft tissue but has a well-defined outline. It is also well-defined within the medullary cavity)
- d/dg ABC (p. 333) and other 'Giant Cell Rich Lesions' (pp. 331–332)

Ewing's Sarcoma
See also p. 58.
- Clin. (fever, ↑ WCC and ESR), radiol ('moth-eaten', 'onion skin') and macro (≈ pus) d/dg osteomyelitis
- SBRCT, indistinct cell borders (syncytial) and bubbly cytoplasm (glycogen), few mitoses
- *Atypical (large cell) Ewing's*: prom. nucleoli, larger cells and mitoses ++ (but prog. is no different)

- Cytogenetics: PNET t(11;22)(q24;p12)(FLI1;EWS) – unlike d/dg DSRCT (see p. 58)
- Immuno: CD99 +ve (membranous), vimentin +ve (dot-like, at least focally), Fli-1 ±ve in 75% (also in PNET and Merkel cell tumours but not other childhood-type SBRCT), S100 −ve, CK −ve
- d/dg:
  - ➤ osteomyelitis: it may require a thorough search to find the Ewing's cells amongst reactive changes of necrotic bone, marrow fibrosis and mixed inflam^n
  - ➤ EM shows no specific organelles in Ewing's: d/dg NB (dense core neurosecretory granules), carcinomas (tight junctions), RMS (sarcomeres), lymphomas (absence of glycogen)
  - ➤ lymphoma: Ewing's is glycogen +ve and LCA −ve with little intercellular reticulin
  - ➤ metastatic neuroblastoma – but neuroblastoma has ↑ urinary catecholamines, fibrillary tissue ± ganglion cells and is NB84 +ve and ≈ always CD99 −ve
  - ➤ PNET and Askin are different differentiation variants of the same entity – see p. 58
  - ➤ small cell osteosarcoma / mesenchymal chondrosarcoma: presence of matrix (e.g. osteoid) excludes Ewing's
  - ➤ other: true (cf. artefactual) nuclear spindling excludes Ewing's
- Prog.: ➤ worse if: systemic Sx, axial site, large tumour bulk (esp. soft tissue extension)
  - ➤ better in tumours with exon 6/7 variant of t(11;22)

Osteosarcoma
- Clin.: usu. arise in metaphysis in immature skeleton or 2° to Paget's disease/radiation. Serum ALP is prognostic
- Macro: assess tumour size, local spread (esp. if through the periosteum into soft tissue – e.g. infiltration of skeletal muscle on Bx samples), skip lesions (intra-osseous mets) and % non-viable tumour (= necrotic + severest form of chemoRx damage)[2] after chemoRx
- Pleomorphic spindle cells (ALP +ve) producing lacy (often basophilic) osteoid/chondroid/cartilage with features of malignancy (see 'General Features in the Differential Diagnosis' p. 332)
- Immuno: vimentin +ve, c-erbB-2 (HER2) ±ve, αSMA ±ve, membranous CD99 ±ve, S100 +ve in chondroid areas, CD56 ±ve
- Grade is determined by histological type: high grade (most types of central osteosarcoma and juxta-cortical osteosarcoma), intermediate grade (periosteal), low grade (parosteal, osteoblastoma-like and FD-like)
- Imprint cytology: many pleomorphic cells strongly +ve for cytoplasmic ALP granules in the correct clinicoradiological setting is diagnostic even if no osteoid/bone on Bx (but ! must exclude d/dg angiosarcoma/other endothelial tumour because endothelial cells are also ALP +ve)
- d/dg: other lesions have ALP +ve cells but are not pleom. (e.g. ABC) or only a small subset stain (e.g. GCT). Also, differentiating reactive callus or osteoblastoma from low grade osteosarcoma may not be possible, so if the cells are not pleom. you cannot make a benign diagnosis using ALP imprints
- d/dg osteosarcomatous component of a de-differentiated chondrosarcoma (q.v.)
- d/dg 1° or 2° leiomyosarcoma: may be a problem in recurrent/metastatic osteosarcoma that shows spindle cells but no matrix because both are αSMA +ve. ALP should still be +ve in osteosarcoma (unless anaplastic)

Central osteosarcoma (Medullary osteosarcoma)
- Mixed osteosarcoma is the usual type and has osteoblastic, chondroblastic and fibroblastic foci
- The more the chondroblastic differentiation, the worse the response to chemoRx ∴ estimate % chondroblastic
- Variants:
  - ➤ Fibroblastic: predominantly fibrous matrix. d/dg fibrosarcoma/MFH rests on ALP +vity and CPC
  - ➤ Chondroblastic: predominantly ① lobules malignant cartilage and ② peripheral spindle cells ± focal osteoid (usu. at the interface between the two). d/dg chondrosarcoma: ALP +ve cells, young age with lack of pre-disposing lesion and evidence of rapid growth (incl. no scalloping or buttressing on radiol) all favour osteosarcoma.
  - ➤ Osteoblastic: predominant matrix is osteoid/bone. Osteoblastoma-like osteosarcoma is a low grade variant of this and is discussed above under d/dg osteoblastoma (p.335)

---

[2] may require use of prolif^n marker immuno; >90–95% non-viable tumour = good prognosis

> Central low grade (= fibrous dysplasia-like): infiltrates around pre-existing trabeculae of bone and does not have typical 'lobster-claw' trabeculae or 'ground glass' radiol of d/dg FD. Pleomorphism is mild and there may be maturation of the bone as in parosteal osteosarcoma

> Small cell – like d/dg atypical Ewing's but with matrix and ALP +ve (! ± CD99 +ve) cells. d/dg mesenchymal chondrosarcoma: this has well-developed lobules of cartilage and any bone is formed by ossification of the cartilage (not by malignant cells as in osteosarcoma)

> Telangiectatic: like d/dg ABC but with *pleomorphic cells*, mitoses ++ and invasion

> Giant cell-rich (Osteoclast-rich): def^n: >50% of the tumour must have many benign GC admixed with malignant bone-forming cells. This is very rare. (see also d/dg GCT of Bone, p. 335)

> Epithelioid: d/dg carcinomas: use ALP and immuno (one instance where immuno is helpful)

> Anaplastic: may be ALP −ve ∴ need focal evidence of typical osteosarcoma +/ typical CPC

High grade surface osteosarcoma (Juxta-cortical osteosarcoma)
- A rare tumour with similar histology and prog. (or worse) *cf.* high grade central osteosarcoma

Parosteal osteosarcoma
- Lobulated, firm tumour usu. on posterior surface of (± invasion into) the diaphysis of long bones
- Superficially: spindle cells (producing collagen, atypia is minimal) and chondroid areas
- Mid-to-deep: bone trabeculae (woven and metaplastic-like) mature towards the host bone cortex (where it may even form lamellar bone and may show signs of remodelling into parallel arrays)
- May have de-differentiated foci which worsens the prognosis ∴ sample well.
- d/dg:
  - ☞ osteochondroma, but
    - ☞ no continuity with the medulla of the bone via a 'cortical gap'
    - ☞ 'marrow' spaces are solid spindles not fatty/haemopoietic
  - ☞ myositis ossificans, but
    - ☞ opposite zonation (spindles and cartilage superficial, bone deep)
    - ☞ no osteoblastic rimming of trabeculae in osteosarcoma
    - ☞ the spindle cells are fibrogenic in osteosarcoma
    - ☞ no 'air gap' sign on X-ray (see Figure 21.1, p. 309)
  - ☞ fibrous dysplasia, but
    - ☞ site: this osteosarcoma is on the bone, FD is within it

Periosteal osteosarcoma
- Peripheral spindling of mod. pleom. malig. cells, slit-like vascular spaces and soft tissue invasion (these *spindle cells* may form 'arcades' ! not to be confused with arcades of *osteoid/bone* in callus)
- Centrally there is malig. chondroid lobules with central maturation, calcification ± ossification
- Osteoid streamers may rise perpendicular to the surface of the host bone
- Macro involvement of the medulla should prompt a re-think to medullary chondroblastic osteosarcoma
- d/dg chondrosarcoma: osteosarcoma cells are ALP +ve, also see under chondroblastic osteosarcoma, p. 336

Extraosseous osteosarcoma
- Usu. in the elderly, in the stroma of a malig. phyllodes tumour or rarely as a 1° in other soft tissues
- d/dg mixed mesenchymoma (= any combination of ≥2 of osteosarcoma, RMS, liposarcoma without MPNST)
- d/dg myositis ossificans: the zonation is reversed and the bone is malignant (see p. 332 and p. 309)

Ecchondroma (Osteochondroma/Osteocartilagenous Exostosis)
- Pedunculated or sessile cartilage-capped bony outgrowth starts at the physis and migrates down the bone, growth stops at skeletal maturity
- May be multiple (= *diaphyseal aclasis / HME* and this has an increased risk of chondrosarcoma)
- Stalk: cortex and medulla (contains fatty/red marrow ± cartilage islands) of the exostosis is continuous with the cortex and medulla of the host bone (in radiology this medullary junction is described as the 'cortical gap')
- Cap: hyaline cartilage covered by perichondrium, <1cm thick in adults and shows endochondral ossification
- 2° chondrosarcoma (usu. low grade): esp. if axial/proximal site, rapid/resumed growth or pain without fracture/bursa
- d/dg parosteal osteosarcoma (*vide supra*), BPOP and subungual exostosis (see under BPOP p. 333)

Enchondroma

- Benign cartilage tumour centred in the medulla, often in the tubular bones of the hands and feet
- *Multiple enchondromatosis*: if predominantly unilateral = Ollier's disease; if bilateral + spindle cell haemangiomas = Maffucci's syndrome (has ↑ risk of 2° chondrosarcoma and 1° visceral neoplasms)
- Typically: solid hyaline matrix without myxoid degeneration, hypocellular, vague clusters of small cells with small single nuclei, lobular arch. ± a peripheral rim of bone
- Arch.: fused lobules ± separate lobules at periphery surrounded by marrow (*does not* imply invasion)
- If multiple or in hands and feet may be ↑ cellular with binucleation ± myxoid (micro) but no invasion
- May de-differentiate (see 'Chondrosarcoma') ∴ prophylactic surgery or F/U may be indicated in the elderly
- d/dg chondrosarcoma (or 2° chondrosarcoma change): microscopic invasion ('permeation' – for definition, see 'Chondrosarcoma', below) and macroscopic myxoid change (if high grade) and CPC/radiol.

Periosteal Chondroma

- Well circ., small chondroid lesion on the surface of tubular bones (rare in hands and feet)
- Causes scalloping erosion of the cortex ('saucerisation') but are not infiltrative
- Very cellular with binucleate and hyperchromatic cells
- d/dg chondrosarcoma: small size and circumscription

Soft Tissue Chondroma

- (Multi-)lobulated, non-invasive, cellular hyaline cartilage lesions in the soft tissues of the hands and feet. See also 'Synovial Chondromatosis' on p. 341

Chondroblastoma

- Centred in epiphysis (or a 2° ossification centre) of long bones; may give rise to benign metastases
- Polygonal cells with well-defined cytoplasm (pale) and oval nuclei (± grooves and small nucleoli); generally bland but with 'random' atypia; mitoses are present but not numerous; scattered giant cells
- Chondroid ± honeycomb pericellular calcification in a 'chicken-wire', 'lace-like' or 'pepper-like' pattern (may be recapitulated on a retic stain in decalcified preparations) ± fragments of normal physis.
- No intercellular matrix (other than the chondroid) ± coagulative necrosis in the mineralised areas
- GC nuclei are similar to polygonal cells' nuclei
- Immuno: +ve for vimentin and S100; ±ve for CK, αSMA, EMA
- d/dg: may have ABC-like areas ∴ see ABC, GCT of bone and 'Giant Cell Rich Lesions', above
- d/dg chondromyxoid fibroma (site and cytology) and clear cell chondrosarcoma (cytology, invasion, CPC)
- d/dg osteosarcoma is invasive with pleom. cells and lacy mineralisation of osteoid (*cf.* honeycomb pericellular mineralisation of chondroid matrix)

Chondromyxoid Fibroma

- Metaphysis, similar age group to chondroblastoma (i.e. usu. teens or 20s)
- Chondroid, myxoid or fibrous *lobules* (more cellular at the periphery) separated by fibrous septa
- Cells are stellate, ovoid or spindled with nuclei of various shapes ± focal worrisome anisonucleosis
- Septa are vascular, cellular ± giant cells, ABC-like areas +/ osteoid
- Immuno: S100 +ve (may help if chondroid differentiation is not obvious)
- d/dg chondroblastoma: some foci may be similar but site and presence of other features help
- d/dg chondrosarcoma, esp. grade 2 (myxoid): age, lack of invasion and constellation of features above

Chondrosarcoma

- Clin.: usu. in proximal/axial skeleton of old people (unless 2° – usu. to ecchondroma/enchondroma)
- Radiol.: shows evidence of slow erosive growth (cortical erosion and buttressing)
- Macro: lobules of chondroid with central coalescence ± myxoid/cystic degeneration, necrosis, Ca^{2+}
- Micro: wide sampling is important to ensure confident diagnosis and grading
- Malig. cells produce hyaline chondroid matrix ± central necrosis/Ca^{2+} ± periph. fibrosis/benign bone (any malig. bone, not part of a separate de-diff area, should change the diagnosis to osteosarcoma)
- Cytological atypia = *plump nuclei* in many cells (with more than occ. binucleate forms) and *giant chondrocytes* (with ≥1 large nuclei ± chromatin clumps)

- Exceptions: ↑ cellularity and cytol. atypia may occur in benign tumours of growing children, small tubular bones of the hands and feet, well-circ sub-periosteal tumours, soft tissue chondromas and chondromas in multiple enchondromatoses. Bland cytology can occur in sternal chondrosarcomas
- Arch.: ➤ invasion (permeation) is the single most useful criterion = 'wall-to-wall' filling of pre-existing marrow space with partial erosion of the lamellar trabeculae (not just occ. nodules separated from the main mass by marrow ± surrounded by lamellar bone as occurs in benign enchondromas)
  - ➤ lack of clonal clustering of cells
- Grading (determines the likelihood of metastasis):
  - G1. lobular hyaline matrix, bland cytology, ≈ no mitoses/necrosis
  - G2. myxoid/necrotic foci, ↑ cellularity at lobule periphery, mild cytol. atypia, mitoses <2/10hpf
  - G3. extensive myxoid/necrosis, ↑ periph. lobule cellularity, obvious cytol. atypia, mitoses ≥2
- *Borderline chondrosarcoma* = clin. and radiol. suggestive but no firm histological malignant features
- Prog: complete excision at 1st operation with clear margins (and no spillage/seeding) gives best hope
- d/dg chondroblastic osteosarcoma (*vide supra*, see also p. 336 and de-diff chondrosarcoma below)
- d/dg degenerative cartilage: radiological signs of degenerative joint disease, joint involvement (rare in chondrosarcoma), clonal proliferations and other features of OA are all evidence against chondrosarcoma
- d/dg chondromyxoid fibroma (*q.v.*): this also has chondroid lobules with peripheral hypercellularity
- d/dg chordoma: usu. a problem at either end of the spinal column, see p. 184

De-differentiated chondrosarcoma

- *Low grade* cartilage tumour *sharply demarcated* from a high grade soft tissue sarcoma (or osteosarcoma)
- d/dg chondroblastic osteosarcoma: but this has *pleomorphic* cartilage that is *admixed* (also age and CPC)
- d/dg mesenchymal chondrosarcoma: but this has a monomorphic Ewingoid sarcoma component

Clear cell chondrosarcoma

- Good prog., teens to old age, assoc^d with epiphysis/diaphysis, radiol: *no* buttressing/cortical erosion
- Cytology: clear cells (glycogen), well-defined cell borders, central nuclei (± binucleate / prominent nucleolus)
- Arch.: vague lobules (± periph. osteoclast-like giant cells or central osteoid/bone)/sheets/trabeculae
- Chondroid is not obvious and foci of typical chondrosarcoma are only present in 50% of cases
- Vascular fibrous septa, ABC-like areas, chondroblastoma-like polygonal cells ± chicken-wire Ca^{2+}
- Immuno of clear cells: S100 +ve, CK −ve, EMA −ve
- d/dg chondroblastoma, osteoblastoma, GCT of bone or ABC
- d/dg metastatic CCC has opposite immuno and lacks the other features

Mesenchymal chondrosarcoma

- Poor prog, young adult, 1° bone (any site), 1° extraskeletal (esp. head and neck), radiol 'popcorn' Ca^{2+}
- SBRCT with islands of low grade chondrosarcoma – the interface may be abrupt or gradual.
- Immuno: CD99 ±ve
- ± Pushing margin (with vascular plugs), a HPC-like vasculature and a fibrillary matrix (! not d/dg osteoid)
- d/dg small cell osteosarcoma (p. 337) and de-diff chondrosarcoma (*vide supra*)
- d/dg lymphoma (matrix and immuno)
- d/dg Ewing's sarcoma: matrix +/ spindling (may occur in mesenchymal chondrosarcoma) excludes Ewing's
- d/dg mesenchymal hamartoma occurs in infants, shows osteoblastic bone formation (not just ossification of chondroid) and does not have malig. SBRCT elements or chondrosarcoma radiol.

Articular Pathology

Differential Diagnosis of Pigments in Joints/Synovium
- Haemosiderin: inflam^y arthritides, trauma, haemophilia, haemochromatosis, haemangioma and PVNS
- Tetracyclines result in brown *bone* (*cf.* cartilage/synovium)
- Osmicated fat in the synovium
- Metal deposits (see 'Joint Prosthesis Pathology', p. 341)
- Ochronosis (polymerised homogentisic acid in articular cartilage in patients with alkaptonuria)

Differential Diagnosis of Neutrophils in Joints/Synovium
- Sepsis (see p. 341 and pp. 375–376)
- Crystals (for details of polarisation analysis, see p. 375):
    - monosodium urate (gout, water-soluble, murexide reaction +ve) deposits in superficial artic- ular cartilage or as soft tissue masses (tophi) with a prominent giant cell reaction; pale pink on H&E (d/dg amyloid) but may contain Ca^{2+} or cholesterol clefts; may occur together with CPPD
    - Ca^{2+} pyrophosphate (CPPD, pseudogout, removed by decalcification, murexide −ve) deposits in the cartilage (in OA and chondrocalcinosis) or the superficial layers of the synovium, basophilic on H&E and may lack a giant cell reaction. Occasionally associated with some metabolic diseases (e.g. hyperparathyroidism), a familial tendency and haemochromatosis
    - Ca^{2+} hydroxyapatite may be seen in Milwaukee shoulder, trauma, hyperparathyroidism, sys- temic malignancies, PSS and CRF
- Acute/active RhA and some seronegative arthritides (esp. Behçet's disease)
- Haemorrhage

Granulomatous Arthritis and the d/dg of Histiocytic Infiltrates
- Bacteria: TB (may be non-caseating in synovium), atypical mycobacteria and brucellosis
- Fungi (thorn synovitis may also show thorn-related foreign body)
- Rheumatoid nodules: rarely occur in the synovium (d/dg hemigranulomas = rheumatoid nodule-like lesions that appear to spill their contents into the joint, seen in OA and some seronegative arthritides)
- Sarcoid (rarely affects joints)   these may also present as non-specific
- Crohn's disease   chronic inflam^n without granulomas
- Foreign body granulomas e.g. detritus synovitis (see 'Joint Prosthesis Pathology', p. 341)
- d/dg histiocytic infiltrates: HX, multicentric reticulohistiocytosis, Whipple's disease

Osteoarthritis and Degenerative/Regenerative Cartilage
- Clin. and radiol. evidence of degenerative joint disease, usu. polyarticular unless $2°$
- Tangential flaking ± vertical fibrillation ± blurred/irregular/duplicated tide mark
- Loss of MPS basophilia esp. in the interterritorial and superficial zones
- 'Clonal' proliferation of chondrocytes → multicellular groups ± dead ('ghost') chondrocytes
- Growth of cellular fibrocartilage over the surface of the articular cartilage from the joint periphery
- Synovium may show a reactive detritus synovitis with villiform hypertrophy and hyperplasia, chronic inflam^n ± haemosiderin (!d/dg RhA, PVNS or infective/other causes of granulomas) ± pseudogout
- Peripheral osteophytes ± concentric osteocartilagenous loose bodies (d/dg synovial chondromatosis)
- Subchondral bone sclerosis/necrosis ± degenerative subchondral cyst formation (ganglion-like)
- d/dg chondrosarcoma (pp. 338–339)

Rheumatoid Arthritis and Other Chronic Inflam^y Arthropathies
- Polyarticular incl. the TMJ and cervical spine (odontoid peg or vertebral bodies → fusion/slippage)
- Villous hypertrophy and lymphoplasmacytic infiltrate and germinal centres (Mφ > T-cells > B-cells)
- ± Giant cells derived from synovial lining Mφ (rheumatoid nodules are rare in the synovium)
- Superficial fibrin (→ rice bodies) and PMN (d/dg infection which can also occur) ± haemosiderin
- Pyrophosphate crystals are *very rare* in RhA (but can occur)
- Cartilage: superficial: Swiss cheese vacuolation (= enlarged chondrocyte lacunae) usu. occurs in cartilage covered by a pannus of granulation tissue and inflamed synovium
    - deep: local undermining by chronic inflam^y tissue in the sub-chondral bone
- Lymphoid hyperplasia in sub-chondral marrow fat spaces
- d/dg: other conditions that may have similar chronic inflam^n to RhA incl.:
    - seronegative arthritis: PSS, SLE, psoriatic arthritis, ankylosing spondylitis (see also 'Behçet's Arthritis', below)
    - Reiter's arthritis (has more PMN and may show vessels plugged by platelets and granulocytes)
    - Lyme disease: stain for spirochaetes (*Borrelia burgdorferi*) which may be found in the walls of synovial vessels, some of which show obliterative changes (unlike RhA)
    - OA (some of the more inflammatory cases overlap with RhA – look for other features of OA)
    - syphilis: a non-specific chronic inflam^y arthritis (± miliary gummas)

Behçet's Arthritis
- Villous hypertrophy of the synovium with surface fibrin ± ulceration
- Underlying vascular and fibrous connective tissue with many PMN and mixed inflam^y cells
- d/dg: sepsis/crystals/active phase of RhA

Joint Prosthesis Pathology (Pathology of the Periprosthetic Soft Tissue Membrane)
- Gradual wear → particulate matter from prosthesis → Mφ and inflam^n → loosening of prosthesis
- At surgery for a loose prosthesis, Bx for FS may be sent to decide:
  - ➤ ? infective → surgeon will remove prosthesis and wait until the infection has cleared before replacement
  - ➤ ? wear debris inflam^n only → surgeon will replace the joint immediately

Type 1 periprosthetic membrane – wear debris inflammation
- Def^n: >20% of the membrane surface is lined by Mφ +/ multinucleate giant cells
- Holes that may be large bubbly spaces or small (≈ 80 μ) round holes (± residual debris ≤ 2μ in ∅ = barium sulphate or zirconium) ± foamy Mφ
- Polymethylmethacrylate bone cement or unreacted cement monomer beads (soluble in solvents but stain with oil red O if preserved in fresh FS. If not dissolved, may show as basophilic grape-like clusters on paraffin H&E with mild birefringence
- Tiny black opaque particles (round/sharp-edged), may show a birefringent halo: metal (e.g. titanium)
- Bluish or transparent, birefringent, may be thread-like: HMW polyethylene/other plastics
- Non-birefringent but oil red O +ve (in paraffin sections): submicronic polyethylene
- Refractile bosselated yellowish material, not birefringent: Silastic®
- Silicone granulomas with birefringent particles: silicone elastomers
- Tiny (≈ 1μ) birefringent grey particles in Mφ but few/no giant cells: ceramics
- Thin black rods of variable length: carbon fibre

Type 2 periprosthetic membrane – infective
- Def^n: >10 PMN/10 hpf (because you don't see PMN with wear debris alone) – useful criterion on FS
- Lower grade infection may not have so many PMN but PMN are present with oedema, fibroblasts and proliferated capillaries
- Small lymphocyte aggregates with assoc^d plasma cells are also suggestive of low grade infection
- Multinucleated giant cells are sparse

Type 3 periprosthetic membrane – mixed wear debris/infective
- ≈ Equal proportions of the membrane are affected by Type 1 and Type 2 morphology

Type 4 periprosthetic membrane – indeterminate reactive changes
- Collagen and fibrosis-rich, cell-poor
- ± Mature granulation tissue (but no sig. PMN infiltrate *cf.* d/dg infective Type 2)
- May have a partial lining of fibrin or synovium (! do not mis-diagnose as Type 1 Mφ)

Synovial Chondromatosis
- A metaplastic process, usu. in a single large joint; radiol. may show erosion of the articular surface
- Nodules of chondroid matrix with 'clonal clusters' of proliferating chondrocytes occurs within the synovium, these eventually pedunculate and break off to form many loose bodies in the joint
- The nodules may display a synovial lining and contain focal Ca^{2+}
- May be hypercellular with binucleate cells and mitoses
- Long-standing loose bodies may acquire outer concentric lamellae of fibrocartilage
- d/dg chondrosarcoma: the clonal clusters are unusual for chondrosarcoma which rarely affects the joint space. Synovial chondrosarcoma is very rare, is solid/myxoid and extends beyond the joint capsule or permeates the bone
- d/dg osteochondral loose bodies in severe/rapid degenerative joint disease: the lack of clin./radiol. evidence of severe degenerative joint disease and the presence of 'clonal clusters'

Pigmented Villonodular (Teno)Synovitis (PVNS) – incl. GCT of Tendon Sheath
- Types: diffuse (large joints, 25% recur)/nodular ('GCT of tendon sheath', small joints, rarely recur)
- Nodular arch. (lobulated contour with fibrous septa) – early nodules may have mitoses ++ centrally with peripheral xanthomatoid 'maturation' (nuclei shrink and cytoplasm gets lipidised)
- ± Stromal hyaline or torsion necrosis
- Pseudoglandular cleft-like spaces lined by synoviocytes (d/dg synovial sarcoma)
- Histiocytoid mononuclear cells (modified synoviocytes) ± occ. bizarre cells

- Multinucleated giant cells (fusion of mononuclear cells) – nuclei are variably open to pyknotic
- Xanthoma cell groups (pale islands)
- Haemosiderin is found throughout the lesion (this is the 'pigment')
- Malignancy in GCT of tendon sheath:
  - ➤ benign GCT with an obviously malignant component (i.e. pleomorphism, diffuse infiltration, mitoses abnormal or >10/10hpf, few giant cells, tumour necrosis, lack of maturation)
  - ➤ GCT with benign histology but malignant behaviour (e.g. metastases)
  - ➤ both are very rare so consider the d/dg before making the diagnosis
- Malignancy in PVNS: lobular invasive growth, necrosis and prominent nucleoli.
- Immuno: mononuclear cells are +ve for CD68 and (focally) desmin
- d/dg ! distinguish PVNS from chronic haemorrhage (which is not Rx by surgery): in haemorrhage the haemosiderin is near the surface of the fronds, in PVNS it is throughout the lesion (which is cellular)
- d/dg: inflammatory myxohyaline tumour (= acral myxohyaline fibroblastic sarcoma) has scattered large bizarre virocytes/RS-like cells; it usu. occurs on the hands – see 'Myxofibrosarcoma' on p. 312.
- d/dg: tendinous xanthoma (multiple, giant cells sparse, cholesterol clefts ++, hyperlipidaemia)
- d/dg fibroma of tendon sheath may have occ. giant cells and foam cells (and is possibly related to GCT)

Adventitious Bursa
- A bursa not connected to a joint cavity but forming over bony prominences
- Fibrous wall ± a synovial lining (formed by metaplasia of connective tissue) with mucoid contents

Juxta-articular Myxoma
See p. 327.

Synovial Fluid Analysis
See pp. 375–376.

Bibliography

Aubert, S., Kerdaon, O., Conti, M. *et al.* (2006) Post-traumatic fibro-osseous lesion of the ribs: a relatively under-recognised entity. *Journal of Clinical Pathology*, **59** (6), 635–638.

Beck, J.S. and Anderson, J.M. (1987) Quantitative methods as an aid to diagnosis in histopathology, in *Recent Advances in Histopathology*, Vol. 13 (eds P.P. Anthony and R.N.W. MacSween), Churchill Livingstone, Edinburgh, pp. 255–269.

Dahlin, D.H. and Unni, K.K. (1986) *Bone Tumors. General Aspects and Data on 8,542 Cases*, 4ᵗʰ edn, Charles C. Thomas, Springfield, Illinois.

Fletcher, C.D.M., Unni, K.K. and Mertens, F. (eds) (2002) *WHO Classification of Tumours: Pathology & Genetics Tumours of Soft Tissue and Bone*, 1ˢᵗ edn, IARC Press, Lyon.

Freemont, A.J. (2003) Joint disease and the pathologist, in *Progress in Pathology*, Vol. 6 (eds N. Kirkham and N.A. Shepherd), Greenwich Medical Media, Ltd, London, pp. 79–100.

Ghadially, F.N. (1998) *Diagnostic ultrastructural pathology: A self-evaluation and self-teaching manual.* 2ⁿᵈ edn, Butterworth-Heinemann, Boston.

Malcolm, A.J. (2004) Ewing's tumour – examplar of defining a tumour. *ACP News* (Winter 2004), pp. 11–12.

Morawietz, L., Classen, R-A., Schröder, J.H. *et al.* (2006) Proposal for a histopathological consensus classification of the periprosthetic interface membrane. *Journal of Clinical Pathology*, **59** (6), 591–597.

Pringle, J.A.S. (1996) Osteosarcoma: the experience of a specialist unit. *Current Diagnostic Pathology*, **3** (3), 127–136.

Reid, R.P. and Catto, M.E. (1987) Some unusual tumours of cartilage and pseudosarcoma of the hand, in *Recent Advances in Histopathology*, Vol. 13 (eds P.P. Anthony and R.N.W. MacSween), Churchill Livingstone, Edinburgh, pp. 68–70.

Revell, P.A. (1987) The synovial biopsy, in *Recent Advances in Histopathology*, Vol. 13 (eds P.P. Anthony and R.N.W. MacSween), Churchill Livingstone, Edinburgh, pp. 79–94.

Rosenberg, A.E. and Nielsen, G.P. (2001) Giant cell containing lesions of bone and their differential diagnosis. *Current Diagnostic Pathology*, **7** (4), 235–246.

Szadowska, A., Sitkiewicz, A. and Jarosik, N. (1996) Mesenchymal hamartoma of the chest wall in infancy—a case report of this rare entity with cytologic findings. *Cytopathology*, **7** (3), 211–217.

Symmers, W. St. C. (ed) (1979) *Systemic Pathology*, Vol. 5, 2ⁿᵈ edn, Churchill Livingstone, Edinburgh.

Weiss, S.W. and Goldblum, J.R. (eds) (2001) *Enzinger and Weiss' Soft Tissue Tumors*, 4ᵗʰ edn, Mosby, St Louis.

23. Infection and Immunity

Introduction

This is a morphological guide for practising histopathologists and not a strict taxonomical classification. Some bacteria e.g. *Gardnerella* and *Haemophilus* are classified as coccobacilli here when a microbiologist would call them short bacilli (and they may indeed grow as proper bacilli under some conditions). Some bacteria here are placed in categories that aid morphological recognition in tissues rather than according to strict taxonomy (e.g. *Yersinia* is placed under 'coccobacilli' when it actually belongs to the coliform group of enterobacteria). Further information on some site-selective infections (e.g. rhinosporidiosis or infective colitis/hepatitis) are provided in other chapters.

      The numerous amoebae, helminthes, flies, etc. that parasitise man are too numerous to do any kind of justice to in a book of this sort. Here I give some morphological features of some of the least rare parasites encountered in UK practice but specialist text-books are an essential tool for those working where such protozoan and metazoan infections occur – see the Bibliography for examples.

Bacteria

Morphological Characterization

Cocci
- Gram +ve   ➢ clusters, (e.g. *Staphylococcus*)
  -       ➢ pairs (diplococci e.g. pneumococcus)
  -       ➢ chains (e.g. *Streptococcus*)
- Gram −ve e.g. *Neisseria gonorrhoeae* and *meningitidis* are 'kidney bean diplococci' usu. within PMN

Bacilli
- Gram +ve   ➢ spore-forming
  - ☞ central spores: (e.g. *Bacillus anthracis* [anthrax] or *cereus* [food poisoning, ophthalmitis])
  - ☞ eccentric spores: (e.g. *Clostridium tetani* [terminal spore], *perfringens* [thick bacilli, no spore[1]], *botulinum* or *difficile* [sub-terminal and free-floating spores])
  - ➢ non-sporulating (e.g. *Corynebacterium diphtheriae* [club-shaped short rods], *Listeria* spp., *Propionobacterium* spp. and *Lactobacillus* spp.)
- Gram −ve   ➢ straight (e.g. coliforms [*E. coli*, *Shigella*, *Salmonella*, *Klebsiella* and *Proteus* spp.]), *Legionella* spp., *Pseudomonas* spp. [may be Gram and Brown-Brenn invisible, so use Brown-Hopps])
  - ➢ curved (*Vibrio* spp., *Campylobacter* spp., *Helicobacter* spp., *Gastrospirillum* spp.)

Coccobacilli
- Gram −ve   e.g. *Bartonella* spp. (some may form chains), *Bordetella* spp., *Brucella* spp., *Calymatobacterium granulomatis* (usu. in pairs and surrounded by a clear 'capsule' on Giemsa within a Mφ to form the Donovan bodies[2] of granuloma venerium[3]), *Haemophilus influenzae*, *Yersinia* spp., mycoplasmas, *Rickettsia* spp., *Coxiella* spp., *Francisella* spp.: use Brown-Hopps, silver or Giemsa
- Gram +ve   e.g. some *Vibrio* spp.
- Gram variable: e.g. *Gardnerella vaginalis*
- *NB*: many coccobacillary species are seen within cells (epithelial, macrophage or PMN)

Filamentous bacilli
- *Actinomyces* (silver and Gram +ve, branching 1μ thick filaments, endogenous organism, forms radiating aggregates (macro = yellow 'sulphur granules'), no ↑ incidence in the immunosuppressed)
- *Nocardia* (Gram +ve exogenous actinomycete, usu. scattered in the tissues and seen in the immunosuppressed)

---

[1] *NB*: spore forming bacilli may not always show spores in tissue e.g. it is rare to see spores in tissue-situated *Clostridium perfringens* but they are seen in soil or cultured samples

[2] not to be confused with the amastigote forms of *Leishmania* spp. (= Leishman-Donovan bodies)

[3] also called *granuloma inguinale* : these are not to be confused with LGV (a chlamydial disease)

Diagnostic Criteria Handbook in Histopathology: A Surgical Pathology Vade Mecum by Paul J. Tadrous
Copyright © 2007 by John Wiley & Sons, Ltd.

- *Tropheryma whippelii* is a very short actinomycete but we don't use Gram stains to diagnose it
- d/dg Actinomycosis *vs.* Botryomycosis:
  - ➤ actino colonies may be surrounded by radiating eosinophilic flares of Splendore-Hoeppli
  - ➤ other bacteria (e.g. staphylococci) can cause a mimicking reaction in tissues (= botryomycosis) so careful high power microscopy of Gram stains should be used
- d/dg Actinomycosis *vs.* Pseudoactinomycotic radiate granules (PAMRAG):
  - ➤ PAMRAG have refractile crystalline strips and irregular granules
  - ➤ PAMRAG stain diffusely Gram +ve (filaments are seen in actino) and are silver −ve

Mycobacteria

- Although Gram +ve (and Giemsa +ve in tissue but −ve image in cytology preps) they may not stain hence the use of ZN or silver (or DPAS for large numbers of atypical mycobacietia). *M. leprae* is weakly acid fast so may not stain with ZN hence the need for a Wade-Fite or Fite-Faraco stain
- 3–5μ long, slightly wiggly ± beaded: e.g. *M. Tuberculosis, M. bovis, M. leprae*
- Slightly longer and thicker: atypical mycobacteria (e.g. *M. marinum* or MAI)
- MAI are more beaded *cf.* TB and tend to be intra-Mϕ, aligned in stacks and assoc[d] with non-necrotising diffuse Mϕ infiltration with few discrete granulomas – the latter usu. only in LN or bone marrow
- ≈20μ long, thicker, more crooked and more beaded/banded: some of the atypical mycobacteria (e.g. *M. Kansasii* which tends to form cords/serpentine coils and is assoc[d] with PMN and well-formed necrotising granulomas unlike d/dg MAI)
- Screening a ZN-stained slide for mycobacteria:
  - ➤ use a thick section (e.g. 10μ)
  - ➤ screen for 20 minutes (after which concentration is reduced) at high power (x40 or above)
  - ➤ focus up and down as mycobacteria may stick up ≈ perpendicular to the plane of the section

Spirochaetes

- Stains: silver methods, basophilic (if numerous) and specific immuno for *Borrelia, Leptospira*, etc.
- *Leptospira* spp. characteristically have one or both extremities bent back (as a shepherd's crook)
- *Borrelia* spp. are characteristically variable in length (upto 40μ) and may show 'elbow bends'
- *Treponema pallidum* (like *Leptospira*) are at the shorter end of the spectrum (upto 15μ)

Chlamydiae

- Gram −ve coccoid intracellular bacterioids, may form variably-sized (≈ nucleus-size) basophilic glyco-genated intraepithelial cytoplasmic inclusions stainable by Lugol's iodine, PAS or Giemsa (granular texture) but specific immuno or EM is more useful for diagnosis
- Plasma cells +/ PMN are the typical tissue reaction in the female genital tract
- Stellate necrotising palisaded granulomas with PMN are seen in the LN in LGV
- Follicular conjunctivitis with central necrosis of follicles and peripheral collagenisation in trachoma

Mycoplasma-associated Diseases
- Pneumonia ('primary atypical pneumonia')
- Meningoencephalitis
- Haemolytic anaemia

Group A Streptococcus-associated Diseases
- Acute follicular tonsillitis/quinsy
- Rheumatic fever
- ADP GN/RPC GN
- Scarlet fever
- Infected skin sores of malnourished children

Mycobacterial Pseudotumour
- LN, bone marrow, spleen, lung, skin
- Storiform spindle cell proliferation
- ± Mitoses ± vascular proliferation – d/dg KS (! but KS may co-exist with it)
- Immuno: +ve for desmin (d/dg a muscle tumour), S100, lysozyme, α_1AT; −ve for CD31 and CD34

Syphilis
- Fibrosis esp. of capsules of organs and also perivascularly
- Chronic inflammation esp. plasma cells
- Acute inflammation esp. PMN infiltrating epithelia
- Vascular damage esp. endarteritis obliterans

Fungi

Morphological Characterization

Yeast forms
- Shape and size: round or oval, with capsule or without, uniform diameter or pleomorphic
- Division: ➤ fission (e.g. *Penicillium marneffei* – useful in d/dg histoplasmosis)
                 ➤ budding: ☞ equal/unequal
                                    ☞ thin-necked/broad-based
                                    ☞ single buds/multiple buds
- Nucleus: single or multinucleated (may not be visible in routine stains)

Hyphal forms
- Thin/thick (uniform/irregular thickness)
- Septate (frequent, rare, regularly distributed or not, constrictions present/absent)/non-septate
- Branching (dichotomous[4] or irregular; consider the branch angles)/non-branching
- Pigmented/non-pigmented/hyaline/poorly-staining
- Presence (often where exposed to air) and type of conidia ± fruiting bodies (conidiophores)

Dimorphic forms
- Most pathogenic fungi are dimorphic but few show both their hyphal and yeast stages in tissues

Candida spp. (e.g. *C. albicans*)
- Dimorphic: budding ovoid yeast (budding is single, thin-necked, unequal and yeasts are ≈ 4µ ∅)
- Thin (≈ 4µ) septate, branching hyphae (also pseudohyphae i.e. yeast buds that elongate and stay attached at constriction points but with no true branching)
- d/dg Histoplasma (*vs.* spore-only Candida): granulomas, intracellular yeasts and lack of pseudohyphae

Cryptococcus spp. (e.g. C. neoformans)
- Budding round yeast (*usu.* single, thin-necked, unequal), can form hyphae and pseudohyphae in the immunosuppressed
- Great variability in sizes (5–15µ ∅)
- Clear halo mucinous capsule (mucicarmine, AB, Hale's colloidal iron → crenated/'hairy' capsule)
- Surrounding 'holes' give the tissue a spongy, 'soap bubble' or 'pseudoadipose' look
- Dry-variants exist (non-encapsulated) and capsulated cells may not be common in ordinary forms
- Small-yeast variants exist (d/dg *Histoplasma*, etc. but only *Cryptococcus* has a mucinous capsule and ≈ 50% of histoplasmosis and blastomycosis show some ZN +ve organisms but cryptococci are −ve)

Histoplasma spp. (e.g. H. capsulatum)
- Clin.: spores occur in soil and in faeces of bats/chickens; causes a cavitating TB-like disease in the immunocompetent and disseminated disease in the immunosuppressed (bones, adrenals, liver, spleen, LN)
- Budding ovoid yeast (budding is single and thin-necked)
- May be intracellular (e.g. aggregates in Mφ)
- Smaller and less variable in size *cf.* Cryptococcus (2–5µ)
- ±Artefactual clear halo (esp. if intracellular) but no true capsule (unlike *Cryptococcus*)
- Large yeast variant (*duboisii*) exists esp. in Africa (d/dg *Cryptococcus*, blastomyces, *etc.*)
- d/dg *Penicillium, Candida* and small-yeast forms of *Cryptococcus, Blastomyces* and *Malassezia*; also *Leishmania, Toxoplasma*, etc. *Histoplasma* stains weakly with PAS (other yeasts stain strongly)

Aspergillus spp.
- Regularly septate, dichotomously branching hyphae of regular thickness (≈ 4µ)
- *Typically* each limb of a branch makes an equal angle to the stem to give a 'Y' configuration where the two upper limbs of the 'Y' are at an acute angle to each other
- Viable hyphae are basophilic, necrotic ones eosinophilic
- Conidia (spores) and conidiophores (fruiting bodies) can form in cavities
- d/dg *Pseudallescheria* spp. (their hyphae are identical to aspergillus but their conidia differ)
- d/dg fusariosis but these usu. make branches at 90° to the stem (as well as 'Y' forms)

Mucormycotic Zygomycosis due to Rhizopus spp.
- Irregularly branching hyphae of irregular thickness (upto 20µ) and irregular orientation

---

[4] 'dichotomous' (from the Greek for 'cut in two') means that both branches are of equal thickness

- Branches often come off at 90° and are thinner than the stem (non-dichotomous)
- Non or pauci-septate (but flimsy and often folded/kinked/twisted and may form 'tangles of sticky tape')
- Weakly basophilic thin walls but empty inside; weak Grocott staining
- Conidia (thick-walled with a deeply basophilic core) may form at the end of hyphae, break off and cluster (! d/dg non-budding yeasts)

Viruses

Morphological Characterization of Viral Inclusions

Site
- Cytoplasmic (e.g. HBV surface Ag, HPV, rabies Negri and lyssa bodies, RSV [usu. paranuclear])
- Nuclear (e.g. HBV core, HDV, polyoma, adenovirus, HSV/VZV, parvovirus) – d/dg nuclear clearing due to biotin (! false +ve immuno) esp. in endodermal epithelia (endometrium, lung, thyroid, etc.)
- Both (e.g. HBV core, CMV, measles)

Shape
- Round/oval (e.g. HBV, CMV nuclear inclusion, rabies [Negri and lyssa bodies in neurons], RSV)
- Irreg. (e.g. measles cytoplasmic inclusions or the 'exaggerated' keratohyaline granules in wart HPV)
- Clear rim or larger halo (e.g. early adenovirus, late HSV/VZV, HBV surface Ag, RSV, HPV, parvovirus and CMV nuclear inclusion)
- Blurred margin (late adenovirus nuclear inclusion = 'smudge cell' [*NB:* the term 'smudge cell' or 'smear cell' is also applied to appearance of some CLL lymphocytes in PB films without viral inference])
- Multinucleation with (e.g. HSV/VZV, measles in epithelial cell nuclei, RSV in alveolar cell cytoplasm) or without (e.g. HIV, parainfluenza, measles Warthin-Finkeldey cells) inclusion bodies

Staining properties
- Basophilic (e.g. cytoplasmic inclusion of CMV, nuclear inclusion of HBV core Ag, adenovirus, polyoma, early HSV/VZV [diffuse stage])
- Amphophilic (examples are as for basophilic; esp. seen in the earlier stages of some inclusions)
- Eosinophilic (e.g. nuclear inclusion of CMV [but this may be basophilic], HBV surface Ag, measles, parvovirus, molluscum pox, RSV, rabies [Negri bodies are well-defined, are upto the size of an RBC and have an inner more basophilic core; lyssa bodies are less well defined and have less internal structure], late HSV/VZV [angulated inclusion with halo])
- Uniform texture/'ground glass': (e.g. adenovirus, HBV, delta, HSV/VZV, measles, early polyoma)
- Coarse granular texture (e.g. cytoplasmic CMV inclusion)
- Reticular texture (e.g. late polyoma inclusion)

Non-inclusion morphology
- Many viruses may not show inclusions but show typical inflammatory (e.g. HCV, VHF), reactive (e.g. HIV) or neoplastic (e.g. EBV, HHV8, HPV) manifestations

HIV and AIDS

AIDS-defining illnesses (ADI)
- Molluscum, CMV, HSV, PML
- Recurrent bacterial pneumonia, TB, MAI
- Severe Candida, PCP, Cryptococcus, Histoplasma, Coccidioides
- Toxoplasma, Cryptosporidium, Isospora
- SCC cervix, high grade B-cell lymphoma, KS
- HIV dementia, HIV wasting syndrome

AIDS and the skin / bone marrow and AIDS lymphadenopathy
See pp. 306–307, p. 100 and p. 119.

AIDS and the GIT
- HIV enteropathy: ➢ villous atrophy of the crypt atrophic or crypt hyperplastic type
   ➢ ↑crypt apoptoses and IELs (d/dg GVHD)
- Opportunistic / other infections ('gay bowel syndrome' is an outmoded loosely-defined term relating to any number of a variety of alimentary tract infections associated with HIV/AIDS e.g. gonorrhoea, syphilis, *Shigella*, *Salmonella*, amoebiasis, giardiasis, *Enterobius*, spirochaetosis, ~~Campylobacter~~, ~~Chlamydia~~, HPV warts and even viral hepatitis have all been included in this 'syndrome')
- Oral hairy leukoplakia, cystic LESA, KS, lymphomas

AIDS-associated malignancies
* Sarcomas: KS and angiosarcoma
* Lymphomas: HL, NHL and multiple myeloma
* 1° brain tumours: gliomas and PNET
* Seminoma
* Others (e.g. anal and cervical SCC) may be common in pre-AIDS HIV but don't have a marked post-AIDS increase in incidence as the above examples do

Parvovirus B19 Related Disease
* Infects erythroid precursors and is present in most people (serum IgG is +ve) being asymptomatic
* Normal hosts may get immune complex mediated 'fifth disease' with a rash in children ('slapped cheek') or arthralgias in adults
* The more proliferative the erythroid line (e.g. in the fetus or in sickle cell disease), the more pathogenic the effect on red cell production culminating in pure red cell aplasia ($\rightarrow$ *hydrops fetalis* in the fetus)
* Micro: giant pronormoblasts ± red cell precursors with clear or eosinophilic [nucleolus-like] nuclear haloed inclusion(s) (but these are not always seen, even in proven infections)

EBV (HHV4) Related Disease
* Non-neoplastc: infectious mononucleosis, cytophagic histiocytic panniculitis
* Lymphoma: HL, Burkitt's, angioimmunoblastic, angiocentric T/NK-cell, DLBCL (−ve for HHV8 except in PEL), extranodal lymphomas in HIV,
* Post Tx lymphoproliferative disorders (PTLD)
* Nasopharyngeal carcinoma

KSHV (HHV8) Related Disease
* KS, multicentric Castleman's, PEL, some plasmablastic lymphomas/microlymphoma and PTLD

Protozoa

Pneumocystis carinii
* Cysts are ≈ size of an RBC and may be spherical or partly collapsed (incl. crescentic)
* Grocott shows thick wall with a dot-like thickening or comma-like inclusions (1 or 2 thereof)
* Giemsa doesn't stain wall but may show tiny dots in (sporozoites) or outside (trophozoites) the cysts

Giardia lamblia
* Trophozoite: a binucleate, amphophilic, DPAS −ve, $10 \times 20\mu$ 'tear-drop' or sickle-shaped flagellate
* Cyst: a $10 \times 8\mu$ ovoid with internal longitudinal linear structures (= axonemes) and rounded structures (= nuclei, upto 4 thereof and crowded into one end)
* The trophozoite is seen in the small bowel and both trophozoite and cyst may be seen in faecal smears

Toxoplasma gondii
* Tachyzoites: fast-growing forms in cells and interstitium are $4 \times 2\mu$, crescentic, haematoxyphil and Giemsa +ve (but PAS and silver [e.g. Grocott] −ve). They suggest lack of immunity and are always pathogenic. Immunity slows them into encysted bradyzoites
* Bradyzoites are haematoxyphil, Giemsa and PAS +ve (DPAS −ve) dots in a well-defined cyst within cell cytoplasm (cyst wall is silver +ve). Pathogenicity cannot be assumed without a tissue reaction
* Bradyzoite cysts may rupture ($\rightarrow$ tissue reaction and bradyzoites become less basophilic) or immuno-suppression (e.g. steroids) may cause transformation into free tachyzoites
* Tissue response (general): lymphocytes, Mφ ± PMN inflam^n with focal necrosis ± vasculitis or endarteritis
* LN (characteristic features useful in d/dg): follicular hyperplasia may be prominent, para/intra-germinal centre microgranulomas (here defined as <25 nuclei), no multinucleated giant cells, sparse (<3 per section) larger granulomas (typically <50 nuclei and non-necrotising), ± sinus B-cell reaction
* Brain: glial nodules (neonates have subependymal lesions with ulceration ± Ca^{2+})
* Placenta: bradyzoites in chorion and decidual cells – usu. without a reaction
* Others: lung (interstitial pneumonitis), GIT (ulceration), bone marrow (cysts), etc.
* d/dg (use immuno to *Toxoplasma* and serology for IgM):
    * ➢ fungi (esp. *Cryptococcus* and *Histoplasma*) – *Toxoplasma* are silver −ve
    * ➢ viruses (CMV cytoplasmic inclusions lack a capsule and are granular rather than distinct dots)
    * ➢ protozoa (*Leishmania*, *Trypanosoma cruzi*, microsporidia)

Entamoeba histolytica
See p. 143.

Cryptosporidia spp.
- Clin.: like isosporiasis (*q.v.*). Biliary/respiratory infection is rare and usu. only if immunosuppressed
- Histology ranges from near-normal to active inflam[n] (or coeliac-like in the SI) ± regenerative changes
- Oocysts (spherical, 5µ ∅) infect epithelial cell cytoplasm and bud onto the lumenal surface being invested in a cytoplasmic coat (hence they appear larger)
- Although deep gland epithelium may be infected, cryptosporidia don't invade sub-epithelial tissues
- Stains: the cysts are basophilic, dark blue with Giemsa and variably acid fast, silver and Gram +ve

Microsporidiosis (Enterocytozoon and Encephalitozoon spp.)
- Oral, ocular or inhalation of spores → infection of epithelial, endothelial, stromal and Mφ cells
- Clin.: diarrhoea, nausea, weight↓, biliary obstruction, cough, maxillary sinus polyps, haematuria, etc.
- Granulomatous interstitial nephritis/prostatitis, diffuse punctate keratoconjunctivitis, etc.
- SI may show variable sprue-like changes with disorganisation of epithelium ± vacuolisation
Spores
- Are ovoid (1 × 1.5µ for intestinal spp., upto 4 × 2µ for corneal spp.) with posterior vacuole and dark nucleus (best seen in toluidine blue semithin sections)
- Form clusters in the cytoplasm (apical in enterocytes and may 'cup' indent the nucleus)
- Staining: usu. basophilic, refractile and variably birefringent (blue with Giemsa, pink with Brown-Brenn and white with Warthin-Starry), Gram +ve ('hourglass' shape) and have a PAS +ve polar body
- d/dg : EM can help; PCR and immunoassays are also available (serology, urine, etc.)

Isosporiasis (e.g. Isospora belli)
- Clin.: watery diarrhoea ± (if immunosuppressed) weight loss, malabsorption, fever, headaches, etc.
- Variable villous atrophy of the crypt hyperplastic type (duodenum/jejunum)
- Enterocytes become disorganised and flatter with loss of nuclear polarity
- Parasite stages are present in the epithelium (usu. closer to the BM): Giemsa, AB, PAS and silver +ve
- One ovoid (schizont) or multiple elongated structures (merozoites) in a cluster (total size is ≈ size of one enterocyte nucleus). This is surrounded by a clear halo (= parasitophorous vacuole)
- Macrogametocyte: an oval cell (just larger than an enterocyte nucleus) with central round nucleus, prominent central nucleolus and surrounded by lipid rich granules in the cytoplasm
- Microgametocyte: (≈ $\frac{1}{2}$ size of a goblet cell's mucin blob) contains many dots (microgametes)
- d/dg: if in doubt, EM can help

Plasmodium spp. (Malaria)
- Female *Anopheles* mosquito injects sporozoites that get taken up by hepatocytes where they multiply to form a schizont (bag of merozoite 1µ dots) that ruptures → merozoites infect RBC and undergo further schizony divisions to form an RBC schizont (via an early signet 'ring form') that matures into a gametocyte (15µ long, banana-shaped and expands the RBC in *P. falciparum*) → taken up by mosquito (→sexual stages →sporozoites). RBC cytoplasm may have stippled or cleft-like densities
- Giemsa stain is best for seeing the nuclear DNA of the parasitic stages
- Infected RBC stick to endothelium (via knobs seen on EM) and may cause clogging/ring haemorrhages
- Malarial pigment in phagocytes: a birefringent porphyrin-globin conjugate from digested Hb
- General: 2° changes of haemolysis, infected RBC, blocked capillaries (*et seq.*) and malaria pigment
- Liver: Kupffer cell expansion with malarial pigment (zone 3 early on but more in zone 1 later)
- Brain: ➤ ring haemorrhages
             ➤ Dürck's granulomas (demyelinated patches and gliosis and infected RBC)
- Kidney: effects of haemoglobinuria and ADP GN/membranous GN/membranoproliferative GN
- d/dg: morphology of RBC stages on thick (haemolysed) and thin blood films: multiple ring forms in one RBC suggest *falciparum* malaria (over *vivax*, *ovale* or *malariae*) as does the banana-shaped gametocyte (others have round ones). Strap-shaped 'band-form' early schizonts suggest *P. malariae*

Leishmania spp. (Visceral Kala-azar and Mucocutaneous Espundia)
- A sandfly injects the flagellate form into man → parasitises Mφ and looses flagellum (= amastigotes)
- They are 4µ ovoids containing a double-dot structure on Giemsa (= nucleus + elongated kinetoplast)
- Inflam[n] in the skin/mucous membranes may be ulcerative, acute, granulomatous or non-reactive (anergic) with sheets of Mφ; viscera are expanded by infected Mφ (e.g. in the sinusoids)
- Granulomas (even necrotising/caseating) may occur in the LN draining mucocutaneous lesions

- d/dg *Toxoplasma*, *Histoplasma*: these lack a kinetoplast (also, EM is diagnostic)
- d/dg TB: apart from ZN, PCR on fixed/fresh tissue can be done for *Leishmania* and TB
- d/dg *Trypanosoma cruzi* amastigotes form similar double-dots when they multiply within smooth muscle, cardiac muscle, Mφ or ganglion cells during Chagas' disease (best seen in early stages)

Metazoa

Enterobius vermicularis (Pinworm/Threadworm/Oxyuriasis)
- Adult worms have two longitudinal lateral pointy alae (wings)
- The eggs are ovoid, have a bilayered shell and are slightly flatter on one side
- *Usually* intralumenal (in the GIT) and not a cause of appendicitis or other GI inflammation
- May cause intra-abdominal granulomas in women (via the genital tract) or genital tract inflam[n]
- Other sites rare and via an intra-lumenal route (e.g. to prostate) – never pathological tissue invasion

Schistosoma spp.
- Clin.: rash, diarrhoea, weight loss, portal HT *et seq.*, haematuria, obstructive uropathy, renal failure
- Eggs hatch in fresh water → ciliated miracidia → multiply in snail → fork-tailed cercariae → penetrate human skin (and loose tail = schistosomulae) → lung/liver (mature into adult trematodes) → settle in veins (thinner, darker-staining female within gynaecophoral groove of male) → eggs
- Symmers clay pipestem fibrosis of liver (PT fibrosis, dilated PT arterial branches, collapse of PT veins but no nodular cirrhosis), cirrhosis, varices, mass lesions (e.g. colonic pseudopolyps, bladder polyps, cystitis cystica calcinosa, fibrous plaques), immune complex mediated (e.g. mesangioproliferative GN) and cancers (e.g. SCC bladder)
- $150 \times 80\mu$ eggs are seen in the gut/bladder/liver/lung/genitals ± 'ectopic' sites e.g. LN/CNS
- ZN +ve shell and spine (lateral in *S. mansoni*, lateral but small/invisible in *S. japonicum*)
- ZN +ve spine only (terminal in *S. haematobium*) [*NB:* 'Bilharzia' = urinary haematobium infection]
- The egg shell is often buckled after fixation and an internal 'horseshoe'/'ring' of nuclei is characteristic (but only seen if cut in the right plane – otherwise there will just be a central mass of nuclei)
- Viable eggs have well-preserved nuclei and lie in cellular granulomas ± eos./ Splendore-Hoeppli
- Dead eggs show variable involution ± fragmentation of the shell/Ca^{2+} and the granulomas become less cellular to form fibrous foci (but live eggs may be present elsewhere ∴ use CPC, smears, etc.)
- Granulomas without eggs may have (Perls −ve) schistosome pigment ± eos. → do levels
- d/dg eggs of Enterobius or flukes are much smaller and lack schistosomal horseshoe string of nuclei

Sarcoptes scabii (Scabies)
- May see eosinophil-containing chronic inflam[n] in the dermis but must see ≥1 of the following for diagnosis
- Egg-shells or eggs (containing larvae) or faecal fragments } all are present in the *stratum corneum*
- Adult mite (female) – seen at the end of the burrow in the *stratum Malpighii* (has an ≈ round body)

Larva Migrans (Toxocara canis, Toxocara cati, etc.)
- Clin.: visceral and ocular larva migrans rarely overlap (cutaneous and neural forms also occur)
- Ocular form may infect retina, choroid +/ vitreous, may form a mass and shows variable amounts of eosinophils (even abscesses), granulomatous inflam[n] and fibrosis ± Splendore-Hoeppli reaction
- For morphology see Figure 23.1 (Baylisascaris occurs mainly in North America)
- d/dg filariform larvae of *Strongyloides* (difficult unless good transverse sections are present)
- d/dg clinically, retinal lesions may be misdiagnosed as retinoblastoma → unnecessary enucleation

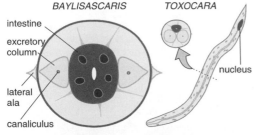

FIGURE 23.1 Larva migrans.

Baylisascaris ($70\mu \varnothing \times 1600\mu$ long) has large (8μ) alae, triangular excretory columns & ovoid intestine (central, laterally compressed & multicellular with prominent granules) *Toxocara* ($18\mu \varnothing \times 400\mu$ long) has small (1μ) alae, ovoid excretory columns & triangular intestine (dorsal/laterally displaced & unicellular with nucleus at anterior, pointy, end of worm)

Cysticercosis (Pork Tapeworm, Taenia soleum, Cysticercus cellulosae)
- Poorly cooked pork with cysticerca is eaten → cysticerca evert and attach to jejunum → grow to adult tapeworm and release proglottid segments bearing eggs into faeces → faecoral egg ingestion → eggs release oncospheres that burrow into tissues to form cysticerca (muscle, eye, brain, soft tissues)
- Cysticercal cyst: a couple of cm in ∅ with one scolex (with hooklets and four suckers)
- Cyst wall has a loose stroma (± small calcispherules) and cellular serrated lining with microvilli
- *NB*: Beef tapeworm (*taenia saginata*) is rare nowadays and rarely causes cysticercal disease in man

Hydatid Disease (Echinococcus spp., e.g. E. granulosus)
- Tape worm in dog → eggs in dog faeces → contaminated vegetation is eaten by man/sheep → eggs hatch in GIT → resulting oncospheres lodge in tissues → cysts
- Cysts may form in many tissues (liver, lung, brain, soft tissues, etc.) with an outer fibrous reaction
- Cyst wall is 1 mm thick, acellular and lamellated with a simple inner lining of cells (= germinal layer)
- Scolices may be seen in the cysts (they have suckers and rows of ZN +ve hooklets)

Strongyloides stercoralis
- Filariform larvae penetrate skin → lungs via lymphatics → mature, migrate up and swallowed → females anchor in proximal SI (males shed into lumen after mating) → eggs containing rhabdatidiform larvae in mucosa → hatch into lumen → passed PR → moult in soil to become filariform larvae
- Autoinfection: a few rhabdatidiform larvae moult in the gut → filariform larvae penetrate gut wall
- Immunosuppression (e.g. steroids, AIDS, HTLV-1): many larvae become filariform → penetrate the gut (and carry bacteria with them) → hyperinfection/superinfection (= larva migrans, multiorgan disease, systemic Sx ± septicaemia)
- Range of GI inflam^n: none; submucosal PMN and ↑ surface mucin (catarrhal enteritis); submucosal oedema with variable fibrosis (oedematous enteritis); severe inflam^n with much oedema and fibrosis (ulcerative enteritis) and may affect the colon to mimic UC (clinically and endoscopically)
- Adult female: 30–90µ ∅, contains a GI tract and paired ovaries (± eggs)
- Rhabdatidiform larva: 25µ ∅, one end blunt and one pointy, bulbous oesophagus, thin intestine
- Filariform larva: 15µ ∅, speckled body, thin intestine, 4 lateral alae (a useful feature for diagnosis but may be hard to see on routine histology preparations)

Some Immunological Disorders

Hypersensitivity (Types I–V)
I   Immediate/Anaphylactic/Atopic: mast cells/basophils coated with Ab generated in 1° response have their receptors cross-liked on exposure to Ag → degranulation → histamine, etc.
II Cytotoxic Ab Mediated: Ag binds to Ab on surface of cells but instead of cross-linkage of receptors and degranulation as occurs in type I, it causes destruction of the cells coated with Ag by antibody-directed cell cytotoxicity, binding and activation of complement or opsonic phagocytosis. Examples incl. Rhesus D isoimmune haemolytic anaemia and homograft Tx rejection (hyperacute and acute)
III Immune Complex Mediated: persistent Ag (chronic infection, autoimmunity, environmental Ag) combines with Ab either circulating (serum sickness) or *in situ* (e.g. Arthus reaction in skin or GN in kidney) resulting in complement activation and inflammation.
IV Cell Mediated Delayed Hypersensitivity: due to cell mediated immunity e.g. chronic Tx rejection, reaction to TB
V Stimulatory/Inhibitory Ab Mediated: e.g. Graves' disease, Myasthenia gravis

Cryoglobulins and Cryoglobulinaemia
- Clin.: ischaemia, Raynaud's phenomenon, vasculitis, GN, ± HCV
- Type I (monoclonal IgM) e.g. Waldenström/myeloma
- Type II 'Mixed' (monoclonal IgM rheumatoid factor) e.g. Waldenström/myeloma/CLL
- Type III 'Mixed' (polyclonal IgM rheumatoid factor) e.g. RhA, SLE, PAN
- 'Mixed' indicates that there are two types of immunoglobulin involved (*viz.* IgM and IgG)
- >90% of mixed cryoglobulinaemia cases have HCV (50% of HCV cases have cryoglobulinaemia)

Common Variable Immunodeficiency (CVID)
- Usu. sporadic (late onset), some are familial (early onset)
- B-cells can't mature to plasma cells (and there is also T-cell dysfunction which may result in the granulomatous form of CVID)
- ↓Serum IgG, IgA, ± IgM; ±↓CD4 count (! d/dg AIDS)

General features
- Lack of plasma cells in tissues (esp. noticeable in the GIT MALT)
- Lymphoid follicular hyperplasia
- ± Granulomas in many organs (d/dg Sarcoidosis, etc.)
- ↑ risk of NHL (incl. MALToma)
- ↑ risk of all types of infection e.g. *Giardia*, Cryptosporidia, viruses, *Haemophilus influenzae*, fungi
- ↑ risk of autoimmune disorders (e.g. AIH)

Specific organs
- LN: follicular hyperplasia ± granulomas, ± NHL
- Lung: LIP ± MALToma
- Liver: viral hepatitis/AIH/granulomas
- Kidney: mesangial and paramesangial immune complexes ± interstitial granulomas
- GIT: nodular lymphoid hyperplasia, villous atrophy, *Giardia*, Cryptosporidia, CMV, *Candida*, granulomas, etc., absence of plasma cells (see also pp. 142 and 148)

Antiphospholipid Antibody Syndrome (Anticardiolipin Antibody or Hughes' Syndrome)
- Def^n: persistent antiphospholipid Abs + TMA/thrombocytopenia ± recurrent IUD
- Due to a prothrombotic (*in vivo*) antiphospholipid Ab (e.g. anticardiolipin) that occur in SLE and other conditions. These inhibit coagulation tests *in vitro* (so also called 'lupus inhibitor'/'lupus anticoagulant') and requires immunosuppression +/ anticoagulant cover (or may be self limited)
- Non-thrombogenic antiphospholipid Abs (which ∴ do not cause the syndrome) occur with many infections (incl. HCV, HIV, bacterial, etc.), drugs (incl. antibiotics and cocaine) and some normals
- Pathology is that of a TMA (see pp. 61–62, p. 71 and p. 207)
- d/dg the vasculitis of CTD/lupus (see p. 71)
- d/dg clinically it may be misdiagnosed as MS

The Concept of Granuloma
- Definition of *granuloma*: 'chronic inflammation in the form of a mass' was the original definition. Some modern student texts prefer 'a collection of epithelioid histiocytes'.
- However, the following terminologies only make sense in the light of the original definition (although some are now known to be neoplastic): pyogenic granuloma, foreign body granuloma, xanthogranuloma (juvenile), eosinophil granuloma (HX), nodular paragranuloma, plasma cell granuloma, Dürck's granuloma, etc.
- Furthermore, *diffuse epithelioid granulomatous inflammation* (= swathes of epithelioid histiocytes), not being a tight collection, may be underdiagnosed by those adhering to the simplistic student-definition of 'granuloma'

Bibliography

Allason-Jones, E. (1987) The Gay Bowel Syndrome. *British Journal of Hospital Medicine*, **38** (5), 397.

Chandler, F. and Watts, C. (1987) *Pathologic Diagnosis of Fungal Infections*, 1st edn, American Society of Clinical Pathologists Press, Chicago.

Chapel, H. and Haeney, M. (1988) *Essentials of Clinical Immunology*, 2nd edn, Blackwell Scientific Publications, Oxford.

Connor, D.H., Chandler, F.W., Schwartz, D.A. *et al.* (eds) (1997) *Pathology of Infectious Diseases*, 1st edn, Appleton & Lange, Stamford, Connecticut.

Cotran, R.S., Kumar, V. and Collins, T. (eds) (1999) *Robbins Pathologic Basis of Disease*, 6th edn, W.B. Saunders Co., Philadelphia.

Duerden, B.I., Reid, T.M.S., Jewsbury, J.M. *et al.* (1987) *A New Short Textbook of Medical Microbiology*, 1st edn, Edward Arnold (Hodder & Stoughton), London.

Eapen, M., Mathew, C.F. and Aravindan, K.P. (2005) Evidence based criteria for the histopathological diagnosis of toxoplasmic lymphadenopathy. *Journal of Clinical Pathology*, **58** (11), 1143–1146.

Goedert, J.J., Coté, T.R., Virgo, P. *et al.* (1998) Spectrum of AIDS-associated malignant disorders. *The Lancet*, **351** (9119), 1833–1839.

Gotuzzo, E., Terashima, A., Alvarez, H. *et al.* (1999) Strongyloides stercoralis hyperinfection associated with human T cell lymphotrophic virus type 1 infection in Peru. *American Journal of Tropical Medicine and Hygeine*, **60** (1), 146–149.

Hale, M.J. (2000) Mycobacterial infection: a histopathological chameleon. *Current Diagnostic Pathology*, **6** (2), 93–102.

Harada, M., Fujisawa, Y., Sakisaka, S. *et al.* (2000) High prevalence of anticardiolipin antibodies in hepatitis C virus infection: lack of effects on thrombocytopaenia and thrombotic complications. *Journal of Gastroenterology*, **35** (4), 272–277.

Jannotta, F.S. and Sideway, M.K. (1989) The recognition of mycobacterial infections by intraoperative cytology in patients with acquired immunodeficiency syndrome. *Archives of Pathological Laboratory Medicine*, **113** (10), 1120–1123.

Lucas, S. (2000) Update on the pathology of AIDS. *Current Diagnostic Pathology*, **6** (2), 103–112.

Mount, S.L. and Cooper, K. (2001) Beware of biotin: a source of false positive immunohistochemistry. *Current Diagnostic Pathology*, **7** (3), 161–167.

Niedobitek, G. and Young, L.S. (1995) Epstein-Barr virus and lymphomas: an overview, in *Progress in Pathology*, Vol. 2 (eds N. Kirkham and N.R. Lemoine), Churchill Livingstone, Edinburgh, pp. 247–264.

Peters, W. and Gilles, H.M. (1989) *A Colour Atlas of Tropical Medicine & Parasitology*, 3rd edn, Wolfe Medical publications, Ltd., London.

Pritt, B., Mount, S.L., Cooper, K. *et al.* (2006) Pseudoactinomycotic radiate granules of the gynaecological tract: a review of a diagnostic pitfall. *Journal of Clinical Pathology*, **59** (1), 17–20.

Roitt, I. (1988) *Essential Immunology*, 6th edn, Blackwell Scientific Publications, Oxford.

Spencer, H. *et al.* (1973) *Tropical Pathology*, 1st edn, Springer—verlag, Berlin.

Youngberg, G.A., Wallen, E.D.B. and Giorgadze, T.A. (2003) Narrow-Spectrum Histochemical Staining of Fungi. *Archives of Pathology and Laboratory Medicine*, **127** (11), 1529–1530.

Winn Jr., W.C. (2000) Demonstration of infectious agents in tissues. *Current Diagnostic Pathology*, **6** (2), 84–92.

24. Cytopathology

Cervix Uteri

Sampling
① cervical scrape with Ayre spatula (best single method) ⎱ combined, these detect 98%
② endocervical scrape with brush/pointed spatula ⎰ of all neoplasia
③ upper $\frac{1}{3}$ vaginal wall scrape (to assess hormonal response – it is more sensitive *cf.* cervix)
④ vaginal vault smear (for follow up of patients who have had the cervix removed)

Staining
- Papanicolaou: Harris haematoxylin, Orange G6, EA50 (= eosin solution with light green)
- Allows you to see through mucin (which stains a pale peach/apricot/grey colour)
- Immature cytoplasmic keratin stains delicate pink but depends on pH and fixation ∴ nuclear morphology is more reliable for diagnosis
- Mature keratin stains orange yellow due to the formation of eosin dimers and has a coarse refractile quality in SCC

Assessing a Cervical Smear

Adequacy
- *A smear is always adequate if abnormal cells are seen.* If sparse dyskaryotic cells are present then call it 'dyskaryosis difficult to grade'. If no abnormal cells are present then consider the following:
- Report as inadequate if you are told that the cervix was not completely visualised or if an inappropriate method was used ('finger smear', etc.)
- Cellularity: inadequate if squamous cells cover $< \frac{1}{3}$ of the slide when evenly spread (except in atrophic hormonal states when other factors should be used to judge adequacy)
- Vaginal smears are inadequate (entirely composed of separated superficial cells)
- Endocervical smear: inadequate if entirely composed of endocervical cells unless the object of the test was to sample the endocervical mucosa
- Visual obfuscation: poor fixation/air-drying, thickly spread, cornflakes ++, blood, debris, PMN (→ infective cause should be sought [e.g. *Trichomonas*, HSV, *Candida*] and advise repeat after Rx)

Quality
- Transparent well-stained cytoplasm (not pale)
- Good nuclear morphology
- Evenly spread, well fixed and lack of air-drying

Cell content
- Squamous/glandular/blood/inflammatory/sperm/seminiferous tubule epithelium
- Microbes/artefacts/unusual tumour cells
- Atrophic cells (? postpartum/postmenopause)

Normal Smear Cytology

'Superficial cells'
- Cytoplasm: 45–50µ ∅, polygonal (angular), transparent
- Nuclear: small, pyknotic ± karyorrhectic
- Other: dissociated cells but nests (squamous pearls) may also be seen

'Intermediate cells'
- Cytoplasm: 35–40µ ∅, less angular, denser cyanophil, folds
- Nuclear: 8µ, clearly defined chromatin network (chromocentres, Barr body)
- Other: tend to clump

'Parabasal cells'
- Cytoplasm: 15–30µ ∅, rounded/ragged/disintegrated, dense cyanophil (unless air-dried)
- Nuclear: $\frac{1}{3}$ of cytoplasmic ∅, granular and occ. chromocentres. Some are pyknotic ± karyorrhectic
- Other: seen postpartum, postmenopause and during regeneration

Diagnostic Criteria Handbook in Histopathology: A Surgical Pathology Vade Mecum by Paul J. Tadrous
Copyright © 2007 by John Wiley & Sons, Ltd.

Metaplastic cells
- May be confused with parabasal cells but can be distinguished by:
    a) the company they keep = superficial and intermediate cells
    b) cytoplasmic vacuolation
    c) angular/pointy processes

Hyperplastic reserve cells
- Bare nuclei forms are common
- Resemble glandular cells in shape but have more solid cytoplasm
- Form supercrowded groups (lack architectural features of glandular neoplasia)

Endocervical columnar cells
- Prone to degenerative changes
- Honeycomb/palisaded sheets or single cells or ciliated tufts
- Tall delicate cytoplasm ± vacuoles and basal nuclei
- Reserve cell bare nuclei may be present
- Endocervical mucus ± mid-cycle ferning

Endometrial cells
- Normal for the first 10–12 days of the cycle and seen with: IUCD, COC, HRT
- Cytoplasm: 5–20μ ∅, cyanophil, delicate
- Nuclear: round, chromatin coarse but not clearly visible (because they are partly degenerate)
- Other: berry-like clusters ± stromal core (= 'top hat' formation)

Histiocytes
- Found during the exodus or with IUCD
- Cytoplasm: 15μ ∅, delicate, foamy/vacuolated
- Nuclear: round/oval/bean-shaped
- Other: multinucleate forms are non-specific esp. postmenopause

Flora
- Döderlein bacilli (lactobacilli)
- *Candida albicans*
- *Gardnerella vaginalis* (overgrowth covers cell → 'clue cell' of bacterial vaginosis)

Contaminants
- Spermatozoa and male epithelial cells, RBC, PMN

Pregnancy
- Intermediate cells: navicular (boat-shaped, thick borders, eccentric nucleus, brown glycogen)
- Cytolysis
- Döderlein bacilli ++
- Endocervical cells ++ (due to ectropion), nuclei may have nipple-like projections

Postpartum
- Glycogen-laden parabasal cells and intermediate cells

Postmenopausal
- Parabasal cells ± karyorrhexis
- Blue blobs (dense basophil mucus plugs which vary in size and lack structure)
- Air-drying and paucicellularity, fragile cytoplasm and PMN
- Multinucleated cells

HPV Changes
- Koilocytes: vacuole is large (*cf.* post inflam^y halo), empty and hard-edged (*cf.* glycogen vacuole)
- Nuclear abnormalities: should be present – borderline at least
- Multinucleation (also seen in inflam^n and HSV but the latter has ground glass nuclei)
- Dyskeratosis: single and in groups (cones/rafts/whorls)

Borderline Nuclear Changes in Cervical Smears (National Cancer Network, BSCC and RCPath, 1994)
- Borderline = 'genuine doubt as to whether neoplastic or not' and usu. occurs in three settings:

① In HPV changes
i) less than overt dyskaryosis in *koilocytes* (*NB*: this criterion will be superseded if the 2002 BSCC Terminology is accepted and all HPV-type koilocytic changes are lumped together with mild dyskaryosis as 'Low grade squamous dyskaryosis')
ii) • Variable nuclear enlargement
    • ↑ NCR   } in dyskaryotic clusters forming cones, rafts or whorls
    • Condensed chromatin

If dyskaryosis is present, report grade of dyskaryosis regardless of HPV cytoplasmic changes.

② In inflammatory changes
- These must include epithelial changes (not just PMN) and must be called 'negative' *unless* there is heavy *Trichomonas* infection on F/U for dyskaryosis
  i) Squamous metaplastic cells:
  - Nuclear enlargement with normal NCR
  - Minor variations in size and shape
  - Smooth, well-defined nuclear membrane
  - Pyknosis/karyorrhexis
  - Bi/multinucleation   } inflammatory changes
  - Speckled, evenly-distributed chromatin and small *round* nucleoli
  - ± Engulfed PMN (also seen in dyskaryosis)
  - Cytoplasmic ruffling/strands ('spider cells')
  - (Perinuclear halo in superficial/intermediate cells)
  - ↑ NCR, mild hyperchromasia, mild coarsening of chromatin   } borderline
  - ± Minimally irregular nuclear membrane   } changes
  ii) Glandular metaplasias (Tuboendometrioid):
  - Small cells with ↑ NCR (very little cytoplasm) in crowded or supercrowded groups
  - Well-defined nuclear membrane
  - Dispersed, finely-granular chromatin
  - *No* rosettes, feathering or pseudostratification
  iii) Endocervical cells:
  - Atypical changes occur in inflammation, IUCD, polyps, MGH
  - Dyskaryosis: ➤ the features are described in 'Glandular Dyskaryosis', pp. 356–357
                    ➤ repeated observation of >1 of those features is required else = borderline
  - Inflammatory: ➤ anisonucleosis with normal NCR and normal, well-defined, contour (i.e. variation in sizes of whole cells – not just nuclei [= *anisocytosis*])
                    ➤ finely granular chromatin
                    ➤ prominent, multiple, *regular* nucleoli (vary in size from cell-to-cell)
                    ➤ normal mitoses
                    ➤ crisp, unilocular cytoplasmic vacuoles indenting nuclei (esp. seen with IUCD – but ill-defined, scalloped vacuoles overlying nuclei with irregular macronucleoli suggests adenocarcinoma, esp. ovarian)
  - Borderline: ➤ 3D groups with disorderly arrangement
                    ➤ irregular 'grainy' chromatin   } in the absence of
                    ➤ variable hyperchromasia [= *anisochromasia*]   } overt dyskaryosis
                    ➤ irregularity of the nuclear membrane

③ In the atrophic smear
- For general features and causes see section on 'Atrophy', p. 358
- In *pregnancy* previous dyskaryotic changes diminish/vanish and sampling error ↑ (due to big ectropion) ∴ borderline changes are *not* taken as evidence of improvement if the F/U smear was taken during pregnancy
- Folate ↓ /Inflam^y changes: ➤ ↑ nuclear size, normal NCR, anisocytosis, fine chromatin, well-defined nuclear membrane
  Dyskaryosis: ➤ individual nuclear enlargement and ↑ NCR
                  ➤ ill-defined nuclear membrane
                  ➤ crowded groups with nuclear overlapping/moulding/mitoses
- Borderline: ➤ orangeophil pattern, ↑ NCR, irregular but degenerate nuclei – unsure of dyskaryosis

Nucleoli
- Are not a feature of squamous dyskaryosis
- Prominent nucleoli are seen in invasive carcinoma
- Irregular/pleomorphic/macro nucleoli are seen in glandular neoplasms
- Identical monotonous nucleoli present in all cells in a group (i.e. a 'clonal' pattern) are also suspicious of glandular neoplasia

- Small nucleoli are typical of normal glandular/metaplastic cells
- Larger nucleoli with some size variation are typical of reactive glandular lesions

Dyskaryosis in Squamous Cells
- ↑ NCR (nuclear diameter of $< \frac{1}{2}$ the cell diameter in mild, $> \frac{2}{3}$ the cell diameter in severe)
- Coarse, unevenly distributed chromatin
- Irregularity of the nuclear membrane
- Hyperchromasia (except pale cell dyskaryosis)

Dyskaryosis Difficult to Grade
- Scant cells/poor preservation (esp. in recurrent CIN after Rx) → Mx as for moderate dyskaryosis
- In invasive SCC cells may be sparse/obscured by exudate

Differential Diagnosis/Pitfalls for Severe Dyskaryosis
- Histiocytes (degenerate ones have dark granular chromatin and denser cytoplasm)
- Follicular cervicitis (chromatin coarse but evenly clumped ± tingible body Mφ)
- Endometrial cells
- Keratinised HPV
- IUCD-irritated endometrial cells (rounded with dense cytoplasm and eosinophilic nucleolus ± multi-nucleated with PMN and karyorrhectic debris in streaks of cervical mucus)
- Adenocarcinoma/ASC (extracervical tumours usu. yield scant cells with a clean background)
- False negatives: small/pale cell dyskaryosis, sparse keratinised dyskaryotic cells in atrophic smears, solid microbiopsies of CIN 3, gland crypt involvement, moderately dyskaryotic groups confused for endocervical cells
- False positives: endometriosis/TEM, lower uterine segment endometrium

Small Cell Severe Dyskaryosis
- Irregularly clumped chromatin (nuclear membrane may be smooth and nucleoli inconspicuous)
- Some may show keratinisation
- Presence of unequivocal lesser grades of dyskaryosis help to make the diagnosis
- d/dg histiocytes, immature metaplastic or parabasal squames

Pale Dyskaryosis (any grade)
- Irregularly clumped chromatin but no nuclear hyperchromasia (paler than PMN nuclei)

Solid Microbiopsies of CIN 3
- Loss of polarity/chaotic architecture
- Mitoses
- Coarse chromatin and ↑NCR
- Presence of scattered dyskaryotic cells elsewhere
- If unsure, call it 'borderline' with immediate referral (i.e. 'borderline, possibly high grade')

CIN 2/3 Involving Gland Crypts
- Groups of mod/severe dyskaryotic cells intimately assoc[d] with endocervical cells
- Groups may have a regular border lined by endocervical cells
- Groups do not have architectural features of glandular neoplasia

Moderate Dyskaryotic Groups confused for Endocervical cells
- Squamous cells have central nuclei and more densely staining cytoplasm

Glandular Dyskaryosis (Result Code 6)
- Crowded/supercrowded 3D groups
- Feathering at the border (loss of cohesion with tapering cytoplasm)/rosettes/pseudostratification
- Elongated nuclei with 'grainy' chromatin, poorly-defined nuclear membrane and anisonucleosis
- Dyskaryosis may vary from cell to cell with some looking normal
- Clonal pattern: regular arrangement with prominent red nucleoli, all the same size (reactive glandular cells may have prominent nucleoli but these vary in size from cell to cell)

- Features suggesting invasion (i.e. 'adenocarcinoma' *cf.* '?glandular neoplasia'): malignant diathesis, macronucleoli, chromatin 'windowing'
- Features suggesting extracervical origin: clean background, few groups, alternative architectures (e.g. 3D balls of vacuolated cells)
- Atypical endometrial cells: larger than PMN and with clearly visible chromatin

Endometrial Carcinoma (Result Code 6)
- Small cells in rounded/oval/papillary 3D clusters
- Coarse cytoplasmic vacuoles, PMN engulfment, 'signet-ring' cells
- Degenerate, necrotic cell debris

Epithelial 'Repair' (Post-surgery, HSV Blistering, etc.)
- Metaplastic cells disorganised with indistinct cell borders and anisokaryosis with an irregular nuclear membrane, coarse chromatin and prominent nucleoli (normal NCR on average)
- Appear within 4 weeks and resolve by 8 weeks
- Advisable to suggest early repeat

Tuboendometrioid Metaplasia (TEM)
- Only an occasional or a few groups
- Pattern 1: supercrowded groups of very small cells with very little cytoplasm
- Pattern 2: columnar cells with denser cytoplasm ± terminal bars (± cilia – but this is not reliable because they are prone to degeneration)
- ± Stratification and 'reversed'[1] rosettes but:
  - ➤ blunt cytoplasmic ends (not tapering feathers as in glandular dyskaryosis)
  - ➤ visible lateral cell borders (*cf.* indistinct in glandular dyskaryosis)
  - ➤ denser cytoplasm (*cf.* fragile in glandular dyskaryosis)
- Well-defined and enhanced nuclear membrane, hyperchromatic but evenly granular chromatin
- Lack architectural features of glandular neoplasia and mitoses
- ± Large casts of endometrial glands
- Pure tubal metaplasia tends to form 'dirty'-looking ragged groups

Lower Uterine Segment Endometrium / Isthmic Endometrium
- Combined epithelial-stromal fragments are extremely unlikely to be neoplastic
- Stroma: tangles of spindle cells and non-polarised thick sheets (!d/dg feathering in glandular dyskaryosis)
- Epithelium: tubular fragments/branching/gland openings/supercrowded cuboidal groups
- Mitoses may be present in glands and stroma
- Esp. seen in high scrape (e.g. after cone Bx or use of a cytobrush)

Microglandular Endocervical Hyperplasia (MGH)
- Denser cytoplasm (*cf.* glandular dyskaryosis)
- Fenestrated ('moth-eaten') sheets
- Well-defined and enhanced nuclear membrane, bland chromatin
- Multinucleation
- No architectural features of glandular dyskaryosis

Acetic Acid Artefact (topical application at time of smear)
- Elongated, mis-shapen endocervical cells (pseudo-fibre cells)

Intra-Uterine Contraceptive Device (IUCD) Changes
- Endometrial cells and histiocytes ± actinomyces
- Irritated endometrial cells (rounded with dense cytoplasm and eosinophilic nucleolus ± multinucleated in a background of PMN and karyorrhectic debris in streaks of cervical mucus)
- Bubblegum cells (crisp, unilocular cytoplasmic vacuole indenting nuclei)
- Brown cells (mis-stained endometrial cells)
- Cockleburrs (small aggregates of Mφ surrounding gunk/haematoidin)

---

[1] i.e. nuclei nearer the centre of the rosette (*cf.* nearer periphery in glandular dyskaryosis)

Atrophy
- Occurs in: pregnancy, postpartum, lactation, postmenopausal, progestational Rx (e.g. POP users) and post ovarian radioRx
- Epithelial 'crazy paving', orangeophilia (inversely proportional to cell size)
- Parabasal NCR but cells have fine chromatin, small nucleoli and well-defined nuclear membranes
- Parabasal predominance, blue blobs, air-drying, inflammation and blood complicate the picture
- Orangeophil pattern: may get many small keratinised cells (similar to but not due to, HPV changes)

Tamoxifen
- ↑Maturation
- ↑Glycogen-laden navicular-like cells
- If endometrial cells are present advise further Ix for:
  - fibrous polyps with metaplasias
  - endometrioid adenoCA
  - oestrogen-independent cancers:
    - CCC
    - pap. serous
    - MMMT

Radiotherapy Changes
- Iridescent two-tone staining (high colour saturation)
- Inflammatory debris
- Cytomegaly, bizarre shapes, cytoplasmic vacuolation (may be fine and non-coalescent)
- Wrinkled hyperchromatic nuclei, prom. nucleoli, multinucleation, karyorrhexis, nuclear vacuolation
- Radiation-induced 'dysplasia' (greater risk of progression than sporadic CIN, esp. if <3 years post Rx)
- Malignancy: ↑NCR, mitoses, (± hyperchromasia) and similar appearances to pre-Rx cancer cells
- If cytology is used to check for recurrent carcinoma post local radioRx, the smear should be done >8 weeks after Rx because cells from the original tumour take this long to disappear with successful Rx

Chemotherapy Changes
- Hard to distinguish from dyskaryosis. Advise F/U

NHSCSP Guidelines 2001
- **Mild dyskaryosis** is an indication for referral on its *second* occurrence *unless*
    a) the woman is unlikely to comply with the repeat (→ refer on first occurrence)
    b) mild follows Rx for CIN (→ manage at discretion of pathologist/gynaecologist)
- **?Glandular neoplasia** (Result Code 6)
    ➢ do NOT use for equivocal changes (use 'borderline, repeat in 6 months with brush as well as smear')
    ➢ should expect *repeated* observations of >1 of the features in the smear to make the diagnosis
- **Normal endometrial cells shed at inappropriate times**
    ➢ age <40 years, ignore
    ➢ age >40 years, call 'negative, routine recall' – but note their presence and possible significance
- **Borderline nuclear abnormalities**
    ➢ a pathologist may recommend gynaecological referral at its *first* occurrence if there is suspicion of an underlying high grade abnormality (e.g. ? solid microbiopsies of CIN 3)
- **Management guidelines**
    ➢ there should be no more than three abnormal smears over any 10 year period without a referral
    ➢ after mild dyskaryosis/BNA: at least three negative smears (at least 3 months apart) should be obtained before returning to routine recall or screening is ceased for reasons of age
    ➢ after Rx for CIN 1: 5 year follow-up with at least three smears
    ➢ after Rx for CIN 2/3: 5 year follow-up (two smears in the first year then annually)
    ➢ gynaecological referral: when changes suggest extracervical disease
    ➢ urgent referral: if ? invasive carcinoma or ? glandular dyskaryosis

Recent Advances in Gynae Cytology (2003–2007)

Uniform approach to screening across the UK
- First call at age 25, then three-yearly till 49, then five-yearly till 64

Introduction of liquid-based cytology (LBC)
- ✓ ThinPrep® and SurePath® give less inadequates because the screener puts the spatula directly into fluid (no smear = no air-drying) and lack of clumping, blood, mucus and inflammation
- ✓ LBC preps are more amenable to automated image analysis

✓ The supernatant can be used for molecular biological studies e.g. HPV subtype testing[2] with hybrid capture/FISH
✓ Detection rate of squamous lesions is increased (and glandular rate is unchanged) *cf.* conventional smears
✓ Can make repeat preps e.g. for immuno or if in need of further haemolysis, etc.
× Criteria for adequacy not yet defined
× Endocervical glandular lesions look different and their criteria are not fully worked out
× SurePath® preps can give rolled edges to squames simulating koilocytes
× LBC makes high grade cells appear smaller and they can be dispersed and rare
× Solid microbiopsies are broken-up or not retrieved ∴ important diagnostic material could be lost
× In non-gynae cytology, valuable background features are lost (∴ LBC may be useful as an *adjunct* to conventional prep) and there is no advantage of LBC over cytospins w.r.t sputa and bronchial washes
× More expensive due to cost of filters
× Can't make air-dried Giemsa preps (because all are OH-fixed as part of the LBC procedure)
× Problems of de-skilling in conventional smears because:
    ① previous smears needing review are likely to be of conventional type
    ② if, after the 5 year assessment period, it is decided to go back to the conventional method

Advanced practitioners
• Autonomous reporting of abnormal smears by specially trained screeners. Their autonomy is subject to guidelines e.g. they must work in a department where at least two consultant cytopathologists are available for showing difficult cases to

BSCC review of guidelines for follow-up of CIN 2 or 3
• The post-cone F/U period is now 10 years rather than the 5 years it was previously

New terminology (BSCC 2002 conference in Manchester, UK)
• The official document is currently (2007) in press – it will be upto the NHSCSP to decide when or if this terminology is to be recommended
• 'Unsatisfactory' – give reasons
• 'BNC' has 3 options:
    ① free text to conclude 'favours reactive' *or* 'favours HPV' *or* 'favours low grade dyskaryosis'
    ② 'high grade abnormality cannot be excluded'
    ③ 'in glandular cells'
• 'Low grade squamous dyskaryosis' (includes mild dyskaryosis and all koilocyte HPV changes but non-koilocytic HPV is still BNC)
• 'Ungraded dyskaryosis' (equivalent to 'dyskaryosis difficult to grade' and usu. refers to the distinction between grades 1 and 2)
• 'High grade squamous dyskaryosis' (= moderate and severe)
• '? Invasive carcinoma'
• '?Glandular neoplasia' (endocervical, endometrial, other specific type or NOS)

Serous Cavities

Mesothelioma Features in Pleural Fluid (vs. Reactive Mesothelial Proliferations)
① Abundant cell aggregates
• Tight and 3D aggregates (flat sheets favour reactive)
• Aggregates vary in size and incl. large clusters (uniform size and small clusters favour reactive)
• ! Abundant cells in non-pleural locations may be reactive (pericardial, peritoneal, hydrocoele)
• ! Papillary aggregates may be benign in hydrocoele
• ! Abundant cells may be seen in reactive pleura if chest drain *in situ*
② Nuclear atypia
• A weak feature (only helpful in 50%) and best assessed on small groups *cf.* single cells
• Reactive mesothelial cells may show hyperchromasia
• Most significant if widespread

---

[2] may be useful in women >30ys old as many younger women have high risk HPV with low grade lesions. Cervical (not blood) HPV testing is considered a possible 1° screening test for these women with only those positive going on to have morphological assessment of smears. Positivity predicts the presence of a dyskaryotic lesion but not its grade. HIV +ve women may also be screened in this way due to their ↑ risk of CIN

- Not present in well diff mesothelioma
- Also seen in radioRx, dialysis, pancreatitis (all reactive)

③ Cell enlargement
- A useful feature, esp. if 'gigantic' forms are seen
- NCR may be preserved
- Not present in all cases

④ Macronucleoli
- A weak feature, but helpful if widespread
- Seen particularly in well diff mesothelioma
- May be seen in reactive mesothelial cells

If still in doubt, do immuno (preferably on cell blocks):
- EMA: thick peripheral membranous staining in malig. *vs.* thin/weak/focal membranous in reactive
- Desmin: +ve in reactive, but 10% of malig. are also +ve
- p53: −ve in reactive but only 50% of malig. are +ve
- CK20: −ve in reactive, +ve in malig. according to some reports (but not an absolute)

Sarcomatoid Mesothelioma
- Effusions are rare and show sparse malignant spindle cells: not specific – d/dg soft tissue tumours/spindle carcinomas (esp. RCC)

FNA of Mesothelioma
- 'Metaplastic'-like cells in flat sheets and 3D clusters; cellular smear
- Central nuclei, elongated cell processes, hyaluronic acid vacuoles (goblet cell-like)
- Sarcomatoid: ① cohesive spindle cell clusters or ② sparse spindle cells with oval nuclei
- d/dg: reactive mesothelium: low cellularity, flat sheets with admixed inflammatory cells, no 3D arch.
- d/dg: adenocarcinoma (esp. BAC) or spindle carcinoma (esp. RCC)

Mesothelial Cells
- Angulated flat sheets with regularly-spaced nuclei (esp. in washings)
- Small groups (<10 cells) with scalloped border/small papillae (± rare psammoma bodies)
- An oblong 'window' (clear space) may be seen between cells in an isolated pair or small group
- Single cells (variable size, dense cytoplasm, fuzzy borders, low NCR, even chromatin)
  - ➤ ± T-cell rosetting
  - ➤ ± mitoses (esp. after chemoRx)
  - ➤ small vacuoles that are perinuclear (*cf.* whole cell in adenoCA) and contain lipid
  - ➤ degenerate → large vacuoles (d/dg signet ring cells, but mucin −ve)
- *Not* 3D clusters/true acini/epithelial mucin. Exception: can get 3D clusters in liver disease ascites
- CK is perinuclear (*cf.* whole cell in carcinomas)
- Immuno: +ve for thrombomodulin, nuclear calretinin (± cytoplasmic), CK5, CK7, CA-125, SM047 (SM047 is −ve in breast carcinoma cells whereas CK7 may be +ve)
- Immuno: −ve for Ber-EP4, TTF-1, EMA and CEA

Eosinophils in Effusions
- Pneumothorax
- Recurrent aspirations/instrumentation
- Rarer: HL, T-cell lymphomas, Churg-Strauss, parasites, etc.

Rheumatoid Arthritis
- Proteinaceous 'messy' background with amorphous purple globules (= immune complexes)
- ± Cholesterol crystals
- Multinucleated Mφ with elongated cytoplasmic extensions
- PMN, lymphocytes, ± a few mesothelial cells

SLE
- Variable inflammatory cell component
- LE cells (PMN with engulfed light magenta globules = nuclear fragment-Ab complex)

Ruptured Oesophagus
- Nucleated squames
- Purulent background

Adenocarcinoma (General Features)
- Large 3D clumps with smooth ('hard') outline (not flat sheets)
- Nuclei: crowded, unevenly distributed, overlapping, anisonucleosis, irregular nuclear membrane, ± prominent nucleoli; NCR is high and variable
- Cytoplasm: sharp borders, mucin (neutral or hyaluronidase resistant AB), lipid in RCC
- Glandular differentiation: acini, papillae, proliferation spheres, solid cell clusters
- d/dg endometriosis/endosalpingosis

Non-Cohesive Tumours
- Lymphoma, melanoma, sarcoma
- Some carcinomas (signet ring, RCC, breast ILC, poorly diff)

Some Features of Malignant Cells
- Intranuclear cytoplasmic inclusions: melanoma, lung, paraganglioma, thyroid, Dutcher bodies
- Round shape except: SCC, TCC, sarcomas, granulation tissue and cells with radiation effect
- Big cells except: breast, stomach, pancreas, lung, SBRCTs, lymphomas
- Mucin vacuoles: neutral/acidic (sialated/sulphated/highly sulphated)
- Pigments: melanin/bile
- Glycogen: mesothelial/mesothelioma, CCC, liver/HCC, RCC, seminoma, Ewing's, RMS
- Crystalloids: Reinke/alveolar soft part sarcoma
- Psammoma bodies: esp. if many – but diagnosis must only be made on cells

Some Features Suggesting Primary Sites for Carcinomas in Effusions

Lung
- Clusters (rarely acini, papillae or psammoma bodies)
- Cytological atypia can vary from severe (adenocarcinoma) to bland (Clara cells)
- SmCC: moulding in single cell columns, angulated nuclei, sparse cytoplasm
Upper GIT
- Dispersed cells ± signet ring forms; can be bland (d/dg Mϕ)
Breast
- Proliferation spheres, dispersed, single files (but nuclei are not angulated/hyperchromatic as in SmCC)
- Targetoid private acini: single vacuole (true signet ring cells are said to have multiple microvacuoles)
- Monotonous cell size and nuclear morphology (CK pattern may distinguish them from mesothelium)
- Lobular carcinoma is more likely to involve the peritoneum *cf.* IDC
Ovary
- Very cellular with large clusters or dispersed cells with prominent vacuolation
- Serous: ➤ cells are pleomorphic to bland, papillae (but, rarely, a dispersed cell pattern is seen)
             ➤ psammoma bodies: brownish on Pap, only its outer rim stains with MGG (d/dg 'vacuole')
- Mucinous[3]: ➤ large cohesive groups of vacuolated atypical cells
             ➤ confirm mucin with stains (because endometrioid can look similar but has glycogen)
- Endometrioid: similar to carcinoma lung/colon, squamous metaplasia helps if present
- Clear cell (CCC): small groups and single cells:
    ➤ Pap: cytoplasmic border accentuation ('vegetable cells'), irregular nuclei and ↑nucleolus
    ➤ MGG: RCC-like vacuolation
    ➤ PAS: glycogen ++
RCC
- Like CCC of the ovary but without vegetable accentuation and the vacuoles also contain lipid
- Immuno: CD15 +ve (for more information, see p. 217)
Other carcinomas
- Colonic carcinoma: ± columnar cells and palisades
- PTC: typical cytology ± psammoma bodies (may also occur in Müllerian metaplasias/malignancy)

---

[3] see 'Pseudomyxoma peritonei', p. 375 – but note that most people currently believe the 1° site of epithelial neoplasia in PMP is the GIT (usu. the appendix) rather than the ovary

- TCC: ➤ clusters of mesothelial-sized cells ± cercaria-like cells (i.e. tadpole with big head and short fat tail)
          ➤ immuno: +ve for Ber-EP4, CK20 and LP34, −ve for CA-125
- Well-diff SCC: ! beware anucleate squames – these may be: contaminants, from a ruptured teratoma, squamous metaplasia of the serosa or from a pleural fistula to the bronchi/oesophagus
- Curschmann's spirals: may be assoc[d] with adenoCA (but are more common in the sputum of COPD)

Lymphoma/Leukaemia
- Highly cellular – macroscopically the fluid may be chylous (i.e. milky)
- Dispersed cell pattern ± aggregates but no cohesive clumps
- Low grade: reactive effusions are mainly T-cell ∴ B-cell predominance suggests lymphoma (do κ:λ)
- High grade: may show many apoptoses (d/dg poorly diff carcinoma/melanoma – do immuno)

Low grade lymphomas
- CLL: monomorphic, coarse clumping of chromatin
- LPL: Dutcher bodies
- FCL: centroblast morphology
- Rarely MALT or myeloma (usu. the high grade plasmablastic myelomas cause effusions)
- T-cell: polylobated nuclei, aberrant T-cell phenotype (to distinguish from reactive)

High grade lymphomas
- Burkitt: cytoplasmic lipid vacuoles
- ALCL (d/dg carcinoma)
- DLBCL incl. 1° effusion lymphoma (PEL) and pyothorax-assoc[d] lymphoma (PAL)
- PEL: B markers −ve; +ve for CD45, CD38, CD138, EMA, CD30, HHV8, AIDS, KS, clonal EBV
- PAL: +ve for pan-B markers, pleural/thoracic mass; −ve for CD30, HHV8, EBV

Hodgkin lymphoma
- Rare in effusions; see typical H/RS cells; eosinophils are scant

Leukaemias
- The effusion may be infective (leukaemic cells get into any serous fluid ∴ you need to see many leukaemic cells to diagnose a leukaemic effusion)
- Chromatin is not as vesicular or clumped as lymphomas
- Cytoplasmic granules may be positive for: MGG, MPO, lysozyme, CD68 (KP1), CAE

Melanoma
- Dispersed, ± multinucleate, prominent nucleoli, vacuolated cytoplasm[4] – d/dg meso, adenoCA, RCC
- Pigment = dust-like melanin: meso has lipofuscin, HCC has bile ∴ do Masson-Fontana or bleach
- Amelanotic *vs.* RCC *vs.* meso (all can be S100 +ve and melanoma can be CK +ve, vimentin +ve)

Sarcoma
- Rare – consider sarcomatoid tumours first (mesothelioma, melanoma, carcinoma)
- Low yield of cells: small round, pleomorphic epithelioid, spindle (pleomorphic/monomorphic)

Germ Cell Tumours
- Seminoma/dysgerminoma: small clusters, pale nuclei, multiple nucleoli, vacuolated cytoplasm, T-cells
- Embryonal carcinoma (MTU): large pleomorphic cells with prominent nucleoli
- YST: eosinophilic hyaline cytoplasmic globules: ! may be confused with adenocarcinoma; AFP immuno is weakly +ve (fluid AFP level may be better)

Ancillary Techniques
- Neutrophil granules are a useful internal control to check adequacy of diastase digestion in DPAS
- CD15 (Lewis[x]) is specific but not as sensitive as CEA for adenoCA (BG8 – Lewis[y] – is also good)
- B72.3 is not generally useful but is positive in serous ovarian carcinoma
- CEA: −ve in meso, RCC, breast, ovarian serous CA; +ve in GI and most other adenocarcinomas
- Ber-EP4: more sensitive for pulmonary *cf.* non-pulmonary epithelia. Most specific if basolateral staining (only) is accepted as +ve
- Adenocarcinoma *vs.* meso panel: CEA, CD15, Ber-EP4, TTF-1, CAM5.2, EMA, CK5/6, calretinin

---

[4] esp. 'balloon cell' melanomas. In melanoma the vacuoles contain glycogen not mucin

- Poorly diff. large cell (carcinoma *vs.* lymphoma *vs.* melanoma) panel: CAM5.2, MNF116, EMA, LCA, S100, HMB45, T-cell markers, B-cell markers, CD30
- Poorly diff. small cell (SmCC *vs.* SCC *vs.* lymphoid *vs.* neuro/nephroblastoma *vs.* sarcoma) panel: CK, desmin, LCA, T-cell markers, B-cell markers, Tdt, CD10, CD99, CD56, NSE, S100
- Spindle cell (sarcoma *vs.* carcinoma *vs.* mesothelioma) panel: CK, vimentin, desmin, EMA, S100, αSMA ± myogenin/MyoD1, CD34, CD31, HMB45, c-kit
- CK is occ. +ve in: synovial sarcoma, epithelioid sarcoma, myeloma, ALCL, leiomyosarcoma, epithelioid angiosarcoma, RMS, chondrosarcoma, melanoma
- S100 is occ. +ve in: RCC, breast carcinoma, mesothelioma. Only 50% of MPNST are S100 +ve

Site Selective Antibodies
- PSA, TTF-1, surfactant, thyroglobulin, GCDFP15, uroplakin III
- CK7 and CK20: if both are negative consider gastric, renal, prostate, HCC
- ER/PgR: ➤ Strong: breast (but a weak or −ve reaction could also occur with breast CA)
              ➤ Weak: sweat gland, endometrium, cervix, ovary
              ➤ Negative: colorectal, lung, HCC

Lymph Nodes

See also 'HIV and Opportunistic Disease', below.

Some General Pointers
- With cohesive cellular clumps on low power, consider: granulomas, histiocytic lesions, carcinomas
- Clumps of histiocytes: check to see if epithelioid else it could be Kikuchi's (look for apoptotic debris)
- Large horrible cells: consider ALCL, HL and metastatic malignancy
- Neck LN: before diagnosing SCC consider squamous metaplasia in a branchial cyst or in metastatic PTC

Epithelioid Granulomas
- Epithelioid Mφ with admixed lymphocytes
- The typical epithelioid Mφ nucleus is slipper-shaped, vesicular, pale-staining ± nucleoli

Hodgkin Lymphoma (HL)
- The background may be relatively hypocellular due to sclerosis
- Features favouring H/RS cells over mimics (e.g. immunoblasts/carcinoma) are:
    ➤ the atypical cells are few and scattered
    ➤ mitoses are rare
    ➤ nucleoli are large and red on Pap (pale blue on MGG)
    ➤ paler, less basophilic cytoplasm
    ➤ reticular chromatin (→ paler nucleoplasm)
- Need to see classic RS cells to make a 1st diagnosis but mononuclear Hodgkin cells suffice for recurrence

Features Favouring Lymphoma over Reactive Lymph Node
- Monomorphic population (or dimorphic in FCL with comma-shaped Cc), but can be mixture in TCL/HL
- Lack of: 'germinal centre structures', tingible body Mφ and admixed plasma cells (germinal centre structures are loose aggregates of a mixture of cells of the types expected in a normal germinal centre)
- Predominance of large cells ± ↑mitoses and apoptotic debris (tingible body Mφ may be seen, e.g. in Burkitt's)
- Although some mixed populations may be present, these are not in 'logical proportions' – i.e. those expected in a benign lymph node including any reactive pattern

HIV and Opportunistic Disease

Indications for FNA of LN in HIV Lymphadenopathy
- LN size >2 cm in any peripheral site *or*
- Tenderness *or*
- Recent ↑size *or*
- Deep-seated (mediastinal, retroperitoneal/peri-pancreatic, etc.)

Common Diagnoses
- Reactive HIV-type LNp (clinical correlate is PGL) – ! d/dg blast-rich reactive LNp *vs.* lymphoma
- Infections (usu. mycobacterial) – ! may only show non-specific inflam^n ∴ take samples for culture:
    - MAI usu. shows foamy Mφ and long, beaded, numerous, intracellular AAFB while TB usu. has granulomas, PMN, necrosis and scant, short, less beaded AAFB but the converse (and *M. bovis*) may also occur – so take samples for culture +/ PCR. For more information, see p. 344
    - finding *Aspergillus* spp. in respiratory samples does not imply clinically significant disease
- Neoplasia (usu. KS or lymphomas)
- Inadequates (*NB:* acellular samples may still culture bugs) and multipathologies (e.g. infection + KS)

Folliculolysis (as part of PGL)
- May see aggregates of epithelioid-like cells with a few admixed lymphocytes but these are the residual FDC of germinal centres and not granulomas. FDC nuclei are round/ovoid (not slipper-shaped) with denser chromatin (not vesicular) *cf.* true epithelioid histiocytes
- Lymphoid cellularity in the background may be low

Cystic Lymphoid Hyperplasia (Cystic MESA)
- Painless fluctuant swelling ± bilateral – usu. restricted to the parotid
- Intermediate or anucleate squames
- Lymphocytes ± lymphoblasts} !/d/dg FCL
- FDC and Mφ
- Similar lesions occur elsewhere (multilocular thymic cyst and multicystic autoimmune thyroiditis)

Kaposi Sarcoma
- Overlapping spindle cell tissue fragments
- Spindle cells (individual or in loosely cohesive clusters) with elongated cytoplasm ± vacuoles
- Nuclei are oval with fine chromatin ± prominent nucleoli (± bare nuclei)
- MGG shows metachromatic stroma
- d/dg granulation tissue, mycobacterial pseudotumour or vascular transformation of LN sinuses

CSF Cytology in HIV
- ↑ Lymphocyte count is non-specific – it could be infective (viral, TB, other) or lymphocytic leptomeningitis (if marked)
- *Cryptococcus* (do Grocott/ABDPAS) – in IRDS you may not see the fungi (just lymphocytosis)
- Lymphoma may be confirmed in the appropriate clinical context
- CSF cytology can't diagnose the following ADI: PML (JC polyoma virus), HSV, *Toxoplasma*

AIDS-Defining Illnesses (ADI) Likely to be Diagnosed Cytologically
- SCC cervix (*NB*: SCC of the anus is not an ADI)
- NHL incl. extranodal high grade BCL, EBV +ve, plasmablastic and PEL (see p. 362)
- KS
- CMV – most likely seen in respiratory samples (esp. BAL) but is uncommon – (unlike in Tx patients)
- PCP – see p. 370 (the granulomatous variant is most difficult to diagnose)
- *Cryptococcus*

Urinary Tract

Cells that may be Present
- Seminal vesicle (lipofuscin), renal tubular, columnar ± cilia (seen in *cystitis cystica glandularis* or ileal conduit samples), endometrial, corpora amylacea

Inflammation
- Reactive single cells ± degeneration (vacuolation, ragged cytoplasm), anucleate squames

Infection
- *Trichomonas, Candida, Enterobius*, schistosome ova, viruses (CMV, BK polyoma, HSV, HPV)

Casts and Crystals
- Red cell casts and dysmorphic RBC are mostly indicative of renal disease
- The term 'granular cast' traditionally refers to a cellular cast not made of RBC (e.g. PMN or tubular epithelial cells that may be seen in pyelonephritis or ATN respectively)
- Hyaline casts are composed predominantly of Tamm-Horsfall protein and are usu. insignificant
- Casts of wide diameter suggest dilated tubules (as occur e.g. in end stage renal disease)
- Oxalate crystals are octahedral ('folded envelopes') and may indicate Ca^{2+} urinary calculi if plentiful
- Urate crystals are fusiform and may be seen in normal urine as well as gout
- Cystine crystals are hexagonal/flower-shaped (seen in cystinuria)

Instrumentation and Calculi
- Instrumented urines / bladder washings: cohesive groups with smooth outline, (normal NCR and chromatin)
- Instrumented/stones: cells often look columnar
- Calculi:
  - papilloid clusters of atypical cells: smooth outline ± mixture (smooth and ragged groups)
  - background of inflammation, RBC, crystals
  - lack of atypical single cells (*cf.* d/dg TCC)

Carcinoma (TCC)
- G1: clusters (ragged outline) of and single mildly atypical cells in clean background
- G2: clusters with more atypia, less cohesion, clean background
- G3: more atypia with prominent nucleoli, less cohesion, cannibalism, malig. diathesis background
- CIS: high grade cells, many single cells, no nucleoli, clean background (50% are diagnosed as G3)
- generally look for *the malignant cell*:
  - dense cyanophil cytoplasm
  - intensely hyperchromatic nucleus (helpful criterion but may be relaxed if other features present)
  - enlarged nucleus with irregular outline and chromatin.
  - NCR should be $\geq 1:2$
- Malignant cells may be sparse and partly degenerate but can still result in a positive report once the pitfalls are excluded. Repeatedly positive cytology (esp. CIS) should result in close F/U even if cystoscopy and Bx are negative as it may precede a clinically detectable cancer by some time and cystoscopy has $> 10\%$ false negative rate. May advise retrograde studies to detect ureteric/renal pelvis/renal parenchymal tumours

Pitfalls (Reasons for False Positive Interpretation)
- Over-interpreting cells with low NCR
- Considering papillary clusters to be a reliable sign of low grade neoplasia
- Calculi/inflammatory/regenerative/degenerative and instrumented changes
- Ileal conduit samples – p. 366
- BK polyoma virus (= 'decoy cells', a term also applied to some degenerative changes) – *vide infra*
- Effects of cytotoxic chemoRx (esp. cyclophosphamide and alkylating agents) or radioRx – *vide infra*
- Seminal vesicle cells

BK Polyoma (Papova) Virus
- Dark homogeneous inclusion, does not replace all the chromatin (some internal strands still present)
- Nuclear outline smooth, ± clear rim between nuclear membrane and inclusion
- Post-infective 'spireme' lacy chromatin

Chemotherapy and Radiation Changes
- Similar to that seen in cervical epithelial cells (p. 358)

3D Clusters
- Endometrial cells: small cells with high NCR and dark nuclei. Consider menstrual contamination or endometriosis if outside the expected range of the menstrual cycle
- Renal tubular cells: more cytoplasm *cf.* endometrial cells, often degenerate, delicate chromatin, slightly bulging peripheral nuclei
- Other causes: instrumentation/calculi/infection/crypts in trabeculated bladder/neoplasia

Ileal Conduit Urine
- Cellularity decreases with time since conduit formation
- ± Bacteria
- Degenerate columnar cells which may shrink into rounded cells with eosinophilic cytoplasmic inclusions ('pseudoeosinophils')
- ± Goblet cell clusters (! don't misdiagnose as adenocarcinoma)

Degenerate Urothelial Cells
- Nucleus becomes darker but also smaller and NCR is preserved
- Nucleus may begin to break up with discontinuous nuclear membrane
- Cytoplasmic changes: fine vacuolation/disintegration ± coarse red granules

Ureteric Brushings
- More cellular (*cf.* voided urine) often with aggregates or sheets of better-preserved urothelial cells
- The cytological principles are similar to effusions: look for a dual population of cells

Secondary Malignancy
- Rare – example primary sites include cervix, colon, melanoma, breast
- The cytological principles are similar to effusions:
  - ➤ palisaded columnar cells: consider colorectal
  - ➤ signet ring cells: consider upper GI (but may also be 1° to the urinary tract)
  - ➤ proliferation spheres: consider breast
  - ➤ squames: consider TCC with squamous differentiation (i.e. 1°) or cervix/lung
  - ➤ small cell morphology: consider SmCC bladder (1°) or lung

Miscellany
- 1° melanoma is rare but urinary melanin pigment may be seen with widespread metastatic disease
- Spindle cells in urine: ➤ inflammatory pseudotumour (commoner than sarcoma)
  - ➤ post laser/diathermy spindling
  - ➤ low grade papillary TCC
- Columnar cells in urine: instrumented/bladder stones, cystitis cystica, ileal conduit, adenoCA (1°/2°)
- Non-cytological detection of cancer (urine immunoassays) for CK20, BTA, NMP22 and a cocktail of Abs against tumour cell surface proteins/sugars (ImmunoCyt™ test)
- MSU (good for microbiology) is not ideal for cytology – a full voided sample is better (because it contains sedimented cells) and this should be a mid-morning sample (to avoid the degenerative effects of overnight stagnation in EMUs)

Biliary Tract (Brushings)

Normal/Reactive
- *En face*: flat sheets of regularly arranged cells, may have cellular projections at edge or spaces
- On edge: cells are thin columnar with terminal ovoid nucleus ('matchstick') without prom. nucleoli
- Some overlapping of cells and small nucleoli can be seen in reactive states (NCR is still low)

Dysplastic and Malignant
- Dysplasia shows moderate cell crowding with overlapping, small nucleoli, moderately ↑NCR
- AdenoCA may show the usual features (3D groups, nuclear irregularity, ↑nucleoli, etc.) but special types (mucinous and papillary lesions) can have bland cytology – look for irregular cell arrangement, 3D clustering, pointy oval nuclei (in papillary lesions) or NE cells (in mucinous lesions) and advise further Ix if present

Thyroid

Adequacy Criteria
- Need at least six groups, of ≥10 epithelial cells per group, on at least two slides
- if colloid ++ but no cells call it 'suggestive of colloid nodule but not diagnostic due to lack of epithelial cells'

Thyroid FNA Grading/Scoring System
Thy1:   non-diagnostic/inadequate
Thy2:   non-neoplastic
Thy3:   follicular lesions
Thy4:   suspicious of malignancy
Thy5:   diagnostic of malignancy

Intranuclear Cytoplasmic Inclusions
- Sharp edged and filled with cytoplasm-coloured material (i.e. not empty vacuoles)
- Thyroid carcinomas: PTC, medullary, follicular, anaplastic
- Malignant melanoma
- Paraganglioma
- Metastatic renal cell carcinoma
- Non-neoplastic conditions
- Radiation effect

Hashimoto's Thyroiditis
- Lymphoid cells assoc[d] with Askanazy cells
- ± Multinucleated histiocytes and epithelioid Mφ
- With age: lymphoid ↓ and Askanazy↑
- May present as a localised nodule

de Quervain's Thyroiditis
- Mixed inflam[y] infiltrate with lots of giant cells ± epithelioid Mφ
- d/dg Hashimoto's disease with occ. giant cells: de Quervain's lacks an intense lymphocytic infiltrate
- d/dg giant cells *vs.* pseudogiant cells (i.c. intact follicles – but these are round with a crisp border)

Graves' Disease
- Moderately cellular, scant colloid, lack of inflammation
- 'Normal' and hypertrophic (Askanazyoid) two-dimensional groups ± intact follicles
- Non-specific signs of hyperfunction: colloid at the periphery of cell groups shows smudged out-pouchings ('fire flares') or bubbles ('colloid suds' and 'marginal vacuoles')

Features Favouring Colloid/Multi-nodular Goitre
- Colloid in abundance
- Flat sheets of cells (but relatively few sheets *cf.* neoplasia/hyperplasia)
- Cell uniformity (regular honeycomb pattern)
- Assoc[d] features: haemosiderin, foamy Mφ, giant cells, stromal fragments, degenerate RBC
- *Dominant nodule*: more cellular with follicular aggregates of varying size (+ features of MNG)

'Cellular Lesion, Advise Excision'
- If not sure whether papillary or follicular – but exclude a hyperplastic focus in a colloid goitre if possible

Features Favouring a Follicular Neoplasm
- Scant colloid
- (Micro) follicle formations, relatively abundant
- Cell crowding and anisonucleosis

Hürthle Cell Lesion or Variant (of some Lesion)
- Lack colloid
- Well-defined eosinophil granular cytoplasm
- Nuclear pleomorphism (usu. less than Hashimoto's)

Papillary Carcinoma (PTC)
- ! Inclusions (and grooves) can be seen in other lesions (they are more helpful if plenty)
- Papilloid/3D groups/flat sheets of 'metaplastic' cells (can be confused with Askanazy cells)
- Single cells with dense cytoplasm (usu. bare in follicular lesions or finely granular in medullary)
- Squamous metaplasia can be widespread (esp. diffuse sclerosing variant) (d/dg thyroglossal cyst)
- Psammoma bodies may be seen in other conditions (e.g. Hashimoto's) but always advise histology because more likely to be from a PTC

- Multinucleated giant cells, microfollicles and thin colloid (with PTC nuclei) favour follicular variant
- Cystic change can lead to false −ve because there are many foamy cells but few diagnostic PTC cells
- 'Chewing gum' colloid (small dense irregular colloid fragments – not specific)
- 'Cellular swirls' defined as 'concentrically organised aggregates of tumour cells in which many of the most peripherally situated cells have ovoid rather than round nuclei that are oriented perpendicular to the radius of the swirl' (Szporn *et al.*, 2006)

Medullary Carcinoma
- Dispersed cell pattern
- Plasmacytoid or spindled with occasional bizarre cells with big nuclei
- NE nucleus (see p. 271), may be elongated in spindle cell forms, ± inclusions
- Fine red granularity to cytoplasm (esp. on MGG)
- Follicular formations can be present (! do not misdiagnose as a follicular lesion)
- Amyloid (irregular globules)

Anaplastic Carcinoma
- Typical Hx: >50ys, M>F, recent rapid enlargement of a prior nodule/goitre
- Large pleomorphic cells
- PMN infiltrate ± necrosis
- Cellularity may be scanty due to fibrosclerosis

Metastatic Carcinoma
- RCC may look like follicular neoplasms and may have nuclear cytoplasmic inclusions
- Other 1° sites: breast, lung, melanoma, colon, lymphoma, etc.

Radiation Atypia (e.g. from Radio-Iodine)
- Cell enlargement with bizarre shapes ± cytoplasmic vacuoles
- Nuclear changes may include hyperchromasia, coarse chromatin, big nucleoli, vacuoles, folds and cytoplasmic inclusions
- Hürthle cell change ± lymphocytes (d/dg Hashimoto's thyroiditis)
- Background features may be consistent with colloid goitre (colloid ++, foamy cells)
- d/dg anaplastic carcinoma (architectural and background features remain benign + Hx of radiation)
- d/dg PTC: cells are too large and bizarre for a PTC that is differentiated enough to show good grooves and inclusions. Cytoplasmic vacuolation, architecture and Hx also help

Salivary Glands

Pleomorphic Salivary Adenoma
- Metachromatic fibrillary background substance
- Dispersed plasmacytoid cells with well-defined cytoplasm
- The epithelial groups may show some atypia/anisocytosis: ! do not mis-call as malignant
- Malignancy: marked pleomorphism, necrosis, Hx of rapid enlargement
- Adenoid cystic-like areas may be present in pleomorphic adenoma

Mucoepidermoid Carcinoma (MEC)
- 'Dirty' background with mucin
- 'Goblet' cells/mucin vacuoles in cytoplasm } low grade
- Intermediate cells: smaller, dark oval nucleus ± vacuoles }
- Squames } can't tell if 1°/2° SCC or high grade MEC } high grade
- Malignant squames }

Warthin's Tumour (and Oncocytoma)
- Mucoid material, fluid, debris, lymphoid cells (absent in oncocytoma)
- Flat sheets of polygonal cells with regular nuclei (3D groups in oncocytoma)
- ± Atypical squames with degenerate/regenerative hyperchromatic nuclei but *never* the true refractile orangeophilia of SCC
- d/dg: ! common misdiagnoses are SCC or MEC[5]

---

[5] if it initially looks like a Warthin's tumour but lacks true oncocytoid features, consider mucoepidermoid carcinoma and look for cells with mucin vacuoles

Adenoid Cystic Carcinoma
- May have lots of dispersed bare nuclei
- Globules of variable size including large ones
- Some cells have nucleoli (not a feature of d/dg basal cell adenoma)
- d/dg basal cell adenoma and collagenous spherulosis: globules are small and uniform in these

Acinic Cell Carcinoma
- Clean background ($\pm$ lymphoid cells)
- Very cellular $\pm$ cell groups on vascular stalks
- Oncocyte-like cytoplasm but fragile and less dense on Pap

Cystic Lymphoid Hyperplasia (Cystic MESA) – see 'HIV and Opportunistic Disease', p. 363

Sialadenosis
- This is hyperplasia of acinar cells, often bilateral, assoc^d with systemic disease (e.g. diabetes)
- Cytology shows numerous groups of plump acinar cells in normal acinar configuration

Mucus Retention Cyst
- Watery viscous fluid
- Mϕ and inflammatory cells in variable numbers (lots if there is $2°$ infection) and debris
- *Few* groups of columnar cells $\pm$ squamous metaplastic cells with inflam^y atypia (d/dg MEC)
- d/dg cystic acinic cell carcinoma, MEC, Warthin's tumour, lymphoepithelial cyst, etc.

Respiratory

Adequacy Criteria in Respiratory Cytology
- If a confident diagnosis can be made, the sample is adequate
- Sputum: need 'plentiful' alveolar Mϕ (i.e. at least an occasional streak of them, not just 1 or 2)
- Brushings: inadequacy may result from air-drying or scant cells
- Washings: need to see alveolar Mϕ
- BAL:
  - ➤ Mϕ out-number epithelial cells
  - ➤ Mϕ count >10/hpf
  - ➤ lack of visual obfuscation (PMN exudate, degenerative changes, etc.)
  - ➤ adequacy is important for assessing cell counts and opportunistic infections

Bronchioalveolar Carcinoma (BAC)

BAC in Sputum/Washings/BAL
- Numerous small 3D clusters, clean mucoid background
- Regular ('clonal') small cells with abundant cytoplasm/mild pleomorphism
- Nuclei: hyperchromatic, irregular border/vesicular, prominent nucleolus
- Dispersed pattern resembles degenerate Mϕ ($\therefore$ only diagnose on well-preserved cells)
- d/dg Creola bodies (3D clusters of benign bronchial cells with goblet mucin $\pm$ cilia- seen in inflam^y disease/COPD)/hyperplastic bronchiolar cells (pneumonia, TB, bronchitis/bronchiolitis) $\therefore$ never diagnose BAC on just a few small groups and be cautious if there is an inflam^y background or Hx of asthma. Reactive conditions resolve within 1 month $\therefore$ wait and repeat may help
- d/dg metastasis esp. if widespread necrosis or tight moulding in 3D (the latter esp. if breast $1°$)
- d/dg reactive glandular aggregates in BAL after DAD (ARDS)

BAC in FNA
- Flat sheets of regular cells (endocervix-like in mucinous BAC) plus 3D clusters
- $\pm$ Papillae / psammoma bodies/nuclear inclusions
- Occasionally a pleomorphic dispersed pattern is seen
- d/dg reactive bronchiolar epithelial cells which have the following characteristics:
  - ➤ fewer, smaller sheets and lack 3D clusters
  - ➤ anatomical border, terminal bar, cilia, goblet cells, nuclear moulding
- d/dg metastases (esp. from prostate CA) and mesothelioma can mimic BAC $\therefore$ CPC is essential

Bronchial Adenocarcinoma

Adenocarcinoma in sputum/washings
- Architecture: aggregates or dispersed (Mϕ-like)

- Nuclear features: ↑size, anisonucleosis, irregular membrane, prominent nucleoli; (hyperchromasia and abnormal chromatin are less important)
- d/dg hyperplastic bronchial cells: anatomical border, cilia, Hx or background of eosinophilia

Adenocarcinoma in brushings/FNA

- Flat sheets ± aggregates
- Rounded nuclei, large central nucleoli in most cells, fragile cytoplasm, mucin secretion
- ± Columnar cells, rosettes, acini
- d/dg monolayered sheet of reactive/'repair' epithelium

Hyperplastic Clusters of Respiratory Epithelial (± Goblet) Cells vs. Adenocarcinoma

- Fewer cells (but can be profuse in pulmonary fibrosis)
- No macronucleoli
- Lack of single cells
- Focal cilia/terminal bar

Features Favouring Reserve Cell Hyperplasia over Small Cell Carcinoma

- Cohesive clusters (not streaks or single cells)
- Nuclei all alike (i.e. less pleomorphic, same degree of degenerative change in all cells)
- Lack of necrosis
- Less moulding and a thin rim of cytoplasm is visible between the moulded cells

Carcinoid

- Partly dispersed uniform cells (rounded or spindled) with NE nucleus
- Some palisades/trabeculae
- Bare nuclei common but no moulding/smearing/necrosis
- Plexiform vascular fragments (not a feature of SmCC)

Honeycomb Bubbly Alveolar Casts suggestive of Pneumocystis carinii Pneumonia – d/dg

① alveolar proteinosis

② amyloid

③ fibrin in early organising pneumonia

- PCP casts are sharp-edged and may show a two-tone staining pattern on Pap

Blue Bodies

- Calcific blue bodies: Ca^{2+} carbonate – central birefringence ⎫ seen in various
- Corpora amylacea: non-Ca^{2+} glycoprotein incl. amyloid ⎬ chronic lung diseases
- Psammoma bodies (calcospherites): laminated, *not* birefringent. Seen in malignancy and benignity

Aspergillus

- Fruiting heads and oxalate crystals seen with aspergilloma (which may develop in a cavity caused by invasive aspergillosis, TB, carcinoma, etc.)
- Septate with dichotomous branching (at 45°, on average)
- d/dg zygomycetes (e.g. mucor): these have broad, non-septate, variable-thickness hyphae ± brown pigment, branching at irregularly-spaced variable angles (incl. 90°) ± tangled cellophane formations

Eosinophils ++ in Sputum

- Occur in: asthma, chronic bronchitis, eosinophilic pneumonia, tumour, parasitic infections
- May also see Charcot-Leyden fusiform eosinophilic crystals of lysophospholipase: stain blue with MGG and have a hexagonal cross section (seen in histological sections)

Miscellany

- Ciliocytophthoria = fragmentation of ciliated cells into rounded fragments, some containing cilia and others a degenerate nucleus which may be swollen with prominent nucleolus and without cilia. It is a potential false +ve pitfall in inflammatory disease (e.g. viral) but may also occur with neoplasia
- Radiation effect: usu. does *not* include ↑NCR and irregular chromatin distribution
- When there is *diffuse* radiological shadowing / Hx of pulmonary fibrosis be cautious in reporting carcinoma because profuse hyperplastic clusters and atypical type II pneumocytes can be present
- In long-standing bronchiectasis you get atypical squamous metaplasia and isolated bizarre squamous cells ∴ need numerous bizarre cells to diagnose SCC with confidence

- Actinomyces are a commensal in the tonsil ∴ small amounts in sputum are probably insignificant
- For d/dg asbestos bodies *vs.* other types of ferruginous body see pp. 85–86. For every 1 ferruginated asbestos body identified there are many thousands of uncoated fibres not visible, ∴ it is significant to mention their presence – even if only 1 is found

Breast

NHSBSP Reporting Categories – Cytology

C1 – Inadequate
- Hypocellular: arbitrary adequacy rule is: <5 epithelial groups of ≤10 cells each. However, samples which are diagnostic in an appropriate clinical context should not be labelled inadequate e.g. lipoma, cysts, abscess, fat necrosis and nipple discharge
- Error in aspiration, spreading or staining: e.g. the smear may have reached adequacy criteria for cellularity but if there is reason to suspect that the lesion was missed the sample should be called C1
- Excessive blood

C2 – Benign
- The sample must be adequate and representative of the clinical lesion (see C1, above, for details)

C3 – Atypical, probably benign
- Most features of benignity must be present but with the addition of any/all the following:
  - nuclear pleomorphism/chromatin abnormalities
  - 3D groups of epithelial cells
  - some loss of cohesion
  - nuclear and cytoplasmic changes resulting from pregnancy/hormones/treatment
  - increased cellularity may accompany any of the above

C4 – Atypical, probably malignant
- Confident diagnosis of malignancy cannot be made due to:
  - scanty malignant cells or poor preservation or preparation artefacts
  - only some of the features of malignancy are present
  - benign bare nuclei are present or mostly benign pattern with occasional definitely malignant cells

C5 – Malignant
- Adequate sample
- More than 1 criterion of malignancy must be present
- Absence of benign bare nuclei

Indications for Cytology on Cyst Fluid
① fluid is blood-stained
② fluid re-accumulates after previous aspiration
③ residual lump is present after aspiration (also do FNA of lump)

General Features of Benignity
- Paucicellular
- Cohesive flat sheets of epithelial cells with a regular honeycomb architecture
- Two-cell type (rounded, more open epithelial nuclei *cf.* oval darker myoepithelial nuclei)
- Benign bare bipolar nuclei in the background (some occur in pairs)

Exceptions to the Above Rules in Benign Lesions
- Increased cellularity occurs in fibroadenoma and HUT
- Dyscohesion occurs with some fibroadenomata and in lactational changes/artefactual overspreading
- Nucleoli may be prominent (although round) in apocrine change and lactation

General Features of Malignancy
- Hypercellular sample
- Common low power patterns: ① irregularly distributed cell groups
                                 ② dispersed cell pattern with few/no groups
- 3D epithelial structures with loss of regular honeycomb architecture and with malignant nuclei

- Dyscohesion with single epithelial cells in the background, retaining their cytoplasm
- Epithelial sheets with a single cell type (! do not confuse degenerating pyknotic malignant cells for myoepithelial cells: = 'pseudo two-cell-type')
- Lack of benign bipolar bare nuclei in the background
- Presence of malignant bare nuclei in the background
- Necrosis and features of specific sub-types of malignancy

Exceptions to the Above Rules in Malignant Lesions
- Lobular carcinoma may be hypocellular with bland cytological detail and be mixed with benign epithelial groups
- Tubular carcinoma may show flat sheets of regular cells (but angulated and single cell type)
- Benign bare nuclei may be present in the background in cases of tubular carcinoma
- Bland cytological detail seen in lobular, tubular and pure mucinous carcinoma and low grade DCIS
- Cohesiveness is prominent with tubular carcinoma and low grade DCIS

Epithelial Hyperplasia (HUT, Papilloma)
- Cellular sample
- Bimodal architecture: sheets and 3D clusters (± staghorn formations)
- Mild variable atypia with retained two-cell type
- Benign bare nuclei in the background
- ± Stromal fragments from papillae ± foam cells

Pregnancy and Lactation
- Cellular sample
- Vacuolation of cell cytoplasm and background material (vacuolation is not always seen)
- Dyscohesion with single epithelial cells – but benign bare nuclei are also present
- Nuclear enlargement with prominent nucleoli but nuclear outline is still smooth and round and chromatin is finely granular and evenly distributed

Duct Ectasia (vs. Comedonecrosis)
- Amorphous debris in the background totally lacking nuclear debris (present in comedonecrosis)
- Chronic inflammatory cells and foam cells
- Occasional monolayered sheets of uniform duct epithelium which may show apocrine change
- The lesion should be close to the nipple (duct ectasia is unlikely in the periphery of the breast)

Fat Necrosis
- Dirty background with granular debris fat and adipose fragments
- Few (if any) epithelial cells
- Foamy Mφ and multinucleated giant cells with bubbly cytoplasm
- Chronic inflammatory cells

Tubular Carcinoma
- Moderately cellular
- Cohesive clusters, tubules and sheets with angulated/jagged contour and lacking a two-cell type
- ± Benign bare nuclei in the background
- Epithelial cells are uniform ± only mild atypia

Lobular Carcinoma[6]
- Cellularity is variable but may be scanty in which case the malignant cells may accumulate at the periphery of the smear
- Dyscohesive plasmacytoid cells ± cords/single files/small 3D collections
- Nucleus: eccentric, mild atypia, ± irreg. shape incl. folds and buds ('noses'), ± mild hyperchromasia
- Cytoplasm may be scanty/missing or may show private acini with a targetoid central red droplet
- Co-existent benign epithelial groups may lead to malignant cells being ignored → false −ve result

---

[6] As infiltrating lobular carcinoma cannot be cytologically distinguished from LCIS/ALH it may be advisable to categorise this pattern as C4, not C5

Mucinous Carcinoma (Colloid Carcinoma)
- Cellular sample
- Mucoid background (= the 'colloid')
- Vascular leashes traversing the colloid (helpful for diagnosis but not necessary or specific)
- Bland cohesive sheets with a one-cell type – more obvious malignant features are said to be characteristic of a mucinous component of a usual-type IDC. Beware pseudo two-cell-type (p. 372)

Conditions that may be Misdiagnosed as Malignant[7]
- Fibroadenoma: for true malignancy with FA expect to see two distinct populations of cells
- Apocrine cells: atypical apocrine adenosis may show spindling of (myoepithelial) cells
- Spreading artefacts (pseudodyscohesion): this should be suspected if there are chromatin trails
- Papilloma: 3D staghorn formations, foam cells, stromal fragments and benign bare nuclei (however, there is overlap with papillary carcinoma which may show palisaded columnar cell groups)
- Lobular neoplasia: cannot distinguish between the types ∴ call C4 (not C5)
- ADH: less monotonous and focally two-cell types (*cf.* low grade DCIS) but difficult
- Columnar cell change: dissociation and lobular CA-like cells. Columnar ones resemble bronchial cells
- Lactation and pregnancy: see p. 372
- Radiation atypia: poor cellularity with highly bizarre morphology and Hx of radiation
- Organising haematoma: poorly cellular. Do not mistake haemosiderin for melanin
- Intramammary lymph node: very cellular with dispersed pattern but shows normal LN cytology incl. lymphoglandular bodies (anucleate cytoplasmic blobs) ± germinal centre structures
- Degenerate cells in a cyst / nipple discharge: especially when apocrine
- Ultrasound gel: can be mistaken for necrosis (amorphous material ± cell lysis effect of the gel)
- Inflammatory/granulomatous conditions and fat necrosis
- Adenomyoepithelial lesions: dissociated pleomorphic myoepithelial cells coexist with cells having obviously benign features
- Collagenous spherulosis: granular purple globules surrounded by spindle cells ! d/dg adenoid cystic carcinoma. Seen in hyperplasia, papilloma and duct adenoma
- Granular cell tumour: dissociated granular cells (apocrine-like cytoplasm) interspersed between benign epithelial cell groups

Conditions that may be Misdiagnosed as Benign
- Tubular carcinoma: tubular structures help when present but are not specific
- Apocrine carcinoma: *uniform* atypia and necrosis help to distinguish from benign apocrine conditions
- Lobular carcinoma: (p. 372)
- Carcinoma with extensive fibroelastosis: these are hypocellular
- DCIS: ➢ impossible to distinguish from invasive with certainty on cytology
        ➢ relatively hypocellular *cf.* invasive
        ➢ high grade DCIS is no problem
        ➢ lower grades have normal-sized cells with ↑NCR and abnormal chromatin
        ➢ architecture of cell groups: rigid and monomorphic ± cribriform
        ➢ lack of two-cell type
        ➢ 'atypical intraductal proliferation, advise Bx' may be appropriate

Rarer Conditions to Consider
- Foreign body reactions: silicone, soya oil, etc.
- Benign stromal lesions: fibromatosis, nodular fasciitis
- Phyllodes tumour: malignant ones have benign epithelial groups with malignant stromal clumps
- Metastases: melanoma, SmCC, ovarian serous carcinoma (psammoma bodies are rare in breast 1°)
- Lymphoma: the dispersed cell pattern and recognition of lymphoid cell types is helpful
- Sarcomas *vs.* spindle cell carcinoma: immuno may help

The Hypocellular Smear – Consider
① radiotherapy effect
② lobular carcinoma

---

[7] this and the subsequent two sections are essentially summarised from NHSBSP Publication Nō 50 (2001) (see Bibliography)

③ carcinoma with extensive fibroelastosis
④ organising haematoma
⑤ fat necrosis, lipoma, etc.

Ovarian Cyst Fluid

General Points
- Only benign cysts should be aspirated
- Contaminants: squames (if PV aspirate), columnar cells (if PR), mesothelium (if transperitoneal)

Benign Cysts and Granulosa Cell Tumour
- Simple cyst: clean background/altered blood
- Fimbrial cyst: foam cells
- Mesothelial inclusion cyst: ➤ proteinaceous/granular background ± RBC
  ➤ ± siderophages
  ➤ sparse small bland cuboidal cell groups
- Functional cyst:
  ➤ granulosa cells: ☞ small cells in tight clusters or loose aggregates
  ☞ delicate cytoplasm
  ☞ round-oval nuclei, coarse pale chromatin ± grooves
  ☞ mitoses
  ☞ no cilia/ciliocytophthoria
  ☞ immuno: +ve for α-inhibin, −ve for Ber-EP4 and CA-125
  ➤ admixed small, dark nuclei
  ➤ ± luteal cells: ☞ polygonal
  ☞ abundant granular/vacuolated cytoplasm
  ☞ anisonucleosis
  ➤ d/dg granulosa cell tumour: tumour has the following features
  ☞ hypercellularity
  ☞ tendency to form microfollicular groups
  ☞ ± round, purple, fibrillar bodies on MGG
- Corpus luteum (luteal) cyst: ➤ blood and fibrin in the background
  ➤ luteinised granulosa cells ++ (including cohesive clusters)
  ➤ siderophages and fibroblasts
  ➤ ↑NCR and prominent nucleoli in pregnancy luteoma
- Endometriotic cyst: ➤ macro: thick brown 'chocolate' fluid
  ➤ blood and siderophages ++
  ➤ ±degenerate endometrial cells (α-inhibin −ve, Ber-EP4 +ve)

Dermoid Cyst
- Macro: thick, pultaceous material
- Most of the material may fall off the slide during preparation
- Debris and occ. squames
- ±Hair shaft fragments, inflam^y cells, foreign body giant cells
- ±Other cell types (respiratory/GIT/thyroid)
- d/dg contaminant vaginal squames

Serous Cystadenoma
- Paucicellular
- Occasional papillaroid cluster of bland cuboidal cells ± cilia
- No prominent nucleoli or mitoses
- ± Psammoma bodies (blue-red in Pap, clear in MGG, not birefringent)
- Immuno: +ve for CA-125, Ber-EP4, WT1
- d/dg papillaroid mesothelial hyperplasia of the pouch of Douglas
- Borderline change (atypia): ➤ cellularity ++
  ➤ nucleoli
  ➤ mitoses
  ➤ psammoma bodies ++

Mucinous Cystadenoma
- Macro: thick and viscous/gelatinous
- Stringy PAS +ve mucin in the background
- Bland columnar cells in a picket-fence/honeycomb architecture
- d/dg rectal epithelial contaminants
- Borderline change (atypia):   ➤ 3D cell clusters and sheets
  - ➤ variably-sized or multiple vacuoles
  - ➤ stratification
  - ➤ ⊥ mitoses

Pseudomyxoma Peritonei (PMP)
- Background: fibrillary metachromatic mucin
- Cellular content: mesothelial cells, fibroblasts ± epithelial cells (usu. scant)
- *NB*: PMP is a clinical diagnosis. The pathologist should report the appearances of the specimen ± whether it is 'consistent with the clinical impression of PMP'. Free mucin should be extensively sampled for epithelial cells (! not d/dg mesothelial groups). If none are seen call it 'acellular mucin'. If they are present, qualify their atypia: 'mucin containing bland/atypical/malignant epithelial cells'
- Most currently believe the 1° mucinous tumour originates in the GIT (usu. appendix) – not ovary

Synovial Fluid

Crystals and Particulate Matter
- Identify the common crystals under 90° crossed polars with a $\frac{1}{4}$ λ plate retarder inserted such that its slow axis (usu. marked on the filter) is at 45° to the polarisers. Note the colour of the birefringence of crystals oriented with their long axis parallel and perpendicular to the $\frac{1}{4}$ λ plate slow axis:
  - ➤ parallel: ☞ monosodium urate: intense yellow
    - ☞ calcium pyrophosphate: weak blue
  - ➤ perpendicular: ☞ monosodium urate: intense blue
    - ☞ calcium pyrophosphate: weak yellow
- Monosodium urate crystals are needle-shaped with strong negative birefringence (defined as above) and are pathognomonic of gout when seen ingested within PMN (but are suggestive of gout in the presence of a PMN infiltrate without ingested forms)
- Calcium pyrophosphate crystals are weakly positively birefringent (as defined above) and elongated rhomboid in shape ('brickets'). They stain with Alizarin red instilled under the coverslip
- These crystals should keep their form and properties for days at room temperature and may be seen on air-dried preparations after Giemsa staining
- Hydroxyapatite crystals are tiny, amorphous (dust-like) crystals that are not birefringent until stained with Alizarin red when they produce birefringent particles
- Diagnostic implications:
  - ➤ urate (= gout esp. if intracellular – *vide supra*)
  - ➤ pyrophosphate (= irrelevant/hypertrophic OA/acute pseudogout if ↑WCC)
  - ➤ hydroxyapatite (= exposed bone due to OA/RhA, Milwaukee shoulder)
- d/dg (i.e. non-crystalline particles): cartilage (look for clustered chondrocytes in hyaline cartilage or curly fibres in fibrocartilage), ligament fragments, prosthesis detritus, debris from plastic containers (artefact), steroid crystals (from injections) can mimic pyrophosphate but they do not react with Alizarin red; cholesterol crystals are square/rectangular with a 'notch' in one corner. Other artefacts include starch and lipid crystalloids that may show 'Maltese cross' or needle-shaped birefringence and lipid may be intracellular

Cellular Content
- Nucleated cells include: PMN, lymphocytes, Mφ (some of which may be cytophagocytic i.e. have phagocytosed apoptotic PMN), mast cells and ragocytes. Malignant cells are rare (d/dg activated lymphocytes or synoviocytes – ! the latter may be CK +ve)
- Ragocytes are cells with cytoplasmic granules (immune complex inclusions) that are larger than ordinary PMN granules and are refractile (reducing the condenser diaphragm enhances this and shows that the granules make a transition from black to apple-green upon focusing up and down)

- Inflam^y pattern: >1000 nucleated cells/mm^3 (normal is <200 and is usu. ≈ 100). Very high counts (>55000/mm^3 i.e. 55 × 10^9 l^{-1}) are usu. due to sepsis, gout, RhA or reactive arthritis
- Septic pattern: >10000 nucleated cells/mm^3 with >95% PMN and >95% ragocytes
- Inflam^y pattern + mast cells: typical of seronegative spondyloarthropathies
- Seronegative pattern: inflam^y pattern with <50% PMN (in the absence of methotrexate Rx)
- RhA: most cases show apoptotic PMN (not within cytophagocytic mononuclear cells) +/ ragocytes; a minority show a seronegative pattern
- Lymphocyte rich pattern: consider SLE/TB
- Mϕ predominant pattern: consider viral infection/Milwaukee shoulder/detritus synovitis
- Cytophagocytic mononuclear cell-rich pattern: consider crystal/seronegative spondyloarthropathies

Bibliography

Andersen, C.E. and McLaren, K. (2003) Best practice in thyroid pathology. *Journal of Clinical Pathology*, **56** (6), 401–405.

Atkins, K.A. (2003) Liquid-based cytological preparations in gynaecological & non-gynaecological specimens, in *Progress in Pathology*, Vol. 6 (eds N. Kirkham and N.A. Shepherd), Greenwich Medical Media, Ltd, London, pp. 101–114.

Coleman, D.V. and Evans, D.M.D. (1998) *Biopsy Pathology and Cytology of the Cervix*, 2nd edn, Arnold, London.

Coleman, D.V. (1975) The cytodiagnosis of human polyoma virus infection. *Acta Cytologica*, **19** (2), 93–96.

Ellison, E., Lapuerta, P. and Martin, S.E. (1998) Fine needle aspiration (FNA) in HIV+ patients: results from a series of 655 aspirates. *Cytopathology*, **9** (4), 222–229.

Freemont, A.J. (2003) Joint disease and the pathologist, in *Progress in Pathology*, Vol. 6 (eds N. Kirkham and N.A. Shepherd), Greenwich Medical Media, Ltd, London, pp. 79–100.

Gray, W. and McKee, T. (eds) (2002) *Diagnostic Cytopathology*, 2nd edn, Churchill Livingstone, Edinburgh.

Gray, W. (1987) Pulmonary Cytopathology, in *Pulmonary Pathology* by M.S.Dunhill, 2nd edn, Churchill Livingstone, Edinburgh, pp. 582–605.

Herbert, A., Buley, I.D., Hasserjian, R.P. *et al.* (1999) Cytopathology of metastatic neoplasia, in *Recent Advances in Histopathology*, Vol. 18 (eds D.G. Lowe and J.C.E. Underwood), Churchill Livingstone, Edinburgh, pp. 109–130.

Kocjan, G. and Miller R. (2001) The cytology of HIV-induced immunosuppression. Changing pattern of disease in the era of highly active antiretroviral therapy. *Cytopathology*, **12** (5), 281–296.

Kocjan, G. and Smith, A.N. (1997) Bile Duct Brushings Cytology: Potential Pitfalls in Diagnosis. *Diagnostic Cytopathology*, **16** (4), 358–363.

McGoogan, E. and McLaren, K. (1995) Fine needle aspiration cytopathology of the thyroid gland, in *Progress in Pathology*, Vol. 1 (eds N. Kirkham and P. Hall), Churchill Livingstone, Edinburgh, pp. 201–211.

McKee, G. (1997) *Cytopathology*, 1st edn, Mosby-Wolfe, London.

McNicol, A.M. (2003) Criteria for diagnosis of follicular thyroid neoplasms and related conditions, in *Recent Advances in Histopathology*, Vol. 20 (eds D. Lowe and J.C.E Underwood), Royal Society of Medicine Press Ltd, London, pp. 1–15.

National Coordinating Network, BSCC and RCPath Working Party (1994) Borderline nuclear changes in cervical smears: Guidelines on their recognition and management. *Journal of Clinical Pathology*, **47** (6), 481–482.

Ng, W-K. (2003) Radiation-associated changes in tissues and tumours. *Current Diagnostic Pathology*, **9** (2), 124–136.

Orell, S.R., Sterrett, G.F., Walters, M.N-I. *et al.* (1999) *Manual and Atlas of Fine Needle Aspiration Cytology*, 3rd edn, Churchill Livingstone, Edinburgh.

Reid, A.J.C., Miller, R.F. and Kocjan, G.I. (1998) Diagnostic utility of fine needle aspiration (FNA) cytology in HIV patients with lymphadenopathy. *Cytopathology*, **9** (4), 230–239.

Rogers, S. (1997) Synovial fluid in health and disease, in *Progress in Pathology*, Vol. 3 (eds N. Kirkham and N.R. Lemoine), Churchill Livingstone, NY, pp. 165–178.

Sanders, E., Asscher, A.W., Williams, J.D. *et al.* (1993) *Nephrology in Colour*, 1st edn, Gower Medical Publishing, London.

Szporn, A.H., Yuan, S., Wu, M. *et al.* (2006) Cellular swirls in fine needle aspirates of papillary thyroid carcinoma: a new diagnostic criterion. *Modern Pathology*, **19** (11), 1470–1473.

Trott, P.A. (ed) (1996) *Breast Cytopathology. A diagnostic atlas*, 1st edn, Chapman & Hall, London.

Young, J.A. (1993) *Fine Needle Aspiration Cytopathology*, 1st edn, Blackwell Scientific Publications, Oxford.

Web sites

NHSCSP (2000) *'The ABC Document' Achievable standards, Benchmarks for reporting and Criteria for evaluating cervical cytology*, 2nd edn, Publication Nö. 1, URL: http://www.cancerscreening.nhs.uk/cervical/index.html (accessed July 2004).

NHSBSP (2001) *Guidelines for non-operative diagnostic procedures and reporting in breast cancer screening*, Publication Nö. 50, URL: http://www.cancerscreening.nhs.uk/breastscreen/index.html (accessed July 2005).

25. Autopsy

Legal and Managerial Aspects

Consent
- Should be obtained within the context of a multidisciplinary bereavement team (MDBT)
- A pathologist should be on the team to:
  - ➤ advise on ethical and legal issues
  - ➤ advise on the content of leaflets
  - ➤ be available to discuss autopsy / results with relatives
  - ➤ help with the induction of new staff
  - ➤ help audit the service.
- Consent (for an adult) may be given by someone nominated by the deceased prior to death or a relation (in order of authority): spouse / civil partner, child / parent, full sibling (if > 1, they must all agree), grandchild / grandparent, niece / nephew, step-parent, half-sibling, long-standing friend.
- A request for autopsy should be declined if the consent or Coronial permission is so restrictive as to make answering the clinical questions impossible (discuss this with the consent-taking doctor first).
- A consented case should be reported to the Coroner if the history or PM findings suggest it may be under his jurisdiction.
- GMC ethical guidance (2007) advises that 'recordings' (photo / video / audio) may be made of internal organs, pathology slides or X-rays without consent and used for any purpose provided they are anonymised (but the Human Tissue Act 2004 makes this illegal for PM tissue unless consented). Apart from those exceptions, written consent is required for any recordings to be used in publicly accessible media regardless of whether you consider the patient identifiable.
- The Human Tissue Act 2004 currently (2007) forbids blood testing for serious communicable diseases (e.g. HIV / hepatitis) unless there is appropriate consent:
  - ➤ even if these diseases may form part of the cause of death sequence
  - ➤ even if someone is injured during the autopsy.

Human Tissue Act 2004 (England and Wales – in effect from 1st September 2006)
- This is only a brief summary – for details and exceptions see the whole Act. Scotland has its own laws.
- It replaces the Human Tissue Act 1961, Anatomy Act 1984 and Human Organ Transplants Act 1989.
- The motivation was concerns over the use of PM baby / perinate tissues without appropriate consent after the organ retention 'scandals' at the turn of the 21st century (retention of all baby organs at Alder Hey and baby hearts at Bristol).
- Excluded from the Act are gametes, embryos, cell lines (and any other human material created outside the human body), things done at the behest of the Coroner and 'existing holdings' (i.e. the Act is not retrospective).
- It concerns the removal, storage and use of tissue, DNA, cell-containing fluids, whole organs, whole bodies and body parts from dead (PM) and living (biopsies and 'surgical waste') persons. (Hair and nail from living people and acellular fluids are not covered.)
- It creates a Human Tissue Authority to licence a 'designated individual' and inspect all sites storing or handling human tissues. Only the 'designated individual', those notified to the HTA by the 'designated individual' or those acting under the direction of the latter two may perform activities on human tissues that fall under the Act.
- 'Appropriate consent' is required for most activities relating to storage / use of PM tissue.
- Consent is *not* required re storage / use of tissue taken from a living person (= Bx / 'surgical waste') for:
  - ➤ deriving diagnostic or scientific information that may be relevant to that person
  - ➤ research: if it is ethically approved and the samples are anonymous to the researcher(s)
  - ➤ education or training relating to human health
  - ➤ clinical audit, performance assessment, QA and public health monitoring.
- Public display of a specimen requires witnessed specific written consent of the patient, not a relative.

Diagnostic Criteria Handbook in Histopathology: A Surgical Pathology Vade Mecum by Paul J. Tadrous
Copyright © 2007 by John Wiley & Sons, Ltd.

Clinical Governance and Autopsy
- Gaining consent for autopsies must be encouraged (see MDBT above).
- Coroners must be encouraged to allow sampling for histology and dissemination of their reports.
- Attendance at autopsy by clinicians and radiologists should be encouraged.
- Autopsy may bring to light an adverse clinical event (see p. 380 under Coroner's autopsy).
- Hold (and minute) regular mortality meetings to discuss clinicopathological discrepancies.
- Audit the quality and timeliness of autopsy reports.
- Participation in an autopsy EQA scheme is part of good Clinical Governance.
- *NB*: the Human Tissue Act 2004 prohibits the use of PM tissue for audit, EQA, education, training or 'performance assessment' without consent.

Autopsy Report Content
- Demographic details, Drs in charge, those present at and conducting the autopsy
- Clinical summary (on a separate sheet for Coronial cases in case the Coroner does not want it)
- External examination (incl. how the patient was identified)
- Internal examination (all organ systems, include negative findings / not examined)
- Ancillary results (histology, toxicology, cytogenetics, microbiology, radiology)
- Summary of main findings and clinicopathological correlation
- Cause of death in ONS[1] format for anyone > 28 days old (special format for perinates). Avoid unqualified words that could result in attracting the Coroner's interest[2] unnecessarily e.g. septicaemia (without giving a specific cause) or accident (as in CVA). Avoid abbreviations. Avoid unqualified modes of dying (e.g. cardiac arrest, asphyxia, shock, uraemia, cachexia, syncope, vasovagal attack, organ failure). 'Old age' is only acceptable for those >80 years old if no other cause is found

Autopsy Report Timing
- Arrange for a member of the clinical team to attend the PM – else phone the result the same day
- Preliminary (or final) report within one week
- Final report as soon as possible after ancillary results become available

Performance Recommendations / Guidance
- Annual pathologist workload should not be < 50 PMs (nor > 300 [DGH] or 150 [teaching hospital])

Cases appropriate for the general pathologist
- Industrial diseases, HIV, non-heart transplants, epilepsy, sickle cell, accidents, suicide, drugs, dementia (non-CJD)

Cases where specialist pathologist input is advised
- Paediatric, child abuse, maternal death, complex cardiac surgery, neuro (esp. CJD)
- Suspicious or criminal cases should be done by a Home Office pathologist

Cases of possible serious communicable disease
- The UK currently lacks official facilities suitable for performing autopsies on cases of some HG4 pathogens (e.g. cases of VHF) so PM should not be done ∴ in suspected cases send blood for testing (prior to doing the PM) to the Specialist Pathogens Reference Unit (SPRU) of the Health Protection Agency (HPA) at Colindale (www.hpa.org.uk; tel: 01980 612224 [during working hours] or 01980 612100 [emergency, out of hours]). See pp. 383–385 for guidance on HG3 agents

Review of Death Certification and the Coronial System

Background
- The *Luce Report* into Death Certification is the basis of the changes made in death certification practice and advised essentially what is described below. *The Third Report of the Shipman Inquiry* (Dame Janet Smith Report) proposed changes to the Coronial system along the lines of a single Medical coroner who would investigate all deaths, order a PM on a random sample of them and, for all, consider – on the basis of facts ascertained with the help of a panel of experts – whether to order a PM, issue a death certificate or open an inquest.

---

[1] ONS = Office of National Statistics, the format is: 1 a) due to b) due to c); 2) disorder 1 and disorder 2 and disorder 3, etc.

[2] If a Dr was in attendance within 14 days of death and knows the cause of death he can sign the death certificate – even if this cause of death is Coronial e.g. cerebral lacerations due to gun-shot wound. It is the responsibility of the Registrar of deaths to report any such suspicious cases to the Coroner. In practice, however, a Dr would refer the case to the Coroner rather than issue such a death certificate.

Death certification
- One-tier system for non-cremations and 3-tier system for cremations[3] is to be replaced with a single
- Two-tier certification system for all deaths preceded by death verification by a health-care worker:
    1. certification of cause of death by the deceased's doctor
    2. a second certifier will scrutinise this certificate – the certifier to be chosen by a Medical Examiner based in a Coroner's office
- This scrutiny may be done by the Medical Examiner (who is to be medically qualified) or delegated to a member of a panel of expert medical practitioners (with differing specialties) on the Medical Examiner's list.
- The second certifier (if satisfied that no Coronial input is indicated) will also issue a disposal order (thereby removing the need for the next of kin to visit the Registrar of Deaths for the customary *viva*) and so speed up the process for those requiring prompt burial/cremation on religious grounds.
- All deaths which cannot be certified or appear unnatural will be referred to the Coroner.
- This process should result in the identification of suspicious Harold Shipman-like trends.

The Coroner's system (Coroner's Reform) for England, Wales and Northern Ireland
- The old 127 jurisdictions of part-time Coroners are to be replaced by 60 full-time, legally qualified Coroners in a single national jurisdiction presided over by a Chief Coroner.
- The old part-time, non-formally trained Coroner's officers are to be replaced by formally-trained full-time Coroner's officers with encouragement towards specialised training in dealing with e.g. child deaths, maternal deaths, etc.
- Coroners also to be supported by Medical Examiners (medically qualified Statutory Medical Assessors) who, in addition to routine death certification duties (*vide supra*) will have a wide panel of medical experts at their disposal to allow a more thorough investigation of deaths establishing natural causes by scrutiny of medical history, etc. thereby avoiding unnecessary autopsies. It is anticipated, therefore, that Coroner's autopsy rates will fall.
- Medical Examiners will have established public health links and be involved in general monitoring and death certification audit.
- Coroners' verdicts are to be narrative to avoid the confrontational short-form legalistic verdicts.
- An advisory Coronial Council and Inspectorate will be set up to promote consistent service standards and disseminate best practice guidelines.
- A Family Charter will be established making it easier for families to raise their concerns.
- The appeals process will be simpler.

Potential problems with pathology practice in the light of the new reforms
- Potential dis-incentives that may lead many pathologists to abandon Coronial work are:
    1. Coronial income might go into NHS departments and Trusts rather than to individual pathologists
    2. defence society subscriptions may rise for those doing Coroner's autopsies in the light of potential problems arising from organ retention and disposal and w.r.t the Human Tissue Act 2004 and the revised (2005) Coroner's rules 9 & 12 (pp. 380–381).
    3. the increased administrative and organisational burden assoc[d] with the storage and disposal requirements of the revised (2005) Coroner's rules 9 & 12 (pp. 380–381).

Guidance for Particular Types of Autopsy

Coroner's Cases
- Is this autopsy a Coroner's case (or should it be)?
    1. unidentified body
    2. no Dr attended during last illness / Dr did not see the person within 14 days prior to death
    3. cause of death unknown ('unascertained') or unnatural (e.g. aspiration pneumonia not accounted for by a natural condition like stroke; or septicaemia not qualified by the causative organism and natural portal of entry)
    4. infant deaths (except hospital deaths where the cause is confidently known)
    5. abortion-related deaths
    6. still-births if there is any doubt as to whether the infant was born alive or not

---

[3] plus, in either case, the usual visit to the Registrar of deaths for a *viva* examination as to the identification of the deceased – prior to issuing of a disposal order permitting burial / cremation

7. death during operation / before recovery from anaesthetic or <24 hours of operation / anaesthetic
8. allegations of negligence
9. accident-related[4]: industrial, domestic or transportation (includes anaphylaxis – p. 382)
10. industrial diseases
11. alcohol / drugs / poisons related
12. suicide or self neglect
13. homicide
14. any history of violence
15. sudden unexpected death or suspicious circumstances
16. death in custody or shortly after release (incl. those sectioned under the Mental Health Act) even if in hospital at the time of death
17. deceased in receipt of an armed forces or industrial disability pension
18. deaths of young foster children or persons in mental institutions ⎫ these aren't strict rules
19. death within 24 hours of admission even when the cause of death ⎬ but should be considered
    is known ⎭

- Giving evidence at inquest:
  - ➤ bring all relevant documentation with you
  - ➤ clarify ambiguous questions before attempting to answer them
  - ➤ avoid jargon and be sensitive in your replies – the family and media may be present
  - ➤ distinguish facts from conclusions drawn from the facts
  - ➤ be prepared to modify conclusions already drawn based on additional information
  - ➤ be prepared to stay in court to hear further evidence / legal representation, and if there is misrepresentation or misunderstanding make this known to the Coroner.
- It is preferable to do the PM in the hospital of the patient – because the notes and clinicians are there.
- Coroner may order PM to be done elsewhere / by a pathologist of different hospital if allegations of clinical negligence are anticipated.
- In perioperative / peri-intervention deaths it may help to invite the relevant clinicians to be represented at the PM and to assist with the dissection (to explain and document complex findings and identify adverse clinical events).
- If evidence of an adverse clinical event[5] is uncovered at any PM and this is considered to be a significant factor in the cause of death – stop, document everything, inform the Coroner (if not already his case) and invite the relevant clinician to witness and discuss the findings.
- If evidence of criminality becomes apparent during any PM[6] – stop and call the Coroner.
- Perform histology in all cases (subject to Coroner's permission) and ancillary tests (e.g. toxicology) where appropriate.
- Do not take tissue / disseminate reports / allow training unless the Coroner gives permission – any action not related to the Coroner's remit (e.g. taking tissue for research) requires, in addition, consent of the next of kin / executor of the deceased's estate.
- Consider retaining material, photos, organs relevant to the cause of death or for expert opinion.
- If the cause of death can only be determined from the clinical details advise the Coroner that he needs to get statements from the relevant clinicians.

A summary of some of the Coroner's Rules (1984, as amended 2005)
- Coroner's Rule 5: PM to be done as soon as practicable
- Coroner's Rule 6: PM to be done by a pathologist with access to lab facilities
- Coroner's Rule 7: relatives have the right to be represented at the PM by a doctor
- Coroner's Rule 8: no representative present shall interfere with the PM examination
- Coroner's Rule 9: the pathologist shall make provision 'so far as possible' for the preservation of material which 'in his opinion' bears upon the cause of death or identification of the body. He must communicate to the Coroner in writing (email is also acceptable) what is retained, the suggested storage period and his reasons for retaining them. The Coroner must then specify the duration for which they shall be stored and, in any case, the storage period expires automatically on the date on which the Coroner's functions cease (it is the Coroner's responsibility to inform the pathologist of when his functions cease).

---

[4] the accident may have occurred any time prior to death – not necessarily immediately
[5] e.g. the misplacement of an intravenous line causing significant haemorrhage or the perforation of a viscus
[6] including those that are already Coroner's cases – because a Forensic / Home Office pathologist may need to be called in to complete the autopsy

The Coroner must communicate to the relatives that tissue was taken and give them the options for subsequent dealings with the material: 1) disposal 2) returned to them or 3) retained for use in research, etc. Upon expiry of the storage period the pathologist must communicate to the Coroner (and retain a record of) how he has dealt with the tissues (incl. who the tissue has been retained for if not disposed or returned). At any stage, the pathologist must tell the Coroner if he thinks the material should be kept for a different period of time than that originally specified by the Coroner.

- Coroner's Rule 10 & 13: report issued to the Coroner only (unless he gives permission for others to see it)
- Coroner's Rule 12: any material used for special examination (e.g. histology) must be stored for a period decided as for Rule 9 and dealt with thereafter according to the details given in Rule 9 (note the implications here for storage/disposal of H&E slides)
- Coroner's Rule 36: 'matters to be ascertained at inquest' are:
  - the identity of the deceased
  - how, when and where the deceased came by his death
  - details necessary to register the death
  - no opinion on any other matter is to be expressed by the Coroner or jury.
- Coroner's Rule 42: the verdict must not appear to determine criminal or civil liability on the part of a named person

Dementia

- Assess the risk of prion aetiology (if present refer to neuropathologist / UK CJD surveillance unit[7]):
  - rapid onset / course (1–2 years from diagnosis to death)
  - ± motor signs (e.g. myoclonus, cerebellar, akinetic mutism)
  - characteristic EEG (not seen in vCJD)
  - prior psychiatric +/ sensory disturbance (esp. vCJD)
  - FHx (in GSS / FFI)
- Aims of the PM:
  - confirm / refute clinical diagnosis of dementia
  - identify the aetiology of the dementia and whether there is an inheritance risk: Alzheimer / familial Alzheimer / mixed Alzheimer and vascular, vascular, Lewy body diseases (e.g. 1° dysphagia), frontoparietal degenerations (e.g. Pick's), rarer (e.g. CJD, metabolic, hydrocephalus, etc.)
  - assess the relation of the dementia to the cause of death sequence: dementia may cause frailty, immobility, falls and disinhibition / lack of co-ordination which may result in thromboembolism, bed-sore septicaemia, bronchopneumonia and contribute to legal liability in fatal accidents. (*NB*: inappropriate Rx of DLB with neuroleptics can be fatal)
- Weigh brain fresh and weigh hemispheres and cerebellum separately after fixation (calculate ratio)
- Exclude cardiovascular lesions and brain infarcts / tumour / infection
- Careful examination of vessels supplying brain (carotids, vertebrals, circle of Willis)
- Sample any focal lesion (cortex, deep white, deep grey)
- Systematic sampling:
  - cingulate gyrus and frontal, parietal and occipital lobes (cortex and deep white)
  - temporal lobe: hippocampus, parahippocampal gyrus, neocortex
  - upper pons (locus ceruleus), upper medulla (hypoglossal nucleus), substantia nigra
  - take spinal cord if there was dysphagia / motor weakness
- Histology (see pp. 181–182)

Stroke

- Establish whether haemorrhagic (SAH or intracranial), ischaemic or erroneous clin. diagnosis.
- Exclude causes with familial risk: CAA, multiple cavernous haemangiomas, familial coagulopathies.
- Exclude potentially treatable causes: e.g. vasculitis, brain tumour (1°/2°), mycotic aneurysm, central pontine myelinolysis.

---

[7] The National Creutzfeldt-Jakob Disease Surveillance Unit, Internet: http:\\www.cjd.ed.ac.uk, Address: Western General Hospital, Crewe Road, Edinburgh, EH4 2XU, UK; Clinical Office Telephone: 0131 537 2128; Pathology Telephone: 0131 537 1980, Fax: 0131 343 1404

- Exclude potentially traumatic causes (these may have medicolegal implications): e.g. arterial dissection or fat embolism (the latter is a cause of ball and ring or pinpoint haemorrhages on histology – also seen in Malaria, HSV-1 encephalitis, acute haemorrhagic leucoencephalopathy and DIC).
- Describe the location and distribution of lesions (remember the boundary zones for watershed infarcts) and 2° effects (ventricular dilatation, midline shift, herniations, etc.)
- Examine: the heart (atria, valves, etc.), aortic arch, carotid arteries, carotid bifurcation, carotid siphon, vertebral arteries, venous sinuses and Charcot's 'artery of cerebral haemorrhage'.

Anaphylaxis
- Causes include: iatrogenic (antibiotics, aspirin, opiates used in the induction of anaesthesia, radiological contrast media – 5min), insect stings (15min) and food (nuts – 30min)[8]
- Mode of dying: shock, asphyxia (laryngopharyngeal oedema or bronchospasm[9]) or both[10]
- Clin.: full medication history / allergies / PMHx / any preparations taken shortly before death
- External: look for insect stings and urticaria
- Internal:
  - laryngeal / pharyngeal / upper airway oedema
  - petechial haemorrhages on mucosal / serosal surfaces in cases of asphyxia
  - bronchial mucus plugging with hyperinflation of the lungs in anaphylactic asthma
  - pulmonary oedema (assoc[d] with adrenaline overdose)
  - signs of resuscitation / ITU pathology (may be the only pathology if death is delayed)
  - cardiac / full PM to exclude other causes
  - in IgG anaphylactoid[11] reactions (e.g. to dextran infusion) there is obstruction of the pulmonary microvasculature with acute dilatation of the right ventricle and pulmonary (rather than laryngopharyngeal) oedema
- Histology:
  - larynx / upper airways: submucosal oedema and infiltration by mast cells and eosinophils
  - lungs: mucus plugging of bronchi with lamina propria oedema, eosinophils and hyperinflation. Chronic asthma changes are usu. absent (BM thickening and mucus gland hyperplasia). Cases with shock show intense congestion and intra-alveolar haemorrhage. IgG reactions show hyaline globules in capillaries (immune complex deposition)
  - heart: contraction bands due to inotropes, ischaemia with normal coronary arteries occurs with anaphylactic shock
  - other tissues: tissue eosinophilia – esp. spleen (red pulp) and liver
- PB (ante-mortem and PM) in plain bottle for mast cell tryptase, IgE levels and specific drug antibodies
- IgE is stable at room temperature for 11 weeks but alone is not proof of anaphylaxis as some normals have ↑ levels and one needs evidence of mast cell degranulation
- Tryptase has two forms – α and β. αTryptase is constitutively expressed and is a measure of mast cell load (↑ in systemic mastocytosis). βTryptase is only expressed during degranulation and is more specific for anaphylaxis. Its half life is >4 days. Very high levels are usu. due to anaphylaxis but those near the borderline may be due to tissue autolysis, 'normal' asthmatics or intracardiac blood sample site (*cf.* femoral). Tryptase may not be ↑ in food anaphylaxis. Tryptase levels peak at 0.5–6.0 hours post allergen exposure so use ante-mortem blood from the acute phase of the illness if death was delayed. Haemoglobin interferes with the assay so spin the sample and separate off the serum (which may then be stored in a freezer)
- d/dg – anaphylactic asthma due to food / aspirin may be misdiagnosed as fatal asthma
- d/dg – anaphylactic shock may be misdiagnosed as MI
- The above differentials are important because anaphylaxis is considered a form of 'accidental' death and measurement of IgE and tryptase may necessitate that a Coroner's inquest be opened. It may also have compensation implications for the next of kin
- Mention the allergen on the death certificate where known

---

[8] times are the average time from allergen challenge to death

[9] bronchospasm = anaphylactic asthma (i.e. due to a systemic – ingested or injected – allergen *cf.* inhaled)

[10] shock does not usu. occur with food anaphylaxis

[11] anaphylaxis requires IgE Ab-dependent cross-linking of receptors on mast cells → release of histamine, tryptase, leukotrienes, etc. Anaphylactoid reactions cause mast cell degranulation without IgE antibody or cause similar symptoms via other mediators without mast cell degranulation. The same agent can cause either anaphylactic or anaphylactoid reactions in different individuals.

Shock (Including Sepsis)
- Causes: **C**ardiogenic, **H**ypovolaemic, **A**naphylactic, **O**ther, **S**eptic
- General shock lesions: microthrombi, haemorrhages, necroses (2° to DIC and underperfusion)
- Shock lung (ARDS): is common in sepsis but rare in non-traumatic hypovolaemia
  - ➤ macro: uniformly solid, airless and dry cut surface with subpleural petechiae
  - ➤ exudative stage: haemorrhage, hyaline membranes, thrombi in alveolar capillaries
  - ➤ regenerative phase: organising pneumonia and proliferation of Type II pneumocytes
- Heart: more common in hypovolaemic/cardiogenic *cf.* septic
  - ➤ subendocardial MI (regional / transmural MI is more likely the *cause* of shock)
  - ➤ focal necroses (esp. in infants / perinates)
  - ➤ epicardial haemorrhages (along the lines of the coronary arteries in perinates)
- Kidney:
  - ➤ ATN: loss of PAS +ve brush border of PCT with dilatation of DCT epithelium and pigmented granular or hyaline casts. Regenerative phase → mitoses and anisonucleosis
  - ➤ renal cortical haemorrhagic necrosis: esp. in perinates ± medullary necroses
- Liver: necrosis is usu. seen after 24 hours; cholestatic changes most common in septic / endotoxic shock
  - ➤ zone 3 necrosis (irregular foci in perinates)
  - ➤ cholestasis, bile ductular proliferation, cholangiolitis (neutrophils) with dilatation and bile concretions at periphery of PTs. Cholangitis may be seen esp. in toxic shock syndrome[12]
  - ➤ old necrosis and fibrosis in stillborns suggest prior cardiovascular collapse *in utero*
- Pancreas: acute haemorrhagic pancreatitis may be the cause of the shock. Infants get islet necrosis without inflammation and with sparing of the exocrine tissue
- GIT: petechial haemorrhages, erosion, acute ulcers in stomach and duodenum. Ischaemic bowel may perforate or heal with stricture and fibrosis. Perinates may show necrotising enterocolitis
- Brain (see also 'Ischaemic Hypoxic Injury' on p. 182):
  - ➤ adults: watershed infarcts, occipital and parietal cortex ischaemic lesions (esp. at the depths of the sulci), Sommer's sector of hippocampus (CA1), cerebellar Purkinje and basket cells
  - ➤ perinates: periventricular leukomalacia and brain stem lesions
- Pituitary: Sheehan syndrome – otherwise apoplexy and haemorrhage are rare without head injury
- Adrenals: lipid depletion of the cortex (affects fetal cortex with sparing of definitive cortex in perinates → 'clear cell reversal pattern' ± pseudofollicular change in definitive cortex). Haemorrhage ± infarction. Thrombi in sinusoids

Sickle Cell Disease
- Causes of death: ACS[13], cor pulmonale, sudden cardiac death 2° to myocardial fibrosis, sickle crisis multi-organ failure, bacterial infections (sepsis, meningitis, pneumonia, osteomyelitis), CRF, stroke, hyperhaemolysis syndrome (post transfusion), drug effects (respiratory depression, fits)
- Children may also die from acute splenic sequestration and aplastic crisis
- Histology (use buffered formalin to avoid artefactual PM sickling):
  - ➤ multiple blocks from: heart and all lung lobes
  - ➤ bone marrow: vertebral sample and femur slice for marrow hyperplasia and infarcts
  - ➤ skeletal muscle for crush injury and any recent operation sites
- Ancillary tests:
  - ➤ microbiology: blood, urine, meninges, lung
  - ➤ toxicology for opiates – specify fentanyl on the request form
  - ➤ blood for sickle test, parvovirus B19 serology and tryptase (if ?anaphylaxis)
- Decide the importance of sickle disease to the cause of death: main cause, contributory or irrelevant

Category 3 Hazard Group Infection Risk Autopsies
- HG3 agents include: HIV, HBV, HCV, TB and CJD, *Brucella* spp., *Salmonella typhi*, anthrax, *Histoplasma capsulatum*, Falciparum malaria, *Trypanosoma* spp. and *Leishmania* spp.

---

[12] due to excretion of staphylococcal exotoxin in the bile
[13] Acute Chest Syndrome: pleuritic pain, cough fever, haemoptysis, leukocytosis – due to sickling in pulmonary vessels ± infarction, infection, thromboemboli, fat emboli, pulm haemorrhage. The commonest cause of death in sickle cell disease.

- Universal precautions:
  - cover all your skin defects and skin and mucosal surfaces (incl. eyes, nose, mouth)
  - waterproofing: scrubsuits, aprons, sleeve covers
  - triple glove (with the middle layer being cut resistant gloves e.g. Kevlar$^{®}$ / neoprene)[14]
  - use a HEPA[15] mask / respirator when TB is suspected – post a notice outside doors when in use
  - use a separate circulator assistant whenever possible
  - all staff must be at an appropriate level of training
  - exclude unnecessary personnel and any with immunosuppression or hands containing open wounds / fresh (i.e. <2 days old) cuts
  - all observers must have the same protection as prosectors and stay at a safe ('splash') distance.
- Handling sharps:
  - instrument tray well laid out, don't have uncapped needles on the tray, don't re-sheath
  - don't point or gesture with sharps
  - don't hand sharps to one another (place them on an intermediary surface)
  - don't hold a container by the hand when introducing a tissue sample by needle
  - remove all sharps from a table immediately after use
  - cover cut ends of bones (e.g. ribs) with padding (e.g. damp towels).
- There must be adequate space, ventilation and lighting
- The undertaker must be notified if a HG3 agent is present.
- Staff should have BCG and HBV vaccinations in cases of HIV, HBV, HCV and TB.
- A separate 'high risk' area is preferable but not essential – do infective PM last on the list.
- Any injury which results in bleeding: wash thoroughly and report to Occupational Health.

HIV
- Risk of infection by inoculation is 0.3% (0.03% by mucosal contamination).
- PM done by a consultant / experienced junior with MTO2 grade technician (and circulator ideally).
- A HEPA filter / respirator is advised and other TB precautions should be taken
- On exposure: stop the PM and report to Occupational Health for testing and prophylactic therapy.

HCV
- Risk of infection by inoculation 3%, respiratory and mucosal routes are not a significant hazard.
- PM done by a consultant / experienced junior with MTO2 grade technician (and circulator ideally).
- On exposure: stop the PM, clean the wound thoroughly and inform Occupational Health.

TB
- Risk is by inhalation of *Mycobacterium TB* (MAI / *M. Kansasii* are not significant risks).
- PM done by consultant / experienced junior with MTO1 grade technician (circulator not necessary).
- A HEPA filter / respirator is essential as standard masks are inadequate. Perform standard dissection of lungs as formalin inflation for next day dissection is not necessary and doesn't sterilise the lungs.
- Send tissue to microbiology for culture, sensitivity and genotyping.
- If known/suspected drug resistant TB: inform Occupational Health and infection control department.
- On exposure (or if an unsuspected case is subsequently diagnosed when TB respiratory precautions were not observed), inform Occupational Health and give a list of all those present at the PM.
- If it is a new diagnosis of TB inform the local consultant of CDC (directly/via Coroner) and the ICD.

CJD
- Risk of infection is by inoculation / mucosal contamination.
- PM to be done by a consultant (only) with MTO2 grade technician (and circulator ideally).
- No one else is to be allowed in the PM room.
- PM to be done in a body bag.
- Use disposable gowns and aprons, standard masks and full face visor.
- Use disposable instruments as far as possible – incl. disposable stapler to close the body.
- Open skull in a polythene bag sealed around the saw and head.
- The spinal cord as well as brain may be needed. Some say limit the PM to brain, others that full PM should be done in case of wrong clinical diagnosis and to document visceral lesions.
- Use of cork, wood or plastic cutting boards is forbidden – cover the PM table in double plastic material to be disposed of afterwards.

---

[14] consider using a chain-mail glove on the non-saw hand when opening the skull
[15] High Efficiency Particulate Air mask / respirator

- 2M NaOH should be used to wipe down tables and soak all instruments. Surfaces should be soaked for a minimum of 1 hour with repeated wetting. Non-disposable instruments are then autoclaved at 120 to 138°C. Disposable ones are incinerated.
- The body should be returned to undertakers in a body bag and undertakers informed of CJD risk.
- Tissues should be fixed in 10% formalin. Blocks for histology should then be decontaminated by immersion in 96% formic acid for at least 1 hour prior to processing. Collect and incinerate any wax trimmings and decontaminate the microtome with 2M NaOH.
- Collect formalin used for fixation, absorb with sawdust and incinerate.
- On exposure: record names of all staff present at PM and retain records for 40 years.

Maternal Death (MD)
- International def[n].: death during pregnancy or within 6 weeks of delivery / miscarriage.
- UK def[n] includes deaths upto 12 months – hence the division into 'early' (≤6 weeks) and 'late' MD – each of these are subdivided by cause as 'direct' (diseases of pregnancy), 'indirect' (pre-existing diseases exacerbated by pregnancy) or 'coincidental'.
- The pathologist should check with a clinician whether the case was reported to the Director of Public Health so the case may be investigated for the triennial Confidential Enquiry into MD (CEMD).
- Record a detailed history and demographics (incl. height and weight).

Direct maternal deaths
- PE: ?FHx, ?evidence of recurrent PE, ?morbid obesity, ?antipsychotic drugs
- PET: placental bed (failure of vascular transformation beyond the decidual / myometrial junction), kidney (membranoproliferative GN, pre-existing disease), liver (periportal zone 1 necrosis, microvesicular steatosis in HELLP), DIC
- Obstetric haemorrhage: placental abruption, *placenta praevia*, morbidly adherent placentae, PPH – estimate blood loss and look for genital tract trauma and examine any recent hysterectomy / RPOC specimens (?fat, ?unusually deep i.e. muscle ++)
- Amniotic fluid embolism (AFE): Lungs contain mucin (from meconium) and squames (34βE12) – do an AB or a Lendrum's phloxine tartrazine alcian green. Examine the placenta and uterus for a tear
- Early MD due to an ectopic (estimate blood loss and gestational age), miscarriage or TOP (?sepsis – search for uterine and bowel perforations, may see blotchy skin marbling with Group A Streptococci)
- Acute Fatty Liver of Pregnancy: (zone 2/3 microvesicular steatosis, perivenular zone 3 necrosis, canalicular cholestasis ± ductular reaction, ± lymphocytic infiltrates)

Indirect maternal deaths
- CVS: pulmonary HT (1° plexogenic ± Eisenmenger's complex [VSD + overriding aorta], Eisenmenger's syndrome [any left to right shunt with subsequent pulmonary HT] or 2° to multiple thromboemboli); cardiomyopathy (dilated and pseudohypertrophic – i.e. without disarray or familial tendency); aneurysms (coronary, splenic, renal)
- Suicide – esp. by violent methods
- Epilepsy – do PM blood anticonvulsant levels and exclude PET
- Malignancy – treatment / diagnosis may be delayed due to pregnancy
- CNS: subarachnoid and intracerebral haemorrhage (exclude PET), *hyperemesis gravidarum* – look for Wernicke's encephalopathy
- Infections: TB / viral – exclude a genital tract site of entry
- Respiratory: acute asthma

Sudden Cardiac Deaths
- Exclude solvent / cocaine / alcohol / illicit drug use
- Only when toxicology and detailed structural examination is negative may SADS be diagnosed
- Coronary artery pathology: ostia may be stenosed or malpositioned (e.g. pulmonary trunk), tunnelling (esp. if >5mm deep)
- Cardiomyopathies: HOCM, pseudohypertrophic (HOCMoid), dilated, restrictive (amyloid, sarcoid)
- ARVD: familial in 30%, assoc[d] with aneurysm or dilatation of RV. Requires interstitial fibrosis in >1 hpf ± inflam[n] [not just fatty replacement]. May be focal and involve LV as well (or solely – contentious)
- Conducting system: see 'Conducting System of the Heart,' pp. 389–390
- Myocarditis: esp. in infants, ! must exclude this before diagnosing SIDS
- Blunt trauma: *commotio cordis*
- SUDEP: no cardiac morphological abnormality and not related to a grand mal seizure

- The Davies criteria for classifying acute cardiac deaths:

    i. demonstrable coronary thrombosis +/ acute MI
    ii. ≥1 coronary artery < 1mm Ø AND evidence of healed MI
    iii. ≥1 coronary artery < 1mm Ø with NO evidence of MI
    iv. no evidence of IHD but features of CCF or significant LVH/RVH and/or dilatation
    v. SADS

Developmental Cardiac Anomalies
- Features that help identify left *vs.* right chambers:
    ➢ atrial appendages (see Figure 25.1): the right is a smooth blunt triangle, the left is a crenellated elongated hook-like sac
    ➢ ventricular muscle trabeculae: coarse on the right, fine on the left
- Coronary artery anomalies (p. 385)
- ARVD (p. 385)
- HOCM (see p. 78)
- Tetralogy of Fallot:
    ① pulmonary (infundibular) stenosis
    ② RV hypertrophy
    ③ high ventriculoseptal defect
    ④ overriding aorta

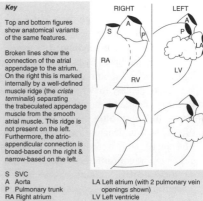

Atrial Appendage Anatomy in the Infant Heart

Key

Top and bottom figures show anatomical variants of the same features.

Broken lines show the connection of the atrial appendage to the atrium. On the right this is marked internally by a well-defined muscle ridge (the *crista terminalis*) separating the trabeculated appendage muscle from the smooth atrial muscle. This ridge is not present on the left. Furthermore, the atrio-appendicular connection is broad-based on the right & narrow-based on the left.

S SVC
A Aorta
P Pulmonary trunk
RA Right atrium
RV Right ventricle

LA Left atrium (with 2 pulmonary vein openings shown)
LV Left ventricle

FIGURE 25.1   Perinatal heart chambers

Cardiac Valves and Other Prosthetics
See Butany and Collins, 2005.

Heart and Lung Transplant Patients
- Contact the Tx centre pathology department for advice and Hx (they may also want you to send the organ): date of Tx, original disease, post op complications, immunosuppression and rejection Hx, etc.
- Assess: infection, rejection, post-op complications, drug and immunosuppression effects, neoplasia, systemic effects
- Sample: suture lines, focal lesions, conducting system, lung periphery (multiple), microbiology

Limited Autopsies (Limitations and Uses)

Needle biopsy and ultrasound scan autopsies
- May miss: PE, MI, whole organs or small lesions and pseudomembranous colitis
- Can sample the brain
- May be useful in infective cases (HIV)

Endoscopic / laparoscopic autopsy
- May miss PE, MI, aspiration pneumonitis and small tumours
- Refrigeration makes insufflation difficult

Plain X-rays
- These are an autopsy supplement rather than an alternative form of autopsy.
- Localise foreign objects (e.g. bullets).
- Identify fractures not visible on gross exam.

Angiography / bronchography
- Angiography in the brain cannot identify old infarcts or distinguish filling defects due to cerebral oedema *vs.* other causes.
- Angiography in the heart is superior to macro dissection, gives a permanent record and gives an accurate estimate of extent of coronary artery stenosis.
- Angiography can identify vascular malformations esp. in perinates.
- Bonchography can confirm lobar aplasia in perinates.

Magnetic resonance imaging (MRI)
- MRI can yield high quality, high resolution images post mortem (because the subject is still)
- Detects CNS abnormalities not seen on gross dissection
- Not good at detecting cardiovascular abnormalities esp. coronary artery abnormalities

- Cannot distinguish clot from thrombus
- Cannot distinguish oedema from inflammatory infiltrate
- A recent DoH report (Feb 2004) recommended 3 year trial of MRI *vs.* conventional PM

Ancillary Tests

Toxicology
- Rescue *in vivo* blood samples from labs before they are discarded as some drug half lives are very rapid and PM blood levels may be misleading
- Femoral vein blood (fluoride bottle), preferably two samples – one from each side
    - ➤ this is for quantitative analysis. For qualitative (screening) purposes central blood (heart / great vessels) may be collected in plain containers
    - ➤ acute alcohol poisoning requires a blood level of 350–400 mg/100ml
    - ➤ for microbiology blood samples, *vide infra*
- Muscle for opioids and carboxymyoglobin (because carboxyhaemoglobin can dissipate as a result of vigorous CPR)
- Urine in a plain sterile container – ! bacterial fermentation can raise urine alcohol levels but careful toxicological analysis may detect if this is the case by looking for by-products of bacterial fermentation ∴ discuss result with toxicologists
- Stomach contents – whole contents collected in suspected overdose
- Hair – in suspected drug abuse or to check compliance e.g. with epileptic medications (get a pencil-thick lock of hair)
- Vitreous
    - ➤ make your needle insertion point well posterior and reconstitute the eye volume with saline
    - ➤ useful for alcohol and glucose levels as blood and urine PM can be unreliable
    - ➤ electrolyte ratio (Na:K) can help determine the time of death
- Request alcohol and illicit drug screen and specify drugs of known interest in case they are not part of the routine screen (e.g. fentanyl is not part of the standard opiate screen)
- Less commonly tissue samples may be useful e.g. liver (100g from right lobe, un-contaminated with bile, for certain complex poisoning cases), lung (100g from apex in sealed jar/bag at 4°C in cases of gaseous toxicity), brain (deep brain substance for e.g. cyanide estimation) and nail and bone samples (useful in chronic heavy metal toxicity)
- Assessing alcohol: quantitative results from vitreous combined with urine and blood levels should be used. Remember potential complications of PM putrefaction / bacterial action
- Assessing glucose: glucose measurement in blood or urine PM are unhelpful (blood glucose falls rapidly PM). Vitreous is better but other tests such as blood glycated haemoglobin (HbA1c) and the presence of acetone in the blood / urine are better indicators of glycaemic control / ketoacidosis respectively

Microbiology
- Take femoral vein blood in a plain bottle for viral serology, an EDTA bottle for Malarial parasites and also in blood culture bottles
- Lung, spleen, meninges: for sepsis. (include liver and CSF in infant / perinate). Take lung samples *before* removing lungs from the body. Get CSF by inserting needle of syringe into 3rd / 4th ventricles

Genetics / Molecular / Metabolic Studies
- Take samples as soon as possible after death
- Liver, skeletal muscle, heart, brain, chorionic villi: frozen for metabolic/genetic defects; also EM
- Skin and chorionic villi for fibroblast culture for cytogenetics: put in culture medium

Imaging
- Photography and babygram or proper skeletal survey if suspected NAI or skeletal anomaly

Other
- Frozen sections / imprint cytology for rapid diagnosis (e.g. to confirm pneumonia)
- Macro histochemistry for amyloid (brown with Lugol's iodine), iron (blue with Prussian Blue), cardiac enzymes (lack of purple in early ischaemic myocardium with nitro-blue tetrazolium [NBT] – ! must be done <12 hours after death), fat (red with Sudan IV), calcium (red with Alizarin Red), etc.
- Blood in an EDTA tube may be used for a sickle cell test

Technical Notes on Specific Dissections

Brain
- An MTO may open the skull. Examine the dura and superior sagittal sinus, incise the dura at the level of the saw cut, cut the falx at the crista galli and reflect it back. Lift the frontal poles to cut the olfactory and optic nerves, pituitary stalk and carotids. Lift the temporal lobes and cut the tentorial attachments. Cut the cranial nerves then transect the brain stem / cord close to the foramen magnum and deliver the brain.
- Fix the brain for 3 weeks in a bucket, suspending it by a cord hooked to the basilar artery.
- An exception to the rule of never examining a fresh brain is in the case of subarachnoid haemorrhage where the blood should be washed out of the basal cisterns and the vessels examined *in situ* before fixation. Look between the frontal lobes and in the Sylvian fissure for berry aneurysms, etc.
- Record whole brain weight fresh and fixed (= wb). Record the weight of the cerebellum + brainstem after removal (= cbs). The fixed weights ratio cbs/wb should normally be ≈ 0.12 .
- After examining the vessels and removing the brainstem (by cutting at level of colliculi to examine peri-aqueductal grey matter and substantia nigra) and cerebellum (by cutting the peduncles), the cerebrum is sliced in two at the level of the mammillary bodies and each half serially sliced using 1 cm thickness guides. Check the cortical ribbons, white matter capsules, periventricular regions and deep grey matter. Remember Sommer's sector (= CA1) of the hippocampus (best seen in the first slice posterior to the mammillary bodies) and other vascular boundary zones for patients with potential hypotensive episodes ($\rightarrow$ 'watershed infarcts'). See Figure 4.1 on p. 36.

Eyes
- ! Relatives should give specific agreement and replacement prostheses should be available.
- Anterior approach: retract lids with an eyelid retractor, incise conjunctiva, hold globe by the cut end of the conjunctiva and tilt to allow cutting of the muscles and optic nerve with blunt-nosed scissors.
- Intracranial approach: chisel around the bony orbital roof, remove it, cut the surrounding muscles and optic nerve and lift globe out to cut the conjunctiva (! take extreme care not to damage the lids).
- For more detail and other procedures see article by Parsons and Start (2001) in the Bibliography

Middle and Inner Ear
- Strip the dura from over the petrous temporal bone with forceps and scalpel.
- Apply chisel to floor of middle cranial fossa to take the top off the petrous temporal bone.
- Alternatively, remove the petrous temporal bone *en block* for decalcification (best method for mid and inner ears).

Vertebral Arteries
- Arise as the 1st branch of the subclavian arteries and enter the foramina of C6
- Open the anterior bony bars of the vertebroarterial canal (of C6 to C2) with snippers or wire cutters
- The arteries deviate laterally on going from C3 to C2 and medially and posteriorly after leaving C1 to enter the cranial cavity through the atlanto-occipital membrane. Open the posterior part of the vertebroarterial canal of C1 and incise the atlanto-occipital membrane to follow them into the skull
- Inspect the intracranial segments from within the cranial cavity and remove them with the brain
- For more detail, see Bromilow and Burns, 1985; and Aggrawal and Setia, 2006

Spinal Cord
- Posterior approach: incise the skin from occiput to sacrum, clear the muscles to expose the laminae and saw down and slightly medially on the lateral parts of the laminae to the vertebral canal (see Figure 25.2). Remove the bony strip, cut the cauda equina and remove the cord in its dural sheath by cutting the nerve roots as you hold the cord up from the inferior end with locking forceps (e.g. arterial clamps). Cut across the cord just below the foramen magnum.
- Anterior approach: remove the brain then cut the dura circumferentially below the foramen magnum from inside the cranial cavity. Clear the paravertebral muscles to visualise the cervical and lumbosacral nerve roots then saw through the vertebral pedicles just anterior to the nerve roots changing the angle of the saw from $\approx$ horizontal in the lumbar region to $\approx$ vertical cervically (see Figure 25.2). Transect the cauda equina and remove the cord as described above.

- Removing the cord within the vertebral column: this method is used if there is a suspicion of spinal cord infarct as it preserves the cord blood supply (but the body must be reconstructed with a broomstick and crossbars). Method is as for the anterior approach but instead of cutting the pedicles you cut through the ribs close to the spine, cut through the sacroiliac region to free the sacrum and dissect the whole spine from the soft tissue severing any atlantoaxial connections. Fix the whole thing then access the cord by laminectomy as in the posterior approach.
- Avoid crush artefacts: whatever method is used, do not kink or sharply bend the cord during removal or fixation (if a long enough fixative container is not available, bisect the cord after making an opening in the dura – never cut through cord and dura together).
- Maintain a knowledge of the levels (by tying a suture to L1 prior to removing the cord, by preserving the dentate ligament when opening the dura at the time of cut-up and by counting back to the distinctive roots of T1 [T1 has the last large roots distal to the cervical enlargement and has unequal-sized anterior and posterior roots, unlike T2, with posterior bigger than anterior and each bigger than the roots of T2]).

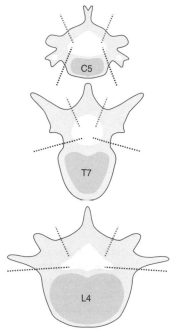

FIGURE 25.2 Accessing the spinal cord

Muscles for ?Myopathy
- Take samples from: digastric (both anterior and posterior belly separately), tongue, larynx / pharyngeal muscles, sternocleidomastoid, diaphragm, biceps / triceps, small hand muscles and vastus lateralis.
- Lay the sample out on a labelled card until they are a little dry (to stick to the card) then fix. Take transverse and longitudinal sections for histology.

Nerves for ?Neuropathy
- Sample the ulnar, femoral and sural ± autonomic ganglia. Fix and section as for muscles (*vide supra*)
- If ? MND take spinal cord, muscles (as above) and examine brain stem cranial nerve nuclei (*NB*: III, IV and VI are usu. spared in MND)

Parathyroid Glands
- These are soft, ovoid and browny-yellow.
- Dissect the posterolateral grooves between the oesophagus and thyroid.
- Upper pair are usu. midway down the posterior border of the thyroid.
- Lower pair are usu. just beneath the inferior margin of the thyroid.

Conducting System of the Heart
- Refer to Figure 4.6 on p. 39 and to the instructions below
- Indications: complete AV block not explained by IHD, suspected congenital conducting system defects, confirmation of tumour/sarcoid involvement (e.g. 1° mesothelioma of the AV node or mets)
- ECG correlation and input of an expert cardiac pathologist is advisable *before* dissection because some specialist dissections may be necessary (e.g. complete radial serial sectioning of both AV rings is indicated in some pre-excitation syndromes – see specialist texts in the Bibliography)
- The basic dissection may be performed on the fresh heart or after intact fixation (flush out blood / clots, stuff chambers with formalin-soaked cotton wool and immerse whole in formalin)
- All the blocks require serial sectioning and stain with Masson's trichrome and H&E → 100s of sections
- Open the right atrium anterolaterally (*do not* join-cut the *venae cavae* as usual) and identify the *crista terminalis* – the internal crest between the ridged anterior atrial muscle and the smooth posterior muscle continuous with the *venae cavae*. Take a rectangular block of the *crista* as it arches over the junction between the atrial appendage and the SVC. The SA node ('pacemaker') is usu. in the anterolateral part but may be more extensive (= 'horseshoe node'). Serial sectioning for histology is done from anterolateral to posteromedial.

- Identify the triangle of Koch (the AV node is within its apex, near the medial attachment of the septal cusp of the tricuspid valve) and membranous septum (it contains the AV bundle of His) – transillumination may help. Take a rectangular block to include these two areas and part of the subjacent muscular septum (containing left and right bundle branches) to include the septal papillary muscle (the latter is usu. a group of little papillae rather than a single muscle). Divide this rectangle into top and bottom halves. For histology, serially section the top half longitudinally (perpendicular to the plane of the valve ring) and the bottom half transversely (across the septum).
- The 'moderator band' is a bridging piece of *trabeculae carnae* near the bottom of the septum that reaches across to the anteroinferior wall of the RV at the root of the anterior papillary muscle. It contains the distal part of the right bundle branch of the conducting system.

Femur
- Incise the skin from medial to lateral across the patella anteriorly and continue up the lateral thigh.
- Transect the patella, clear the muscles from the femur inferiorly and divide the medial, lateral and cruciate ligaments of the knee joint.
- Clear the muscles upto the hip, incise the hip joint capsule around the femoral neck and swing the femur laterally till the head pops out of the acetabulum. The femur can now be removed.
- Slice the femur longitudinally to reveal extent of red marrow. Alternatively, chisel segments from proximal mid and distal parts by cutting parallel vertical slices mid way into the shaft at these points and then chisel across to give a semicircular segment from each location (this may be done without having to remove the femur completely).

Biliary Tract
- Open the lateral duodenum and squeeze the GB to locate the ampulla and demonstrate patency.
- Mobilise the GB and cut down on the cystic duct then open it to the CBD.
- Open up the left and right hepatic ducts and continue down the CBD.
- Remove the intact GB and open it into a clean container – don't spill the bile.

Air Embolism
- ! Consider this *prior* to PM: it alters the order and nature of dissection to avoid artefactual air bubbles.

Venous
- Open the abdomen first, fill it with water and inspect IVC for bubbles.
- Make a surgical window in the chest to expose the praecordium (avoid removing the whole sternum or cutting the 1st rib because this will damage the subclavian).
- Open the pericardial sac, inspect the epicardial veins, fill the sac with water and insert the needle of a water-filled syringe body (no plunger) into the RV – look for bubbles.
- Frothy blood in the right heart may occur with large air embolism.

Arterial
- This may follow thoracic surgery (e.g. CABG) or any trauma to the pulmonary veins.
- The key is to demonstrate bubbles in the vessels of the meninges (*in situ*) or base of brain.
- The cranium must be opened without damaging the meninges.
- The internal carotid and basilar arteries must only be cut after clamping them – then remove the brain.
- Inspect the vessels of the circle of Willis for bubbles (while immersing the brain under water).

Others
- Oesophageal Varices: tie the oesophagus high in the chest before cutting it. Remove oesophagus in continuity with stomach. Open the distal stomach, remove its contents and insert grasping forceps into the stomach (via this incision) to the top of oesophageal portion then grasp and pull the oesophagus down into the stomach to evert it and inspect for varices.
- Renal disease / Hypertension: look for accessory renal arteries.
- Hiatus Hernia: you need to keep the diaphragm intact to demonstrate this.
- Small Intestine: always check the 1st part of the duodenum for ulcers.
- Intestinal ischaemia / embolism: dissect down to the superior mesenteric artery to inspect its branches.

Normal Weights and Measures in Adults

TABLE 25.1   Normal values in adults

Weights (g)	Male	Female
Heart*	290–440	230–390
Pericardium	20–50 ml	20–50 ml
Right Lung[†]	420–900	340–750
Left Lung[‡]	370–800	290–640
Pleura (each)	50 ml	50 ml
Liver	1280–2070	1110–1840
Kidneys (each)	120–200	100–170
Testis (each)	20–30	–
Prostate	15@20 yrs to 40@80 yrs	–
Spleen ($\propto$ age)	70–240	60–220
Pancreas**	100–180	90–160
Adrenals (each)	6–8	6–8
Thyroid[††]	10–40	10–30
Parathyroids (all together)	116–124 mg	137–147 mg
Brain	1200–1600	1100–1500
cbs/wb	0.12	0.12

* for males the heart is 0.45% body weight (0.4% for females). Formalin fixation increases heart weight by $\approx$ 6%
[†] older sources for the right lung weight suggest 400–500g (M), 350–450g (F)
[‡] older sources for the left lung weight suggest 330–450g (M), 300–400g (F)
[×] PM splenic weight range is wide: upto 350g being acceptable with physiological atrophy down to 40g
** older sources for pancreatic weight suggest 70–100g (M), 60–90g (F).
[††] the lower end of this range occurs in the very young and the very old.

- Table 25.1 was compiled from various sources (see Bibliography). Values for heart, lungs, liver, kidneys, spleen, pancreas and thyroid were calculated from recent data by Lorin de la Grandmaison *et al.* (2001) on Caucasians who died within 1 hour of injury and had no detected disease.
- The range shown in the table is $\pm$ 1 SD about the mean, rounded to the nearest 10g. For Normal distributions, 95% of cases lie between 1.96 x SD either side of the mean so the actual ranges are very wide indeed.
- I have tried to illustrate variation between sources in the footnotes. Variation in lung weights may be due to differing amounts of agonal pulmonary oedema in otherwise healthy patients.
- Heart weights were not found to correlate with height in females (contrary to older data) but many organ weights depend on BMI (as measured post mortem), age, exercise history, etc.
- All these complexities should be considered when interpreting your findings, especially when your conclusions have medicolegal implications.
- See tables 25.2 and 25.3 for cardiac measurements

TABLE 25.2   Cardiac wall thickness

Cardiac Wall	Thickness
Right Atrium	2–2.5 mm
Left Atrium	2–2.5 mm
Right Ventricle (1cm below pulm. valve, at conus)	2–3 mm
Left Ventricle (1cm below posterior leaflet of mitral)	12–15 mm

TABLE 25.3   Cardiac valve circumference

Valve	Circumference[‡‡]
Tricuspid	11–13 cm
Pulmonary	8–9 cm
Mitral	9–11 cm
Aortic	7–8 cm

[‡‡] measured linearly with valve cut open

Fulton's Method for Separating the Left and Right Ventricle
- Demonstrates isolated ventricular hypertrophy (esp. RVH) and ratios may be esp. useful where interpreting total heart weight is difficult (e.g. in some paediatric / perinatal settings) – Figure 25.3

① cut off the atria and all valves (scissors)
② trim and scrape all the epicardial fat off
③ with broad-bladed scissors place one blade on the septum and cut the RV off the septum as shown in the figure without leaving a ridge of muscle behind. Also cut off all muscle protruding from the septum into the RV cavity. The free wall of the RV and any protruding

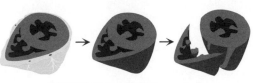

FIGURE 25.3   The Fulton method

muscle thus trimmed constitute the RV mass (RVm). The LV and septum constitute the LV mass (LVm). The RVm and LVm are weighed separately and used to assess Fulton's criteria for normality/hypertrophy as below[16].

---

[16] Fulton's series was small, none were >65 years old and M & F data were pooled. However they are considered reasonable (*NB*: large/active – but healthy – people may have higher values).

Normality: requires all of the following: ① $(LVm + RVm) < 250g$
                                                     ② $RVm < 65g$
                                                     ③ $LVm < 190g$
                                                     ④ $LVm:RVm$ is between 2.3:1 and 3.3:1
RVH: $RVm \geq 80g$ or, in isolated RVH, $LVm:RVm < 2:1$
LVH: $LVm \geq 225g$
Pomerance and Davies (1975) report normal ranges for: ➤ $LVm = 84–195g$ (M); $73–181g$ (F)
                                                          ➤ $RVm = 26–73g$ (M); $24–65g$ (F)

Perinatal Autopsy (a Procedure)

In practice, the precise method varies depending on the clinicoradiological Hx and any suspected anomalies.

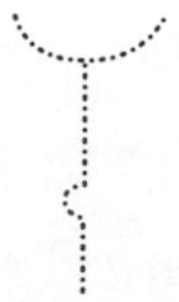

1. external examination, weights and measures, babygram +/ specific radiography
2. skin incision (see Figure 25.4 – take section of cord, measure subcutaneous fat thickness)
3. check for pneumothorax[17]
4. check internal connection of cord vessels:
   a) check umbilical vein then cut it
   b) incise skin around other side of cord then lay it caudally with umbilical arteries and urachal remnant attached
5. check rotation of gut and identify gonads. If sex differs from the request form phone this result through urgently so parents can be informed (for correct naming on the gravestone, etc.)
6. remove plastron at cartilages anterior to the costochondral joints from bottom up. Take the thymus
7. Is there blood-stained fluid in the serous cavities? (a sign of maceration)
8. remove intestines and take samples of rectum, ileum and jejunum for histology
9. check the venous drainage of the lungs into the heart *in situ* and the inferior veins into the IVC
10. neck – sample part of tongue in mouth
11. Rokitansky removal of organs (i.e. thoracic and abdominal organs removed together *en bloc*)
12. probe the oesophagus into stomach, open the oesophagus and strip it off
13. separate the heart and lung block
14. dissect the heart (samples for histology should include septum and papillary muscle):
    a) join-cut the IVC – SVC
    b) cut along the AV border
    c) examine the fossa ovalis and coronary sinus (see Figure 25.5)
    d) cut down the septum on RV and examine the tricuspid
    e) probe up the pulmonary artery into the ductus arteriosus
    f) cut along the pulmonary artery to examine the pulmonary valve
    g) connect the pulmonary veins on the left atrium and cut along the AV border
    h) cut down septum into the LV and examine the mitral valve
    i) probe up aorta and cut along the probe to examine the aortic valve
    j) remove the heart and weigh it
    k) take a *longitudinal* section of right and left ventricle to include papillary muscles
    l) take a transverse section of septum
15. cut down the tracheobronchial tree
16. remove, weigh, examine and sample lungs (combined weight is used for lungs:body ratio)
17. cut the trachea at the level of the thyroid
18. remove the diaphragm (and sample it) – take care not to destroy the adrenals
19. separate the kidneys from the liver-spleen-stomach
20. remove and weigh the adrenals (together) and sample them
21. weigh the kidneys (separately)
22. sample the psoas muscle

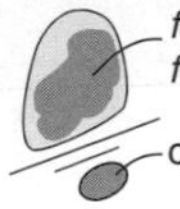

FIGURE 25.4 Perinatal body incision

fossa ovalis ±
foramen ovale
coronary sinus

FIGURE 25.5 Medial aspect of Rt atrium

---

[17] incising the thoracic cavity under water works but allows any pleural fluid also to escape and allows water in to dilute and contaminate intrapleural contents should microbiology be required. To overcome this, use a sterile needle and syringe partly filled with sterile water. Insert the needle into the cavity and pneumothorax will cause bubbles to rise in the syringe. A babygram (whole body X-ray) may also give warning of pneumothorax

23. sample the left and right lobes of the liver
24. sample the stomach, spleen and gonads
25. sample a costochondral junction (and sample some other growth plates if ? skeletal dysplasia)
26. remove the brain and examine the cranium, falx, venous sinuses and meninges
    a) coronal skin incision from ear to ear over posterior fontanelle, reflect to eyebrows and base
    b) make longitudinal nicks in the dura at the lateral aspects of the anterior fontanelle
    c) extend nicks to create bilateral bone flaps – bend back and cover edges with a wet towel
    d) examine the tentorium and falx cerebri (use gravity and wet scalpel handle to shift the brain)
    e) remove the central strip of bone

Weight ratios

① fetal:placental – for IUGR (normal values are 1:1 at 14/40 to $\approx$ 7:1 at 40–44/40)

② brain:liver – for asymmetric IUGR (defined as ≥ 5; normal range is 2.5–3.5)

③ lungs:body – pulmonary hypoplasia is ≤ 0.015 before 28/40 or < 0.012 after 28/40 (in the absence of complicating factors like hydrops, general IUGR, pneumonia, etc.), radial alveolar counts also help (count the nõ. of alveoli or septa transected by a line from a resp. bronchiole to the nearest acinar margin – see Cooney and Thurlbeck, 1982).

Bibliography

Aggrawal, A. and Setia, P. (2006) Vertebral artery dissection revisited. *Journal of Clinical Pathology*, **59** (9), 1000–1002.

Becker, A.E. and Anderson, R.H. (1983) *Cardiac Pathology: An integrated text and color atlas.* 1st edn, Churchill Livingstone, Edinburgh.

Benbow, E.W. and Roberts, I.S.D. (2003) The autopsy: complete or not complete? *Histopathology*, **42** (5), 417 423.

Bromilow, A. and Burns, J. (1985) Technique for removal of the vertebral arteries. *Journal of Clinical Pathology*, **38** (12), 1400–1402.

Butany, J. and Collins, M.J. (2005) Analysis of prosthetic cardiac devices: a guide for the practising pathologist. *Journal of Clinical Pathology*, **58** (2), 113–124.

Cooney, T.P. and Thurlbeck, W.M. (1982) The radial alveolar count method of Emery and Mithal: a reappraisal 1 – postnatal lung growth. *Thorax*, **37** (8), 572–579.

Cooney, T.P. and Thurlbeck, W.M. (1982) The radial alveolar count method of Emery and Mithal: a reappraisal 2 – intrauterine and early postnatal lung growth. *Thorax*, **37** (8), 580–583.

Cotran, R.S., Kumar, V. and Collins, T. (eds) (1999) *Robbins Pathologic Basis of Disease*, 6th edn, W.B. Saunders Co., Philadelphia.

Cotton, D.W.K. and Cross, S.S. (1993) The Hospital Autopsy. 1st edn, Butterworth Heinemann, Oxford.

Davies, M.J., Anderson, R.H. and Becker, A.E. (1983) *The Conduction System of the Heart*, 1st edn, Butterworths, London.

De Paepe, M.E., Friedman, R.M., Gundogan, F. (2005) Postmortem lung weight/body weight standards for term and preterm infants. *Pediatric Pulmonology*, **40** (5), 445–448.

Department of Health (2003) Families and Postmortems. A code of practice. *DoH Publication 31518.*

Department of Health (2003) The use of human organs and tissue. An interim statement. *DoH Publication 31520.*

Esiri, M.M. and Oppenheimer, D.R. (1996) *Oppenheimer's Diagnostic Neuropathology: A Practical Manual*, 2nd edn, Blackwell Science Ltd., Oxford.

Evans, T.J. and Krausz, T. (1994) Pathogenesis and pathology of shock, in *Recent Advances in Histopathology*, Vol. 16 (eds P.P. Anthony, R.N.M. MacSween and D.G. Lowe), Churchill Livingstone, Edinburgh, pp. 21–47.

Gallagher, P.J. (1994) The investigation of cardiac death, in *Recent Advances in Histopathology*, Vol. 16 (eds P.P. Anthony, R.N.M. MacSween and D.G. Lowe), Churchill Livingstone, Edinburgh, pp.123–146.

Gresham, G.A. and Turner, A.F. (1979) Post-Mortem Procedures (An Illustrated Textbook). 1st edn, Wolfe Medical Publications Ltd., London.

Hardin, N.J. (2000) Infection control at autopsy: a guide for pathologists and autopsy personnel. *Current Diagnostic Pathology*, **6** (2), 75–83.

Hasleton, P. (2003) Wither the Coroner? *ACP News*, (Winter 2003), pp.13–18.

Ince, P.G. (2000) Autopsy in dementing disorders of the elderly. *Current Diagnostic Pathology*, **6** (3), 181–191.

Ironside, J.W. (1999) New variant Creutzfeldt-Jakob disease, in *Recent Advances in Histopathology*, Vol. 18 (eds D.G. Lowe and J.C.E. Underwood), Churchill Livingstone, Edinburgh, pp. 1–22.

Johnson, S.J., Sheffield, E.A. and McNicol, A.M. (2005) Examination of parathyroid gland specimens. *Journal of Clinical Pathology*, **58** (4), 338–342.

Lorin de la Grandmaison, G., Clairand, I. and Durigon, M. (2001) Organ weight in 684 adult autopsies: new tables for a Caucasoid population. *Forensic Science International*, **119** (2), 149–154.

Lowe, D. (2001) A practical approach to the autopsy in dementia, in *Recent Advances in Histopathology*, Vol. 19 (eds D. Lowe and J.C.E. Underwood), Churchill Livingstone, Edinburgh, pp. 163–179.

Lucas, S.B. (2005) Could this be ebola? Serious communicable disease: How to approach the autopsy and satisfy all the interested parties. *ACP Yearbook*, 48–49.

Lucas, S.B. (2005) Autopsy practice should be an essential part of postgraduate training in pathology – Against, *Journal of Pathology*, **207** (Supplement), 60A.

Millward-Sadler, G.H. (2003) Pathology of maternal deaths, in *Progress in Pathology*, Vol. 6 (eds N. Kirkham and N.A. Shepherd), Greenwich Medical Media, Ltd, London, pp. 163–184.

Parsons, M.A. and Start, R.D. (2001) Necropsy techniques in ophthalmic pathology. *Journal of Clinical Pathology*, **54** (6), 417–427.

Pomerance, A. and Davies, M.J. (eds) (1975) *The Pathology of the Heart*, 1st edn, Blackwell Scientific Publications, Oxford.

Royal College of Pathologists (1995) HIV and the practice of pathology. Available from RCPath directly.

Rezek, P.R. and Millard, M. (1963) *Autopsy Pathology: A Guide for Pathologists and Clinicians*, Charles C. Thomas Publisher, Springfield, Illinois, U.S.A.

Roberts, I.S.D., Benbow, E.W., Bisset, R. *et al.* (2003) Accuracy of magnetic resonance imaging in determining cause of sudden death in adults: comparison with conventional autopsy. *Histopathology*, **42** (5), 424–430.

Roberts, I.S.D. and Pumphrey, R.S.H. (2001) The autopsy in fatal anaphylaxis, in *Recent Advances in Histopathology*, Vol. 19 (eds D. Lowe and J.C.E. Underwood), Churchill Livingstone, Edinburgh, pp. 145–162.

Rooney, C. (2005) Instructions for doctors certifying cause of death. *ACP News*, (Summer 2005), pp. 25–29.

Sheppard, M.N. (2003) Sudden adult death and the heart, in *Progress in Pathology*, Vol. 6 (eds N. Kirkham and N.A. Shepherd), Greenwich Medical Media, Ltd, London, pp. 185–202.

Solcia, E., Capella, C. and Klöppel, G. (1995) Tumors of the Pancreas, fascicle 20 in *Atlas of Tumor Pathology*, 3rd series, AFIP, Washington D.C.

Sternberg, S.S. (ed) (1997) *Histology for Pathologists*, 2nd edn, Lippincott Williams & Wilkins, Philadelphia.

Tansey, D.K., Aly, Z. and Sheppard, M.N. (2005) Fat in the right ventricle of the normal heart. *Histopathology*, **46** (1), 98–104.

Toner, P.G. and Crane, J. (1994) The pathology of death in pregnancy, in *Recent Advances in Histopathology*, Vol. 16 (eds P.P. Anthony, R.N.M. MacSween and D.G. Lowe), Churchill Livingstone, Edinburgh, pp. 189–211.

Tranberg, H.A., Rous, B.A. and Rashbass, J. (2003) Legal and ethical issues in the use of anonymous images in pathology teaching and research. *Histopathology*, **42** (2), 104–109.

Wainwright, H.C. (2006) My approach to performing a perinatal or neonatal autopsy. *Journal of Clinical Pathology*, **59** (7), 673–680.

Wigglesworth, J. and Singer, D.B. (eds) (1991) *Perinatal Pathology*, 1st edn, Blackwell Medical Publishers Inc, Boston.

Web sites

City Hospital Birmingham (2004–2007) *Guide to Toxicological Sampling from the Regional Laboratory for Toxicology*, http://www.toxlab .co.uk/postmort.htm (accessed September 2007).

GMC (2006) *Ethical Guidelines incl. use of Recordings and Consent*, http://www.gmc-uk.org/guidance/a_z_guidance/guidance_list/list_p.asp (accessed September 2007).

GMC (1997) *Guidance on Serious Communicable Diseases*, http://www.gmc-uk.org/guidance/current/library/serious_communicable_diseases.asp (accessed September 2007).

GMC (2007) *Important note for doctors: Update to Serious Communicable Diseases guidance – Non-consensual testing following injuries to health care workers*, http://www.gmc-uk.org/guidance/news_consultation/update_to_serious_communicable_diseases_guidance.asp (accessed September 2007).

King's College Coroner's Law Resource (2004) http://www.kcl.ac.uk/depsta/law/research/coroners/contents.html (accessed September 2007).

Special Pathogens Reference Unit HPA Porton Down (2004) *Specimen Referral Guidelines and Service Information Pack*, http://www.hpa.org.uk/cepr/specialpathogens/SPRU_brochure.pdf (accessed September 2007).

Index of General Terms

Diagnostic Criteria Handbook in Histopathology: A Surgical Pathology Vade Mecum by Paul J. Tadrous
Copyright © 2007 by John Wiley & Sons, Ltd.

Index of Molecules

Diagnostic Criteria Handbook in Histopathology: A Surgical Pathology Vade Mecum by Paul J. Tadrous
Copyright © 2007 by John Wiley & Sons, Ltd.

Index of Eponyms

For more on medical eponyms, including those not found in this book, try this web site by Ole Daniel Enersen www.whonamedit.com (last accessed 25 November 2007)

Diagnostic Criteria Handbook in Histopathology: A Surgical Pathology Vade Mecum by Paul J. Tadrous
Copyright © 2007 by John Wiley & Sons, Ltd.